1 MONTH OF
FREE
READING

at

www.ForgottenBooks.com

By purchasing this book you are eligible for one month membership to ForgottenBooks.com, giving you unlimited access to our entire collection of over 1,000,000 titles via our web site and mobile apps.

To claim your free month visit:

www.forgottenbooks.com/free786350

ISBN 978-0-483-52426-2
PIBN 10786350

This book is a reproduction of an important historical work. Forgotten Books uses
state-of-the-art technology to digitally reconstruct the work, preserving the original format
whilst repairing imperfections present in the aged copy. In rare cases, an imperfection in
the original, such as a blemish or missing page, may be replicated in our edition. We do,
however, repair the vast majority of imperfections successfully; any imperfections that
remain are intentionally left to preserve the state of such historical works.

SOUTHERN

MEDICAL AND SURGICAL JOURNAL.

EDITED BY

L. A. DUGAS, M. D.,

PROFESSOR OF SURGERY IN THE MEDICAL COLLEGE OF GEORGIA.

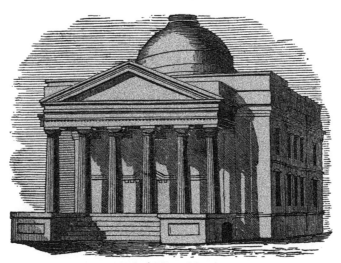

Medical College of Georgia.

" Je prends le bien où je le trouve."

VOL. VIII.—1852.—NEW SERIES.

AUGUSTA, GA.

JAMES McCAFFERTY, PRINTER AND PUBLISHER.

1852.

SOUTHERN
MEDICAL AND SURGICAL
JOURNAL.

Vol. 8.]　　　NEW SERIES.—JANUARY, 1852.　　　[No. 1.

PART FIRST.

Original Communications.

ARTICLE I.

The Pathology of Phlegmasia Dolens. By H. V. M. MILLER, M. D., Professor of Physiology and Pathological Anatomy in the Medical College of Georgia.

Milk leg, White leg, Swelled leg, Puerperal tumid leg, Anasarca serosa (Cullen), Bucknemia sparganosa (Goode), Phlegmasia lactea, Œdema lacteum, Phlegmasia dolens, Crural phlebitis. These various names, by which this disease has at different times been called, indicate to some extent the changes of opinion which have taken place in relation to its pathology.

It has been observed, and imperfectly described, by older writers, more distinctly by Mauriceau, and its history still more accurately sketched by Puzos in the year 1759. These all concur in the opinion that it is caused by a deposit of milk in the affected part; and to prevent the metastasis upon which it was supposed to depend, many practitioners kept the child constantly to the breast, in order to determine the secretion of milk in its appropriate organ. Puzos, however, occasionally resorted to much more energetic treatment, from which it appears that he regarded the disease, at least in its subsequent progress, as highly inflammatory; but, notwithstanding the energy of his treatment, he bewails the loss of some of his patients in terms which would do no discredit to the renowned

Sangrado himself. "J'ai eu le malheur de perdre plus d'une malade malgré toutes les saignées que j'avois pu faire : non que les saignées eussent été contraires ; mais elles avoient été insuffisantes pour ces cas las, parceque le mal étoit plus puissant que le remède et qu'il n'y en avoit pas d'autre."

This view of its pathology is still perpetuated in the popular belief of this and of most of the countries of Europe, but has long since been discarded by the profession: first of all, perhaps, by Dr. Hunter, who, although he published nothing on the subject, and advanced no new theory of the disease, constantly in his lectures denied the correctness of the old.

In 1794, Mr. White suggested the opinion that the disease depended upon obstruction or some other morbid condition of the lymphatic vessels and glands of the affected part. This hypothesis, or the modifications of it, proposed by Mr. Tyre and by Dr. Ferriar, one of whom thought the lymphatics were ruptured, and the other that they were acutely inflamed, became generally prevalent.

In the year 1800, Dr. Hull attempted to show that many of the circumstances attending the disease could not be accounted for upon the supposition that the lymphatics were alone affected. He contended that there existed a general inflammatory condition of the limb, involving all of its textures, but having its primary seat in the muscles, cellular membrane and cutis. In accordance with these views, he gave to the disease the name by which it is still most generally designated—Phlegmasia dolens.

The general adoption of the name proposed by Dr. Hull is not to be regarded as a measure of the favor with which his pathological opinions were received : to these there were many objectors. It was not, however, until 1823, that appearances observed in post-mortem examinations were appealed to for the purpose of elucidating this topic. During that year, M. Bouillaud, and Dr. Davis, of London, published accounts of dissections of the bodies of persons, dead of this disease, which, if they did not enable them satisfactorily to explain all the phenomena which it presents, constituted something solid and tangible upon which to base subsequent pathological enquiries, and demonstrated the superior value of even a few facts, in such investigations, over the most ingenious speculations.

In none of these cases, nor in any which have since been published, did the lymphatic vessels or glands appear to have been primarily affected, and in most of them, in no other way than by slight tumefaction, such as frequently attends œdema of the extremities from other causes. In a few, they seem to have participated to some extent in the inflammatory condition of the neighboring parts, and in but one were they found in a state of suppuration.

In recent cases, the veins of the affected limb were uniformly found to be more or less firmly and completely plugged up with a coagulum of blood, which adhered to the sides of the vessels, the inner coat of which was of a deep red color, produced, it was supposed, either by contact with the coagulum, or by inflammatory action. In cases of longer standing, the vessel was found obliterated by the organization of the coagulum, or of the coagulable lymph which had been effused from its walls. These appearances were co-extensive with the disease, involving the vessels of one or both extremities, or extending some distance up the vena-cava, and implicating its communicating branches to whatever height the plugging and obliteration might have gone.

In accordance with the pathology which these observations were supposed to establish, the disease was called Crural phlebitis, and its proximate cause asserted to be "a violent, destructive inflammation of the iliac veins and their contributary branches, including, in some cases, the inferior portion of the vena-cava." Pressure upon the veins of the pelvis by the gravid uterus, during gestation, Dr. Davis thought, predisposed to the disease, and upon the sudden removal of it by the consummation of parturition the phlebitis was developed.

The facts, detailed in these publications, have never been controverted; but the explanation of them has been deemed so unsatisfactory by many persons as to create a doubt whether the cases described by Bouillaud and Davis were to be considered as examples of genuine phlegmasia dolens, or to be viewed as essentially different diseases, analagous in their nature to those formidable attacks of phlebitis which are sometimes consequent upon venesection, or succeed to accidental injuries. Even Mr. Lawrence, who made the post-mortem examination

in the first of the cases which threw any light upon the nature
of the disease, became subsequently fully satisfied that phlegmasia dolens did not arise from inflammation of the iliac and
femoral veins.

That inflammation in those veins had existed in the cases
submitted to examination was undeniable; but in what way it
was established, or how connected with parturition, or with the
condition of the uterus, subsequent to delivery, had not been
very clearly made out. If, as was said, it was produced by
pressure upon the veins of the pelvis, why was it not developed
during gestation; if, by the removal of the pressure, why was
its appearance delayed, always for some, and often for many
days after delivery?   •

Dr. Robert Lee has subsequently attempted, by numerous
dissections, to demonstrate that the inflammation acknowledged
to exist in the large veins, is in all cases propagated from the
vessels of the uterus in which he thinks it originates. His
publications furnish abundant testimony of the accuracy and
faithfulness of previous observers, and of the fact that the cases
submitted to examination were ordinary examples of phlegmasia dolens. They also prove, that in many instances the veins
of the uterus are in the same condition as those of the lower
extremity, but he has utterly failed to show why that condition
should originate in the veins of either, or in what manner it
may be extended from the one to the other. Other observers,
indeed, and among them Dr. Locock, her Majesty's accoucheur,
deny the universality of the diseased condition of the uterine
veins, as contended for by Dr. Lee. But supposing this condition always to exist, will it account for all the phenomena
which phlegmasia dolens presents, or are we, with Dr. Churchill,
to conclude that some further information is necessary before
we can fully comprehend its true theory?—and with Hasse,
that the subject demands further investigation?

It is a fact, confirmed by universal observation, that the
veins do not readily take on inflammatory action. They may
be bruised, cut, torn, stretched, and injured in a variety of
ways, without the exhibition of greater liability to inflammation than other tissues of the body; and when in common with
the contiguous structures they have assumed this condition,

how seldom is it that the formidable and rapidly fatal symptoms, characteristic of what is called phlebitis, are presented. It cannot be denied, that in every instance in which any organ of the body is inflamed, the veins participate in that condition, and yet there is no propagation of the inflammation in either direction along their walls. There is nothing, in fact, in. their structure which would favor such propagation, or lead us to suppose it possible, independently of the extension of the inflammation in the surrounding tissues. Their nutrition is independent of the blood which is contained within them, and is ministered to, solely by the *vasa vasorum* which are derived from the arteries, distributed to and serving for the nutrition of neighboring parts. Inflammatory action, which depends upon a perverted action of the nutrient vessels, cannot therefore exist in the veins alone, without being extended to or from the adjacent tissues, not along the course of the vessel, and certainly not with the rapidity observed in cases of phlegmasia dolens, for such is not the course of the nutrient vessels, and such is not their mode of vascular connexion. If, however, in defiance of well established physiological laws, we were to concede the possibility of the extension of inflammatory action along the coats of the veins, from any point where it might be established, as for example, in the vessels of the uterus, in what manner would we account for the peculiar direction which it takes, and for the effects which it produces. Upon this supposition, it would follow the route of the circulation until it arrived at the veins from one of the lower extremities, and then the reverse direction, until it had implicated all the vessels in communication with them, when it would capriciously extend its influence some distance along the vena cava and seize upon the veins of the other lower extremity, and terminate by obliterating the cavities of them all, and by the establishing of purulent deposits at one or several points in their course.

. It will not remove the absurdity of the hypothesis to suppose, with Dr. Davis, that the puerperal condition establishes a predisposition to inflammation sufficient to account for every physiological absurdity, for the disease has been observed in females who were not in this condition, but affected with cancer of the uterus, simple ulceration, or other diseases of this or other of the pelvic viscera which result in suppurative action ; and also in persons of the male sex, suffering from hemorrhoidal, vesical, or renal inflammations.

..In view of these difficulties, it is not surprising that, while due credit is awarded to the gentlemen who have with praiseworthy zeal investigated this subject, and perfect credence is given to their descriptions of post-mortem appearances, many persons have hesitated in the adoption of all their deductions, and of the names by which they choose to designate the disease, as indicative of its true pathology, and have preferred, with Dr. Churchill, to retain the older appellation while awaiting the further information necessary to the perfect theory of the disease.

It is not improbable, that the desired information has been delayed by the preconceptions of pathologists and their too close adhesion to the exclusive solidism which has supplanted the humoral pathology of older writers.   The changes of structure in solid parts are readily appreciated by the senses, and are better calculated to arrest the attention and to furnish facts of indisputable authenticity, by which a solution of the various symptoms of a disease may be obtained, than the more mysterious and uncertain alterations to which the fluids of the body are subjected.   It is difficult also to trace these alterations, from their origin to their ultimate results, with the precision and accuracy which are demanded by the rigid analytic philosophy of the present time ; and hence in the investigations of the origin and nature of diseases the solid parts of the body have received a very disproportionate share of attention.

The extension of pathological knowledge has more recently in theory at least, led to the rejection of the exclusive claims of either fluidism or solidism, and to the concession that the animal structure is composed of parts, every one of which, may not only partake of disease, but under certain circumstances become the cause of it ; and has induced enquirers to engage in the tedious and difficult task of tracing the different changes which the blood undergoes in its circulation, and the effects of agents upon it, whether these are the retained material of normal, or the product of morbid secretions, or foreign substances introduced from without.

Much is to be anticipated from the further prosecution of these investigations, and already it is probable that they justify us in advancing one step in the pathology of the disease at the head of this article, and if the deductions are not erroneous, will lead to a fuller understanding of phlebitis in all its forms.

The conclusions to which they would lead are, that phlegmasia dolens or phlebitis is caused by the introduction of diseased matter, usually pus, into the blood—that inflammation of a vein is not an essential part of the primary affection, which precedes constitutional symptoms, *even when morbid matter has found its way into the circulation through a vein,* and that when the veins are inflamed, it is an effect, and not the cause of the reception of diseased or foreign matter into them.

John Hunter showed that admixture of pus with blood caused its coagulation. If but a little of it be mixed with recently drawn blood, the latter will coagulate round the globules of pus and form a mass which will adhere to the first surface with which it comes in contact, and it is not until the coagulum thus formed, is broken up or dissolved, that its elements can circulate with the blood.

Mr. Henry Lee, of London, has recently shown that this change is produced in blood out of the body in two minutes, while fifteen minutes are required for the coagulation of unmixed or healthy blood.

The following experiment performed by him, proves that pus will cause the coagulation of blood more rapidly within the vessels than out of the body:

" The right jugular vein (of an ass) having been opened, two fluid ounces of pure healthy pus were injected and propelled in the course of the circulation, by pressure upon the vein externally, the vein became tense during the operation, and sensibly resisted the attempts that were made to propel its contents toward the heart, *even forcible pressure was not sufficient to overcome the resistance offered to the return of the blood,* symptoms of constitutional irritation followed, the vein was felt thickened as far as the sternum, and the animal was destroyed about nine days afterwards.

Post mortem appearances. * * * * On the right side an abscess had formed in the course of the vein, and for two inches the whole of the parts were imbedded in a confused mass of pus and lymph, in which it was impossible to distinguish the structure of the vein. Both above and below this for several inches, the vein was filled with coagula, which effectually obliterated it. These coagula extended for several inches in the course of the circulation; but beyond, in both directions, the vessel was pervious."

In a number of other experiments, "so sudden was the effect, that the mixture of blood and pus coagulated before it could traverse the jugular vein, as indicated by the induration and cord-like feeling of the vessel."

The immediate effect then of the introduction of pus into the veins is the coagulation of the blood within them, and the degree to which it may take place, will depend upon the extent of the injury and the degree of healthiness of the blood, and may vary from a small coagulum, such as re-unites the edges of a punctured vein to the prolonged plug which precedes its obliteration.

The object of the coagulum so formed appears to be to isolate the purulent matter, and thus prevent its introduction into the general circulation; and it is only when this intention is frustrated, by the large amount of pus, the mechanical disturbance of the process or the loss of the coagulability of the blood, that the grave and often fatal constitutional symptoms are manifested.

The blood coagulated within the vessels is in the same condition as if it were effused into a serous cavity, and becomes organised in the same manner, or as coagulable lymph would do in the same position, the only difference between them being the presence of the red particles in the former; and there is no sufficient reason to suppose that they would cause fibrin, which contains them to comport itself differently from that which is free from them.

The coagulum adhering to the sides of the vessel becomes a bond of union between them, a pellicle of lymph forms around it which increases in thickness, and finally becomes vascular and so firmly united to the sides of the vein, as to be inseperable from them. Inflammation is not necessary to the completion of this process; it is an example internally, of "union by the first intention," which is so frequently observed, and al-

ways desired in external injuries, and doubtless in many instances accomplishes the sequestration of the vessel or the insulation
of the pus without the accompaniment of symptoms of constitutional irritation, or other changes in the surrounding structures
than would result from the obliteration of a vein from the application of a ligature.   But if the amount of pus be considerable,
or the adhesive process be from any cause interfered with, additional phenomena are presented, characteristic of the farther
progress of the disease.   The pus, though cut off from the general circulation, may fail to be absorbed, and like other foreign
matter, be discharged externally by the ulcerative process.   Inflammation of the vein and of its communicating branches may
be thus excited at one or many points, by the presence of the
pus within it, or by the congested state of the capillary vessels,
consequent upon its obliteration.   This is precisely what is observed in disease, and what is produced by experiment.

"On the 23d of November, 1848, about an ounce of perfectly
pure pus (previously warmed,) was injected into the right
jugular vein of an aged ass; the vein immediately became corded, and the blood appeared to have coagulated in the vessel.
26th, the *wound in the neck began to suppurate,* and an abscess
subsequently formed in the course of the vein about midway
between the opening and the sternum."   Several abscesses
had also formed in the neighborhood of the external opening.
(H. Lee.)

Cruveilhier produced similar effects by injecting ink into the
veins of animals, the tannic acid of which would here seem to
coagulate the blood as quickly as pus would do; thirty-six hours
after, the large veins were distended with adherent coagula of
blood, a number of bloody patches or congested spots were found
in the muscles and cellular tissue of the limb, which, if the animal were allowed to live, subsequently suppurated.

These experiments certainly explain several of the circumstances occasionally attendant upon phlegmasia dolens.   They
account for the obliteration of the vessel which is known to
precede inflammation of it, for the conjestion of its communicating capillaries, for the exemption of those which have some
collateral anastamosing branches, for the tumefaction of the
limb, for the subseqent establishment of inflammation and for the

occurrence of suppuration at one or several points of the affected vein.

If any mechanical or other cause disturb the reparative process, the coagulum béginning to be formed, or an additional
amount of purulent matter may be propelled in the course of
the vein, ahd the same process be recommenced at another.
point, or if the occlusion of the vessel be not complete, the passage of successive portions of pus would seal up the cavity for a
still greater distance in the direction of the heart, and thus, if
the pus had its origin in the uterus, might successively implicate as has been witnessed, the vena cava and all the vessels
emptying into it as high as the hepatic vein.

· It generally happens, when the provisions to prevent the
passage of this poison into the veins which are known to exist
at the seat of suppuration, have been inoperative, that it will
be arrested by the immediate effect which it produces on the
blood.   It is perhaps only when there exists some morbid condition of the circulating fluid induced by previous disease, the
purperal condition, hemorrhage, or some vice, of constitution,
that pus is permitted in any dangerous quantity to go the round
of the circulation, and even then there exists a farther provision
for its arrest and ejection from the body, not as has been supposed by the mechanical arrest of its larger globules in the capillary vessels, but by the repetition in them (with diminished
force, but more favorable conditions of adhesion,) of the same
phenomena that attend its first introduction.   Under these
circumstances, when the mass of the blood has become infected,
are developed, the well known symptoms of constitutional irritation during which different organs of the body may be simultaneously attaçked and various isolated spots in them will become
rapidly disorganised, while the surrounding textures remain unaltered either in structure or color.   The final effort to stay
the progress of the poison is made in the capillaries and hence
they are the seat of pathological appearances which vary according to the condition of the blood at the time.   If it still
retain coagulating force, though much impaired, one or more of
the capillary vessels will become obstructed and the ordinary
changes follow, local inflammation will be developed by the
irritation of the poison and pus will be formed at the seat of the

congestion, and not translated thither from the original injury. In fact, in persons of enfeebled habits and where the blood is in a depraved condition at the outset of the disease, these distant abscesses are observed sometimes to occur without any apparent evidence of a previous attempt to circumscribe the poison, and even so early as scarcely to allow the supposition that pus could have been fully formed at the original point affected. But it is not difficult to comprehend how coagulation and arrest of circulation may be produced in the slow moving minute columns of blood in the capillary vessels, by causes insufficient to affect larger streams or even those in the normal and healthy state of the circulating fluid.

It is scarcely-necessary, if the limits of this article allowed it, to exhibit proof of suppurative action in some organ having always preceded attacks of phlegmasia dolens. This has been abundantly furnished by persons who have sought to establish its necessary connexion with inflammation of the veins. In no instance has it occurred in persons, not in the puerperal condition, where purulent matter was not found in some organ from whose veins its transmission into the larger vessels would account for the phenomena, as in the left leg, after amputation of the right, after ulceration of the kidney, uterus, any of the pelvic viscera, or of hemorrhoidal, tumors, &c. In every case of parturition, the resemblance of the vascular condition of that portion of the uterus to which the placenta was attached, to a recent wound, or amputation, has been long the subject of remark, and will account for the production of purulent matter in cases which terminate favorably, without the accompaniment of metritis; and in most of the instances of a fatal character pus has been actually found in the veins, insulated by coagula in the same manner as in experiments on animals.

It is not intended to extend this notice to cases of phlebitis occurring in other parts of the body, but it is evident that if the conclusions expressed are not erroneous, they are referable to the same cause, as they unquestionably present similar phenomena. They occur most generally under circumstances which favor the ready introduction of pus into the veins, as when some of the larger veins have been wounded, and the process of union has been disturbed; when some portion of bone has been involved in the original lesion, as in amputations or injuries of the head, in which the closure of the vessel is prevented by its firm attachment to unyielding surrounding structures. But in no part of the body is the same facility afforded for the occurrence of this accident as in the uterus. The intimate union existing between its muscular fibres and veins, renders the contraction and dilatation of the latter dependent upon the permanent contraction of the former, and consequently upon every relaxation of the uterine fibres, the coagula which close the large venous trunks are liable to be displaced, and no obstacle would be offered to the access of purulent or other offensive matter into them. And to this facility of entrance is perhaps to be attributed the fact that, in phlegmasia dolens, the coagulation and obliteration of cavity do not always begin in the uterine veins, which are sometimes found pervious and healthy, while the ordinary effects of the disease are manifested in the larger vessels.

These instances are much more readily accounted for upon this supposition than by attributing them to inflammation originating in the uterus and propagated along the walls of the veins. The healthy condition of the vessels in the supposed seat of the original lesion, forbids the idea of any such propagation, and leaves but the plain inference that the cause of the appearance is to be sought in the character of their contents.

Fortunately, the contraction of the muscular fibres of the uterus and the tortuous condition of its veins render the coagula so firm as usually to prevent the introduction of pus, from the surface of the uterus or when it may be formed in its substance by inflammation of the organ, and it is only in exceptional cases that phlegmasia dolens makes its appearance. Any cause which will relax this contraction or by other means disturb the coagula, will favor its production: hence hemorrhage, which would not be likely to excite inflammation, is not an unfrequent precursor of it, and in almost every instance it makes its appearance some days after delivery, when by the ordinary process of reparation the coagula are being separated from the mouths of the vessels by absorption or by the spontaneous contraction of their fibrine.

The study of the post-mortem appearances in cases of phlegmasia dolens and of so called phlebitis in other parts of the body, by whomsoever published, (but which cannot be here reproduced) will strongly tend to confirm the pathological views imperfectly sketched in the preceding pages, and if established they should so far modify the treatment as to avoid the danger of breaking up the adhesions and interfering with the process by which nature seeks to repair the injury, while combating an inflammatory condition which, when it exists, is but the effect of a pre-existing cause, and is never to be regarded as the origin or essence of the disease.

ARTICLE II.

Additional Remarks upon the value of Veratrum Viride. By W. C. Norwood, M. D., of Cokesbury, S. C.

We have been endeavoring for some time to awaken and interest the profession in the powers and properties of Veratrum Viride. We now venture again, and the third time, to call aloud! We have been cautiously, and, as we believe, judiciously, using the above article, alone and in various combination, for the space of eight years, which ought to allow us to speak with some confidence, and should be a reasonable warrant for what we may assert in the sequel. After various trials and combinations, we unhesitatingly assert that we verily believe we have adopted that form of combination which is *the best.* We gave to the public, in two former numbers of this Journal, (see June No. for 1850 and January No. for 1851,) a portion of our experience, with a statement of what were the powers and properties of the article; and we give this in farther addition. Its powers are perhaps more strikingly manifested in the speed and certainty with which it relieves and cures pneumonitis typhoides. Its culminating curative powers stand out in all probability more strikingly in this than in any other disease. We fearlessly assert, that it is as much of a specific in pneumonitis as quinine is in the treatment of intermittent fever, and that it will cut short and break up at the first outset of the attack as many cases—due allowance being made

for the violence of the attack and the importance of the organs
affected—as quinine will, of intermittent. We challenge the
world to produce its equal, either singly, or in any combination of remedies. Again: it is the sheet-anchor in typhus and
in typhoid fevers. It is the only remedy that has ever been
found to arrest the above fever or fevers, and to rob them of
the terror and dismay they are known so universally to produce. It not only cures cases beyond the reach of any known
remedies, in the last stage of the disease, but it breaks up many
cases at the outset, and cuts short others that are fully formed,
and in full and perfect progress. Farther: we have found
nothing that arrests convulsions in children, accompanied with
high febrile symptoms, from one year old and upwards, with
any thing approximating such certainty and speed. In hooping
cough, it stands unrivalled and alone, as a remedy that may be
relied on when accompanied with high febrile excitement.
Dr. J. A. Stewart, in writing to us in relation to its powers,
states thus:—"I know of no remedy worth mentioning, save
yours. Having seen cases of pertussis every day for ten
months, and used your remedy every few days, I cannot recommend it to that notice it deserves without being considered as
an enthusiast in its use." We hasten on to notice, farther, that
it is a powerful and reliable agent in the treatment of typhoid
dysentery: that with it we can readily manage that fearful,
malignant and mortal disease.

The next class of diseases we shall notice, and briefly illustrate its powers in by a couple of cases, is the certainty and
speed—we mean undoubted certainty—with which it cures or
relieves the pain and febrile excitement occasioned in mumps,
by a metastasis to the testicle.

Case 1st, Mr. A.—Found him with the testicle much swelled
and intensely painful; great pain in the head; skin hot and dry;
pulse 110; tongue thickly coated. Commenced with eight
drops every three hours, the dose to be increased one drop
every portion till nausea or vomiting occurred. The third
portion excited free emesis. The pulse was reduced to 65
pulsations per minute, the skin became cool and moist, and
there was perfect relief of the pain and all unpleasant febrile
symptoms were subdued and removed, and by continuing the

remedy in small portions, so as not to sicken, there was no return of either pain or febrile symptoms. The symptoms of Mr. S., in the second case, were similar to the first, being free from pain, in the head excepted. He was treated in the same manner precisely. - The third or fourth portion vomited freely, on the occurrence of which the pulse was reduced to 60 beats per minute, which before commencing was upwards of 110, with an entire removal of all pain and febrile excitement.

In traumatic lesions we have tested its powers sufficiently to warrant us in asserting that it will control and regulate any arterial excitement produced thereby. We fully tested that fact in the New York emigrant's hospital. Who can calculate its value and importance, by the ease and certainty with which it controls and subdues high arterial excitement after capital operations? How many cases run down and perish from high sanguineous excitement alone, without any other appreciable cause, after well executed operations? We feel confident that in the above we can afford the surgeon a remedy that will quiet his fears and remove his apprehensions in such cases, and that he can control at will inflammation, arterial and general sanguineous excitement, that so often supervene and defeat the successful result of the most skilfully executed operations in surgery.

We feel fully assured, that we can confidently offer to the world the desideratum so long sought and wished for, namely, an agent that will certainly and undoubtedly control and subdue morbid arterial excitement, the great frequency of the contractions of the heart and arteries, so especially belonging to all acute diseases, and the removal of which has been as difficult as its presence was universal in all severely acute diseases. Dr. Bass, writing us on the subject, observes, "It seems to act directly upon the heart and arteries, as manifested by a diminution of the force and frequency of the pulse; it relieves irritation, congestion and inflammation—establishes the equilibrium of the circulation—excites free diaphoresis and expectoration, which well adapts it for the treatment of pneumonitis, pneumonia typhodes and asthma—in which diseases I have used it effectually, or in other words, with unparalleled success."

Dr. J. Branch, in writing us on the same, states, "I will simply

say, I regard it as one of the most important articles of the
materia medica.   You never made a more just and appropriate
remark, than you did when you said,. it would say to "the
pulse thus fast shalt thou beat and no faster." I have used it
in many cases of the severest sort of typhoid fever, with the
happiest effect; it will cool the surface, reduce the *frequency*
of the pulse, while at the same time it does not diminish its volume or strength.   Indeed, I have sometimes thought that the
volume and strength of the pulse was increased, in atonic cases,
under the use of this article.   The following will serve as an
illustration of its use and effects:—When called to a case of
typhoid fever—with a hot surface, frequent pulse, great restlessness, in a word, with all the symptoms of such a case—if
the patient be an adult, I commence with giving him 8 drops
of the article every two hours, and increase the dose a drop or
two at every succeeding dose, until slight nausea is produced,
never fearing but that when this effect is produced I shall have
a cool surface, an infrequent pulse, and an absence of all febrile
excitement.   I then continue more or less of the article, until
the case is broken up."   Dr. J. A. Stewart, in a letter on the
same subject, writes thus: "I do not believe any remedy or
combination of remedies possesses the same powers in pneumonia or pleuritis as yours—it not only lessens the frequency
of the pulse, but exerts a curative influence on the disease, and
with regard to its lessening the frequency of the pulse, I unhesitatingly say, without fear of successful controversy, that it will
control the pulse in *any* and *every* case where it is morbidly excited. I regard your "remedy" as peculiarly adapted to the
treatment of pneumonitis, pleuritis, pneumonia typhodes, pertussis, typhus fever with increased action of the heart and arteries. Mr. Rodgers, in whose family you practice, was attacked with typhoid pneumonia about the time you left home,
and Drs. Agnew and Traynham attended him, and when all
hope of his recovery was lost, his family recollected that some
of them had been rescued from an untimely grave by your
remedy—urged the physicians to give the "drops." Neither
of the physicians having the medicine, they determined to send
to me for it; and, with only ℨij of the tincture, both of the
physicians assured me they had saved Mr. Rodgers, and would

not take less than five dollars for the remnant of the two drachms."

We have every confidence that it will cure scarlet fever, also that it will be a valuable remedy in puerperal fever. We are waiting an opportunity to test its powers in the treatment of yellow fever. If we should succeed in curing yellow fever or materially lessening its fearful mortality, who will not hail it the master discovery of the age?

Above we have given a brief outline in addition to what we have heretofore published. We intend shortly to give a full detail of the powers of the article and our entire experience. We challenge the world to discredit the above. We pledge ourselves, and stand ready to demonstrate the powers and effects claimed. We have staked our reputation for veracity and medical skill on the above, and we are perfectly willing to abide the verdict of a liberal and enlightened profession and an intelligent community. Truth is omnipotent. The above was not got up in a day, or a corner, but is the result of years of laborious investigation, and of time and money spent to prove and test the certainty and correctness of our experience, and the conclusions reached, the world can either receive it or reject it.

[The preparation of Veratrum Viride used by Dr. N. is the Saturated tincture of the root.—Edt.]

ARTICLE III.

Report of a Case of Phimosis, with Remarks. By Juriah Harriss, M. D., of Augusta, Ga.

Phimosis differs very much in character and form, according to the circumstances under which it occurs. It may be temporary or permanent, and the latter kind, which alone requires an operation, may be congenital or accidental.

Permanent accidental phimosis may be the consequences of chancres, vegetations, indurations of the prepuce, herpes, and adhesions of the prepuce to the glans penis. All of these causes induce phimosis, and frequently to such an extent as to render an operation necessary. When the deformity is con-

genital, it of course requires an operation. Ricord observes,
that when the adhesions between the prepuce and glans penis
are intimate and of long standing, they should not be dissected
up, but only a portion of the prepuce should be removed, sufficient to allow free micturition. The old operation of slitting
the prepuce above or below the glans, is very objectionable.
It was first proposed and performed by Celsus; after prevailing a considerable time, it fell into disuse, but was revived and
extolled by M. Cloquet. Since this, it has been the process
preferred by the profession generally.

A very serious objection to this operation is, that it substitutes one deformity for another. It removes the phimosis, it
is true, but there remain two flaps, which destroy the symmetry of the organ and constitute an impediment to coition.
The operation of simple circumcision is decidedly preferable
to the old plan of Celsus. The wound heals as rapidly, and
leaves a much prettier result. Ricord's operation, which is in
effect but a circumcision, is more neat and much to be preferred
to either of the above modes. I will give his manner of operating, by detailing a case.

A boy, about eight years of age, being presented for examination, I discovered a very long prepuce, with a small tumor
upon its lower margin. The tumor was situated just beneath
the skin, in the subcutaneous cellular tissue. It felt very much
like an adipose tumor. Its position and size lessened very
much the perputial orifice and rendered micturition somewhat
difficult. I deemed it advisable to circumcise the child, as by
so doing I would relieve him at the same time of the tumor
and phimosis; moreover, the wound would not be any larger
than that required for the extirpation of the tumor, and this
might result in a permanent phimosis which would itself eventually necessitate another operation.

Ricord divides his operation into four stages: 1st. An ink
mark is made two lines in front of the base of the glans : this mark
is of course oblique and serves as a guide to the forceps. 2d. A
long needle, with its point covered with a ball of wax, to prevent pricking too soon, is then passed between the prepuce
and glans and made to transfix the upper portion of the prepuce
a line or two in front of the mark, at the base of the glans

penis. 3d. The phimosis forceps are then applied to the prepuce in front of the mark and behind the point of the needle.
4th. The needle is next seized and pulled upon to extend the
prepuce. 5th. The bistoury is, lastly, passed between the needle and forceps, and the protruding prepuce is excised. The
operator should be careful to cut against the forceps, which
have a smooth edge which serves as a guide and secures a
regular surface.

After the section, and before the forceps are removed, a
sufficient number of sutures are to be passed through the
groove in the jaws of the instrument, and thus entirely through
the two sides of the prepuce. The forceps are then removed
and the sutures severed in the middle and tied upon either side.

I performed the operation according to the plan of Ricord, except that I did not apply the sutures, but made use of the ser-
refines, or small wire forceps of Vidal de Cassis. These forceps
close of themselves and are very useful in slight wounds.
They retain the parts together, and may be removed at any
time without pain.

Upon dissection of the tumor, after the operation, I found
that it was not adipose in structure, but was an encysted tumor. It was composed of a sack containing a soft substance,
resembling rich cream. This matter I placed under the microscope, and found an abundance of rhomboidal crystals of chol-
esterine. These crystals were disseminated through the mass,
and were in some points agglomerated together and overlapped
each other. There were also an abundance of fatty granules
or cellules (grumeaux graisseux.) There were but few elementary granulations, which is rather unusual in such tumors.

The cyst was composed of fine cellular tissue and a number
of small cells, some with and some without nuclei. The cyst
appeared to the naked eye delicate, pearly and semitranspar-
ent. The French style this kind of tumor a *cholesteotome.*
Cold water dressing was applied to prevent hemorrhage and
too great inflammation.

I performed the same operation upon an adult, sometime
since; but owing to a strong syphilitic taint, the wound has not
healed properly, and the patient is consequently not yet well.
I may give a report of this case at some future time, with additional remarks upon phimosis.

PART II.

𝕰𝖈𝖑𝖊𝖈𝖙𝖎𝖈 𝕯𝖊𝖕𝖆𝖗𝖙𝖒𝖊𝖓𝖙

Cod-liver oil; Superiority to any other single remedy in phthisis; Illustrative instances of its value; Different kinds compared; Collateral remedies sometimes useful, often unnecessary; Effect of its introduction into the system by friction; Mode of action; Important practical generalizations derivable from a knowledge of its mode of action; The appreciation and use of facts. By THEOPHILUS THOMPSON, M.D., F.R.S., Physician to the Hospital for Consumption, &c.

THE great object, gentlemen, of all our researches is to attain to the successful treatment of disease. With this conviction I propose to devote the present lecture to the consideration of the effects of a remedy which you will have observed is very largely employed at this hospital, even to the extent of more than 600 gallons annually.

The records of the hospital give you an opportunity of comparing the effect of treatment conducted on general principles, irrespective of the use of this remedy, with treatment in which the administration of this medicine has occupied an important place; and the more carefully you institute the comparison the more will you be convinced of the value of this substance in the treatment of phthisis, when appropriately administered, and combined with the use of such other measures as any special circumstances in the individual patient may require.

But you will like to see examples of its use. I first introduced M. A. F., a female aged thirty-two. The expansion of the two sides of her chest at the upper part is not perfectly equal, although a practised eye may be required to detect the difference; in the left sub-clavicular region inspiration is interrupted; in the right subclavicular region the expiratory murmur is prolonged. The disease is at a very early stage, and cod-liver oil has been given in the hope of improving her strength, and thus warding off further disease. Her progress is encouraging; the pulse, in the last six weeks, having gone down from 116 to 80, and her weight increased five pounds,

The next patient, A. S., is a tailor, who has suffered much from confinement in close workshops. The principal physical signs at the time of his admission were, dulness on percussion and extensive moist crepitation over the upper half of the left chest. Softening of tubercular deposit was obviously proceeding rapidly, and this is the period in phthisis when the influence of remedies is usually least satisfactory. The patient looks very delicate. The pulse has remained about 100 for the last seven weeks, notwithstanding the administration of the cod-liver oil, and his general aspect is unpromising ; still some good effect has been produced, and there is an addition of five pounds to his weight.

The next patient, L. D., a young woman aged twenty-one, came into the hospital on' the 31st of October, with moist crepitation at the apex of the right lung, and gurgling in respiration and cough on the left ; phthisis existing in the second stage on one side, and the third on the other. The pulse, as in the previous patient, remains as yet unaltered, but there is an improvement of strength, a subsidence of night perspirations, a regular state of bowels, which were previously relaxed and, in the three months of her use of the oil, an increase of weight to the extent of six pounds. The local signs also indicate amendment. The expectoration is much diminished, and a dry, blowing respiration has taken the place of gurgling.

E. M., the patient now before you, under the judicious care of my colleague, Dr. Cursham, has acquired so ruddy a complexion that you would not suppose her an invalid. There is, however, cavernous respiration at the apex of one lung ; still, the cough is subdued ; the expectoration, once profuse, has ceased, and she has gained no less than fifteen pounds weight in about twelve weeks. It is right to mention that she has had spermaceti mixture and compound hemlock-pill for her cough ; and of late, in addition to cod-liver oil, the following mixture : Twenty-four grains of ammonio-citrate of iron ; two drachms of spirit of nutmeg ; six ounces of infusion of calumba ; an ounce twice a day.

Here is another patient, S. G., aged twenty-five, who is fattening, and the catamenia, long interrupted, have returned— a circumstance of great significance and promise. You find a little cavernulous rhonchus, only, where there was formerly extensive gurgling ; and a marked flattening in the subclavicular region indicates the process of contraction of a cavity. Her weight, which was seven stone thirteen pounds on her admission, in July, has steadily increased, and now, at the end of February, it is nine stone, two pounds, and the concurrent symptoms of vomiting, palpitation, and œdema, with which this patient was for a time harassed, have entirely disappeared. In addition to cod oil she had syrup of iodide of iron, and counter-irritation has occasionally been established by the application of a liniment made according to the following prescription : Take of iodine, and of iodide of potassium, each an ounce ; of rectified spirit, two ounces: mix.

I must have the satisfaction of introducing one more patient, whose case is highly gratifying. This young woman, M. B., is, I am informed, the only remaining member of a large family all of whom have died of phthisis. She was admitted five months since, with dull percussion at the right apex; at the left, gurgling in respiration, and cough. Her case was examined and recorded by two other medical gentlemen before I explored her chest, and my account corresponded with theirs as to the existence of cavity in the left side. To-day two of my colleagues have examined her, and agree with me in the opinion that no sign of cavity can now be detected in that situation. Let me describe the progress of her improvement: The extent of the gurgling gradually lessened, then dry cavernous respiration was the principal sign; this was superseded by blowing, and then bronchial breathing, and at present I detect nothing wrong except a little flattening of contour, slght dulness on percussion, and wavy inspiration. The catamenia have returned; the pulse has sunk from 112 to 80 Her weight five months since was seven stone twelve pounds and a- quarter; we will try it again: it is now nine stone five pounds and a quarter.

You may wish to form an opinion regarding the comparative efficacy of the different kinds of cod-liver oil. In my early trials of the remedy, six years since, forty or fifty cases-were treated with the coarse kind, resembling what is used in preparing leather, and the average benefit derived did not materially differ from that effected by the purest varieties subsequetly employed. At a later period I had the curiosity to try these different kinds, combined with liquor potassæ, and peppermint oil, giving alternately the coarse and the purified cod oil, and recording the report of the patients; and it is a curious fact that the majority actually gave the preference to the mixtures in which the coarser oil was introduced. Objections have been made to this combination as complicating the treatment with the addition of a medicine by some persons supposed to be inappropriate; but my experience is favourable to the use of liquor potassæ, especially in the early stage of phthisis, and theoretical arguments might be advanced in its favour. In scrofulous affections, if Dr. Hughes Bennet be correct in his hypothesis, there is probably undue acidity of stomach, unfavourable to the solution of albuminous materials. The alkali of the salivary and pancreatic fluids, being neutralized, fails to convert the carbon into oil. The lungs not having enough carbon to excrete, local congestions arise; the blood is overcharged with albumen, and the albuminous exudation being deficient in fat, elementary molecules are not formed so as to constitute nuclei capable of development into cells, and tubercular corpuscles are the natural result.

Cod-liver oil probably tends to obviate the series of derangements just described, by combining with the albuminous element of chyme, so as to form the healthy chyle-granules which feed the blood, and, for the reason above named, is probably better introduced in scrofulous subjects when combined with an alkali. It is a curious fact, that when, about seventy-five years since, cod-liver oil was largely used at the Manchester Infirmary, chiefly in the treatment of rheumatism, the medicine was ordinarily given combined with alkali; Dr. Percival's favourite prescription being twelve minims of soap lixivium, an ounce of cod-liver oil, and half an ounce of peppermint water. The practice of administering a little lemon-juice afterwards would not necessarily interfere with the action of the alkali, and is worthy of incidental notice in connection with the recent valuable suggestions of Dr. G. O. Rees in the treatment of rheumatism with the acid of lemons. Occasionally, although not frequently, the stomach rebels against the oil, however purified, and in whatever combination; and I have been accustomed in consequence, under such circumstances, to introduce the oil endermically.

Three years since I was requested to see a gentleman from the country, confined to his bed, emaciated, hectic, and apparently failing rapidly, with a cavity at the apex of the right lung. There was considerable diarrhœa; and thinking the internal use of cod-oil unseasonable, I ordered an ounce, combined with oil of lavender, to be rubbed into the chest night and morning. This gentleman gradually rallied, and returned to the country, where he advanced much in strength and weight, and rode about on horseback. I examined him last year, and judging from the physical signs, found the size of the cavity materially reduced.

J. S., a patient under my care for the last two years, with softened tubercle in the left lung, notwithstanding the adoption of a tonic regimen, and the internal administration of cod oil, got gradually worse, and in the four months preceding August, 1850, her weight was reduced from 105 to 97 pounds. I then prescribed, as a liniment, three ounces of cod oil; an ounce of sal volatile; half a drachm of oil of lavender; five grains of opium: half to be rubbed in night and morning. In a fortnight improvement commenced, and in two months her weight had risen to 104 pounds.

M. A. W., a patient lately in the hospital with cavernous respiration at the summits of both lungs, and who had weekly lost on an average a pound in weight for twelve weeks, rallied, gained a little weight during the first month of using the same liniment, and left the hospital somewhat improved. But I will not multiply examples. It is enough to say that satisfactory results have been sufficiently frequent to authorize the measure, sometimes as an auxiliary to the internal use of the oil, but more especially as a substitute when the stomach revolts at its internal administration.

I am indebted to Dr. Glover, of Newcastle, for a reference to some observations of Dr. Klencke, of Braunschwig, confirmatory of the results just described. In a memoir on the Therapeutical History of Cod Oil, Dr. Klencke says,—" I shaved some young dogs, and rubbed them with cod-liver oil twice daily for three weeks. At the end of this period they were in as good conditon as dogs to whom oil had been internally administered ; their bile was found as rich in fat, and their chyle equally charged with corpuscles without nuclei." Klencke adds that similar changes were observed in the bile and chyle of a cat bathed twice a day for some time in the same remedy, and that some oil was discovered in the urine of the animal, proving its free absorption by the skin.

You will naturally ask me whether there are any disadvantages incident to the use of so valuable a remedy ? and you may repeat questions I have occasionally heard : Does it often produce diarrhœa ? Does it tend to increase hæmoptysis ? As respects the latter question, it might be sufficient to mention that the average frequency of the occurrence of hæmoptysis, as recorded by Louis and other observers, was fully as great in phthisical cases before cod-liver oil was introduced as it has proved in those cases statistically reported at this hospital in which this remedy has been perseveringly used. When hæmoptysis is active, as characterized by phenomena described in my second lecture, it is, indeed, easy to imagine that a remedy which increases the fulness of the pulse might aggravate the spitting of blood ; under such circumstances the fish-oil should be discontinued, and the removal of blood by cupping may be desirable. When, however, as is frequently the case, the hæmorrhage is passive, means which tend to enrich the blood are calculated to lessen the hæmorrhagic tendency, and its occurrence is by no means an adequate reason for the suspension of the oil.

As respects diarrhœa, a malady which the remedy under consideration has been supposed occasionally to aggravate, my own impression is that no such influence is evinced unless a state of erethism of the mucous membrane is present, in which case measures should be used to obviate such condition prior to the administration of the oil. Many of the patients take the oil unmixed, or, when such combinations are appropriate, floated on nitro-muriatic acid mixture, or on lemon-juice. The addition of creasote occasionally makes the stomach more tolerant of the remedy.

An ounce and a half of cod-liver oil, four drops of creasote, two drachms of compound tragacanth powder, and four ounces and a half of aniseed water, form a suitable mixture, of which an ounce may be taken thrice daily.

Those who take the oil unmixed, may cover the taste by eating dried orange peel, or by introducing a little dinner-salt into the mouth before and after the oil.

You will observe from the cases tabulated in the preceding page, all of which you have had an opportunity of seeing,— and the conclusion is in harmony with more extended observations,—that if the use of cod oil has any influence on the condition of the bowels, that influence is rather astringent than laxative.

I believe the fact to be that this medicine has no direct influence on the intestinal action, but that by improving the general health it tends indirectly to restore a natural condition of the bowels, whilst it expands the pulse, lessens the expectoration, moderates the night perspirations, and in many instances supersedes the necessity for the use of any other remedy.

You will say the evidence adduced of the powers of cod oil is strong, but that the remedy was formerly highly estimated and yet fell into disuse, and you may inquire whether it may not exhibit the fluctuations of fashion, and again sink into oblivion. The best way to secure for any remedy its proper place in therapeutics, is to determine its mode of action ; and with this view I have from time to time endeavoured to obtain an analysis of the blood of patients who were in the course of improvement under its use : as an example, let me show you the analysis of the blood of a phthisical man in the Le Blanc ward, who had gained fourteen pounds weight in three months and had essentially improved under the cod-oil treatment.

Dr. Snow did me the favour to make the analysis. I place by the side, for comparison, the analysis of the blood of a healthy male, as given by Becquerel and Rodier :—

Analysis of Blood of a Healthy Male.	Of a Phthisical man after three months Treatment with Cod oil.
Water................................ 779·0	.... 770·6
Blood-globules.................... 141·1	.... 143·5
Fibrine............................... 2·2	.... 4·0
Albumen.............. 69·4 ⎫ 76·2	.... 81.5
Extractive and salts.... 6·8 ⎭	
Fatty matters...................... 1·6	.... 0·4

The interest of these analyses is increased by their harmony with the observation of Simon, who recorded an increase of blood corpuscles and diminution of fibrine under the use of cod oil ; and their importance becomes more obious when they are viewed in reference to the facts stated by Andral and Gavarret

who, having analysed the blood in twenty-one cases of phthisis
found their maximum of fibrine, 5·9, their minimum 2·1, and
that the amount of corpuscles approximated to the normal
standard in only two instances, in which it was represented by
122·1 and 120·4.   Frequently, indeed, the amount was below
100, and the decrease of corpuscles was almost always accompanied with a corresponding increase of fibrine. (Simon's " Animal Chemistry," vol. i., p. 281, Sydenham Soc. edit.)

You see that, in the patient just referred to, the proportion
of blood corpuscles pretty closely corresponds with that characteristic of health, and Mr. Rodgers reports a similar result
from the examination of the blood of some other patients to
whom we have given the oil.   As far as I am aware, however, chemical observations lead to the conclusion, that in phthisis deficient proportion of blood-corpuscles is the usual peculiarity.   Struck with this circumstance, I took pains to collect,
chiefly from Simon, analyses of the blood in different diseases,
and I have placed before you averages of the proportion of
blood-corpuscles and albumen in certain diseases, with a view
to compare them with phthisis.

Average Proportion of some Constituents of Blood.

	Albumen.	Corpuscles.
In health..............	76	130
Pneumonia..........	80	122
Phthisis..........	100	78
Rheumatism..........	100	74
Diabetes............	105	80
Chlorosis........ ....:	72	56
Bright's disease.........	103	50
Carcinoma........	45	55
Erysipelas........	—	100

You will observe that there are two diseases which present
a peculiar similarity to phthisis, in their proportions of albumen
and of corpuscles.   These are rheumatism and diabetes.   Now
it is a remarkable fact, that rheumatism is the malady for the
treatment of which cod-liver oil was first introduced into this
country, and for which it has been so largely and successfully
employed elsewhere.   The variety of rheumatism in which it
was most effectual is that in which the impoverished condition
of blood is most likely to occur.

Dr. Percival, half a century since, (see Works Literary,
Moral, and Medical, by Dr. Thomas Percival, vol. 4, p. 354,)
observes,—" Men and women advanced in years, whose fibres
may be supposed to have acquired a degree of rigidity, find
surprising effects from it (cod-oil.) Some who have been crip-
ples for many years, and not able to move from their seats,
have after a few weeks' use of it been able to go with the as-

sistance of a stick, and, by a longer continuance, have enjoyed the pleasing satisfaction of being restored to the natural use of their limbs, which for a long time before had been a burden to them. Two cases occurred lately in which the oil had an extraordinary effect, even on young persons, whose ages did not exceed ten years. Guaiacum, calomel, blisters, &c., were tried on both these patients, but with so little benefit that opiates were given merely to procure temporary relief. Their lower limbs seemed to be a burden to them, and they had such an appearance of distortion, that no hopes of relief could be well entertained. In compliance with the particular request of their parents, the cod-oil was given. The one obtained a perfect cure, the other nearly so ; the latter having a little distortion in his back, is prevented the use of his legs. So general (adds Dr. Percival) has been the use of the oil with us, that we dispense fifty or sixty gallons annually ; and the good effects of it are so well known amongst the poorer sort, that it is particularly requested by them for almost every lameness. Except bark, opium, and mercury, I believe no medicine in the materia medica is likely to be of more service, and I should wish for a more general use of it in order to prove that the above account of its good effects is no exaggeration."

I am strongly impressed with the value of the remedy in diabetes. It is true that this. disease involves an additional element, which it is not easy to suppose amenable to such a remedy as fish-oils, but the benefit derived in many respects is often remarkable.

In the month of April, 1848, a patient came under my care who had been affected with diabetes for some months, and had taken creasote and other medicines with little advantage. At the time I first saw her the quantity of urine passed in twenty-four hours, amounted to ten pints.

The following table will show the progress under the cod-liver oil treatment ;—

Dates.	Remedies.	Urine.	
		Quantity.	Specific Gravity.
1848.			
April 1	Cod-oil, two drachms three times a day.	Ten pints.	
" 13	Ditto.	Six pints.	
" 20	Ditto.	Four pints.	1·040
" 27	Cod-oil, four times daily.	Six pints.	1·042
May 4	" five times daily	Three pints.	1·042
" 11	Ditto.	Three pints.	1·037
" 18	Ditto.	Two pints and quarter	1·020

Subsequently this patient passed unavoidably into other care and owing to a misunderstanding, did not resume the cod-liver oil, which had been, from temporary causes, intermitted. She took a variety of remedies, including sulphur, hydrochloric acid opium and alkalies. Drachm doses of carbonate of soda for a time acted favourably, but on the whole she retrograded. Her weight, which in Juue, 1848, was 107 pounds, had fallen, by December, 1849, to 88 pounds. Her appearance was haggard and there was threatening of pulmonary disease. The cod-oil was resumed, and even then with temporary advantage, but she ultimately relapsed and sank.

The theory which I have now proposed in explanation of one mode of action of the oil is in harmony with the fact that its good effects are specially produced in women and children, for in them the relative proportion of corpuscles is stated by chemists to be small.

I may state that the remedy has afforded me most satisfactory results in neuralgia and sciatica, when associated with anæmia. Whenever arterial or venous murmurs indicate such a condition, a rapid improvement may be expected to follow the administration of the oil, even without the assistance of ferruginous medicines. In some disturbed manifestations of the nervous system which may appear more moral than physical, the presence of a weak, small pulse, has sometimes led me to give the oil, and with signal success. Do not think that I dwell on this subject from any love of fanciful hypothesis. When the light issuing from a certain number of facts seem to converge towards a particular point of explanation, it is useful to try the applicability of that explanation to analogous facts, and thus to entertain, I do not say to adopt a theory—a sort of tentative theory, or "*prudens quæstio.*" If the theory prove universally applicable, we obtain a law; if the explanation be found incorrect, it is yet seldom fruitless: indeed the proof of its inadequacy serves to narrow the field of inquiry, and to increase the probability that the next step may be in the right direction towards the attainment of truth. Time is sometimes lost in the laborious accumulation of miscellaneous facts. Numerism is productive only by the amount of "*lumen siccum,*" intellectual intuition,— applied in the selection and appreciation of facts. There is an aristocracy in facts as well as races, and the mind should be taught to discern their prerogative dignity. "The naturalist who cannot or will not see that one fact is often worth a thousand, as including them all in itself, and that it first makes all the others facts—who has not the head to comprehend, the soul to reverence, a central experiment or observation, (what the Greeks would perhaps have called a protophænomenon,) will never receive an auspicious answer from the oracle of Nature."

To apply these observations to our immediate subject, let

me remark that changes produced on the blood by diseases or remedies may fairly be placed amongst the cardinal facts. It can scarcely be doubted, that if a professor accomplished in chemistry were officially connected with every hospital, such facts might be so collected as to render the discoveries of this important science available, in a remarkable degree, for the advancement of practical medicine.

Should further observation confirm what has been suggested in this lecture regarding the influence of fish oils on the composition of the circulating fluid, we shall discover more than the reason of their usefulness in phthisis; we shall show that they have no exclusive adaptation to that disease, but that they may be given with equal promise in various diseases associated with analogous conditions of the blood; and thus we may come to establish a therapeutical law so widely applicable as to simplify our principles, extend our resources, and consolidate our system of practical medicine. Such a generalization would commend itself to my mind by its freedom from complication and obscurity; for I am sure you will agree with me as to the evidence afforded in the noblest triumphs of philosophy, that although shallowness and obscurity are continually associated, yet that the ocean of truth is clear as well as deep, and that in proportion as we approach the truth, we shall attain to simplicity.   [*London Lancet.*

On a rarely observed, but very fatal Effect of Gastro-intestinal Revellents; especially of the Tartrate of Antimony and Potassa, and particularly in the treatment of Pneumonia. By Wm. M. Boling, M. D., of Montgomery, Alabama.

There are but few articles of the Materia Medica which exercise so certain a control over any serious morbid state or action, as the tartrate of antimony and potassa does, over inflammation of the pulmonary parenchyma. Its efficiency, I may say, is universally admitted. Unfortunately, however, its value as a remedy in pneumonia, or any other disease indeed in which its protracted use may be required, is diminished by the circumstance of its occasioning in many instances, violent disease of some of the abdominal viscera, which often leads to a fatal result. It is in pneumonia, however, according to my own observation, that the effect referred to is most frequently produced by it, and developed in the most violent and rapid manner; probably, it is but reasonable to suppose, because in this disease its protracted administration is more frequently practiced than in any other. As generally administered, it is not improbable, that the remedy, even in cases in which the ultimate result may be favourable, produces by its contact, more or less irritation of the gastro-intestinal mucous membrane, which gradually subsides, after its suspension, during convalescence. Its visible effect upon the skin, when used locally, might lead to such an inference, and indeed appearances somewhat analogous to this are sometimes observable, not only after death, in the gastro-intestinal mucous membrane, but during life, in the mouth and fauces, as a result seemingly of its use. In fact it is to a revellent effect, resulting from this local irritant action, that its efficacy in pneumonia and other diseases, is attributed by the advocates of the physiological doctrine. It is not, however, this local action, *merely as spoken of and described by the generality of writers*, to which it is my object to call attention at present, but more particularly to an array of symptoms of a much more violent and sudden character, connected seemingly with a metastasis of morbid action, from the thoracic (when administered in the diseases of this cavity), to the abdominal viscera; the result, it may be, of an exaggerated influence of the character mentioned. Whatever the correct explanation, however, as to the mode in which the effect is produced, the condition itself is one of extreme danger.

There is reason to believe, however, that though in the treatment of pneumonia, the state in question is more frequently induced by the use of tartar emetic, than by anything else, a similar condition is occasionally brought about by other agents administered to such an extent as to produce a high degree of irritation of the gastro-intestinal mucous membrane; and I believe that it is with more certainty developed, under a combination in the treatment, of calomel with the antimonial, than by the latter alone.

Supposing the remedy to have been continued several days, the phenomena referred to, are developed much in the following manner. The patient may seemingly be doing well under the continued use of the remedy; the dulness on-percussion, and the frequency of the pulse diminishing; the skin perhaps becoming moist, and the respiration improving. Suddenly in some cases, in others somewhat gradually, the patient becomes restless, the thirst is augmented, the discharges from the bowels are more numerous and thin, the abdomen becomes tympanitic and perhaps tender, the tolerance is lost, and though he may not have done so for several days, he vomits or makes frequent efforts to do so; the tongue becomes dry and pointed; there is jactitation present, anxiety of countenance, delirium and perhaps stupor a short time before death. Occasionally jaundice supervenes, and in a few cases the matter vomited bears a close resemblance to that ejected in yellow fever. During the progress of the change, the pulse becomes more frequent, hard, concentrated, small and thready.

The rapidity with which the symptoms mentioned are developed varies a good deal in different cases. I have known instances in which death has taken place in about six hours from the time of the first evident unfavourable change; in every respect, up to that time, the progress of the case being apparently favourable, and the graver symptoms subdued. Oftener the case is protracted to ten or twelve hours, and sometimes to a longer period.

Simultaneously with the changes above spoken of, or, as it were, preceding them rather, a more or less rapid disappearance of the signs and symptoms of the primary disease takes place. From a state of almost complete solidification of an entire lung, with dulness on percussion, and bronchial respiration; in the course of four or five hours, I have found the pulmonary tissue permeable, and the chest resonant and yielding a healthy respiratory murmur; a corresponding improvement in the cough, thoracic pain, difficulty of breathing, &c., proceeding at an equal rate. The rapidity with which this change in the condition of the lung takes place is proportionate to the violence and rapidity of the newly developed abdominal disease.

In any case of pneumonia under the antimonial treatment, although the patient may seemingly have been doing well, the supervention of the slightest tympanitis, with augmented thirst and a tendency to diarrhœa, may be regarded with suspicion, as the probable precursors of a very grave condition; and I am now led to regard my patient's doom as almost settled, when, in addition to these symptoms, there is a *rapid* instead of a gradual removal of the dulness on percussion, *unattended with the crepitant rale of resolution.* Where a case is closely watched the latter will be found to precede somewhat the former symptoms of the progressing change; and I have more than once surprised, not only the relatives of patients, but professional gentlemen in attendance with me, by announcing a coming change for the worse, basing my opinion on the physical sign just stated, where everything otherwise seemed favourable; the patient comfortable, and apparently, perhaps, convalescent.

This termination of pneumonia, under the administration of antimonials, especially when given in what would be considered anything like adequate doses by the advocates of the doctrines of Rasori, I am led to believe cannot be of very rare occurrence in the south; for I think that I have seen almost as many patients die of the superinduced or substituted affection as of the primary. And yet the largest quantity for the twenty-four hours, in which I have been in the habit of prescribing the tartrate of antimony and potassa, falls far short of what would be considered a medium dose for the same time, by the generality of physicians of the contrastimulant school. Under the supposition, however, that it not unfrequently occurs, it is somewhat strange that we find so little in the works of authors who have written on pneumonia, especially as treated with antimony according to the contrastimulant doctrine, in which anything like a distinct reference is made to it, much less an accurate account of the condition. Neither in the French nor Italian writers of the contrastimulant shool accessible to me have I been able to find any account of it, though in many we find allusion to the mere local irritant action of the agent in question upon the gastro-intestinal mucous membrane. This is more especially, however, the case among the advocates of the physiological doctrine, by whom the curative influence of the remedy in question, in pneumonia, is ascribed to a revellent operation. The condition spoken of by the followers of Rasori as a loss of the tolerance, resembles it in many respects, and I have sometimes suspected that in their descriptions they may have had in view a state identical with that to which I now have reference. If so, however, their delineation is incomplete in several important particulars ; and I would especially mention the sudden subsidence of the original disease, with the occurrence of the new train of alarming symptoms. Moreover no one, I imagine, who has ever observed a well-marked case of the state to which I have reference, even under the influence of a favourite doctrine, could see in it *merely* a general depression of the vital powers somewhat below the standard of health ; and, in short, could suppose that the phenomena manifested were not the consequences of actual local lesion of the viscera of the abdomen.

I have been disappointed in not finding an account of it in such of the writings as I have met with, of the Italian followers of Rasori ; because, not only from the immense doses in which they are in the habit of administering the antimonial preparations, but from the similarity of their climate, and diseases generally to our own, in their hands especially, I had been led to suppose it must frequently occur. Owing to the fact, that in the north, the susceptibility of the gastro-intestinal mucous membrane to irritant impressions is less than in the south, it probably occurs less frequently there than with us. One rather mild, but unqestionable case, I find recorded in the *American Journal of Medical Sciences* for April, 1848, by J. F. PEEBLES, M. D. of Petersburgh, Virginia, in a paper calling attention to certain unfavourable effects of tartar emetic. Two other cases are given by B. R. JONES, M. D. of Montgomery Alabama, in the *New Orleans Medical and Surgical Journal* for September, 1850; in which he particularly refers to it as a result of the operation of antimony.

My own attention, several years ago, was forcibly drawn to this unfavourable action of the tartrate of antimony and potassa in pneumonia, especially, and it was alluded to in a paper on the treatment of the inflammatory affections of malarious districts, which I published in the *American Journal of Medical Sciences* for July, 1844. Two cases are there given, among others of a different character; and, in regard to one of them, the following remarke is made. "In this case, an occurrence took place, which is by no means unusual with us here, in the treatment of acute thoracic diseases, particularly when tartar emetic or calomel is used to any considerable extent, and more especially when they are used in combination; viz., the super-vention of gastro-enteritis about the time, or *soon after a con-siderable amendment has taken place in the original disease.*"

But, though I have been able to find nothing, or but little, that can be regarded as having allusion to the accident in question, where most I expected to find accounts of it, viz., among authors of the school of Rasori, in speaking of the use of tartar emetic in pneumonia, a graphic description of a similar state produced by the continued administration of calomel may be found in the work of Golis on hydrocephalus. "Many times," he says, "I saw, under these large and long-continued doses of calomel, the hydrocephalic symptoms *suddenly* disappear, and inflammation of the intestines arise, which terminated in death. Still oftener, I have observed this unfavourable accident, from an incautious use of calomel in croup; viz., where all the fright-ful symptoms of this tracheal inflammation, which threatened suffocation, would *vanish suddenly*, and enteritis develop itself, which passed rapidly into gangrene and destroyed the patient."— (*Davis, on Acute Hydrocephalus.*)

Although it is probable, that it is through a local irritant ac-tion of the antimonial upon the gastro-intestinal mucous mem-brane, that the effect in question is brought about; the manner and circumstances of its development lead not unreasonably to the inference, that a real metastasis takes place; that in addi-tion to that irritation, which the remedy, probably, in almost every instance produces, where it is long used; that, for instan-ce, which it would produce in a healthy subject; there is a superadded morbid action, transferred upon the abdominal vis-cera, in lieu of the pneumonia, which has suddenly disappeared. It will be remembered, that, generally, it is not till after a par-tial subsidence of the pneumonic symptoms, that evidences of the gastro-intestinal irritation are manifested. It partakes, then, more of the character of metastasis than revulsion, though an irritant action may have determined it.

Why the morbid action, from which the patient was, probably, to all appearance in no great danger, in the lungs, should prove so frequently fatal when transferred to the abdominal viscera, is a question which naturally suggests itself. Perhaps it may be the suddenness of the invasion. Perhaps the translated morbid action, operating in conjunction with a morbid state, which had already been developed in a high degree in the gastro-intestinal mucous membrane by the remedy, but which, up to the moment of the metastasis, had remained latent, in consequence of the preponderance of the pneumonic inflammation. Perhaps, a greater depression of the vital powers results from an equal degree of morbid action in the gastro-intestinal mucous membrane, than in the pulmonary parenchyma.

Notwithstanding this occasional unfavourable influence of the tartrate of antimony and potassa, I have felt reluctant to dispense with its use entirely in the treatment of pneumonia, in which, otherwise, its efficacy is so great ; and, for some time, it has been an object with me to devise some plan of administration, by which, while its favourable operation might be secured, the former effect might be entirely, or in a great measure avoided.

Without entering into any detail or discussion of the various and somewhat contradictory views entertained by different physicians, or sects of physicians, as to the modus operandi of the tartrate of antimony and potassa, I think it may at present be safely assumed that, while its sedative or contrastimulant influence is exerted, after its absorption and commixture with the circulating mass, the unfavourable effects resulting from its adminstration, to which reference is here made, are consequences of its direct local action upon the gastro-intestinal mucous membrane. To be sure, according to experiments of Magendie it would appear that its *emetic* operation is secondary to its absorption, and the result of a special affinity for, or action upon the stomach, while in its transit through the vascular circle ; but it would seem a visionary refinement in toxicology, to refer the effects of which I have been speaking to an influence thus exerted, aware, as we already are, of its irritant action upon the mucous and dermoid tissues, when locally applied.

It is not at all improbable, however, that in some rare cases, the revulsive operation of the remedy on the gastro-intestinal mucous membrane may prove favourable, according to the views of Broussais ; but, knowing as we do, that other gastro-intestinal revellents exercise no such special control over the phlegmasiæ of the thoracic viscera, as the agent in question, as a general rule, his explanation of its modus operandi will, I am inclined to believe, be deemed incorrect. On the contrary, when the local effect on the gastro-intestinal mucous membrane is developed in any considerable degree, recovery, even when it follows, is retarded rather than advanced by the circumstance; not only by the additional febrile disturbance, but by the diminished absorption which results in consequence ; and that when it occurs in a high degree, it occasions in pneumonia the train of alarming, and so often fatal phenomena.

Assuming then that the sedative effect of the remedy through which its curative influnce in pneumonia is brought about, is produced by that which is absorbed ; and the deleterious effects under consideration, by that which, remaining unabsorbed, or which is not for a considerable time absorbed—remains long applied in contact with the gastro-intestinal mucous membrane—by what indeed may very properly be deemed a redundancy of the article—that over and above what can be readily acted on by the absorbents, it is manifest that to secure the former and avoid the latter, no more of it should be prescribed than it is probable will be promptly taken up by these vessels, and its administration regulated in such a manner as best to secure this end.

With this object in view, I at first commenced to diminsh the dose, although in no case had I ever given it in anything like the quantity recommended by many physicians of the contrastimulant school; nor did I find the efficacy of the remedy less when I had fallen back upon about the quantity advised by many before the rise of the contrastimulant doctrine : say three, four, or at most six grains in the twenty-four hours, than when I gave it in doses twice or thrice as large ; but its mischievous effects were infinitely less. It does not necessarily follow because in many cases the larger doses of the ultra contrastimulists are tolerated for the time, and generally without any manifest ulterior mischievous effects, that they are really required.

Besides this reduction of the dose, say for the twenty-four hours, to the smallest possible quantity capable of producing a sedative influence, I have also adopted the plan of giving it in small portions, frequently repeated, so that not more will be swallowed at a time than may be promptly, at once indeed, acted on by the absorbents, rather than in larger portions at longer intervals, by which the mucous membrane would be of necessity subjected to a longer contact with a part of each portion swallowed. The method has seemed to me a bad one, of giving the quantity intended for the twenty-four hours at lengthened, though equally divided intervals throughout this period ; but still wors e the plan followed by Laennec, in some cases, of giving the entire quantity intended for the twenty-four hours, in but three or four portions, at short intervals, and then omitting it for the remainder of the day.   By this method the local or revellent influence of the remedy is induced in the highest possible degree, while the sedative influence is obtained in a degree, perhaps, proportionably lessened.   Generally, I give from three to six grains, according to the extent of the inflammation and the grade of febrile excitement present, in the twenty-fours, dissolved in six ounces of water.   Of this solution, I give, during the day, a teaspoonful every half hour ; but, if the patient is disposed to sleep, that his rest may not be too much disturbed, twice the quantity every hour during the night.   I have not found, as we are led to believe would be the case by some of the followers of Rasori, that the tolerance of these smaller doses is less readily established than of the larger. In some cases, where the attack is violent, in connection with blood-letting and other appropriate measures, with the view of bringing the system as speedily as possible to some extent under the influence of the agent, I venture to give at first one or two doses, say of a third or half a grain each, of it.   To favour its rapid absorption, by all means the remedy should be administered in perfect solution, in water alone; and the plan of administer-ing it in combination with mucilage, as of acacia, flaxseed, elm, &c., is eminently calculated to lead to the result it is intended to obviate.   Instead of sheathing the gastro-intestinal mucous membrane, or at least of protecting it in this way against the local irritant action of the remedy, such substances favour the latter effect, by retaining the salt for a long time in contact with the mucous surface, in consequence of the obstruction to its ready imbibition, which they present.   That absorption should take place, it is manifest that contact is necessary ; con-sequently, nothing can be gained by placing either the absorb-ing surface, or the remedy to be absorbed in such a condition as to protract the process.   Neither do I think the plan is a good one, of giving such fluids in the intervals ; though from the universality of the practice, popular prejudice is so strongly set in its favour, that the physician who prohibits them entirely is in danger, in case of a fatal result, of censure from the pa-tients' friends, for the omission.   The pilular is also a very ob-jectionable form of administration ; being calculated to lead to a slow absorption, and a protracted contact of the remedy, with a limited portion of the gastro-intestinal mucous membrane ; favouring thus a concentrated local action, and the develop-ment rather of its topical irritant, than of its general constitu-tional influence.   The form of administration in complete solution, in as large a quantity of water as it is probable will be entirely absorbed in the intervals between the doses, I regard as important.

Although I have had reason to be gratified with the method above recommended of administering the remedy in question in pneumonia, it is more than I am willing to assert, that its noxious operation can be thus, in all cases, entirely obviated.

More recently, with the same object in view, in some cases I have adopted the plan of administering the tartrate of antimony and potassa, in the form of enema, under the impression that its local irritant action upon the rectum, would be unimportant, in comparison with that on the stomach and duodenum ; hoping the while, that in adequate doses its general sedative operation might be as well secured. In the use of the remedy, after this method in pneumonia, I generally give about three grains every third hour, with fifteen or twenty drops of the tincture of opium in an ounce or two of warm water ; and its controlling influence, where the enemata have been well retained, has not appeared to me appreciably less, over the febrile excitement and local morbid action, than when I have administered it by the mouth.

Although the results of my practice from this method of treatment have been highly favourable, one case stands on record in my case book, in which it was principally adopted, calculated to cast a doubt upon its invariable innocuousness. Determining in the commencement of the attack to treat the case principally with the antimonial enemata, I ventured—as I thought I might do with safety, having this intention in view, and as the attack was a very violent one—upon a more free administration of the remedy by the mouth, during the first eighteen hours, than is my common practice ; and it is not improbable that it was to this, in conjunction with the action of mercurials administered occasionally by the mouth during the progress of the case, that the metastasis was in reality attributable. Still I could not entirely divest myself of doubt on the subject ; but even admitting in this instance an unfavourable operation from the enema treatment, I still rest satisfied of its comparative safety, in contrast with the usual method of administering the remedy by the mouth.

In the case in question, up to the evening of the fifth day, the patient was apparently doing well ; the febrile excitement regularly moderating, and the organic disease gradually subsiding. At this time a *very slight* tendency to tympanitis was discoverable, and a more rapid removal of the thoracic dullness on percussion had taken place, than between any two of my previous visits. The patient expressed himself better, however and the general symptoms were apparently favourable. It was consequently with no slight surprise on the part of the patient's friends, as well as of a professional friend who, on this occasion, visited the patient with me, that my intimations were received of a probable speedy fatal termination. The signs and symptoms of pneumonia rapidly disappeared; the tympanitis increased; diarrhœa, thirst, restlessness, jactitation, delirium followed by incomplete stupor of short duration, came on, and in ten hours from the time of the first symptom of the approaching change, he was dead.—[*Amer. Journ. of the Med. Sciences.*

On Ovarian Irritation. By FLEETWOOD CHURCHILL, M. D. T. C. D. & E., and M. R. I. A. Read before the College of Physicians of Ireland.

The following description relates to an affection which, although very common, is but very little noticed in books. This has probably arisen from its having been placed among the symptoms of other diseases, although it is quite distinguishable from them.

It resembles most closely the disease described by Dr. Tilt under the name of subacute ovaritis; but the cases that I have seen have led me to differ from that very intelligent writer, and to conclude that the affection to which I refer is not inflammatory. I have, therefore, preferred the term *Ovarian Irritation.*

I have met with it in women of all ages between the commencement and cessation of menstruation, so that I do not think age has much influence in the production of the disease; but I am quite certain that it is most frequent in women of a delicate, nervous temperament, though by no means confined to them.

The chief characteristic symptom is an uneasiness, amounting in the greater number of cases to pain, and in some cases to very severe pain, to one or both iliac or inguinal regions, but most frequently in the left, which Professor Simpson seems to think is owing to the propinquity of the left ovary to the rectum, and the exposure to any irritation thence arising. This pain may be a constant dull aching, or it may be acute and occuring in paroxysms; it is greatly aggravated by standing, and generally by walking: indeed, in the severer cases, I have known the patient quite unable to walk.

There is generally some complaint of fulness about the iliac region, but upon careful examination I have rarely been able to satisfy myself that this was more than a sensation: I certainly never felt anything like a distinct tumor. There is, however, always considerable tenderness, which in some cases is extreme to the slightest touch. When the irritation is great it may be extended to the bladder, giving rise to a desire to evacuate its contents frequently, and causing great pain in doing so. Hysterical paroxysms are by no means unfrequent. In two of the most violent cases of hysteria that I have seen for some time, there was extreme tenderness of the region of the left ovary and pressure there aggravated the hysterical paroxysm.

If we make a vaginal or rectal examination, we shall most frequently discover nothing unusual, neither heat nor tenderness nor swelling ; in a few cases, however, I have found that moving the uterus laterally caused uneasiness in the side affected. When speaking of a rectal examination in subacute ovaritis, D. Tilt remarks, that the ovaries are more or less painful on pressure, and that they are from twice to four times their original size. This I have not found in the affection now under consideration, and it constitutes one reason for my doubting that it is the same disease, as that described by Dr. Tilt.

These are the principal local and direct symptoms I have observed ; they vary much in degree, and are in some cases so intense as to resemble an attack of acute ovaritis. They differ also more or less according to the circumstances in which the attack occurs ; and in order to elucidate this point, I shall briefly enumerate the circumstances.

1. In patients who suffer occasionally from amenorrhœa, it is not uncommon to find ovarian irritation at these periods, and not altogether confined to them. Whether the ovarian irritation be the cause of the suppression of the catamenia, or merely a symptom, is a question not easily decided. In many cases I think it is probably the primary affection, but in some others it appears to be the reuslt of the amenorrhœa. The suffering is often considerable, and may be prolonged until the next catamenial evacuation ; if that be full and free, the pain and tenderness generally disappear.

2. Upon the sudden suppression of menstruation, it is not unusual for the ovaries to be almost instantly affected, either by the form of disease I have described, or by an acute inflammatory attack, which is more rare.

3. In dysmenorrhœa there is more or less ovarian irritation. If we examine the patient minutely as to the seat of the pain during the period, we shall find that it is principally in the region of one or both ovaries, and often accompanied by tenderness on pressure. In the majority of these cases I am inclined to think that the ovaries are secondarily affected.

4. In menorrhagia, the ovaries may apparently preserve their integrity for a long time ; but if the attacks be frequent, I have generally found that these organs, one or both, become affected, and that the irritation frequently continues long after the discharge has ceased.

5. I have repeatedly seen this ovarian irritation accompany congestion and erosion of the cervix uteri, but it most frequently comes on after the latter disease has persisted for some time or after it is nearly or quite cured. The ovarian irritation, however, in these cases, very soon subsides.

6. I have already mentioned its occurrence in hysteria, both when the latter is evidently dependent upon catamenial disturbance, and when the periodical discharge is quite correct.

7. In some few cases I have recognised ovarian irritation in cases where the uterine and ovarian monthly functions were apparently accurately performed, but the patients were of a highly nervous temperament, in delicate health, and without offspring.

These various classes include, I think, all or nearly all the examples of the diseases which have come under my observation. In many cases it requires care to separate the ovarian symptoms from those caused by the concurrent disease, but in other instances this distinction is quite obvious. When uncomplicated, the disorder rarely gives rise to any general or constitutional symptoms. Many of the subjects of it are delicate and weak, and of course this attack keeps them so ; but ordinarily, the pulse is not quickened by it, and there is neither heat of skin nor thirst. The appetite is seldom good, but it is not worse than usual, and the bowels are generally irregular. I have examined the urinary secretion, and have repeatedly found it scanty, acid, and occasionally mixed with mucus.

As to the *pathology* of this affection, there are several points of considerable interest.. I think we can entertain no doubt that the ovaries, one or both, are the seat of the irritation ; the peculiar and fixed locality of the pain, and its frequent connexion with the ovarian function of menstruation, all confirm this view. But the next question is more difficult to decide positively, viz: Is the disorder an inflammatory affection of the ovaries, either acute or subacute ? The disease described by Dr. Tilt certainly presents characteristics of inflammation, which I have never observed in the present disorder. The absence of tumefaction generally, and of a distinct tumor always, the negative results of an examination *per vaginam* and *per rectum,* the intermitting and paroxysmal character of the attack, the absence of all the ordinary results of inflammation (as abscess, accumulation of fluid, &c.), even in the several cases, and the success of a certain line of treatment, are all, to my mind, very strong arguments for the non-inflammatory nature of the disease. In most of these particulars, it differs from the subacute ovaritis of Dr. Tilt. I have certainly seen some cases in which the point seemed doubtful, and it is probable that the one form of disease may, under certain circumstances, merge in the other; but I cannot resist the conviction, that the affection I have described is essentially neuralgic and not inflammatory.

Again, it may be asked, is this ovarian irritation the cause of the menstrual disorder or its effect, or merely a concomitant symptom? No one acquainted with the present state of ovarian physiology could deny that the integrity of the menstrual function must be largely influenced by the condition of the ovaries. If this ovarian irritation always preceded the catamenial period, I should be inclined to attribute to it the subsequent distress; and in many cases it appeared to me that I could so trace it as the chief cause. But, in some cases, the ovarian irritation distinctly followed the menstrual disturbance or came on towards the termination of the monthly period; and lastly, in other cases, the irritation existed with no catamenial derangement at all. Without doubting, therefore that ovarian irritation may disturb the menstrual functions in various ways, I cannot agree with those who think it invariably does so, nor yet with those who are inclined to attribute all menstrual disorders to deviations from the normal condition of the ovaries.

I need not occupy time by enumerating many *causes* for its production; all those which act either upon the uterus or ovary and disturb their functions, may be considered as causes of ovarian irritation, and among these the most frequent, probably, is cold.

I believe that, in many cases, excess in sensual intercourse has given rise to it; and I am also inclined to think, that in a few cases I have known it originate from the entire deprivation of that stimulus. For some valuable remarks upon this subject I shall refer my readers to Dr. Tilt's excellent work, a review of which appeared in a late number of this journal; all that he says upon this point is, I think, equally applicable to ovaritis and ovarian irritation.

The circumstances under which the attack occurs, I mean its relation to the menstrual functions, the symptoms, and the peculiar locality of the pain, render the *diagnosis* tolerably easy in most cases. It may, certainly, be mistaken for intes-

tinal irritation ; but, in general, there are no other symptoms
than the pain to justify such an opinion. The bowels, even if
irregular, are free from irritability.

It will, however, require a little more trouble to render it
certain that there is not acute ovaritis, which the tenderness
might lead us to suspect. But this tenderness is *generally
much greater than that resulting from inflammation;* it is a
kind of a nervous tenderness which shrinks from the weight of
a finger as much as from severe pressure. Moreover, in
acute ovaritis, the organ is always swollen and enlarged, and
it can generally be felt distinctly to be so by an internal examination.

In phlegmonous inflammation of uterine appendages, or
pelvic abscess, as it has been termed, the hard and painful
tumefaction is quite plain at the brim of the pelvis, and, therefore, it cannot easily, be confounded with the present disorder.

I shall not enter at any length into details of the *treatment*
of this disease, inasmuch as I have only my own experience
to which I can refer. The choice of remedies will be governed, to a certain extent, by the health, strength, and state of
constitution of our patient. With strong, healthy women, I
have tried leeches to the ovarian region, with some benefit, but
not complete success, nor in all cases ; from six to twelve may
be applied at once, and repeated, if necessary, after an interval.
Poultices after leeching are of use ; and indeed, when no leeches have been applied, I have seen much comfort and relief
derived from repeated poulticing. With delicate women,
and they are frequently the subjects of this disease, bleeding
in any form has appeared to me rather injurious than beneficial.

I have tried the repeated application of small blisters with
better results than leeching. The irritation of the surface certainly relieves the pain in many cases, and, if continued, may
finally cure it ; but, I must confess, I have seen it fail repeatedly.

Anodyne liniments and anodyne plasters occasionally seem
to afford relief, but they are often of little or no use ; I tried
anodyne enemata several times with partial success.

In two or three cases I used the tincture of aconite, applied
liberally to the iliac region, but I confess the result disappointed the expectations I had formed.

Having failed in affording relief in two or three obstinate
cases, I determined to try the effect of opium applied to the
upper part of the vaginal surface. I accordingly ordered some
balls or pessaries to be made, somewhat in the mode of Dr.

Simpson's medicated pessaries, each ball to contain two grains of opium, half a drachm of white wax, and a drachm and a half of lard. The whole, when mixed'together, formed a ball about the size of a large marble, and I placed it at the upper end of the vagina by means of the speculum, leaving the patient in bed for the rest of the day. The success was quite beyond my expectation ; the relief was very speedy, and in most instances complete. Even-when the pain did return after a few days, a second application removed it. The tenderness disappeared with the pain, and no unpleasant consequences have resulted in any instance.

I have now tried this remedy in a considerable number of cases, and with almost invariable success. I have rarely found it necessary to bleed or blister since I first adopted this plan ; and I recommend it, with considerable confidence, to the profession. I may add, that I have tried these pessaries in cases of dysmenorrhœa, applying one the day before the catemenia were expected, with decided benefit.

It is hardly necessary to say that, in this disease, the bowels should be regulated, and gently freed by medicine when necessary. If the appetite is bad, vegetable bitters may be given, and I have generally found it useful to combine some alkali with them.—[*Dublin Quarterly Journal of Medical Science.*

History of a case of Congenital Ovarian Tumor with Cysts, Fatty Matter, Hair, and Bone, in which Ovariotomy was proposed. By ROBERT LEE, M. D., F.R.S.

I was requested by Mr. Gaskell, in November, 1842, to see Miss F——, about twelve years of age, who had not long before suffered from an attack of mumps, followed by pain and enlargement of the abdomen. The whole abdomen, and especially the hypogastrium, was large, hard, and irregular. It was supposed by the mother of the patient that sufficient attention had not been paid to the regular evacuation of the bowels while at school, from which she had recently returned. The catamenia had not appeared, and'there were none of the symptoms of puberty present. Active cathartics were given, but the enlargement and hardness of the abdomen continued after' the bowels had been thoroughly evacuated. I saw the patient with Mr. Gaskell thrice at short intervals, and formed the opinion that some obscure organic disease, not glandular, existed.

Dr. Merriman was then consulted, and I am indebted to his kindness for the following account of the case from the 22nd December, 1842, till the month of May, 1843 :—

"On first seeing this young lady, I was sensible of a fluctuation low in the cavity of the abdomen, and a feeling of tightness within the pelvis, which led me to believe that the pelvic viscera were involved in the disease, and I ordered diuretics as principal remedies. Miss F—— was from time to time brought to my house; and on the last day of her paying me a visit, the opinion I gave of the case was so unfavorable as to induce her parents to wish that Dr. Paris's opinion should be taken. Dr. Paris met me, and a plan of treatment was adopted and acted upon for about a week. Meantime her parents had been urged to consult the late Mr. A. White, who saw her with me January 23rd, 1843, and on this occasion a tumor, evidently ovarian, was distinctly to be seen emerging out of the pelvis. She was now put upon a course of hydriodate of potash, which, together with change of air and more advanced season, appeared to improve her general health. Throughout the month of March her health remained much the same, but the tumor did not diminish, and in April Mr. Aston Key was called in. He continued to give the hydriodate of potash, and had the parts fomented, without much benefit. She was brought to me in the month of May, and, I believe, went to the sea-side."

About the end of October, 1843, nearly a year having elapsed from the time I first saw Miss F—— with Mr. Gaskell, her parents again consulted me respecting her, and as the abdomen was then greatly distended with fluid, I recommended that she should be tapped, and that Mr. Aston Key, under whose care she had been for some months, should be requested to perform the operation. This was done on the 2nd of November, and a quantity of dark-coloured, gelatinous fluid, evidently the product of an ovarian sac, was drawn off. As no case of ovarian dropsy at the age of thirteen had ever before come under my observation, and before the appearance of the catamenia, I had been led to conclude that the fluid was contained in the sac of the peritonæum, and that the case was not one of encysted dropsy. After the fluid had been drawn off, the lower part of the abdomen was still hard and irregular, and a solid mass about the size of a hen's egg, was distinctly felt the day after the tapping in the epigastric region.

From the 3rd of November, 1843, to the 7th of February, 1845, I was never consulted by the parents of Miss F——, nor obtained any information respecting the state of her health. On the morning of the 7th of February she was brought to my house by her father and mother. The abdomen was again largely distended with fluid. I was informed by them that they had been induced to consult Dr. F. Bird, and that he had given it as his opinion that their daughter's case was in all respects most favorable for the operation of ovariotomy. They further stated that Dr. Locock had been consulted the day before, and that he considered the case highly favorable for the operation, and urged its immediate performance. It had, in fact, been determined, before they came to me, that the operation should be performed, and they seemed confident that their daughter would speedily be restored to perfect health. Apparently their purpose in calling upon me, was not so much to obtain my sanction to the proceeding as indirectly to reproach me for not having long before recommended or performed an operation which they believed to be so efficacious and devoid of danger. Instead of offering any observations on the propriety of the operation, I took down Vol. xxvii. of the *Medico-Chirurgical Transactions*, and turning to Mr. B. Philips' Table of "Operations for the Extraction of Ovarian Tumors," begged them to run their eyes along the column of results. In this they saw the word "death" repeated twenty-eight times, thrice three times running, and once four times without any intervening case of "cure" or "recovery." Nothing further was said respecting the operation on that day.

On the 16th of July, 1845, I was requested to meet in consultation, Dr. S. and W. Merriman, Dr. H. Roe and Dr. F. Bird, to consider the propriety of the operation of ovariotomy in this case. I pointed out the necessity of having the patient again tapped, and the condition of the ovarian cyst and tumor, and of all the pelvic and abdominal viscera, carefully determined before any operation was attempted. After some opposition, I succeeded in obtaining the acquiescence of all to this proposal. During the tapping, the canula being obstructed, the fluid ceased to flow, and on inquiry into the cause of this, it was discovered to have arisen from a quantity of fatty matter and long hair. It was at once obvious that the dark-coloured viscid fluid was not escaping from an ordinary ovarian cyst, but from a cyst containing, along with the fluid, long hairs and fatty substance, and probably a jaw-bone and teeth, as in numerous recorded cases of congenital malformation of the ovaria. After the fluid, fat and long hairs had been drawn off, a large irregular mass remained in the hypogastrium, and the small tumor in the epigastric region was still to be felt. At this consultation "it was the opinion agreed to, that the operation was not immediately necessary, and might with propriety be deferred three or four months." Dr. W. Merriman made this memorandum the same day.

To the best of my recollection I never saw the patient again, and, until about the end of August, 1846, could not learn what had become of her. I was then accidently informed that Miss

F—— had died at Ramsgate, but after much trouble I have not succeeded in ascertaining precisely when this took place. The body was, however, brought to London, and a post-mortem examination made by Dr. H. Roe, Dr. F. Bird, and Mr. B. Holt. Mr. Holt did not preserve any notes of the morbid appearances, and does not know the date.

On the 6th of September, 1846, Dr. F. Bird very kindly gave me the following description of these, which I took down in writing in his presence, and the same day copied into my journal of cases, from which it is extracted.

"Abdomen greatly enlarged. On opening the integuments, adhesions equal to a space of six inches, the centre where the puncture had been made, from which the adhesions radiated. No other adhesions elsewhere. Slight attachments above to the omentum. A great ovarian sac came into view, connected with the right ovary, involving the whole of it, the pedicle formed by the broad ligament and Fallopian tube, which was eight inches long; the chief vessel was the spermatic; the anterior half of the tumour presented a spherical outline, but, posteriorly, nodulated throughout; the sac an inch thick anteriorly, whereas, behind it was extremely thin, like tissue paper; within this a soft vascular mass, which had ulcerated, and this had poured out a great quantity of blood; the sac having given way, hæmorrhage had also taken place into the peritonæum. On laying open the sac, it was multilocular, but one large cyst, with a number of small ones; patches of inflammation on the lining membrane. One large and hard mass existed on the left side, where we felt the hardness traced up on the left side, eight inches long, four wide, and two in thickness; consisted of numerous small condensed cells, having a centre of bone, with hairs—not yet examined."

I obtained permission to examine this mass, by making an incision into it. The structure was that usually termed by pathologists malignant disease of the ovary. The tumor had interspersed throughout its substance numerous long hairs and pieces of bone.*

A case in some respects analogous to the preceding occurred several years ago in the United States of America, in which the operation of ovariotomy was performed, and was followed by a fatal result. I am not aware that any other case resembling this has yet been recorded.—[*Londun Lancet.*

---

*Had a full examimation of all the parts of the tumor been made, it is probable that teeth would likewise have been discovered.

On the use of Fat in the Animal System. By Prof. Draper.

There is deposited in certain parts of all animals a substance insoluble in water, fusible at a low temperature, combustible, and, though of variable constitution, known under the general designation of fat.

I shall direct your attention to the nature and functions of this substance. It discharges an important duty in the economy.

Fats are secreted from the blood, in which they pre-exist, by the adipose cells, which sometimes occur sparingly scattered through the areolar tissues, or, when clustered, constitute the adipose. The primary form of these cells are spheroidal, though, as is often the case both in plants and animals, this form is departed from through the influence of pressure, and polygonal forms are assumed. Between the cells of adipose tissue a net-work of blood-vessels ramifies, for the double purpose of furnishing to the cells the fat they are to secrete, and likewise water; advantage being taken of the proverbial insolubility of all oily material in this liquid, and so long as the walls of the cells are kept moist, the contents cannot escape by transudation.

The adipose tissues occupy an intermediate position between the tissues that are constant and those that are variable. They do not necessarily exhibit that extreme proneness to change so characteristic of the muscular or nervous. With some insignificant exceptions, which will be discussed hereafter, no oily substance ever escapes from the system until it has undergone change. These bodies being insoluble, in water, cannot be removed in the urine.

It is not alone in animals, but also in plants, that we find fat. In the leaves of various grasses, in seeds, and fruits, it can be detected, by resorting to proper chemical processes. In those articles that are used as food by the herbivora, it constitutes a very appreciable part. One hundred pounds of Indian corn contain about nine pounds of a thick oil, and one hundred pounds of dry hay contain about two pounds of fat.

What is the purpose for which nature resorts to this substance? I may answer that question by asking another. Why do men resort to it? Why do they go in ships, and brave the winter of the Polar Seas, encountering the perils of the whale fishery? Why, in some parts of the country, are animals raised, as much for their fat as their flesh? What is the object of all those inventions which transmute the lard of the hog into a pure and cleanly body, approaching in quality spermaceti or the wax of the bee? It is for the purpose of availing ourselves of the combustion of this tribe of bodies, which experience has shown are the best of all sources of heat. Fat is burnt in lamps and candles, because it is the most compendious source from which a high temperature can be obtained. Nature resorts to the combustion of this substance in the interior of the system, for the same reason that we do in domestic economy.

The constitution of the common fats is that they contain carbon, hydrogen, oxygen; the two former in great excess. During their oxydation a very large amount of heat is set free, because the heat-giving powers of hydrogen are brought into operation. When a fat burns, if there be an abundant access of air, the carbon turns into carbonic acid, and the hydrogen into water; but if the supply of air be limited, and this is a remark which should be borne in mind from is constant-physiological application, the hydrogen burns away first and leaves the carbon. In our experiments, we often witness this; it gives origin to the dense black soot or smoke that arises from smoky lamps. When the combustion of an oil or fat in the system is complete, the products arising, carbonic acid and the vapor of water, are so constituted that they can escape through the lungs; and advantage is taken of this incident to effect the grand process of the introduction of atmospheric air. These bodies thus ministering to the functions of respiration, we speak of them as elements of respiratory food.

Two opinions have been entertained respecting the origin to the fat thus deposited in the tissues of animals. 1st. That it is manufactured in the system by certain vital or chemical metamorphoses from the food, in which it is not found to any great extent. 2d. That it is simply extracted from the food, in which it occurs naturally, being fabricated, in the first instance, by plants.

There are many facts which seem to show that fatty bodies can be formed from other organized substances. Several years ago it was discovered, on opening one of the burying grounds in Paris—the Cemetery of the Innocents—for the purpose of removing the dead bodies that had accumulated there, that all those which were below a certain depth had become converted into a fatty substance, now known under the name of adipocire. The muscles, the hair, the brain of these bodies appeared to have been entirely changed, giving origin to this substance, which has received its name from a resemblance it possesses to wax and fat.

But, as respects the case of the cemetery of the Innocents, and the production of adipocire generally, Chevreul has established its nature by showing that adipocire contains the same constituents as human fat, partially saponfied by ammonia. A mass of flesh, placed in a current of water, will, under certain circumstances, change into adipocire, but not more truly fatty matter can be obtained in this way, than could have been ex-tracted directly from the flesh by the action of sulphuric ether. So we conclude that, whenever the change takes place, it is not a production or generation of fat, but the muscular and other tissues decaying away, the fat is simply set free, and becomes saponified by the ammonia, arising during the putre-faction.

In a former lecture it was stated, that both waxes and fats occur in the leaves of plants. These substances possess such a relation to one another that all the oily bodies may arise in succession from wax by a series of partial oxydations. Under the influence of the sunlight, the leaves effect the decomposi-tion of carbonic acid, causing its oxygen to be evolved and its carbon to be fixed in their tissues. There can be little doubt that one of the starch family of bodies is the first to make its appearance. The formula of those bodies shows that, by par-tial oxydation, they can be converted into fat, a result that we witness every summer. The sap which has a sweet taste in the stem, loses its sweetness in proportion as oily matters form in the fruit.

From plants, animals derive the oleaginous substances they fix in their tissues. The vegetable world obtains them from the carbonic acid and water of the air,—the animal returns them back to the atmosphere as carbonic acid and water again. And, indeed, in this manner, all the carbonaceous atoms of which our bodies are composed, vibrate as it were backward and forward from the inorganic to the organic world. Now they reside in the air, and are tossed about by winds and currents —now they are organized as vegetable forms, and, after serv-ing awhile for the sustenance of animals, are cast back by pro-cesses of oxydation into the atmosphere, to run their race again.

The general mode of accumulating fat is by collection from the food, both in the case of carnivorous and also herbivorous animals,—the food in which it occurs most commonly to a suffi-cient extent. But the animal system can, when forced thereto, transmute both starch and sugar into the condition of oil, in the process of duodenal digestion.

I have so often incidentally referred to the physiological uses of this important body, its destruction by oxydation in the inte-rior of the system, for the purpose of sustaining animal heat, so often pointed out the great superiority it possesses over other bodies in this respect, by reason of the large amount of hydro-gen it contains, that it is scarcely necessary to dwell on those points in detail. In fevers, where there is an abstinence from food, we see how quickly the fat disappears, a general emaciation setting in, and from those deposits where it has been so carefully stored this combustible body is removed.

For the accumulation of fat, whether it be incidental, as in the human species, or purposed, as in the preparation of cattle for the market, there are obviously two conditions. The accumulation will depend—1st. On the quality of fat presented in the food. 2d. On the slowness of its consumption in the system. Now, there are several circumstances which bear on this latter condition, and which here require to be pointed out.

1st. Whatever checks the respiratory process, or the introduction of oxygen into the system, will aid in the deposit of fat. Quick respiration implies quick oxydation ; for the air introduced must have its affinities satisfied. To promote the accumulation of fat, an animal must be so situated that its respiration shall be slow.

2d. The higher the surrounding temperature the less is the loss of heat from the body by radiation and contact of the air, and the system is not required to develope so much heat, and consequently the destruction of fat is less. A high external temperature tends, therefore, to the accumulation of this body.

3d. Rest, or quiet. All movements taking place in the muscular tissues tend to the accleration of the respiratory act. A man runs, and he quickly begins to pant. Large quantities of air are introduced, and the destruction of fat is the consequence. For this reason, of all the conditions under which an animal can be placed, sleep is by far the most favorable for the accumulation of fat. The respiration is tranquil and slow, there is a great freedom from muscular exertion, and usually the temperature is higher than when we are exposed in the pursuits of active life to the open air.

These things have been long understood by persons interested in the fattening of animals before their significance was detected by physiological chemistry. In certain places, where an inordinate obesity is given to animals for special purposes, each of these conditions is carefully observed. When geese are fattened for the sake of their livers, a delicacy much sought after by epicures, the process is to cram the bird with as much Indian corn, or other oily food, as possible, to tie its wings and feet, to ensure quiet, to place it in the chimney corner, or other warm situation, where the temperature is pretty high. Under these extraordinary conditions the bird sleeps profoundly, breathes slowly, introduces little air, destroys little fat. But the absorbents are busily engaged in taking it up, and an amazing accumulation is effected at last.

We sometimes see at agricultural exhibitions, hogs in a state of prodigious fatness. The form of the animal is altogether gone, if its feet touch the ground they are of no use as organs of locomotion, the snout barely projects beyond the rotundity of the face, the tip of the tail looks as if it were at the bottom of a pit. This forced condition of things has been produced by resorting to the precepts just laid down. The animal has been kept in a dark, warm place, crammed with oily food, in quiet, and asleep. Every thing is done to lower the respiratory process, and abate the destruction of fat.

When we come to discuss the functions of the liver, we shall find that the secretion of that gland, the bile, stands in a certain relation to the respiratory function,—bile, the predominating constituents of which, carbon, hydrogen, sulphur, are all combustible bodies. In cases where there is an interference with the respiratory functions, as in phthisis, and where less oxygen than usual is introduced into the system, these combustible bodies cannot be got rid of in the usual way, by converting them into carbonic acid, water, &c., and a reflected action is thrown upon the liver, which, unable to discharge its duty, often becomes engorged with fat. In this respect the condition is not unlike that artificially produced in the goose, as above mentioned.

I am persuaded, also, that these things are intimately connected with those embarrassments of the action of the liver, and hepatic diseases generally, which are so constantly encountered in hot climates, and in the warmer portions of our own country, in the hot seasons of the year. The high temperature of the surrounding air, often at a point near that of the animal system, prevents any great loss of heat, either by radiation or by contact; the dew point, too, is commonly very high, and loss of heat by evaporation goes down to a minimum. In this semi-febrile condition, a man instinctively abstains from every thing that can raise his temperature, he avoids violent or perhaps even moderate exercise, he sleeps in the heat of the day, and as far as he can diminishes the activity of the respiratory functions, and the quantity of air introduced. But as the consequence of this, the lungs are unable to discharge their appointed duty, an embarrassment is thrown on the liver, the carbon and hydrogen since they can be no longer burnt, fall under the action of that gland, which is overtaxed with the unnatural task.

It is for this reason that men in warm climates instinctively abhor all oily and fatty food, and choose fruits and watery diet. In these the amount of combustible materials is small—the use of them, therefore, leads to the evolution of little heat, and the disturbance I am dwelling on is to an extent avoided. How different with the man who lives in the cold north regions ; an orange or pine-apple is but a poor tempation to a Laplander or Esquimaux. He wants tallow and train oil. The cold air that surrounds him keeps his temperature down, so that he has hard work to keep it up. He wraps his greasy person in furs of warmest kind and consoles himself with the belief that in another and happier world the righteous shall feed on the blubber of whales.

What, then, gentlemen, is the result at which we arrive from a full consideration of the subject ? We conclude that man and all other animals under ordinary circumstances find in their food all the fat they require ; that these have been made in plants by the all-pervading influence of the sun ; but, under special circumstances, we are constrained to admit, that if fat does not occur in the food to an extent sufficient for the wants of the system, the system by resorting to processes of sub-division, which we can artificially imitate, can manu- facture it : that introduced by the lacteals, but not by the veins, the fats are either destroyed by gradual oxydation for the production of heat, one fat after another appearing in succes- sion, as these partial oxydations go on, and carbonic acid and water being developed at last,—or the excess is stored up in the adipose tissues for the future wants of the system, or, in the female, it passes into the secretion of the mammary gland, and is a constituent of milk. But whether it is thus stored up or thus secreted, its final duty is the same, it is to be burnt for the sake of the caloric it can evolve, and thus translated into car- bonic acid and water is restored to the atmospheric air, ready under the influence of the sunshine to be metamorphosed by plants back again into fat.

From these general views we now descend to particulars, and I shall proceed to offer you rigorous proof that both in her- bivorous and carnivorous animals the fat deposited is not made in the stomach, but collected from the food. We shall then ex- amine the system followed on the great scale by those who are interested in the fattening of cattle for the market, and also the production of milk, one of the main constituents of which is butter, this will furnish us with striking illustrations of the principles under consideration. Next, we shall see how all oily bodies when once introduced into the system begin to undergo change, and evolve caloric, and how, in order to regu- late and control this, a special mechanism is resorted to, in which the cutaneous and respiratory surfaces and the malpi- ghian bodies of the kidney discharge an important duty.

[*N. Y. Med. Gazette.*

A Case of Sciatica treated successfully by Inoculation with Sulphate of Morphine. By CHARLES BRACKETT, M. D., of Rochester, Ind.

The following, if you think proper, you may publish. It is concerning a case of Sciatica, (I like the shorter, and full as expressive term, in lieu of the Neuralgia Femero-Poplitæ,) of long standing, which I treated by inoculating the skin over the course of the nerve with Sul. Morphine, made into a thin paste with Croton Oil.

This was a case of some years duration, and had been treated in this country and New York without an appearance of benefit.

The patient Wm. R., aged about fifty years, of a spare habit but large and muscular frame, and active disposition, had suffered for the past ten or fifteen years with occasional rheumatic attacks, affecting generally his upper, though often his lower extremities and back. The pain, and weakness in his back, and in the course of the sciatic nerve for the past two years, had been persistent, so that he needed the aid of a cane when walking; for the past few months he had been confined to his bed, suffering such pain as only the victim of neuralgia has a knowledge of. I have tried most of the medicines which I thought could give him relief, both in the form of internal and external medication; at length I concluded to try this plan of inoculation, although I had not a remote idea of deriving *permanent* benefit from it, yet I could not bear the idea to give him up to the perpetual use of morphine, from which alone in large doses he found relief.

I began about the origin of the nerve, and inoculated the paste above mentioned about every four inches, down to his heel, which was as far as he felt any pain. That night he rested better than he had for a long time previously, the pain being entirely removed along the track of the inoculations; towards morning the pain attacked the Anterior Tibial Nerve, where previously it had never existed, and where it became as acute as it ever had been on the posterior part of his leg. I followed this pain up with my scarifications, putting in as much of the paste as I dared do in from four to six punctures made with a point of a thumb lancet at each place of inoculation. At this time I made my points of inoculation about three inches apart from the knee to the middle of the dorsal surface of the foot, so far as the pain existed; it ceased, and at my next visit it had appeared in the Plantar Nerves. I scarified and inoculated the sole of his foot, and from that time till his death he never suffered from any pain about that leg.

This patient, a robust Virginian, suffered more I think than any one I ever saw. Judging from his appearance, I thought it must be truly *perfect agony* he suffered.

He lived about a year after the cure of his Neuralgia, when he died from complicated disease of the Spleen and Liver, chronic in its character. As a *post mortem* was not allowed, I cannot give the exact condition of the viscera.

Though there is nothing remarkable about this case as respects the originality of its treatment, which I do not claim for it, yet the rapid and almost magical effects of the inocculation, together with the total and permanent disappearance of the neuralgic disease, I think probably ought to place it among the first remedies to be used in this disease, the treatment of which (through necessity from an absence of a knowledge of its existing causes) so often assumes an empirical tendency. At any rate it is to be considered a valuable adjuvant to other treatment.—[*North-western Medical and Surgical Journal.*

Quinine in Cholera Infantum. By G. W. BOOTH, M. D., of Hardin county, Tenn.

I have for some time intended to call the attention of my professional brethren to the quinine mode of treating cholera infantum. I have practised in Mississippi and Tennessee for several years—regions where that disease annually makes its visitations. I have had an opportunity of seeing much of it, and treating a great number of cases. I believe its remote cause to be identical with that of our common autumnal fevers.

It prevails at the same period of the year, and in the same locations, and I have found it amenable to the same treatment, aided by the usual remedies for the local complications. There are in all the cases that have fallen under my notice distinct remissions, if not intermissions. During this subsidence of the symptoms, I give quinine liberally, and, in fact, in many cases I give it, regardless of fever, throughout the disease. I can confidently recommend this mode of treatment as pre-eminently successful, after testing it for many years. I have seen many cases recover under the use of the sulphate, that I should have despaired of without its aid. I write this simply to get you to call the attention of the profession to the use of quinine in this disease. I have never written an article for the medical press ; and this is not intended for the public eye.* I do not expect that any, or at least many, will adopt my mode of treatment

[*We insert it nevertheless, in the hope that Dr. B. and others of what are called country practitioners will be encouraged to write for the medical press.—ED.]

differing from what is usual, on the recommendation of an obscure practitioner—one entirely unknown to fame.   As this is the season for the prevalence of cholera infantum in your city, I request you to give it a full and fair trial; and if you find it successful, then send it abroad under the prestige of your Gazette. I use the quinine in every stage of the disease, in what would by many be considered large doses.   Occasionally I defer its use for a short time, to relieve some of the most urgent symptoms —such as excessive gastric irritability, and cerebral affections.
[*New York Medical Gazette.*

Abstract of a Paper on the Variations of the Sulphates and Phosphates excreted in Acute Chorea, Delirium Tremens, and Inflammation of the Brain. By H. B. Jones, M.D.

Having determined the variations of the sulphates in the states of health when different diets, amount of exercise, and medicines were taken, the variations of the sulphates in disease were examined.   At the same time the total amount of alkaline and earthly phosphates was determined, partly in order to see whether the amount of sulphates and phosphates bore any relation to one another, and partly to test the conclusions which were drawn in the author's previous paper on the variations of phosphates in disease.   The cases were thus classified:

1st. Acute and chronic diseases, in which the muscular structures were chiefly affected, as chorea.

2d. Functional diseases of the brain, as delirium tremens.

3d. Acute inflammatory diseases of the nervous structures, as inflammation of the brain.

4th. Chronic diseases of the nervous structures.

5th. Acute diseases, in which neither the nervous nor the muscular structures were chiefly affected.

6th. Chronic diseases, in which neither the muscular nor the nervous structures were chiefly affected.

The three last classes gave only negative results.

In illustration of the first class, three cases of most intense chorea are detailed; the urine was examined frequently, from the third to the eleventh day.   The phosphates were found to be diminished.   The sulphates were found to be in very great excess.   The urine was found to be so loaded with urea, that nitrate of urea, chrystalized out before the urine was concentrated.   The specific gravity of the urine was as high as 1036 in one case, 1035 in another, and in the third, 1031.

In illustration of the second class, three cases of delirium tremens are given.   The urine was examined from the fifth to the

fourteenth day of the disease. The phosphates were not found
to be so remarkably as in the cases reported in the previous
paper. The sulphates were found to be exceedingly increased.
The amount of urea was so great that nitric acid caused an
instantaneous crystallization. The specific gravity also was
in one case, 1041; in another, 1037; and in the third, 1027.
In other words, there was the most remarkable correspondence
between the state of the urine in acute chorea and in delirium
tremens.

In illustration of the third class, four cases of acute inflammation of the brain are given. The urine was examined from
the fourth to the twenty-sixth day. Though the inflammation
in these cases was not so intense, as in those which were recorded in the author's previous paper referred to, yet they
confirm the statement that in inflammation of the brain, the
phosphates in the urine are increased; they also lead to the
conclusion that the sulphates are at the same time increased
in the same degree.

In conclusion, the author states the phenomenon common to
acute chorea and to intense delirium tremens is increased and
unceasing muscular action. The muscles are highly complex
organic compounds, in which sulphur exists in an unoxidized
state, and the muscular action of oxygen, which, among other
results, gives rise to the formation of sulphuric acid and urea,
the amount of oxidation being proportioned to the intensity of
the muscular action. The result produced is an increase of
the sulphates and of the urea of the urine, just as in health they
would be increased if continued strong exercise were taken.
The increased amount of urea does not constitute a disease resembling diabetes, but it is only an evidence of the changes
which are taking place within. The increase of sulphates and
phosphates in inflammation of the brain, is also an evidence of
increased oxidation of the nervous structures. These simultaneous variations depend on the fact that the amount of sulphur
in the brain is nearly the same as the amount of phosphorus.
Thus at one time we have evidence of increased oxidation of
the elements of the nervous structures; and we may thus arrive at the conclusion, that at one time the function of the nerves,
and at another that of the muscles, is inordinately increased.

[London Lancet.

Intermittent Fever, affecting only one half of the Body.

Dr. M. L. Knapp has given in the September number of the
New York Journal of Medicine, the history of a case of fracture
of the tenth dorsal vertebra, with other injury to the spine, which

resulted in complete paralysis of sensation and motion of the lower half of the body. While in the state of paraplegia he was attacked with intermittent fever and strange to relate, only the part of the body *above* the fracture suffered the lower half that was paralysed retaining its ordinary temperature.

Dr. Knapp goes on to say:—"The peculiar condition of the patient, however, under a paroxysm of fever is full of interest, and arrests the attention in a remarkable manner, filling the mind with a kind of awe. One half of the body of the man had a perfectly developed ague, and the other half had none ! Who ever heard of or saw the like before ? Who ever will look upon the like again ? Does it establish the nervous pathology of fever ? The distinctive symptoms that go to make up an intermittent fever, were strongly marked, and observed their regular succession in all parts of the system above the injury where the cerepro-spinal influence was maintained ; but the parts below were completely exempt from all febrile phenomena—neither cold, nor heat, nor pallor, nor rubor, nor sudor l

If this case does not prove the nervous pathology of fever, it proves at least that parts cut off from direct and healthy connection with the spinal axis are exempt from the phenomena of fever ; and the inference is that these nervous phenomena are consequent on the primary impressions made on the cerebrospinal system by the malarious poison circulating in the blood. The altered and vitiated secretions of the stomach, liver, etc., for which oceans of mercurial cathartics have been given in malarious fevers, aimed at the primary cause of the disease, are but secondary phenomena.—[*Charleston Med. Journal.*

On the Constitutional Origin of Erysipelas, and its Treatment.

Dr. A. J. Walsh has furnished the Dublin Quarterly Journal, (Aug. 1850) some remarks on this subject, with cases, which are worthy of consideration. The following is a summary of his remarks :—

1st. That erysipelas is a constitutional disease, depending solely on a morbid state of the blood; and that the eruption and fever are the means that nature takes to get rid of this poison.

2d. That, for all practical purposes it is only necessary to divide the disease into idiopathic and traumatic.

3d. That tartar emetic seems to act specifically in erysipelas, by assisting nature in her efforts to throw off the disease.

4th. The best method of administering this medicine is by dissolving one grain in a quart of any bland fluid ; the solution to be taken in the twenty-four hours.

5th.   That as soon as the tartar emetic has acted sufficiently, sulphate of quina, or some other tonic is to be administered.

6th.   That, if the patient is debilitated, we must administer tonics at the same time that we give the tartar emetic.

7th.   That under this treatment the erysipelatous inflamma. tion may spread, but not with the same violence, nor to the same extent, as if the disease were left to itself.

8th.   That we shall often require to give aperient medicine during the course of the case, as it is absolutely necessary to keep the bowels free.

9th.   That local applications are unnecessary, and often inju. rious.

10th.   That incisions are not necessary, except in the third, or suppurative stage : and if the antimonial treatment be early resorted to, it very rarely occurs that suppuration takes place.

[*Amer. Jour. Med. Science.*

On Anasarca in Disease of the Heart.   By M. Chomel.

The progress of infiltration is ordinarily slow and progressive in affections of the heart ; but, nevertheless, nothing is more common than to meet with individuals among the working-classes, who, while presenting the appearace of health, and without having manifested any sign of disease, are seized with anasarca, the physical and material signs of cardiac alteration not being present, or only, at all events, to a very slight degree. This is because there are causes prevailing in this class of society—such as excess of labour, fatigue, watchings, misery, drinking—which, in a measure, precipitate the course of the disease.   These causes come in addition to the natural influence of the disease ; and the anasarca appears at a period when without these it would not have manifested itself.   So, when these causes are removed, and the patient is kept at rest, and sheltered from the unfortunate conditions that have given rise to so serious a complication, the œdema diminishes daily, and the patient soon leaves the hospital believing himself cured. Few exposures to excesses, fatigue, or misery, reproduce the anasarca, which may be again dispersed, and that for several times ; but after a certain number of such attacks, it in the end becomes permanent.

Frequently the appearance of an acute anasarca throws a ray of light on obscure and embarrassing cases, indicating in the great majority of cases an acute disease of the heart. Doubtful endocarditis and pericarditis are often thus revealed to the observer by general œdema.   M. Chomel thus considers that in the case of anasarca coming on, when we can discover neither change in the blood nor albumen in the urine, we are authorized in admitting the existence of disease of the heart, or large vessels, even when all material signs of this affection are completely absent.—[*Brit. and For. Med. Chir. Rev.*, from *L' Union Medicale.*

Cases in which there was unusual Difficulty in the Diagnosis of Pleuritic Effusions. By T. A. BARKER, M. D. (Proceedings of Royal Med. Chirurg. Society, May 27, 1851.)

The first case related by the author was one in which there was extensive emphysema of the left lung, which had encroached greatly on the right side of the chest, pushing the heart and mediastinum beyond the mesial line. The right lung, which was closely adherent to the costal pleura, was reduced to about a fourth of its usual size, was exsanguine, and contained no air, resembling a lung compressed by effusion in the pleura. In consequence of these changes, no respiration could be heard in the right lung during life : the right side of the chest was universally dull on percussion, and the patient could only lie on the right side or sit erect. Along with these symptoms were others closely resembling those which usually attend hydrothorax; and the dyspnœa and symptoms of approaching apnœa being very urgent, the author thought himself justified in having a very fine trocar introduced into the chest, in order to ascertain positively whether there was fluid. No inconvenience resulted from the operation, and the symptoms were soon afterwards explained by the discovery, on post-mortem examination, of the very unusual state of parts above described.

The next case was one in which, without any of the general symptoms of pleuritic effusion, it was discovered, by auscultation, &c., that there was no respiration going on in the posterior third of the left lung. In four days the person died. The lungs were healthy ; but there was extensive effusion, confined to the back part of the chest by a very narrow line of adhesion extending from the upper and back part of the chest to the diaphragm, half way between the ribs and the sternum. The author referred to three other cases which he had seen, in which the pleuritic effusion had been limited by adhesions in the same position and precisely similar ; only one of these had been seen by him during life, and in that the symptoms closely resembled those in the case last related. Two other cases were shortly alluded to, in which there was emphysema to a considerable extent ; but respiratory sounds could be heard in every part of the affected sides, in consequence of the lung being kept partially in contact with the ribs by mucous adhesions, forming several separate cavities in which the purulent matter was contained.—[*Lond. Med. Gaz.*

ﬃﬃﬃscellany.

A new Method of preventing Fats and Fixed Oils from becoming Rancid.—By CHARLES W. WRIGHT, M. D , of Cincinnati.—In company with one of the early settlers of this part of the United States, the conversation turned upon the history and habits of the Indians formerly living in this valley, and among other things he mentioned the curious manner in which they preserved bear's fat from becoming rancid, of which the following is a brief account : In the early part of winter the fat is removed from the body of the animal and subjected to the *trying-out* process, as it is termed ; that is, it is subjected to a degree of heat sufficient to coagulate and separate the azotized matter which subsides to the bottom of the vessel, and the oil is drained off. After this operation is completed, it is melted again with the bark of the slippery elm tree, (*ulmus fulva*) finely divided, which may be used either in the fresh or dry state. The proportion is about one drachm of the bark to the pound of fat. When these substances are heated together for a few minutes, the bark shrinks and gradually subsides, after which the fat is strained off and put aside for use.

The bark communicates an odor to the fat that is hardly to be distinguished from that of the kernel of the hickory nut.

Thinking this might be turned to account in the preservation of the fatty matters, I subjected many of them to experiment, and in every instance the result was alike successful. One specimen of butter, (an article which is well known becomes rancid sooner than any other kind of fat,) prepared in this way more than a year ago, is as sweet and as free from disagreeable odor, as the day it was made, having been exposed all this time to the atmosphere and changes of temperature.

Hog's lard may be preserved in the same manner.

This fact will be of much importance in the preparation of cerates and ointments which can be thus protected from rancidity.

In the lubrication of delicate machinery an acquaintance with this fact may be of benefit by preventing the injury that results from the use of rancid oil.—[*Western Lancet.*

Free Medical Education.—The class at the University of Michigan, numbers 151 bona fide *under graduates.* If the physicians who are availing themselves of the free lectures were included in the catalogue, as is the fashion elsewhere, the aggregate would exceed 200. The course of instruction in this school is thorough, and the standard of qualification for the doctorate elevated, so as to challenge comparison with the best colleges in the country. At present there are 5 Professors, shortly to be increased to 7. Such provision for free medical teaching, must prove a blessing to the state, which has so liberally endowed their University and set the example of a free Medical College.

It must not however, be supposed, that free medical education is exclusively to be had in Michigan, else injustice would be done to other schools, every where in the country. To go no farther back than last year, we know two Colleges, which in the aggregate on their catalogues, numbered 641 students, viz. 411 * and 230, † respectively, and yet the highest number of tickets paid for, numbered 140 in the former, and 151 in the latter. By this it is apparent, that *free medical education* was extended to 271 in the one, and 79 in the other, being an aggregate of 350 free students in these two colleges! The difference lies in the fact, that in Michigan this liberality is extended by the State, while in New-York, the credit is due to the Professors in these schools, and to the very natural ambition of excelling each other in the numbers of their students. Many gentlemen who can afford it, would doubtless rather lecture to large classes for nothing and find themselves, than to be paid for teaching small classes. The title and position is sought, rather than the emoluments of professorships; and if such men are capable and faithful to their trust, they are worthy of double honor, and to them should be awarded the merit of making medical education free, at their own expense. They may not thank us for depriving them of the prestige they derive from the hypothetical receipts of their chairs ; but it may serve to reconcile restless aspirants for high places to learn that they do not pay at all, in the proportion which they seem to do, from the statistics of college catalogues, which are *signa fallacissima.* Let such learn to be content with the emoluments derived from diligent practice, and seek to make their private station a post of honor, for such it will be, when they shall inspire public confidence in their integrity, skill and success. Such practitioners secure both dignity and emolument beyond the modicum of either, which they can hope to reach as public teachers.—[*NewYork Med. Gaz.*

Professor Gorini.—This gentleman, who is professor of natural history at the University of Lodi, made, before a circle of private friends, two nights ago, a very remarkable experiment illustrative of his theory as to the formation of mountains. He melts some substances, known only to himself, in a vessel, and allows the liquid to cool. At first it presents an even surface, but a portion continues to ooze up from beneath, and gradually elevations are formed, until at length ranges and chains of hills are formed, exactly corresponding in shape with those which are found on the earth. Even to the stratification the resemblance is complete, and M. Gorini can produce on a small scale the phenomena of volcanoes and earthquakes. He contends, therefore, that the inequalities on the face of the globe are the result

---

* University of New York ?

† College of Physicians and Surgeons, New York ?

of certain materials, first reduced by the application of heat to a liquid
state, and then allowed gradually to consolidate. In another and
more practically useful field of research the learned professor has developed some very important facts. He has succeeded to a most surprising extent in preserving animal matter from decay without resorting to any known process for that purpose. Specimens are shown
by him of portions of the human body, which, without any alteration
in their natural appearance, have been exposed to the action of the
atmosphere for six and seven years; and he states that at a trifling
cost he can keep meat for any length of time in such a way that it
can be eaten quite fresh. The importance of such a discovery, if on
a practical investigation it is found to answer, will be more readily
understood when it is remembered that the flocks of sheep in Australia
are boiled down into tallow, their flesh being otherwise almost value-
less, and that in South America vast herds of cattle are annually
slaughtered for the sake of their hides alone.—*Times.*

Kate Dresser, 36 years old, of Schuylhill Co., Pennsylvania, has had
more children than most women. The first child was born in 1826,
and the last in February, 1851. She had twins five times, and in
February, 1848, had four children at one birth ! making twenty-one
children in twenty-one years, and *six* children in the space of *eighteen
months !* The four children at a birth were apparently healthy and
well formed. One lived about four weeks, another eleven months, the
third a little over a year, and the fourth, a fine boy, is still living.
There are now twelve of the whole number living, seven boys and
five girls !—[*Bsston Med. and Surg Jour.*

Distribution of Prizes to Idiots.—The French periodicals contain
the details of a singular exhibition at the *Salpetriere* Hospital of Paris.
This is the great asylum for aged and incurable females, and contains
a great number of idiotic and epileptic inmates, who are incited to
cleanliness, industry and good behaviour, by the distribution of prizes
to the most meritorious in these particulars. The scene is represented as having been exceedingly interesting.

Quarantine Laws.—A convention of some of the most distinguished physicians of Europe, has been for some time sitting in Paris for
the purpose of maturely considering the quarantine regulations in
force, and of recommending to their respective Governments such
modifications as they may deem proper under the more enlightened
views of the age. The result of their labors will be very interesting
to all commercial communities.

Scrofulous Ophthalmia and Granular Lids.—These intractable affections have been treated with great success by Dr. Isaac Hays, of

Philadelphia, with cod-liver oil. The testimony of a practitioner of such well established reputation cannot fail to secure to this plan of treatment a fair trial.

Suicide with Chloroform.—We perceive that Dr. Reyer, chief physician of the Imperial Hospital at Vienna, has recently committed suicide by fastening a bladder filled with chloroform to his mouth and nostrils by means of adhesive plaster.

Death of distinguished men.—It is our painful duty to record the deaths of several of the most distinguished members of the profession in this country. Within the last two months we have lost Professor Granville Sharp Pattison, of the University of New York, one of the ablest lecturers on anatomy we have ever heard; Dr. John Kearny Rogers, long known as one of the best surgeons of New York; Dr. James R. Manley, one of the most aged and respectable physicians of the same city; Dr. E. De Kay, a distinguished naturalist; and Dr. Nicholas Hard, the able professor of anatomy in the Medical College of Iowa.

We are indebted to the authors for quite a number of pamphlets, which we regret not having room to notice more at length. Among them are:

A Lecture on Sanitary Reform, by Lewis Rogers, M.D., Professor in the University of Louisville. It is an able and strong appeal upon the subject, and will be again noticed by us.

Two Lectures, by Professor Jackson, of Philadelphia—the one showing that "Medicine is a Science and not a mere Art"—and the other upon the "Vital Forces." Both are full of interest, and in the distinguished author's most captivating style. The latter is especially valuable as bearing upon practical principles of great importance.

An Appeal to the Legislature of Alabama, for the establishment of a State Hospital for Lunatics and Idiots; prepared by order of the "Alabama State Medical Association." This paper is from the pen of Dr. Lopez, of Mobile, and is one of the most interesting of the kind we have seen. It is to be hoped that the philanthropic efforts of the association may be favorably acted upon by the Alabama legislature.

The Transactions of the first annual meeting of the Kentucky State Medical Society, held in the city of Frankfort. Being its first meeting, nothing more was done than the appointment of committees and the adoption of a constitution.

Proceedings of the organization of the Physicians' Society for Medical observation of Greene and adjoining counties, Georgia. We wish this society every success, and hope it may lead to the formation of others like it.

An Address on the Hygienic and Medicinal uses of Alcoholic Stimulants; by F. M. Robertson, M. D.—being No. 10 of a series of addresses delivered before the Charleston Total Abstinence Society. An excellent address, full of valuable truths to the physician as well as to society at large.

Report of the Committee appointed on Mrs. Willard's theory of Respiration, by the New York State Teachers' Association.—Mrs. Emma Willard, so well known as a teacher of young ladies, is ambitious to enlarge the field of her inculcations, and to enlighten physiologists and pathologists in relation to respiration, circulation, and the treatment of diseases. The reporters "beg leave to state that they believe the theory to be *true*." "This theory affirms that the motive power, which causes the circulation of the blood, is created by an expansion of the volume of the blood in the lungs, produced by the combustion of the carbon of the venous blood, caused by the oxygen of the air introduced by breathing." Since the publication of her Treatise on the Motive Powers, &c., Mrs. W. has issued another work, entitled "Respiration, and its Effects; more especially in relation to Asiatic Cholera and other sinking diseases." Truth is valuable, from whatever source it be derived, and if our fair country-woman can aid us in its discovery, let us not be slow to award her all merited praise.

Dr. R. D. Arnold, the worthy President of the State Medical Society, has been recently elected Mayor of Savannah.

There are now three or four Female Medical Colleges in the United States. It is not stated whether the Graduates are to adopt the Bloomer costume or not.

Colleges of Dental Surgery are being multiplied. We see another recently established in Syracuse, N. Y. We believe that no institution of this kind exists in Europe—a singular fact.

Kossuth and Sir James Clark.—Sir James Clark has waited on the distinguished Hungarian refugee, and kindly proffered his professional services. We do not know whether the offer was accepted.—[*London Lancet.*

[We hope that this contemptible way of seeking notoriety will not be adopted by any respectable practitioner in our country.]

SOUTHERN
MEDICAL AND SURGICAL JOURNAL.

| Vol. 8.] | NEW SERIES.—FEBRUARY, 1852. | [No. 2. |

PART FIRST.

Original Communications.

ARTICLE IV.

Fractures of the Clavicle. By L. A. Dugas, M. D., Professor of Surgery in the Medical College of Georgia.

The relative frequency of fractures of the Clavicle and of other portions of the human skeleton, may be deduced from a series of two thousand three hundred and twenty-five cases, collected by M. Malgaigne, from the records of the Hotel-Dieu, of Paris, as having been treated in that institution in the course of eleven years. Among these there were—

623 fractures of the Fibula, with or without the tibia.
544 do. " " Tibia, with or without the fibula.
310 do. " " Humerus, including those of its neck.
303 do. " " Femur, do. do. do.
267 do. " " Radius, with or without the ulna.
262 do. " " Ribs.
225 do. " " Clavicle.
145 do. " " Ulna, with or without the radius.

From the above statement we may work out the following table of proportions:

Fracture of the Fibula,   •   •   •   1 in $3\frac{3}{4}$
   do. " " Tibia,   -   -   -   1 " $4\frac{1}{2}$
   do. " " Humerus,   -   -   -   1 " $7\frac{1}{2}$

Fracture of the Femur,			-	-	-	1 in 7⅔
do.	"	"	Radius, not quite	-		1 " 9
do.	"	"	Ribs,	-	-	1 " 9
do.	"	"	Clavicle,	-	-	1 " 10½
do.	"	"	Ulna,	-	-	1 " 16

The inmates of the Hotel-Dieu being adults, these data do not apply to children in whom fractures of the clavicle are probably more common. It appears that males, children as well as adults, suffer this injury more frequently than females; a fact which does not depend so much upon any peculiarity of conformation as upon the circumstance that boys and young men are, by their habits and occupations, more exposed to accidents and violence than girls and young women. These fractures are said to be comparatively rare in the aged of both sexes. Among the 225 cases above enumerated, there were 31 in persons beyond sixty years of age. But it should be remembered that the number of inhabitants thus advanced in life in any community, is small when compared with that of younger adults.

The liability of the clavicle to fracture may be explained by reference to its form, its exposed position, its connections and its office. Its curvatures and the inequality of its diameters add to its fragility, from whatever direction the force applied may proceed, for whilst a straight shaft would more effectually resist the many shocks to which it is exposed by falls, or blows upon the shoulder, a more uniform diameter would lessen the danger of fracture from forces applied between the extremities or to its body. Moreover, it is unprotected by muscular coverings, superficially situated, and peculiarly exposed to blows sustained in conflict. Again: being the only medium of bony connection between the trunk and the upper limb, which is instinctively called upon to avert the injurious effects of falls, it has very often to sustain the weight of the body in addition to the impetus derived from the accident. Finally, it may be broken by muscular efforts, as in lifting or throwing heavy objects, pushing bodies forward, &c.

Fractures of the clavicle, like those of other bones, may be complete or incomplete, simple or compound. Any point of the clavicle may be the seat of fracture, and this may be either oblique, transverse, or comminuted. When occasioned by forces applied, directly or indirectly, to the shoulder, they are usually found to be oblique, and to exist about the middle of the bone. The transverse fractures are less common, and the comminuted still more rare. These result generally from direct blows received in front, and are therefore not so uniformly confined to any particular portion. They are also more often complicated with contusions, laceration, displacement, and injury to the adjacent parts than the former or oblique fractures.

Fractures of the clavicle may be most advantageously studied by dividing them into those which implicate the body or shaft of the bone, and those which occur at the acromial and sternal extremities.

Fractures of the body of the bone constitute the great majority of cases, and may be occasioned by direct blows, by falls upon the shoulder, arms or hands, or by violent muscular efforts. They may be transverse, oblique, or comminuted, including fragments of various dimensions between the two extremities, and sometimes constituting really a double fracture. They are occasionally found to be *incomplete,* the bone appearing to be merely bent at an angle more or less obtuse. In these cases there is only a portion of the diameter of the bone broken, and consequently only a partial laceration of the periosteum. Crepitation cannot therefore be induced without completing the fracture, as is sometimes done in endeavoring to straighten the shaft.

If a *complete fracture* be transverse, with jagged or serrated edges interlocked, there may be neither displacement nor crepitus perceptible, unless the fragments be drawn asunder and rubbed against each other. This variety is therefore sometimes confounded with the incomplete fracture. In a clean transverse fracture of the shaft, the acromial fragment will be dragged down by the shoulder, and may slide beneath, before, or behind the other, according to the position of the shoulder. Such a displacement will be much more readily detected than that attending an oblique fracture, for the obvious reason that the obliquity of the fracture will lessen the diameter of the ends which overlap each other. In either case, the shoulder is drawn forward by the muscles, and there is observed upon the anterior aspect of the bone, a depression at the seat of fracture, which will disappear measurably by pressing back the shoulder. The *obliquity* of fractures of the clavicle varies very much, and has been known to be two inches in length. Its direction is usually from the acromial to the sternal portion, and from the front to the rear. There are exceptions, however, in which this direction is reversed.

The *degree of displacement* consequent upon complete fractures of the shaft of the clavicle varies necessarily according to the *direction* of the solution of continuity. There is usually less apparent displacement in oblique than in non-serrated transverse and comminuted fractures. Yet, if the direction of the obliquity be such as to offer no resistance to the dragging down of the acromial fragment by the weight of the shoulder, the displacement may be equal to that in transverse fractures. It is evident that if the direction of the obliquity be from above downward, and from the sternal to the acromial portion, the acromial fragment will still rest upon the sternal, and thus prevent any downward displacement. The displacement of either of the fragments *may* then be found upwards, downwards, forwards, or backwards, although the distal fragment is that most frequently found displaced downwards and backwards.

Fractures of the shaft are those in which we might reasonably apprehend injury to the adjacent blood-vessels and nerves. Yet this is of very rare occurrence. These fractures are usually detected without much difficulty. The pendulous limb, depressed shoulder, and the inability to use the arm or to carry the hand to the opposite shoulder or to the head, without more or less pain about the clavicle, added to the history of the violence sustained, will be sufficient to direct attention to this bone. If the fracture be *incomplete*, the bone will seem to be bent, and the angle will be detected by passing the finger along the surface of the bone, but no crepitus will be observed unless the fracture be completed as already suggested. If the fracture be complete, the displacement evident to the eye and felt by the finger, the crepitus produced by moving the shoulder in various directions, the local tenderness upon pressure, &c., will leave no doubt as to the nature of the injury.

By *fractures of the acromial extremity* we understand those existing between the articulation and the sternal edge of the coraco-clavicular ligaments These result most frequently from blows upon the top of the shoulder, but may, like those of the shaft, be occasioned by falls upon the shoulder or out-stretched arms. They are much more rare than those of the shaft, though more common than those of the sternal extremi-ty. They are usually transverse or at a right angle with the axis of the bone, but may present various degrees of obliquity. Although formerly thought never to be attended with displace-ment, it is now well established that this sometimes occurs to a very considerable degree. When no displacement exists, it is probable that the fragments are maintained in situ by the coraco-clavicular ligaments, or by the periosteum, or by both, in consequence of their having escaped laceration. The liabili-ty to displacement is increased by the obliquity of the fracture. Being, however, generally attended with very little pain, and often with neither manifest displacement nor crepitus, fractures of this portion of the clavicle may escape detection. The surgeon cannot, therefore, be too guarded in his diagnosis, although even under such circumstances a careful examination, especially if there is not much tumefaction, will usually reveal a slight groove and feeble crepitus.

Fractures of the sternal extremity are so rare that very few cases are to be found on record; hence the discrepancies in reference to the existence of any displacement of the frag-ments—some authorities insisting that none occurs, whereas Malgaigne refers to two cases in which the external fragment was drawn downwards and forwards. In children, the ster-nal epiphysis may be separated so as to simulate a partial dislo-cation, and to render the diagnosis much more obscure than it is, even in those cases in which the fracture exists between the costo-clavicular and sterno-clavicular ligaments without dis-placement.

The *treatment* of fractures of the clavicle has taxed the inge-nuity of surgeons as much, if not more, than that of any other class, so that a mere enumeration of the various plans proposed would far exceed the limits of this paper. They may all, however, be classed under three divisions—viz: those consisting of a cushion or pad in the axilla, and a roller bandage passed around the chest in various directions, of which Desault's may be considered the type ; those consisting of loops passed around the shoulders for the purpose of drawing them backwards; and those consisting of a sling bandage.

In cases unattended with displacement, it is evident that nothing more is required than the maintainance of the limb and shoulder in a state of immobility, so as to prevent subsequent displacement and to favor adhesion. A simple sling, with a bandage thrown around the thorax and elbow so as to keep this firmly applied to the side, will therefore be all sufficient. But when there is a displacement of one or both fragments, this must not only be reduced, but the apparatus used must be such as will effectually secure the reduction until a callus be formed—say from three to six weeks.

The indications to be fulfilled are, in most cases, to carry and to fix the shoulder upwards, backwards, and outwards. In some instances it becomes also necessary to exercise a certain degree of compression upon the sternal fragment. These indications were studiously met by Desault, in the very complex bandage which bears his name. Although still recommended by high authority, it appears to me exceedingly objectionable. In the first place, the cushion placed in the axilla for the purpose of forcing the shoulder outwardly when the elbow is drawn against the side, must necessarily exercise a degree of compression upon the blood-vessels and nerves, which few, if any, patients can endure ; yet, unless the pressure be sufficient to throw out the shoulder the object of the cushion is not secured. Indeed, I must confess that I have never been able to succeed in having it borne by any one to whom I have applied it with a view to this end. Again : the numerous circles of the roller bandage around the chest, offer an impediment to respiration which is often intolerable. Finally, the facility with which the whole apparatus becomes displaced, however skilfully applied and carefully pinned and stitched, requiring frequent readjustment, is, of itself, an objection of sufficient importance to lead us to its total rejection.

A radical objection to the padded loops by which the shoulders are drawn back, is that by this plan we attain only one of the indications pointed out as usually to be fulfilled. The shoulder is neither carried upwards nor outwards. Besides this, they rarely fail to produce chaffing to a greater or less extent.

The sling bandage is that to which I have given a decided preference for the last fifteen or twenty years. It is unnecessary to describe the numerous modifications of this simple bandage, proposed by surgeons of all countries, and I will therefore proceed at once to describe the one I habitually use, without, for a moment, pretending to originality, lest, perhaps, some book-worm might discover that *precisely* the same had been proposed by others.

The displacement having been carefully reduced by movements of the shoulder in various directions, according to the particular case, and by direct action upon the fragments themselves, let an aid maintain the reduction by placing the ends of the fingers of the affected limb upon the top of the opposite shoulder, by bringing the elbow against the side, and by pressing up the elbow so as to carry the shoulder upwards, outwards and backwards, as will be done under those circumstances. The next step will be to secure the limb in this position. For this purpose, I procure a square yard of cotton fabric, (unbleached shirting, for example, as this is softer than the bleached, which is usually starched,) and cut it diagonally, so as to obtain a triangular bit, to the acute angles of which should be sewed slips three inches wide and three or four yards long.

Apply the middle of the base or long side of the triangle beneath the elbow, leaving a margin of about four inches behind, and carrying the obtuse angle towards the fingers. One of the acute angles, with its strip, will now be carried between the arm and chest, up to the fractured clavicle, around the back of the neck, over the sound shoulder, in front, and beneath the axilla, and, finally, around the chest, including the arm just above the elbow. The other end and strip will be carried in front of the fore-arm, up to the sound shoulder, behind and beneath the axilla, and around the chest and arm, so as to meet its fellow, and to be tied to it firmly. The margin left projecting behind the elbow should then be elevated, doubled, and so secured with stitches as to prevent the elbow from sliding out of the sling in that direction. The portion of the triangle situated along the fore-arm should be also folded around it, and thus secured.   Lastly, the strips encircling the chest and arm should be stitched, to prevent their upward or downward displacement.   If it be necessary to press down the sternal fragment, this can be effectually done by interposing a little pad between the bone and the bandage which passes over it.

The advantages of this bandage are to be found in its perfect adaptation to the necessities of the case, in its great simplicity, in the facility with which it may be made secure, and in the very slight inconvenience to which it subjects the patient. Children, as well as adults, bear it without a murmur ; and if it becomes necessary, for purposes of cleanliness, to remove it, any intelligent mother or nurse may re-apply it, if the physician be not accessible.   Whilst it cannot be denied that, under any plan of treatment, there will occasionally remain some unevenness or deformity at the seat of fracture, I must say that I have very rarely seen any thing of the kind in cases treated on this plan, notwithstanding the fact that I have not unfrequently, after applying the bandage once in presence of the mother, left the subsequent management entirely to herself.

ARTICLE V.

A Case of Adherent Fœtuses. By JOSEPH A. EVE, M. D., Professor of Obstetrics, &c., &c., in the Medical College of Georgia.

A remarkable case of adherent fœtuses occurred in my practice on the 19th of October, some account of which may not be altogether devoid of interest to the readers of the Southern Medical and Surgical Journal, especially to those who may be fond of natural curiosities, or feel disposed to study Nature in her sportive freaks.

Mrs. S., a German lady, 21 years of age, was taken in labor, October 19th, 1851, about 4 a. m.   When I was called to her, she had been in labor about eleven hours.   The head of a child had been expelled three or four hours before I saw her ; her pains were violent but ineffectual.   I succeeded, with the greatest difficulty, in bringing down one arm and shoulder, and then the other ; after which the delivery being still retarded, I apprehended an enlargement of the abdomen or some other species of deformity. Directing the patient to bear down with all her strength, and in concert with the uterine contractions, making such traction as I deemed safe and proper, I succeeded in delivering her of two female foetuses, united by their breasts and abdomen as low down as the umbilicus; the amount of force employed in their delivery was by no means excessive. The midwife in attendance stated that the head expelled before my arrival was at first alive—that the lips moved when a finger was inserted into the mouth. I have no doubt from the appearance of the foetuses, that both were alive when labor commenced. The death of the first might have been determined by the long continued violent labor, or by tractions made on the head, or, it may have been consequent upon the death of the second, which must have occurred while the head of the former was descending, as the head of the latter was unavoidably thrown back, and the cervical vertebræ dislocated; the death of one must necessarily have involved the death of the other, as there was but one heart common to both.

The difficulty in the delivery is attributable to their mode of union, and not to their bulk, as they were premature by a fortnight at least, and both together only weighed $10\frac{1}{4}$ pounds, whereas it is not very uncommon for children weighing eleven or twelve pounds, to be born after comparatively easy labors. The foetus that presented first is somewhat larger than the other. The smaller resembles the mother, the larger the father. They are united breast to breast from the neck to the umbilicus. The umbilical cords unite as they pass out, and form one cord, diverging again within an inch of the placenta. There was but one placenta, with nothing peculiar in its appearance.

Mrs. S., was in a very comfortable state, a slight headache excepted, for an hour and a half after the delivery, when she was seized with convulsions, which continued to recur at irregular intervals, averaging about forty-five minutes until she had eleven. By copious blood letting, chloroform, and morphine, with some measures of minor importance, the convulsions were moderated, and finally, arrested, after which her convalescense was as favorable as could have been reasonably anticipated. The patient had applied a bandage firmly around her neck to compress a goitre, fearing that it might become enlarged by her violent efforts during labor ; this of course, was removed as soon as it was discovered : whether this had any agency in determining the attack of convulsions will be considered, differently, according to the theory entertained of the causation of convulsions: in my opinion its influence was by no means inconsiderable, although it must be admitted that much may be fairly attributed to the violence and long continuance of the labor.

That these fœtuses were dead-born was certainly a blessing to themselves, and to their parents, a kind and merciful dispensation of Providence, as life would have been a heritage of misery and mortification.

They were so extensively and strongly adherent that it is difficult to understand how their safe delivery could be effected, without a coincidence of the most favorable conditions, and advantageous circumstances. Had their connection been by the abdomen, admitting of greater mobility, as in a case quoted by Burns, or by a distinct band, as in the Siamese Twins, —had they been more premature, or smaller, the feet or knees presenting, the maternal pelvis very capacious, with the soft parts thoroughly relaxed, they might have been expelled alive, without the interference of art, or the delivery might have been assisted and rendered safer, by gently drawing upon the feet of one, thereby to cause the head of that one to descend a little in advance of the other, and prevent their simultaneous descent into the pelvis, which would most probably cause destructive compression.

Since the commencement of the present course of lectures in the Medical College of Georgia, an examination was made by Dr. H. F. Campbell in the presence of Professors Means and Miller, Dr. R. C. Campbell, and myself. The united cord on section, exhibited three arteries and two veins,—it was examined with a microscope. Each fœtus has a distinct stomach and intestinal canal and set of lungs. There was only one heart and one liver, common to both ; there are two sterna, one on either side, united at their upper extremities, each appertaining as much to one fœtus as to the other, constituting the principal media of junction between them; - the sterna, accordingly, instead of being in the median line in front, having an anterior and a posterior face, are so placed, one on each side, that they face each other from right to left. ·

Before this examination, from a superficial view, they appeared to be distinct fœtuses united by their sterna. The examination could not be extended farther without mutilating and destroying the appearance of this truly interesting and wonderful lusus naturæ, which has been preserved with great care in the College Museum; indeed as it was kindly and generously given to us by the parents for that purpose, we did not feel at liberty to pursue the anatomical investigation farther than might be compatible with the perfect preservation of its original form.

There is in the same Museum, another very similar instance of monstrosity which occured some years ago in the practice of Dr. R. D. Moore, of Athens, and which he kindly presented to the Medical College, through our friend Dr. Wm. E. Dearing of this city.

I requested Dr. Dearing to write to Dr. Moore for an account of this monstrosity, that both might be included in the same communication, but I regret that it has not yet been received.

In Dr. Moore's case of adherent fœtuses, the attachment is not so extensive; the adhesion is chiefly by the abdomen, being separate from two to two and half inches below their necks. They are black, both females; they appear to have arrived at full term. They were taken from the jar in which they are preserved, but they had been so eviscerated during the delivery, or upon subsequent examination, that we could determine nothing satisfactorily respecting their internal organization. We hope Dr. Moore will still furnish for this Journal a particular description from notes taken at the time.

Instances of multiple adherent fœtuses, are, we believe extremely unfrequent in their occurrence.

Dr. Churchill, who is doubtless as well acquainted with the history and statistics of Obstetrics as any author living, or dead, has the following paragraph in the last edition of his "System of Midwifery," edited by Dr. Condie of Philadelphia:

"Double monsters are very rare, and may create great difficulty in the delivery, although there are cases on record of the
children having been born alive. Dr. Burns quotes several
such : ' In the seventh volume of the Nouv. Journ. p. 164,' he
says, 'is a case where two children were born at the full
time, united by the inferior part of the belly, from the centre
of which came the cord. The vertebral columns almost touched
at the lower part. The two children, who were of different
sexes, lived, we are told, twelve days, but nothing is said of
the labour. In the Bulletins for 1818, p. 2, two children, who
were joined by the back at the sacrum, are stated to have been
born, and lived till the ninth day. The first child presented
the head, but the midwife could not well tell how the second
got out. There is another case, at page 32, of a woman who,
after many days of labour, bore a monster double in its upper
parts. The spinal column was united from the sacrum to the
top of the dorsal vertebræ, then the cervical vertebræ divided
to form two necks. The midwife finding the head to present
along with the cord and a hand, tried to turn, but could discover nothing but superior extremities. She, therefore, let
her alone. The head was afterwards expelled, but neither nature nor art could deliver the body. M. Ratel finding the head
and two arms already almost separated from the body, cut
these parts off, then introducing his hand, he found another
head, turned the child, and brought away the whole mass.'
"There is a skeleton in the Royal College of Surgeons of
Ireland, of a double monster, the children being joined by the
lower part of the sacrum, and I believe they were also born
alive. The Siamese Twins is another instance of the kind."

One of the most remarkable and curious laws, appertaining
to the developement of monsters, is that of symmetry. However strangely and variously two or more fœtuses may be united, intermixed, amalgamated, fused or welded together, similar
parts are always found united. We never observe an arm attached to a leg, or a leg to a hand, a side to a back, or a back
of one to an abdomen of another, but similar always to similar
parts, and symmetrically and evenly, appearing to verify the
correctness of Serres' doctrine of evolution.

The most remarkable peculiarities of the internal organization of this monstrosity, consist firstly, in the unity of the heart,
and consequently intercommunion of the circulation, the aorta
soon after its origin divides into two branches, one distributed
to each fœtus. Secondly, in the singleness of the liver, there

being one common to both.   Thirdly, in having one thoracic
cavity common to both, the lateral boundaries of which are
constituted by the sterna, being situated latterally one on either
side, instead of anteriorly. From the fact that there are only one
heart and one liver common to both, while each has a distinct
stomach and intestinal canal, may we not infer that the principal office of the liver is accessory to the heart, whether it be
regarded as a diverticulum or a depurator of the blood.

ARTICLE VI.

A Case of Chorea treated by Chloroform.   By WM. A. MIL-
NER, M. D., of Union Parish, Louisiana.

I believe it is generally admitted that but little more is
known of the nature of this disease, than that it is a functional
derangement of the nervous system.   It is therefore not my
design to advance pathological views upon a subject so imperfectly understood by abler and more experienced practitioners,
but merely to give the treatment of a single case, which will,
perhaps, not be uninteresting.

I am aware, too, that the prognosis of uncomplicated chorea
is generally favorable, there being instances of spontaneous
recoveries; nevertheless, it is a very ugly, and I may say
formidable, disease, and one which excites the greatest interest
and solicitude on the part of friends and parents.

June 5. My attention was called to the daughter of Mr. L.,
aged 9 years.   She was able to run about, but there was irregular motion of the hands, and some slight twitching of the
muscles of lips and face; she was yet able to feed herself—
complained of some headache.   She was taken from school
two months previous to my seeing her, from complaining of
headache and general, but slight, indisposition. ` Prescription—
Active purge of rhei. colocynth and calomel every third night.
Being rather anæmic, put her on Valet's ferruginous pill, three
times per day.

June 8. Bowels are well acted upon; but the case has grown
rapidly worse. It seems that every voluntary muscle in the
whole system is in motion; deglutition is performed with great

difficulty—requires two persons to hold her up. Average sleep in twenty-four 1 to 2 hours, in very short naps. *Prescription*—$\frac{1}{4}$ gr. sulph. morph., repeat every hour until sleep is induced; applied blister, $2\frac{1}{2}$ by 6 inches, over dorsal region; sulph. zinc, 1 gr., three times per day.

June 10. My patient has eaten nothing of consequence for two days; stomach very irritable; the zinc was rejected—repeated, and rejected, for two days; morphine seems to aggravate, even in 1 gr. doses, instead of quieting and inducing sleep. Blister drew well, and is considerably irritated from the incessant motion, which makes me regret having put it on. *Prescription*—Oil and turpentine to move the bowels; stop the zinc, and gave comp. tinct. gentian ʒj., and ℥j. infusion snake root, three times per day, with 1 gr. ext. hyoscy. at night, and repeat once, in an hour, if required.

June 11. Patient rested better last night, stomach is quieted, and desires to eat. Continued same treatment.

June 12. Patient passed a restless night; has some erysipelatous spots on hands and feet, which I attribute to hyoscy., having taken 2 grs. last night. The stomach is quiet; eats soup or gruel with difficulty; takes nothing solid. The muscular disturbance is still very great; no appreciable amendment.

I now proposed to Mr. L. to use chloroform, since the anodynes had ceased to have the desired effect, of inducing sleep, &c., but it was strongly opposed by the family, from the abominable prejudice existing against what I consider a God-sent blessing.

I refused to treat the case farther, without consultation, upon which Dr. Calderwood, of Monroe, was sent for. He arrived in the evening of the 13th. We immediately used chloroform, and kept the patient under its influence for an hour. She slept quietly for about an hour after the anesthesia subsided, but aroused up into the same incessant motion. We again put her under its influence, and used it every time she waked during the night.

June 14. Patient seems more quiet while awake this morning. *Prescription*—Use chloroform at 9 o'clock, A. M., and at 4, P. M., with 1 gr. hyoscy. ext. at night, and chloroform every time she wakes during the night. Commenced sulph. zinc in $\frac{1}{6}$ gr. doses, three times per day, gradually increasing the dose.

June 17. Patient has improved rapidly; can sit alone in a chair; slept all last night without chloroform. Continue same treatment.

June 20. Patient can walk alone, feed herself, and speak tolerable distinctly; has knitted a little. She is now taking as much as 1 gr. zinc, three times per day; has slept without chloroform at night, since the 17th. Continue same treatment. Chloroform once per day. Bowels keep regular without physic, since using hyoscy., and left off morphine.

June 30. Patient has continued to improve; the muscular disturbance is very slight, with short but distinct intermissions; her color is quite sallow; tongue clean, but red: circulation rapid, with good appetite. Have increased zinc to 2 grs., stomach will not tolerate more. *Prescription*—Discontinue hyoscy., and continue chloroform once per day, and zinc as before.

July 5. Patient is quite clear of all symptoms of chorea, but is in a very anæmic condition. *Prescription*—Discontinue other treatment, except the occasional use of chloroform, when wakeful at night, and put her upon an iron tonic, which has had its desired and usual effect in such cases.

Dec. 1. Up to this time my patient has had almost uninterrupted good health.

The speedy and successful treatment of the above case, is attributable, in my humble opinion, almost, if not entirely, to chloroform, having used zinc, silver, copper, ammonia, and the thousand and one remedies, in other cases, before the discovery of chloroform, with bad success.

PART II.

𝕰𝖈𝖑𝖊𝖈𝖙𝖎𝖈 𝕯𝖊𝖕𝖆𝖗𝖙𝖒𝖊𝖓𝖙

On Cancers. Read before the Medical Society of St. Louis, July 27th 1851. By Charles. A. Pope, M. D., Professor of Surgery in the Medical Department of the St. Louis University.

Mr. President:—In whatever light we may regard them, tumors constitute a most important and interesting part of surgery. Whether in their mode of origin, their growth, their local and constitutional effects, their classification, diagnosis or treatment, they are of exceeding interest. Their diagnosis often presents the greatest difficulty, and this is of itself important, for they are not all to be treated alike; as is the diagnosis, so is the operation. The method by exclusion, as applied to the discrimination of tumors, has, in not a few instances, led to results in diagnosis, unparalleled in the annals of surgery. I allude, among others, to the case of the fœtal tumor, removed from the scrotum by Velpeau. But of all tumors, the malignant merit most attention. The very name of cancer carries with it ideas of suffering and of death. The subject then is one of the deepest interest; and having met with the thesis of M. Broca, of Paris, wherein are so clearly and succinctly stated the views of M. Lebert, I have thought it worth while to lay them before the Society in our own tongue. It is, perhaps, proper to state that they have not yet met with that general adoption to which they are entitled, and which a wider knowledge of them will ensure. So far as my own limited experience and observation go, they fully coincide with the doctrines of Lebert, and I have, for several years taught in accordance with them.

M. Broca has ably defended the microscrope, if, indeed, it needed defence. The defects often attributed to the instrument, are oftener due to those who use it. Muller has said that "microscopical and chemical analysis can never become a means of surgical diagnosis; it were ridiculous to desire it or to suppose it practicable." As to the desirableness of such a result, but few, perhaps, will concur with the distinguished physiologist. But although of little or no benefit in the diagnosis of tumors, yet if after removal it show to us whether the growth be benign or malignant, prognosis will be benefitted, and satisfaction result both to the surgeon and the patient. Where else, indeed, are we to look for certainty in this respect. All other tests have heretofore failed. Mere physical characters, although described by the most minute and skilful anatomists are yet insufficient. Their chemical constitution varies it is true, but not to an extent desired by the systematic writer or practical surgeon. Fat and gelantine are the proximate principles usually found in the benign, as albumen constitutes the chief bulk of malignant tumors. This, however, is not enough. Up to the time of Lebert's researches even the microscope had proved ineffectual. Before his efforts, nothing more than the elements which characterize the simplest tissues, had been found in growths avowedly malignant. Thanks, however, to the labors of this distinguished micrograph; the question has at length been solved. Although Muller led the way, yet Lebert found the key. The specific cancer cell has been seen and recognised. Though varying like men's faces, they still bear a sufficient resemblance to be referred to the same generic type.

Proficiency in the use of the microscope is not, as many suppose, of easy attainment. Time and study are requisite; and for this very reason we would urge its repeated employment in order to derive that invaluable aid to be afforded by this wonderful instrument

The observations of M. Broca upon 52 cases of true cancer, are all in favor of his propositions. They embrace a period of six years. Many of the patients were subjected to several operations. He has followed them all, and but one of the whole number was living at the beginning of 1850. He had been operated on eight times by M. Blandin, and within a few weeks after the last operation the disease re-appeared with every probability of a fatal result.

The author is still pursuing his observations, and his researches cannot fail to prove of great value to the profession.

I am glad that this subject has attracted the attention of the American Medical Association, as among the reports to be made at its next meeting is one on the "Results of Surgical Operations in Malignant Diseases." The name of Prof. Gross to whose able hands this report has been confided, affords every assurance that it will redound to the reputation of its author as well as the good of medicine.

A few propositions on the so called Cancerous Tumors.

["Anatomia verum medicinae lumen."—Morgagni.]

I. It is impossible to give a definition of what is generally understood by the term *cancer.* This is not a single affection, but a group presenting merely some marks in common.

II. Pathological anatomy, as it existed prior to the employment of the microscope, has thrown no light on the nature of the different tumors denominated cancerous. The differences

which the most skillful observers had recognized in their structure by no means corresponded with their clinical study.

The microscope has substituted science for hypothesis and
opened the way for exact and fruitful observation. Every observation, past or present, which has not been subjected to the
microscope, should be considered as irrelevant.

III. The juice extracted by scraping or pressure, from the
different so called cancerous tumors, always presents an innumerable quantity of nucleated cells, in different stages of developement. Muller, who discovered them, has pointed out
their various forms; but having seen tumors only, and no patients, he has continued to confound affections which at the
present day are distinct. M. Isaac Mayor has well described
the elements of epidermic tumors, although he did not venture
to separate them from the class of cancers. Lastly, M. Lebert
has studied them both anatomically and clinically, and it is he,
who has the honor of having first divided the so called cancerous tumors into three distinct species, each characterized by a
special histological element.

IV. These elements are :

1. *The cancerous element* properly so called, without analogue in the economy.

2. *The fibro-plastic element,* for a long time supposed to be
without analogue in the economy, but recently found by M.
Robin, in the uterine mucous membrane.

3. *The epidermic,* or better, *the epithelial element,* identical
with the normal elements of the epidermis and epithelium.

V. Hence three kinds of tumors:

1. *Cancerous tumors* properly so called, the only ones which
should henceforth be designated by the name of cancer.

2. *Fibro-plastic tumors.*

3. *Epidermic,* or better, *epithelial tumors.* I prefer the latter denomination, because the epidermis is but a species of the
genus epithelium, and especially, because the dried layers of
the epidermis, in accumulating the one upon the other, may
give rise to inert tumors (corns, warts) very different from
those I am now considering.

VI. The pure fibro-plastic tumors may exist wherever there
is cellular tissue; they seem to be the result of certain chronic
inflammations. Although disposed to increase, and even to
ulcerate, they may sometimes get well without an operation;
they almost always do get well when completely excised.
They should be stricken from the class of malignant tumors.

VII. It being possible for the fibro-plastic element to be developed wherever the cellular tissue is the seat of any chronic
affection, it is consequently often met with in epithelial or can-

cerous tumors; but it is only adventitious, and does not modify either their nature or progress.

VIII. There are no mixed tumors, composed partly of the epithelial, and partly of the cancerous element.

IX. Epithelial tumors can only originate on surfaces covered by epithelium. They are often attributable to mechanical causes; they increase, generally, more slowly than the real cancerous tumors; they ulcerate sooner or later, then grow more rapidly, invade adjoining tissues, and may even penetrate bone; but the ulcers to which they give rise, do not become the seat of hemorrhage; the engorgement of corresponding lymphatic ganglia, takes place very rarely; no general infection is produced, and death occurs only from the exhaustion which is inseparably connected with protracted suppuration. In a word, these tumors are essentially local; they never return, when completely removed. When they re-appear after ablation, it is always *in situ*, because they were not entirely extirpated; they do not return, but merely continue.

Almost all the affections called *cancers of the skin*, particularly, the *noli me tangere*, and the pretended chimney sweep's cancer, nearly all the tumors of the lip, many of those of the tongue, the soft palate, the penis, vulva, vagina, the neck of the uterus, for a long time considered as cancers, are nothing more than epithelial tumors. I have once met with this affection at the pylorus; M. Lebert has found it in the parietal arachnoid of man, and M. Robin in the internal membrane of the iliac veins of the horse.

X. A tumor which does not actually contain cancer cells, has no more chance of becoming cancerous, than any part soever of the body of the individual who bears it. The theory of the degeneration and transformation of tumors is an hypothesis without foundation. It is refuted inasmuch as nothing confirms it. Thus far, nothing proves that a tumor may pass from the benign to the malignant state.

XI. Glandular hypertrophies, already contra distinguished from cancer by Sir A. Cooper, have again been confounded with them by inattentive observers. Cancer cells have been mistaken for the epithelial cells which line the glandular *cul-de-sacs*. M. Lebert has also overthrown this error. The distinction between cancer properly so called and glandular hypertrophy is always possible for those who are acquainted with the intimate structure of glands.

XII. Hypertrophied glandular tumors may seem to re-appear after extirpation, because a still healthy portion left by the operation, may in its turn become hypertrophied; but however numerous the returns, the disease remains always local, and is sooner or later cured by a final operation.

XIII. We have no right to say that a tumor is cancerous merely because there is re-appearance. We should call *cancerous* those tumors only, in which the microscope has shown the existence of the cancerous element.

XIV. The cancerous element is composed of free nuclei, and of cells with nuclei similar to the free nuclei. The uniformity and regularity of the nuclei contrast with the varieties of form and size presented by the cells. Sometimes the number of free nuclei is greater than the cells and sometimes the contrary. The cells may be wanting, but the free nuclei are never absent. I have observed that in returning cancers, the cells were very small and not numerous; on several occasions I have not found them at all.

XV. Genuine cancer may be produced wherever there are vessels. These tumors are developed without a known cause; the influence of hereditary disposition even is far from being demonstrated. They grow generally more rapidly than epithelial tumors; cause always sooner or later in the corresponding lymphatic ganglia engorgements which assume the character of cancer; produce, always subsequently to the ganglionic involvement, a general infection of the system, known as the *cancerous cachexia.* Lastly, at a subsequent period, they often give rise to a great many secondary cancers, called *metastatic.* These may occur anywhere, but they bear a marked predilection for the glands and ganglions. This is a freqent occurrence; I have observed it nine times. It would probably always occur, if the patients lived sufficiently long.

XVI. It is only after having maturely reflected, after having collected numerous observations and followed patients for a long time, that I venture to make the following proposition:

When, after an operation, the microscope has shown the removed tumor to be really cancerous, *the tumor always returns after a greater or less length of time,* either in or around the cicatrix, in the corresponding lymphatic ganglia, or more rarely in some other part of the economy.

XVII. Tumors which have returned, progress both locally and generally more rapidly than the original tumors; if removed, repullulation is more prompt than at first.

Reproduction takes place usually in the six months following the operation, but sometimes much later. I have never seen it postponed longer than two years.

Most of the preceding ideas are now entertained by men who are engaged in general anatomy and clinical study: they are all developed in the work of M. Lebert. He it is, I repeat, who has effected the revolution of which I have shown

myself the partisan.   Having had the good fortune to be timely notified of the structure of tumours called cancerous, I have
been enabled to study a great number during my residence
(internat) in the hospitals.   I have followed, for a long while,
the patients who bore them, and profitably observed the disease and its various terminations.   It is thus that I have come
to the hopeless conclusion, that *real cancer never forgives.*   A
few unimportant details aside, this proposition is among those
above formulated, the only one which belongs to me; but it
has appeared sufficiently grave to be here cited.   In order to
sustain it, it were well to begin by an exposition as rapid as
possible, of microscopical discoveries.

These discoveries are in opposition to classic theories; they
make a clean sweep of what has until now been said by the
most celebrated surgeons; and nevertheless, after having verified, it seems to me proper to adopt them, without being ac-
cused of presumption, and want of respect for one's masters.
Indeed, I am happy to acknowledge that neither talent, perseverance, nor philosophical ideas were wanting to our predecessors, the chasm which they have left, and the errors which
they have committed, are solely due to the insufficiency of their
means of investigation.

It is, in fact, only within a few years, that the microscope
has opened an entirely new era in the science of organization.
This wonderful instrument, long abolished from severer studies,
and given up to the cabinets of the curious has now become
one of the most solid bases of anatomy.   It has revealed to us
the mysteries of embryonic formations, and the admirable structure of the tissues, arrived at their complete developement;
it alone could serve us in the still more difficult study of the
innumerable alterations to which these tissues are liable.

In reading the preface of the first book of Morgagni, we are
struck with the analogy, which exists between his times and
our own; then, pathological anatomy still in its infancy, ran
counter to the humoral theories and empirical doctrines.   In
presence of an impending revolution, with which medicine was
threatened, a violent reaction arose against the youthful science, which attacked two equally redoubtable forces: tradition
and routine.   The struggle was long and angry, but truth must
always triumph: victory was in favor of pathological anatomy.

So at the present time, the study of the ultimate elements,
which compose diseased tissues, has sudenly enlarged the boundaries of pathological physiology.   The microscrope has already upset more than one theory, and ruined more than one
hypothesis, but it has also provoked an obstinate resistance.

The microscope has therefore escaped neither calumny, nor

injustice ; it has been said that it was a faithless instrument, a source of illusion and of error ; that in its confused images, one might, at will, find the most varied forms. A few contradictory results met with in authors, have been opposed to each other, and disdainfully rejecting every new idea, the would be obser- ver has thrown it aside.

The microscope so unjustly discarded, has, in fact, the right to defend itself. Once for all, we should put an end to these trifling accusations, which everybody repeats without having sufficiently thought on them.

The microscope, it is said, gives false images. This unfor- tunate objection recoils heavily on those who make it. Let them follow a course on physics ; they will learn of the pas- sage of luminous rays through superimposed lenses. It is clear that the microscope exhibits what exists, and nothing more nor less.

The microscope, it is also said, is a frequent source of illu- sion. In proportion as the magnifying power is increased, so are the images more obscure, and their outlines more indis- tinct. Optical illusions are favored by this species of twilight, as they occur in reality, towards dark, in the landscape of dis- tant objects. One may, at pleasure, figure these ill defined shadows which his imagination seeks.

This objection has some foundation, but what does it prove ? That real observers should never employ powers capable of rendering images indistinct for want of light. In the present state of the opticians's art, every power which exceeds 1200 diameters (800 diameters according to the new calculations of M. Robin) is a source of confusion. Below this limit, images are sufficiently distinct, and in a given preparation every one should find the same elements.

But whence the innumerable contradictions of which every one speaks ?

First of all the contradictions are more apparent than real ; they bear rather upon the interpretation than on the form of histological elements ; moreover they are, in fact, rare, and ex- ist only in a few accessory-details. Is there even a mediocre observer, who at the present day denies the existence of the globules of the blood, of lymph, of pus, of spermatic animalculi, or of the osseous corpuscles ? Certainly not. It has been asked only, whether the spermatozoa are or are not animals, whether the lymph globules are changed or not, into blood glo- bules, whether the osseous corpuscles are or not, in communi- cation with the large vascular canaliculi, by the intermedium of the small calcareous canaculi. But I ask, is there a point in simple anatomy, on which there has been no discussion ?

Without mentioning the disputes between Vesalius and the Galenists; without recalling the canal of the spinal marrow, the articular glands, the hepatico-cystic ducts, the canal of Cochwitz, and so many other anatomical mystifications : without opposing Sabatier, who gives to the urethra a foot in length, and M. Malgaigne, who allows it only six inches ; shall we find any two anatomists who agree upon the aponeuroses of the groin and perineum ? Should we require of microscopic researches a greater precision than in anatomy, visible to the naked eye ? Is it not more than evident that the miscroscope is quite as innocent of the errors of microscopists, as the scalpel is of those of anatomists ? It is a reflection not generally made particularly when we find ourselves mistaken, because we like better to blame an instrument, than blame ourselves.

But the cause of the microscope is able to triumph even whilst making concessions. I am willing to grant that there are in micrography a number of inexact and contested facts. But what does this prove ? Merely that there are good and bad observers ; that we are too hasty in publishing the result of our researches, and especially that we think ourselves skilled in the use of the microscope, at a period when we should be content to learn and verify what others have said. When we have looked two or three times through a microscope, we see images as distinctly as after prolonged study : we describe and even figure them, and then say : here is what I have seen ; my eyes are as good as those of another ; if any one sees differently from me, it is the microscope that deceives. But this is not so.

The world of the infinitely minute, is a world by itself; most colors have disappeared, perspective is a novelty ; objects seen by transmitted light, seem reduced to but two dimensions, and all elements comprised in their thickness, seem situated on the same place. What habit, what education is required, to bend the sight to these wholly new observations? The infant, although possessed of touch to rectify his errors extends his arms to grasp the moon. Ideas of perspective are only gradually acquired. Such is the case in the first attempts of the student of the microscope. And then, how many precautions are neccessary not to admit into the preparation any foreign element. A filament of any kind, a grain of sand, a bubble of air, have often deceived the tyro.

In the simplest tissues may be found globules of blood, fat and fibres of cellular tissue. It is then a study requiring time under the direction of a master. We should proceed from the simple to the complex, and never venture to give an opinion about a morbid tissue, before we are thoroughly acquainted with normal histology. Ordinarily the reverse is the case.

We make our first essays on diseased tissúes, before having
even read a treatise on general anatomy. Is it any wonder
then that so many reject the micoscrope, disappointed by an
unsuccessful beginning ; that as many others, more culpable
still, refusing to become students again, heap error on error,
contradiction on contradiction.

By a happy initiative, at which the friends of progress should
rejoice, the Faculty have felt that the histological should be
early begun, and carried on simultaneously with other medical
studies. The establishment of a microscopical laboratory
promises splendid results for the future.—[*St. Louis Medical
and Surgical Journal.*

On the Diagnosis of Diseases of the Stomach. By HENRY
KENNEDY, A. B., M. R. I. A., Fellow of the King and Queen's
College of Physicians in Ireland.

There are few medical men who have been engaged in practice, for even a limited period, but must have been struck with
the fact, that the most serious and threatening symptoms of
stomach disease may exist, and be even persistent for a considerable time, and yet in the end the case may turn out to be
one of functional disease merely, and the patient get quite well.
And, on the other hand, a patient may labour under the most
formidable organic disease of this organ, and yet scarcely present a single symtom indicative of its presence. These two propositions it is essentially necessary to keep ever in mind ; and
it may be doubted whether they are yet sufficiently recognised.
Before proceeding farther I shall illustrate them by the following cases, briefly narrated :—

CASE I. Some time back Mr. Cusack exhibited to the Pathological Society a specimen of disease of the stomach of an
extraordinary extent. Literally three-fourths of the organ
were converted into malignant disease. All the coats were
involved, and the mucous membrane presented one sheet of
fungoid disease. But what was extraordinary was, that the
individual from whom it was taken had been able to take his
food, and made no complaint until within a very few days before his death.

CASE II. A medical gentleman, about fifty-five years of
age, had long been what might be described as delicate. He
had been in the army, and on his way home from Jamaica, was
obliged to use, for some weeks, bread of a very inferior quality.
This disagreed with him even more than common, and before
he landed he was suffering daily from dyspepsia of a severe
character. On reaching home the symptoms did not abate,

and shortly afterwards he was invalided. From that period until his death, which took place some months later, he was never free from suffering, referred to the stomach. He was seen by several eminent gentlemen; the symptoms he chiefly laboured under were constant pain, nausea, loss of appetite, and occasional attacks of pyrosis. On one occasion he threw up a considerable quantity of blood; but at the time there were some doubts as to its source. He had some cough, which, with expectoration, increased towards the end; and he finally sank, reduced to the very last degree of marasmus, and never having lost the symptoms referred to above. I assisted Dr. Kirkpatrick to make a *post mortem* examination. On first view the stomach appeared perfectly healthy, and it was only after a very minute inspection that we were able to detect two small ulcers, each about the size of a split pea, existing close to each other, in the great extremity of the organ. The coats, too, of the stomach appeared thinned, having probably partaken of the general marasmus. In the lungs was found some tubercular matter, in large masses, but not occupying any particular site.

CASE III. Mr. ——, a professional gentleman, began to suffer from pain in his stomach, chiefly after his meals, and more frequently after his breakfast than at any other time of the day. He was at this period twenty-six years of age, of tall stature, and had been, though subject to occasional headaches, previously healthy. He had always, however, been inclined to constipated bowels. The attacks, in the first instance, were slight, and were more of the character of painful digestion than anything else; for at a certain period after each meal he felt more or less uneasiness. By degrees, however, they became more severe; and as they did, their character somewhat changed. They were now, in a very marked degree, periodic; that is, the patient would be six weeks, or even longer, free from any suffering, and then an attack would occur very suddenly. On many occasions he went out on his ordinary business in the morning, and would return in an hour or two suffering from the attack. He always referred its commencement to a point opposite the pylorus, from which the pain would spread, but not to any great extent.

I am quite unable to describe these attacks.* They were perfect whirlwinds while they lasted, which they usually did from four to six hours; and the patient's sufferings seemed to be agony itself. He frequently expressed himself as if he should

---

* Any one who will call to mind the story of the " Martyr Philosopher," given with such grapic effect in the " Diary of a Physician," will have a good idea of the patient's sufferings.

die in consequence of them. While the fit was at its height vomiting took place, but never of any large quantity of fluid; and as it passed off, the stomach began to secrete air, which it would then do in enormous quantities, and was always considered by the patient himself as a good sign. It is only necessary to say further of this case that he has been completely free from these fearful attacks for a period of upwards of four years.

Though other cases might easily have been given, these appear to me quite sufficient to show what difficulties surround the question of diagnosis in diseases or affections of the stomach. The well-known fact, too, might be adduced here in further proof of this position :—that the disease known as chronic ulcer of this organ has frequently led to a fatal result from perforation, without any complaint having been previously made by the patient; and their usual condition would seem to bear out this view, for many of these cases present all the signs of the most robust health.* But if we come to inquire why such difficulties exist, the reason appears to me to be in great part explained by the fact, that both the functional and organic affections of this organ give rise to the same series of symptoms; and this will be made evident, if we try to place the signs of organic disease in one column, and those of functional derangement in another; for we shall then find that both lists will contain very nearly, if not exactly, the same series of symptoms. Pain, nausea, vomiting, flatulence, sense of distention, pyrosis, throwing up more fluid than what has been taken, hematemesis of different kinds, and other symptoms, are each and all common to either state. Hence, I repeat it, the difficulties which so frequently arise in arriving at an accurate diagnosis. † But it will be asked here, are there no signs which may be considered as absolutely indicative of organic disease? And this leads me to notice more particularly two symptoms, on which many have placed an entire reliance. I mean the symptom known by the name of the black vomit; and secondly, the presence of a tumor of the stomach itself.

As to the first of these, it appears to me too much stress has been laid on it as diagnostic of organic disease, and, for this simple reason, that it occurs in cases where we have positive evidence there is none. For, what is this black vomit? Nothing, I believe, but an exudation of blood, altered somewhat by the secretions of the mucous membrane of the stomach; and this, I presume, few will assert, can only take place where

---

* An interesting paper by Dr. Lees, on Perforation of the Stomach, will be found in the tenth volume of the New Series of this Journal.
† A similar line of observation has, I find, been pursued in the " Bibliotheque du Médecin-Praticien," edited by Fabre. 1851. Vol. ii. p. 490.

there is ulceration or fungoid disease. Hemorrhage from the stomach we know can occur where there is no morbid change whatever in the mucous membrance, as in some cases of enlarged liver. I have seen instances of this nature, where the first blood thrown up was of a bright red colour; but as the attack passed off, it got gradually darker, and finally put on all the characters of black vomit.* Yet, in these cases, the mucous membrane was found healthy, though congested. But further, many acute diseases exhibit this symptom in a very marked degree, and a most serious symptom it ever is. I have seen it in bad cases of scarlatina, of fever, small-pox, and of puerperal fever; also in a case of ruptured† uterus; and on examination of such cases I have found no organic change in the mucous membrane. The yellow fever, too, of warm climates very generally presents this symptom. Hence, the conclusion appears to me a fair one: that this particular symptom may occur in the more ordinary affections of the stomach, where nothing but functional derangement exists; and before these remarks are concluded, I hope to prove it.

The second symptom I have alluded to, the existence of a tumor, is one of more moment, and it must be allowed that in the great majority of instances it will lead us to a correct diagnosis; yet even this sysmptom, palpable though it be, may deceive us; and I would call particular attention to this fact, for, after having made some research on the matter, I cannot discover that it has been hitherto noticed. The point I would observe upon is this, that a tumour may exist in the stomach, which in the progress of time, may entirely disappear; or, at least, get into a state in which it may not be palpable on external examination. I believe two distinct circumstances may give rise to such a state of things. Before noticing these, however, I would just observe on the much greater facilities which some subjects present for the detection of tumours than others; and it is a point always to be kept in mind. There are, I presume, few who have not met instances where all the symptoms would lead one to look for the presence of a tumor which did in reality exist, but which no external examination could detect. As far as I have seen, this difficulty has been in great measure due to the natural depth of the chest, rather than to any other single cause, such as the thickness of the abdominal parietes, or the site of the tumor. So that it may be safely stated, that the absence

---

* Something very like this may also be seen in cases of hemorrhage from the lungs.

† The occurrence of the black vomit in this case would appear to be important to notice, for it points out a state of the system which cannot be considered healthy, and which may predispose the uterus to an alteration of structure that may lead to its rupture.

of all external sign of a tumour would not justify us in asserting that none existed.

. But, further, there is a state of some of these tumours which
I am not sure has been hitherto noticed, I mean their mobility,
not from external handling, but by the act of respiration. In
a case which I saw, through the kindness of my friend, Surgeon
Neville, of Brunswick-street, it was most remarkable. At
every inspiration the tumour moved fully one inch and a half,
and, what is of more importance, this sign was the means of
settling a question which had previously been raised, namely,
as to whether the tumour was an aneurism or not, for it had a
very strong pulsation.* Whether the mobility was, in this
particular instance, more than ordinary I cannot say, but it is
worthy of remark that the patient was of unusual stature, for,
though he was a tailor, he was six feet four inches in height.
This mobility, then, even granting that it is not always present,
appears to me a symptom which ought to be looked for in this
class of cases.†

It has been already stated that a tumour which has been
palpable to the touch may disappear, and this may, I believe,
occur in either of two ways. In the first the tumour, so far
from enlarging as the disease advances, lessens. This we know
to be common in cases of malignant disease, as in cancer of the
breast when ulceration is going on, and the same may occur
when a similar disease exists in the stomach. This has happened twice under my own observation, and in one instance it
was so marked, that a doubt was thrown on the accuracy of a
previous diagnosis. An examination, however, after death,
solved the difficulty, by disclosing a large ulcerated surface,
with some traces of tumour still remaining. Thus, then, I believe, and it is comparatively well known, our diagnosis may in
one way be rendered obscure. Before describing the second I
shall give some details of the following case :—

CASE IV. Miss ——, about 30 years of age, unmarried,
suffered from a sharp attack of English cholera, in August,
1849. She was of the sanguineous temperament, but of a listless habit of body. The menstrual function was quite healthy.
From the attack of cholera she does not appear to have completely recovered, for shortly afterwards, within a month, she

---

* The *post mortem* examination of this case disclosed a tumour of a malignant character, which formed a complete circle on the mucous membrane of
the stomach, close to the pylorus. It was exhibited at the Surgical Society.

† Through the kindness of Dr. Lees I have very lately seen a case of abscess
of the liver, in which the tumour presented to the right of the epigastrium, and
was very distinctly moved downwards by the act of inspiration, a point of some
importance to determine, as it showed that at the time no adhesions had taken
place. This subject seems worthy of further investigation.

began to throw up a small portion of each day's dinner.   This gradually increased, until, in the course of four months, every thing taken in the way of food came up, though, curiously enough, medicine did not.   With this state of stomach the patient complained of a fixed pain, which she referred exactly to the pylorus, and where, when she was examined in bed, a distinct tumour could be felt.   It was circumscribed, and painful on pressure, and was recognised by Sir H. Marsh, who, at this period, saw the patient with me.   What she threw up at first was merely her food unchanged.   In the course of a month, however, a large quantity of clear fluid, mixed with saliva, came up.   This fluid she described as being salt, bitter, and burning by turns.   Such was what might be called the persistent state of this patient until the latter end of January, and beginning of February,1850; that is, about six months from the time she began to throw up her food.   At this period, attacks of a much more serious character were superadded.   These attacks were wonderfully periodic, taking place regularly each second day, between five and eight o'clock in the evening. They were preceded by shivering, paleness, and great anxiety of countenance; at the same time that the pulse, which commonly beat between 80 and 90, rose to 130, and even 140.   In this state the sense of burning, from which she was never free, became very much aggravated, and she described it as extending from the stomach to the throat; which latter part was constantly excoriated from the nature of the fluids vomited.   With these severer attacks she now also began to throw up a quantity of stuff having the characters of black vomit.   It was of a dark brown colour, and was always attended with a much larger quantity of fluid than what the patient had taken.   On several occasions now, too, what came up was tinged with blood.*   It will be easily understood that from the violence of these attacks and their constant recurrence, the general health must have suffered severely; and such was the fact.   Loss of flesh went on with great rapidity.   She became reduced to a skeleton, being quite unable to leave her bed, and symptoms again and again threatened that her sufferings would be aggravated by stripping.   During the period she was so reduced,

---

* The microscope was not used in this case, there being nothing in what was rejected to lead us to suspect that anything of either an animal or a vegetable organization existed in it.   There can be no doubt, however, that the instrument can afford most valuable assistance in some cases; as proof of which I would refer to a late number of the Medical Times, where a case of great interest is given very fully by Dr. Jenner of London; and also to Dr. Todd's papers in the London Medical Gazette.   Cases also, illustrating its application, have been brought before the Dublin Pathological Society by Drs. M'Dowel and Lyons; but they have not been yet published.

Dr. M'Donnell, whose valuable assistance I then had, felt with me the tumour repeatedly.

It is unnecessary to pursue the history of this case further; it occupied many months more; suffice it to say that the patient has perfectly recovered, *and that now no tumour can be felt.* It must be allowed, however, that at one period of the case the prognosis was gloomy in the extreme.

This case I have given at some length, as it appears to me to be one of considerable interest. The patient certainly presented a series of symptoms from which few have recovered. She had all those which are thought to mark the presence of organic disease, including the black vomiting, the throwing up of much more fluid than she had taken, and the presence of a tumour. Of the exact nature of the case I do not profess to offer anything like a positive opinion. In the first instance it would appear to have been an example of the affection so well described by Sir H. Marsh; while at a later period there were strong grounds for supposing that actual disease had taken place, possibly some form of ulceration. This, however, is only conjecture, though it is borne out by the extreme emaciation which the patient at one period presented. This symptom is, I believe, amongst the most constant of those attendant on organic disease; and yet it does not always exist, as some of the cases of chronic ulcer fully confirm.

But how are we to account for the tumor and its subsequent disappearance? It will be recollected that it was felt by Sir H. Marsh, and repeatedly by Dr. M'Donnell and myself. My conviction is, that at no period of the case did any morbid growth exist but that what was felt due to an irregular action of a portion of the muscular coat of the stomach itself.

Any one in the habit of opening bodies must have been often struck with the varieties which the stomach in its general aspect presents. In one subject it will be very large, and apparently dilated; in another it is found contracted to a remarkable degree, and its coats, to all appearance, thickened; while in a third it presents an example of the hour-glass contraction, described so long since by Sir Everard Home. The other hollow viscera, too, we know, take on at times this irregular action of the muscular coat, as may be seen in parts of the intestines, and still more strikingly, perhaps, in the uterus. In subjects favourable for examination, I have myself felt portions of the intestines, knotted, as it were, so as to afford distinct evidence of irregular action going on; and which has all disappeared with the cause which gave rise to it.

So I take it to have been in the case just given. The irritation, which there can be no doubt of existed in the mucous membrane of the stomach, caused a spasctic state of contraction of a part of the muscular coat, and this, in its turn, caused a thickening, a temporary tumor so to speak, which it was possible to feel through the thin abdominal walls. As the irritation lessened, however, this spastic state gradually subsided; and hence we have an explanation of the disappearance of the tumour, and the recovery of the patient. To suppose that there existed in the stomach a tumor caused by organic disease which subsequently disappeared, would be a straining of experience farther than any case on record would justify.

Much might be said on the treatment of these cases, for it would appear to be anything but yet settled. For the present, however, I must confine myself to one remark. At the period, in the case last given, when there were good grounds for supposing that some ulceration existed, I carried into effect an idea which had been long in my mind, viz: that in such cases we might give medicines for the express purpose of healing the ulcerations, in fact of acting locally on them, as if we had an ulcer on the surface of the body to deal with. With this view creasote was given, to the amount of three drops, three times a day; and, as I believe, with advantage. Nor do I see any reason why other medicines as well might not be administered with this intention, and in cases where it would appear to be too common to consider them as being beyond the resources of our art, as, for instance, the disease known as the chronic ulcer of the stomach. In this disease there is no evidence of anything of a malignant character, and, of course, nothing (amounting, I mean, to an impossibility) to prevent its healing. We know there is proof on record of such an occurrence having taken place; and consequently our efforts should be directed, not merely to pallitate, but to cure, difficult though its attainment may be. But where is there not difficulty in medicine? With this object in view, then, I venture to make this suggestion.

[*Dublin Quarterly Jour. of Med. Science.*

On Chronic Inflammation, and other Morbid states, of the Corpus Cavernosum. By HENRY JAMES JOHNSON, Esq., formerly Lecturer on Anatomy and Physiology, and lately senior Assistant Surgeon to St George's Hospital.

I venture to lay the following cases and observations before the profession, in order to direct attention to a subject which has not hitherto engaged it. I trust that this imperfect notice of what, I should imagine, is a rare affection, may lead to communications of greater value from others.

In a work of mine, which the Lancet recently did me the honour to review, will be found a brief account of "Chronic Inflammation of the Corpus Cavernosum." That account comprised in a solitary case all I had then witnessed. By one of the coincidences which make railway accidents come in a crowd, and cumulate in a week those unfrequent operations at a hospital, which the calculation of chances *should* spread over months, I have seen in the short time which has elapsed since the publication of that work, three distinct instances of the disorder. I shall therefore take the liberty of laying the entire group before your readers, to exhibit at one view their points of similarity and of difference.

CASE I. "A barrister of something more than middle age, had led from early years a dissolute life, and had experienced more attacks of gonorrhœa than he could enumerate or I remember. He managed the majority of these himself, and his principles of treatment were simple. He took capivi till he got well, however long he might be in doing so; and as he did not care to restrict himself in living, he came at last to think that gonorrhœa was almost his normal state, and that it little mattered whether he had it or not. But Nemesis, though lame, still catches her victim, and this gentleman found that the 'gods' do really

"Make scourges of our pleasant vices."

"Some six months before he consulted me, which was in the summer of 1845, he began to experience lancinating pains in the body of the penis, just anterior to the scrotum; the organ was tender on erection, and it gradually assumed a sort of spiral twist, which was neither comfortable nor prepossessing.

"When I saw him, this sort of torsion was considerable, and gave an irresistibly ludicrous appearance to the part, which looked somewhat like the appendix vermiformis, or a pig's curly tail. On examination it was obvious that the cause resided in the corpus cavernosum, the fibrous wall of which was irregularly indurated, while thickening and consolidation invaded the erectile tissue within. The character of the affection more nearly resembled that of the palmar fascia in watermen, than anything with which I can compare it. Erection had become as insupportable as imperfect, and the suffering was positively great.

"I prescribed leeches, blisters, mercurials, tartar-emetic and iodine ointments, fomentations, poultices, cold lotions, even ice, with calomel and opium, salines, iodide of potassium, and sarsaparilla, the liquor potassæ—all the remedies, in short, which would naturally occur to me in the management of such a case.

Their good effects were limited to the removal (and that extremely tardy) of the tenderness and pain.   Beyond that they
had no influence.   The induration remained, the contraction
rather increased, and erection, if no longer attended with actual suffering, was a source of profound discomfort.   In the early
part of 1846, he consulted, I believe, several other hospital
surgeons, and one (he was no anatomist) recommended division of the cavernous body.   It *could* do no good, as it was *not*
attempted.   I have not seen the patient since 1847, and I understand that he remains in nearly the same state as when he
quitted me."

CASE 2..   A respectable tradesman, fifty-one years of age, of
pale complexion, and of nervous temperament, married, but
separated from his wife, had from youth been addicted to
venereal indulgences.   On three or four occasions he had suffered, in early life, from gonorrhea, and he once had syphilis,
eight or ten years ago.

Five or six months prior to my seeing him, he felt, in the
act of connection, an acute pain in the penis.   It was a week
or more before it totally subsided.   Gradually, however, he
became aware that, in erection, the organ was curved upwards,
and that the spot where he had experienced pain was the seat
of distinct uneasiness.   These symptoms increasing, he applied
to me in May of the present year.

· On examination of the penis, I discovered, on its dorsum, immediately anterior to the pubes, a hard nodule, about the size
of a small horse-bean, but not so perfectly defined.   It could
only be distinctly felt on pinching up the corpus cavernosum,
between the finger and the thumb, and I found, or fancied that
the induration was rather in its fibrous envelope than in its
substance.   It was slightly tender when compressed.

The corpus spongiosum was of its usual form and density,
and the course and stream of urine were not the least impeded.

I was disposed to imagine that the case was one of chronic
inflammation, occasioned by the rupture, in coition, of some of
the fibres of the cavernous sheath.   The possibility of such an
accident may be readily admitted, when we reflect on the frequency of partial rupture of the tendo-Achillis, and aponeurotic
fibres of the gastrocnemius.*   But I confess that I was not
without a suspicion that there *might* be incipient scirrhus.

---

* It is generally, I think, supposed that rupture of the tendo-Achillis is a not
uncommon occurrence.   The injury that is looked upon as such is anything
but rare ; but I have never myself seen the whole tendon torn.   When we consider its extreme strength, it is most unlikely that it should be so.   What really
happens in the great majority of instances is this : either some of the outlaying
fibres of the tendon, or some of those of the aponeurotic lamina which dif-
fuses itself over the gastrocnemius, or some of the muscular fibres of the latter,

The patient being then averse to local depletion or blistering, I prescribed the mercurial ointment, with belladonna, which was to be constantly applied.

On the 10th of June he called on me again. The induration was rather less, but the lump was more diffused, and had extended somewhat to the left. He now assented to more active measures, and I gave him Plummer's pill, with opium, at night, and the liquor potassæ, with the iodide of potassium and sarsaparilla, twice daily. At the same time I directed him to blister the penis resolutely.

He had done so thrice when he paid me a visit on the 14th of July. There was little change for the better, in fact, although the hardness had diminished, the superfices of the morbid deposit had increased. There was also a greater degree of tenderness, which he attributed, probably with justice, to the blisters. I requested him to rub in, night and morning, an ointment composed of the iodide of potassium, belladonna and camphor, and not to discontinue the general treatment, which agreed with him particularly well.

On the 18th of August, I saw him for the last time. The induration was still on the decline, and the margin of the swelling was less defined ; but it was more diffused. It was obviously limited to the wall of the cavernous body, which crumbled when pinched, like a piece of parchment. The tenderness had again subsided, and there was little uneasiness in erection, or, indeed, in *coitu*, which, contrary to my express injunctions, he now confessed he had indulged in. The penis, however, on those occasions was twisted to the left side, an alteration due to the extenison of the thickening in that direction.

I advised his taking the mercurial pill every second instead of every night, and in other respects I left the treatment as it was. I have already stated that he has not subsequently called upon me.

CASE 3. A gentleman residing in one of the Channel Islands, between forty and fifty years of age, of florid complexion, and of healthy constitution, consulted me last June, under the following circumstances :—

---

give wav in a sudden effort. Perrot, the celebrated ballet-dancer, was said to have met with this accident. He was forced to retire altogether for a year or two; and, when he returned for a while to the stage, he was compelled to confine himself to pantomime. Now, it so happened that I was called to Perrot, and the tendo-Achillis was *not* ruptured; a few of its fibres had snapped, and that was all. I may take this opportunity of making one other observation. Almost all the cases of this description which have occurred to me were in persons of a gouty habit. The fact is not unattended with interest, and I should be glad to learn if my experience is confirmed by that of others. If it be so, I conceive that the physiological explanation is not difficult, and that some practical conclusions might be drawn from it.

Though long married, he had "intrigued freely," till within the last few months, when he found that, in erection, the penis was curved upwards, and that to a painful extent. The uneasiness, in the act, was seated in front of the pubes, where a spot was tender upon pressure. He applied to a medical friend in the island, who told him that he often saw cases of that sort, and prescribed severe counter-irritation. This was of some service to him, but, coming to London to witness the Exhibition, he had been recommended to me.

On examining the penis, I found, half an inch anterior to the pubes, a perfectly defined and regular induration, situated in the median line, upon its dorsum. It was scarcely so large as a small horse-bean, flat, imperceptible to the naked eye, and distinguishable only on pinching up the corpus cavernosum between the finger and the thumb. It was evidently seated in the wall of the cavernous body, and did not extend into its interior. It was tender on firm pressure, and the seat of discomfort in erection, when the curvature of the penis was so pronounced as to have compelled him to abandon all connubial intercourse.

I prescribed, during his stay in London, when sight-seeing rendered counter-irritation inadmissible, the application of the iodide of potassium in the form of ointment, and its internal use in combination with sarsaparilla and with the liquor potassæ. I also recommended him, on his return home, to pursue an active course of blisters. I have not heard of him since.

CASE 4. A country gentleman, between fifty and sixty years of age, florid, stout, and healthy-looking, had always been addicted to the gratification of his passions. In early life he had attacks of gonorrhœa, but none for many years. Some eighteen months, or thereabouts, before his visit to me, he had felt, in connexion, a sudden though not a violent pain in the penis, immediatly contiguous to the pubes. For some time aftewards, he experienced in erection a sense of inconvénience, which gradually passed away. Eight or nine months ago, he began to observe that the organ, when distended, became curved towards the abdomen, and that sexual intercourse grew difficult on that account. He applied to an eminent physician in his neighborhood, who assured him that it was a matter of no importance, and that he had had the same thing himself! What he prescribed (it was *not* counter-irritation) was unproductive of benefit, and, matters growing worse instead of better, he came to town for advice. He went to an eminent hospital-surgeon, who introduced a bougie, and seemed to regard the case as one of stricture. As the patient found no impediment to the free passage of his urine, this opinion was unsatisfactory, the more so as the instrument rather increased the irritation. On the 23rd of July he consulted me.

I found on the dorsum of the penis, near the pubes, inclining rather to the right side, but spreading over the centre, a flattish, ovoid, defined, but not absolutely regular induration, three lines and a half in its long diameter, and two and a half in its short, the former being from side to side, the latter from before backwards. Its characters were best appreciated by pinching up the corpus cavernosum, in the parietal lamina of which it was seated, immediately beneath the skin. This was unadherent and unaffected; but the hardness (I imagined) extended slightly into the substance of the cavernous body. There was trifling tenderness on pressure, still more in erection, and, in that condition, the incurvation of the organ towards the pubes rendered sexual intercourse extremely irksome, if not actually impossible.

I prescribed the same remedies as in the previous cases, and I have not seen nor heard of the patient since.

The following appear to me the most obvious inferences which the facts warrant us in drawing.

1. A regret that the facts themselves are so imperfect. With the exception of the first, a sufficient length of time has not elapsed to decide the issue, or admit of a positive conclusion. I should be equally condemned by logic and experience, if, under such circumstances, I dared to dogmatize. But I write with the hope of obtaining information, not with the pretence of giving it. That is my apology.

2. One feature is common to all the cases; the subjects were immoderately given to venery. Whoever abuses the functions of an organ, accepts a blank bill upon the future. It may run for a longer or a shorter date, but it *must* come due. • That the sheath of the cavernous body should suffer from excesses of this description is easy enough of comprehension; submitted to sudden and violent distention, the web of which it is composed may very readily be damaged. The chronic inflammation of the palmar fascia, which occurs in watermen and smiths, is a strictly analogous instance, the organic tissue being the same, and the cause of mischief not dissimilar. The respective ages of all the patients were very nearly alike. Each had attained, and one had passed, the middle period of life, when the vital and elastic powers of the organs are declining, and the fibrous membranes exhibit a proneness to disease.

3. In the second and the fourth case, a sudden pain was experienced in connexion, where the induration subsequently formed. It is natural to imagine that this was due to a laceration of some fibres. The correspondence of the phenomena with those exhibited in partial rupture of the tendo-Achillis requires no further demonstration.

4. In the first case only, was there any ground for attribu-

ting the affection to gonorrhœa. I should, *a priori*, anticipate that. The uretha is tunnelled in the spongy body, with which the cavernous is in little more than contact. Gonorrhœal inflammation, when so intense or so erratic as to travel beyond the mucous membrane, would naturally invade the contiguous structure, the erectile tissue of the corpus spongiosum. Such we find to be the fact. Acute and chronic inflammation of *it*, is a common consequence of gonorrhœa.

In the case where the exception to this general rule occurred, the circumstances were themselves exceptional. Debauchery was carried to its extremest limit, and the indulgence of the passions was crowned by the abuses of the most empirical treatment; and perhaps it will not escape observation, that, as the causes were in a great measure peculiar, the result was also different. In the place of a small circumscribed deposit in the fibrous envelope of the cavernous body, a more extensive and more serious alteration implicated its interior.

5. I conceive that this is a rare affection, partly because I have seen it rarely, but principally because I know of no description of it. I imagine, too, that the profession is, in general, imperfectly acquainted with it. For, in my first case, an hospital surgeon proposed to divide the wall of the cavernous body; in the third, the medical attendant protested that he witnessed the disorder frequently; and in the fourth, a physician pooh-pooh'd the thing, *because* he had had it himself: while a London surgeon looked on it as stricture, and treated it with the bougie.

6. To whoever saw, and to some, perhaps, who may read these cases, a suspicion of schirrhus might occur. A candid review of all the circumstances tends, I think, to dispel it; but it would require more time than has elapsed, and indeed more confidence than I possess, to decide, *ex cathedrà*, against the *possibility* of malignant action.

7. The principles of treatment are unhappily more simple than their application is successful. The removal of inflammatory action would be sought, of course, in local depletion and active counter-irritation, while absorption of the lymph would be promoted by the application of iodine or mercury, and by their internal use. The success which may reasonably be expected from such measures would not appear to be extraordinary, although I may observe that the nature of the tissue, as well as the functions of the organ, must naturally discourage the idea of speedy benefit. Few complaints, I imagine, demand more persistence on the surgeon's part, or more steady resolution on the patient's.

In a future and not remote contribution, I shall advert to some other morbid states of the cavernous body, more or less allied to the preceding.—[*London Lancet.*

On the premonitory signs of severe Cerebral Disease and
their importance. By Dr. Devay.

[We have considerably curtailed this valuable essay, but
have endeavored to omit nothing of real utility. The author
introduces the subject by remarking on the extreme difficulty
in arriving at an accurate diagnosis in cerebral affections, the
symptoms being induced by lesions of various kinds—the same
difficulty exists in the interpretation of the premonitory symptoms, which are, nevertheless, excellently demonstrated in the
following observations:]

I. *Premonitory signs, furnished by the intellectual and moral
faculties.*—Almost all authors of repute have mentioned, without always attaching much importance to them, the disturbances
of intellect which precede attacks of severe cerebral disease.
Insanity has its period of incubation, its premonitory symptoms;
and frequently it is found that the first act of insanity, which
caused alarm, has been preceded by several symptoms which
had escaped observation, and sometimes the first phenomenon
of the disease has been taken for its cause. The insane often
combat their false ideas, before the disorder of their reason, and
the internal contest which precedes the explosion of their mad-
ness, are perceived. The most general precursor of every severe affection of the brain is a state of *cerebral lassitude,* presenting much analogy to that state of intellectual torpor which
follows severe or pestilential fevers. There is observed in the
habitual gesture of the patients, in their attitudes and movements
a total absence of what may be called the consciousness of action. The brain seems to have lost its *balancing* power over
the *ensemble* of the functions of the life of relation. These patients are often in a constant state of slight habitual vertigo,
which they call *weakness of the head,* and which is frequently
accompanied by debility in the limbs.

The *memory* is frequently impaired in the precursory period
of cerebral affections. Thus, patients have forgotten the names
of their friends, or of the most common things. In conversation
they have difficulty in finding proper words to express their
meaning, and are obliged to make us of circumlocutions. More
rarely, the memory becomes more powerful; it seems to take
a new flight, and reproduces, to the great astonishment of the
patient and his attendants, events which had seemed to be entirely forgotten. The curious and inexplicable fact of *reminis-
cence* corresponds to the exaltation of the special sensibility of
certain senses. It is sometimes observed after a slight attack
of apoplexy.

Next to the impairment of the memory, and also of the atten-

tion, which is fixed with difficulty, or not at all, on objects presented to the notice of the individual, the most striking change
is in *volition*, which is diminished. The man who has hitherto
been most firm, who has shown most tenacity in his views, who
has pursued the plan of his life with great determination, becomes, in a measure, like the toy of a child; those who are
about him, even his inferiors, can command him. Human de-
pravity has often taken advantage of this moral decadence for
culpable ends; and the man who has hitherto most rigorously
and carefully managed his affairs, is all at once spoiled of his
goods, either by extorted donations, or by burdensome expenses. The public see in these cases *bizarreries* of cháracter;
the physiologist and the physician see in them the first expression of a pathological condition. This weakening of the will,
which, according to our observations, is chiefly connected with
those cerebral lesions which lead to lunacy, or to paralysis of
the insane, necessitates an alteration of the judgment. . . .
This will is the result of the other faculties; and it is not because it is wanting in the idiot, or lunatic, that they are irres-
ponsible; but rather because they are ignorant of the rules
which should direct it.

There is but a slight transition from this to *perversion of the
moral faculties*—one of the most mysterious points in psycho-
logy.

The abrupt changes which may occur in a man's tastes, in
his inclination, in his manner of living, in a word, in his social
aspect, are worthy of attention. Modifications of this nature,
when they do appear in a slow and progressive manner, do not
arise from the action of moral influences, and can only arise
from a change in the nervous system. Thus it has long been
remarked, that unusual gaiety in a habitually grave individual
may denote the approach of an attack of apoplexy. It is the
same with those who suddenly seek for noise and bustle, after
having loved retirement and quietness for a great part of their
life. We have known a man, aged 57, who, having up to that
led a grave and even austere life, gave himself up to the pursuit
of amusements unsuited to his age, and was a few months after
seized with sudden and complete apoplexy (*apoplexie foudroy-
ante.*) A complete change in the turn of the ideas, when it is
not the result of advanced age, when it manifests itself in a
short period of time, and when it cannot be traced to the action
of moral influences is very suspicious. We have known a young
physician who exhibited this phenomenon in a very marked
manner, and who a short time after, was seized with paralysis
of the insane. When we knew him three years before, he was
very free in his assertions, and inclined to exaggerate; but he

had become discreet, and wary in his speech.   His former condition, and the medium in which he had lived, showed sufficiently that this change could not be the effect of *progressive amendment;* we considered that there was some disease, and our
opinion was ultimately confirmed.

It is conceivable, that the same psychological perturbation
which changes the moral sentiments may likewise impair the
sentiment of self-preservation ; and hence that *suicidal melancholy* may mark the commencement of a severe affection of
the brain.   The disease is, moreover, very-often conjoined
with a lesion of the intellectual and affective faculties.

II. *Premonitory Signs furnished by the Sensorial Functions.*—Most of these are furnished by the sense of *vision.*   We
will merely mention dimness, the appearance of objects as if
coloured red, photophobia, &c., which may indicate threatening meningitis, as well as cerebral hyperæmia ; these symptoms bear an especial relation to acute diseases of the encephalon.   These signs may exist several years before the explosion
of the disease.   Before attacks of apoplexy, impairment of vision sometimes exist in a high degree without being known to the
patients, especially when, as is most commonly the case, it is not
sufficient to prevent them from seeing those who are about them.
The mistake is the more easy, as this symptom may be limited
to one eye ; the other compensating for the weakness of its
fellow.   Amblyopia is a frequent symptom ; sometimes there
is a complete blindness, as in the case of the Baron Hornestein,
cited by Wepfer (*Anatomia Apoplecticorum,*) who became
blind three weeks before a fatal attack of apoplexy.

A valuable sign, belonging in some degree to what may be
called the expression of the eyes, consists in a want of parallel-
ism in these organs ; it is not squinting. nor is it the look of
hallucination.   It seems pretty well defined by the following
expression : *The eyes are not in the axis of the reason.*   There
may be certain defects in this relation pointed out between a
material object and a moral fact ; but those persons who are
accustomed to scrutinize the human look, and to see reflected
in it the different passions will easily understand me.

The phenomenon of exaltation of special sensibility, as a
precursory sign of a severe encephalic lesion, is sometimes met
with.   It is in this case, as in other circumstances in which it
is observed, one of the most mysterious problems for the physiologist.   It is well known that hearing often becomes excessively acute before attacks of apoplexy.   The patients, incom-
moded by the least noise, become irascible ; they perceive
distant sounds which are unheard by those who are with them.
The fineness of hearing must be distinguished from the percep-

tion of strange and imaginary sounds, which is nothing but a sensorial hallucination.

The sense of *hearing* may present the same modifications as that of vision. Some persons are tormented with drumming in the ear, with continued or intermittent tinkling. Some believe that they hear the most strange noises. These hallucinations are by no means the constant precursors of an encephalic attack; they may be connected with simple perversions of the sensorial function.

Premonitory Signs furnished by the Organs of Motion and Sensation.—The alterations of the *muscular functions* present great variety, from the simple hesitation which we have already noticed, to paralysis which is complete, but which, on account of its nature and its seat we shall denominate *irregular paralysis.* It is not uncommon to observe a state of general languor which makes the patients seek for rest—for the *far niente.* Van Swieten has remarked, in treating of apoplexy: *Primo oritur languor et amor quietis et otii.* At other times those who are about to be attacked with cerebral disease are much agitated, and expend a great amount of activity in their movements. Dr. Tessier has lately attended a lady, aged 60, who from the critical age, has been subject to attacks every month, at the period when she used to menstruate. She loses consciousness; and after having recovered her senses, is paralysed on one side of the body, with great embarrassment of speech. These symptoms continue some days, and gradually leave her to return at the fixed period. But some days before the new attack, this lady, though usually quiet and peaceable, exhibits much agitation; she cannot remain in her place, and those who are about her always know what this sign means. In this case we recognize an example of *periodic nervous apoplexy.*

Impairment of muscular motion is exhibited in various degrees. It is especially remarked in the lower limbs, which seem to bend under the weight of the body, and render the gait rather unsteady. The debility is the more striking if the person be young, and has no apparent cause for it. Portal was able to prognosticate an attack of apoplexy in a gentleman apparently in perfect health, from observing a slight fixedness in the left eye, and a slight weakness in the leg of the same side. *The dignitus semi-mortuus,* noticed by Dr. Marshall Hall, is one of those instances of *irregular paralysis,* of which it is so important to determine the true signification. Some time ago, we saw the following case:—A man, aged 54, one day called on us. In conversation, he jokingly noticed a sort of deadness which he felt in the little finger of the left hand, while the rest of the hand was able to perform its ordinary functions. We advised him to put himself under treatment : he neglected this advice, and some days after was seized with cerebral conges- tion, which left his faculties remarkably weakened.   The *digi- tus semi-mortuus* has shortly since been noticed in a valuable communication from Dr. Gillet de Grandmont. .

Irregular paralyses, which seem to arise from exhaustion of the sources of the sensitive and motive powers, may appear under circumstances in which they do not constitute a symp- tom of such great importance.   Such are those which some- times follow hysterical convulsions, lead-colic, venereal abuses, &c.   Here, these phenomena are connected with *transient* mo- difications of innervation.   The suddenness of the attacks, their frequent isolation from other symptoms, their seat in parts dis- tant from each other, while those lying between preserve the integrity of their movements, constitute the exceptional charac- ters of those palsies which are connected with a latent alteration in the nervous centres.   We must not lose sight of the difficul- ty of deglutition which some patients experience some time before being attacked ; as well as the semi-paralysis of the vo- cal cords and tongue, giving rise to stammering or aphonia. The paralysis of the upper eyelids, which become œdematous, is also a sign of great value

General sensibility may be abolished, simply diminished or exaggerated.   The first two forms almost always follow mus- cular paralysis ; but they may exist alone.   Sensibility may be exaggerated in two forms.   The patients may present hyper- æsthesia, or exquisite sensibility of the whole cutaneous surface ; so that the least touch troubles them.   This is an increased anormal sensibility—an exaggeration of the sense of touch, cor- responding the exaltation of the sensorial faculties which we have already studied   Sensibility may also be exalted in the form of pain ; and this merits our most careful attention.   Vio- lent pains, precursory of a severe cerebral lesion, have often been mistaken for neuralgia.   The same is the case in treating cephalagia, supposed to be dependent on dyspepsia : and this error is more readily fallen into, as the stomach is often disor- dered.   The diagnosis in these cases is sometimes difficult ; but the duration and violence of the pain will lead to the sus- picion, that there is something more than ordinary headache ; and that, although the functions of the stomach are troubled at the same time, the headache is often too intense to be accounted for by the state of that organ.   The patient cannot in general endure a warm room, nor the noise made by persons about him, nor even the fatigue of agreable conversation, without suffering an aggravation of his headache.   The paroxysms are sometimes accompanied with vomiting, and sometimes with violent beating in the head. If with these symptoms we remark paleness of face, and weakness of pulse, and if active measures have been employed without benefit, we are led to suspect the presence of organic lesion.* Painful cramps are not unfrequent. Portal has seen patients who suffered severely from cramps in the legs before an attack of apoplexy.

Cutaneous sensibility presents other singular modes of perversion. A case is related of a man who, several months before being attacked with apoplexy, experienced from time to time an absolute loss of sensibility on five or six isolated points of the skin of the thorax, each of about the size of a five-franc piece. Here the skin might be pinched without causing any pain ; beyond, the sensibility was perfect. The partial abolitions of sensation were not constant. On some days there was not the least diminution of sensibility ; then suddenly, and simultaneously, it was annihilated in the isolated portions. Such unusual modifications of functions directly dependent on the brain, ought to furnish us with arguments in favor of the possibility of moral and instinctive perversions, and of their dependence, not on the corruption of the moral faculty itself, but on a latent pathological condition of the organ. Hence arises the doctrine of irresponsibility.

It is in the life of relation that indicatory signs are especially to be looked for. At the initial period of severe cerebral disease, organic life reveals few or no disturbances. The symptoms which may exist under this head only acquire value in connexion with those which are derived from the life of relation. The brain must be much affected to produce changes in the nutritive function. Excepting sleep, which is one of the confines of animal and organic life, there is not in the latter any essential functional disturbance. In the initial period, most patients have lost the power of sleep ; or, if this function be performed, it is rather a fatiguing drowsiness than refreshing sleep. The digestive functions present no other special disorder than obstinate constipation, which is often difficult to be overcome by drastics. The eyelids sometimes becomes œdematous ; and, in some subjects, attacks are preceded by small effusions of blood, even in the tissue of the conjunctiva. The secretions are but little altered. The urine is sometimes highly albuminous ; but this is a subject for further researches.

[*Ranking's Abstract.*

---

* Abercrombie. Diseases of the Brain, p. 453.

Pathological Relaxation of the Symphyses of the Pelvis, and its treatment. By M. Ferdinand Martin.—(Translated for this Journal.)

After parturition, there sometimes exists a relaxation of the various symphyses of the pelvis; this is ordinarily produced by the patient leaving her bed too soon. As it is accompanied by various and grave sympathetic phenomena, as also by other co-existent lesions, it is not surprising that it is frequently, even by the most experienced physicians, sometimes mistaken for a uterine engorgement, and sometimes for a retroversion of the organ.

In women effected with relaxation of the symphysis pubis, the erect posture is particularly difficult, sometimes even impossible. The patients then feel an acute pain in the sacral region, with a numbness in the whole extent of the abdominal members. Generally, after making ten or a dozen steps, they are obliged to sit down. It frequently happens that the motion at the symphysis pubis, caused by walking, produces a tension of the tissues surrounding the urethra, and provokes a pressing and painful desire to urinate.

The diagnosis is rendered more certain by the following examination :—If the physician holding the iliac crests makes the patient walk a few steps, he perceives that the os innominatum upon which a small portion of the weight of the body rests, rises very sensibly, whilst the other bone sinks notably. Further, if by the aid of both hands it be attempted to produce movements in an inverse direction to the iliac bones, it is plainly perceived that there is a great want of the normal solidity of the symphysis.

Finally, if it is ascertained that the impediment to standing or walking began during the latter stages of pregnancy, there can be no doubt but that it is a permanent relaxation of the symphysis pubis, and the efficacy of appropriate treatment renders the diagnosis certain.

M. Martin has always observed that the retention of the iliac bones against the sacrum restored to the patient, in a very short time, almost the entire freedom of motion. The apparatus which he always used with success, consists of a large belt of steel, padded on the inside, embracing the entire pelvis, passing over the external iliac fossa in the space between the great trocanter and the crest of the ilium. The belt should be tightly drawn. With this apparatus, a lady who could not go up twenty steps without stopping two or three times, was enabled, after wearing it two days, to walk about a large garden alone. This, however, is not always the case. One of M. Martin's patients could walk with the aid of the belt, but as soon as she would lay it aside progression become very fatiguing. M. Martin was of opinion that another pregnancy would produce a permanent cure, providing the patient wore the belt during the time and kept her bed for at least two months after confinement, without leaving off the apparatus. This plan succeeded, and two years after M. Martin saw his patient, when the longest walk could be taken with ease.

It is proper to state that, the disease here described is not always so grave as in the cases cited by M. Martin. He chose the worst, to show in a clearer light the character of the infirmity to which he has called the attention of his colleagues.
[*Journ. des Con., Medico-Chirurg.*

Experiments with the Ligature on Animals.

DOCTOR HESTER:

Dear Sir—At your requests, I give you a succinct description of experiments made by me on living animals. The following is a faithful and correct account of said experiments, with their bearings on the actual state of Physiology and Pathology, etc.

Some years ago (I was then a student in the Charity Hospital of New Orleans) I noticed repeatedly, that patients dying in the very last stage of Phthisis Pulmonalis, offered at post mortem examination, strong thick cords crossing the cavernous hollows made by the progress of the disease. Upon close examination, I found that these cords were the pulmonary arteries obliterated in that part of the lungs. Such a pathological fact suggested the idea of applying this natural process of obliteration of the arteries in the cure of aneurisms. During my stay in Mexico, I have been able to make experiments on living animals, and such experiments have confirmed the views I entertained on the subject.

On three living sheep, I took up one after the other the following arteries: The two carotids, and the two femoral.

After the first week, I noticed in all three an accelerated process of cicatrization, without any apparent suppuration, although the wounds had not been united by sutures, or any other means. At that time (8th day) I dissected in one the part where the ligature had been applied. Here I must say, that instead of using the ordinary silk ligatures employed in the operation of aneurism, and instead of tying the arteries (as is usually done in the operation of aneurism) tight enough to cut their inner coats, I used the common tape, and pushed it loosely round the artery, as is done in the case of a seton.

After a minute dissection, I noticed there was no perceptible pulsation at the distal side of the artery. I withdrew the ligature quite easily, as it did not press strongly on the artery. I could not perceive as yet any circulation in the above mentioned portion of the artery. I then cut the artery across, and observed that it was completely blocked up by a thick coagulated blood (the clot observed after tying an artery in the usual way.) Withdrawing the clot, a jet of genuine arterial blood came out.

The week after, (16th day) I dissected the neck and leg of the second sheep, and found that the wound was completely cicatrized. There was, as in the first case, no perceptible circulation in the artery below the seat of the ligature. Withdrawing the ligatures, there was no pulsation; cutting the artery, no blood came out; the clot was firmer, and adhered to the walls of the artery. I detached the clot with a little more difficulty than in the first sheep, and arterial blood came out.

In the third sheep, (on the 22d day) the clot was more strongly attached to the walls of the artery, and more firm, than in the two first instances.

In none of these three sheep could I notice any suppuration.

Thinking that some inflammation and suppuration would hasten the obliteration of the arteries, and render it more perfect, I performed successively the very same operation on two more sheep, three dogs and one calf. Instead of using simply the tape line, as I had done in the first cases, I applied to it some strong precipitate ointment, and took a great deal of care in bringing daily a fresh portion of the tape line in contact with the artery, and the parts surrounding it: It was with difficulty that I produced inflammation and a little suppuration in the sheep, but readily produced it in two dogs and in the calf.

After the 17th day, the obliteration of the arteries was perfect in all the sheep, the dogs, and in the calf.

Now, what is the bearing of these experiments in the operation for aneurism—especially in the large arteries? Evidently, if performed on the human being, as I performed it on the living animals, there is not the slightest risk of secondary hæmorrhage; which, consequently, adds considerably to the chances of success, considering that in man inflammation and suppuration is more easily produced than in animals; such inflammation would, at the same time, be propagated to the different coats of the arteries, and, consequently, promote much quicker the obliteration of the arteries.

Yours, respectfully,   J. Piernas, M. D.
San Luis Potosi, Mexico, 1851.

[*New Orleans Med. and Surg. Journ.*

On Scutellaria Lateriflora.

To the Editor of the American Journal of Pharmacy.

Respected Friend,—The article in the last No. of the Journal, page 370, by C. H. Cleaveland, M. D., on Scutellaria lateriflora, calls to mind some of my experience, coinciding with his, which I offer in hopes it may prove a benefit to some of the afflicted ; and because a remedy which is not much known, or has but little reputation, requires testimony in its favor to call it into notice.

About twenty-five years ago my wife had quite a severe attack of tic doloureux on one side of her face, and as the scullcap had been a good deal spoken of as a remedy for hydrophobia, I determined to try it in this case, supposing its influence to be exerted on the nervous system. By the use of two or three pints of infusion, made with an ounce of the herb to a pint of boiling water and taken in doses of a wine-glass full three or four times a day, the disease appeared to be entirely relieved : in the course of a week or ten days, however, it returned, when the scullcap infusion was again resorted to, and continued several weeks, after which there was no return of the disease on that side. A few years after this period my patient was attacked on the other side of her face, but the diligent use of the scutellaria, as before, soon relieved her, and she has, ever since, remained free from that painful disease.

I have advised this remedy in other cases of tic doloureux, and it has had equal success in some, while in others it has failed. I have also given it in cases of tremor, from the abuse of alcoholic drink, with happy effect, and in one case of great depression of spirits produced by dyspepsia. As to the after effect of this nervine, my observation corresponds with that of Dr. Cleaveland.   Respectfully,

WM. STABLER.

Alexandria, Virgina., 10*th mo.* 18*th,* 1851.

Fracture of the Acromion.

All physicians are aware of the difficulty of making a prompt and correct diagnosis of many injuries of the shoulder, and of the unmanageable character of fractures of the acromion, and of fractures and dislocations of the clavicle. In previous numbers of the Transylvania Journal, I have spoken of the plan adopted by Prof. B. W. Dudley in the management of fractures and dislocations of the clavicle. I now propose to explain his views in relation to other injuries of the upper extremity, and I shall dwell more particularly on those, concerning which there is an acknowledged imperfection in surgery.

Fracture of the *acromion process* is more common than a similar injury of any other portion of the scapula. It is caused by a blow on the point of the shoulder, and may be recognized by the flattening of the deltoid outline, and by observing that the broken fragment of bone returns to its position when the arm is extended at right angles with the body. By pressure, exercised along the spine of the scapula towards the acromial extremity with the arm extended, a crepitus may generally be produced. When the arm hangs by the side, more or less pain is produced by the dragging of the central fibres of the deltoid muscle upon the fractured process. Extension of the arm, by relaxing the deltoid and permitting the broken fragment to retreat into the proper position, affords relief, and restores the natural relations of the acromion. The treatment would seem to suggest itself, after a knowledge of these facts in the history of the injury. The complete relaxation of the deltoid muscle is the only means of securing the coaptation of the fractured process, and it is perfectly evident, that the dressings recommended by surgical authors do not tend to produce such relaxation. Dessault's bandage is worse than useless; Sir Astley Cooper admits that his method will not procure ossific union, and John Bell is strangely in error when he directed the arm to be bound to the body and pressed upwards so as to render the shoulder more prominent. The effect of this treatment may be readily inferred from the fact that the shoulder is thereby rendered more prominent. The pressure of the head of the os-humeri upon the central portions of the deltoid muscle can have no other effect than to draw the fractured acromion farther out of its place, and thus defeats the prime object of treatment.

If the fracture results in ligamentous union, a long time is required for the restoration of the perfect functions of the arm. In one case that I had an opportunity of observing, the patient could, with considerable difficulty, raise his arm at right angles with the body after the expiration of 12 months; and it was not until long after that period that the perfect and ready use of the member, in those movements requiring the extending power of the deltoid muscle, was recovered.

If that gentleman had submitted to a confinement of three weeks duration, upon his couch, with the arm extended so as to relax the only muscle that tends to displace the broken bone, he would have arisen with a perfect limb.

It is necessary to secure the arm in the extended position in order to maintain the advantage while the patient sleeps. To depress the limb at any time prior to tolerably firm provisional union, is a backward movement to the starting point. By this simple resource, a fractured acromion may be perfectly cured, and with no sacrifice on the part of the patient, except a confinement of 15 or 20 days. At the expiration of two weeks, if the extended position has been carefully maintained up to that time, the provisional callus will be strong enough to admit of the cautious depression of the limb ; but it would be unsafe to use the limb before the expiration of the fourth week subsequent to the fracture. This treatment is founded upon the mechanical impossibility of adapting any contrivance which will keep the fractured bone in position—exclusive of the extension of the arm—and upon the demonstrable proposition that by removing the traction exercised upon the acromion by the central fibres of the deltoid muscle, the broken fragment will be drawn back into proper position by the trapezius muscle and the coraco-acromial ligament.

Fracture of the coracoid process, requires no other treatment than the application of an ordinary sling, which will sustain the arm drawn forwards into an easy position in front of the chest. This position relaxes the coraco-brachialis, biceps, and pectoralis minor muscles, and permits the fractured process to retreat into its proper position.

It is remarkable that Mr. Skey barely mentions fracture of the acromion in his Operative Surgery, and says not a word in relation to the treatment. The subject of Fractures and Dislocations does not enter, at all, into Malgaigne's treaties on Operative Surgery. These are sad defects. There is no subject of more interest to practitioners generally, and in relation to which plain and simple directions would be of more service. Fractures and dislocations are presented in the every day practice of physicians while capital operations are rare.

[*Transylvania Medical Journal.*

Hints on Cancerous Affections. By Professor W. STONE.

In the October number of the "Register," I called the attention of the profession to the use of the phosphate of lime and nitrogenous diet in depraved states of the system in scrofulous diatheses. Now, as it is believed that true cancer never occurred in decidedly scrofulous subjects, it is fair to infer that an opposite course of diet is more appropriate ; and it is very probable that by directing our attention to the subject, we may be able to fix upon some agent that will aid in arresting the progress of this dreaded disease. Experience has shown that the least nitrogenous diet is best in this disease. In the memoirs of the celebrated Nathan Smith, written some twenty years ago by his son Nathan R. Smith, of Baltimore, are found the views of this remarkable man, which were based purely upon observation, without a chemical idea to theorise upon. His diet for this disease was vegetable; and of this he thought green corn the best. A case is related of a lady on whom he operated for a very large cancerous breast, involving the glands of the axilla. It was in the season for green corn, and the patient was put upon this article of diet. Sufficient was gathered when in the milk, and dried, to last until the season returned, and this made soft by boiling, and used with little or no seasoning. He states that whenever she attempted to return to her usual diet, she experienced shooting pains in the part, but finally, after two years, she gradually changed her diet. The notice of this case was given seven years after the operation, and there was no appearance of a return of the disease. Corn in this State contains, I believe, more phosphorus than any other vegetable, but whether this renders it more suitable to this disease, I am not prepared to say. Professor Bigelow, of Boston, relates a case in which diet kept a cancerous affection dormant, at least, for many years, or rather he states that it was gradually getting well. This was the case of the late distinguished surgeon Amos Twitchell, of Keene, N. H., with whom I was well acquainted. I dined with him in 1848; he furnished a good dinner for his guests, but dined himself on milk and berries. Vegetables of the blandest kind constituted his main food, but I do not think he confined himself to any one article. The disease was seated in the inner canthus of one of his eyes, was removed many years ago with the knife, but the cicatrix soon took on the same degeneration, and he relied upon diet; and although it might appear to a gourmand a very meagre diet, he was able to undergo more fatigue at the age of 64 than many young men. I mention these cases not as being remarkable in themselves, but because they illustrate the effects of diet, and at the same time cover the views of two medical men, remarkable for their powers of observation.

As a remedy to be given in aid of diet, I think arsenic, with our present knowledge, is the best. There was an able article in the London Lancet, I think in the fall of 1849, on the use of arsenic in lupus and canceroid diseases, which was interesting because it showed how it should be given to be useful. The preparation used was Fowler's solution, in doses of from two to five drops, and continued for a long time. The writer also called attention to the fact that instead of increasing the dose after long use, it should be diminished. I have always contended that alteratives, to be useful, should be given in such doses as will not disturb the natural functions. The solution is advised in such doses as will permit its use for an indefinite length of time, without producing any manifest specific effects. I have great confidence that this, together with diet, will exercise a very salutary influence over this dreaded disease.

                         [*New Orleans Med. Register.*

Dislocation of the Femur downwards, reduced after two months. By Professor W. STONE.

Mr. B., a very athletic man, was received into my Infirmary August 21st. He stated, that on the 22d of June, in Western Texas, while taking shelter from a storm, the house was blown upon him causing him serious injury, which confined him over a month, when he was able to move, by the aid of crutches, and finally made his way to my Infirmary. The thigh was greatly abducted, slightly flexed, and lengthened to an unusual degree ; apparently four or five inches, and it gave great pain to move it to any extent. The reduction was effected by making exten- sion and counter extension, in the usual way, to dislodge the head of the bone. The patient was placed upon his back, and the extension made in the direction in which the limb was found. When it was deemed that sufficient extension had been made, lateral force was applied to the upper part of the thigh, by means of a sheet, of which I took one end, and two strong men the other. The body was carried laterally, the knee being fixed by the extending band. until the limb was on a line with the body, or perhaps a little adducted, when I put my foot against the crest of the ilium and gave one strong pull, nearly to my full strength, when it yielded with a sound as if lacerating a firm tissue. The limb could be adducted and moved in any direction, but as soon as the effect of chloroform subsided, there commenced more pain on the inside of the thigh, and in the course of the obturator nerve than in the joint, which lasted several days. After the patient was put in bed, the limb appeared, in some positions of the body, to be an inch or more longer than the other ; indeed about as much lengthened as is usual in dislo- cation into the thyroid hole. As soon, however, as the pain and soreness subsided, so as to allow the limb to be straightened, a careful measurement, from fixed points, showed that it was the same length as the other ; the apparent lengthening being produced by the obliquity of the pelvis, caused by walking upon crutches and leaning to the sound side, to maintain the centre of gravity. The limb was slow in recovering strength, but the patient at the present time, walks about the city with the aid of a cane.—[*Ibid.*

Subnitrate of Bismuth in large doses in Typhoid Fever. By
M. ARAN.

M Moneret had previously noticed the good effects of subnitrate of bismuth in choleriform diarrhœa, and in the diarrhœa
of children.   M. Aran had administered it in a case of obstinate diarrhœa following typhoid fever; its success was rapid,
and in twelve days the patient was convalescent when the subnitrate was administered, and that the completion of the cure
was delayed only by this diarrhœa, which continued with much
obstinacy.   The case, therefore was one of that diarrhœa which
almost always accompanies typhoid fever towards its termination, and which is most frequently connected with lesion of
Peyser's plates, and with an irritated state of the intestinal
mucous membrane; for at this period, the utility of alvine evacuations is indisputable, purgatives having the property, if not
of abridging its duration, at any rate of preventing or rendering less intense the complications of other organs.   But because
this diarrhœa, while it continues within certain limits, does not
present any special indication, at least of active interference, in
the earlier stages of the typhoid fever, it does not follow that it
should be disregarded when it lasts beyond its ordinary term,
during recent, or not yet complete convalescence.   Sometimes
indeed, after a few days fever, appetite returns, fever diminishes, the tongue becomes moist, the meteorism disappears, the
stomach is indolent, and yet the stools continue liquid and frequent, and the patients cannot bear the slightest nourishment.
In this state amylaceous lavements containing a few drops of
laudanum are ordinarily employd, but often without success.
The physician is thus puzzled to raise the strength of the patient;
if he allows food, he has to fear enteritis; if he leaves his patient to absolute diet, his strength, instead of increasing, diminishes daily; he should then have recourse to subnitrate of bismuth as a powerful auxiliary.—[*Bulletin General de Therapeu-
tique. Stethoscope.*

Diuretics in Diseases of Children during Dentition. By G.
W. GARLAND, M. D.

There never was an age when the human mind seemed to
run riot in, as well as out of our profession, amidst the maze of
metaphysics and speculation, so completely as the present. No
sooner is a suggestion made, than the idea is thrown into the
laboratory of science, and undergoes an immediate test. And
of all the subjects upon which the minds of Pathologists have
been let loose, towards the perfecting of none have their energies

been more praiseworthily employed, than in acquiring accurate knowledge of the character or properties of the renal secretion in disease, and in pointing out the revulsive action of diuresis in various conditions of the system.

Observation has taught us that the effect of irritation, both general and local, is to diminish intestinal and urinary secretion; that we have immediately following this, a febrile state, which if allowed to continue may quickly produce alarming symptoms and in young subjects cerebral disturbance is among the earliest. One of its most prolific sources is the irritation produced by dentition. We may safely affirm, however, that there is but little danger from dentition so long as the kidneys act freely, however distressing the symptoms may be. The same remark will hold true in most cerebral affections of children, produced from sympathy.

When there is scanty secretion of urine, the circulation and all the energies seem clogged and oppressed. And who has not witnessed the almost instantaneous relief following a free discharge of urine ? The mind, as well as body, becomes more light and vivacious.

We learn then, by our own feelings, to anticipate the results which must attend the stimulation of the kidneys in many diseases.

Physicians do well, therefore, to pay particular attention to the condition of the kidneys in all febrile and irritative diseases, especially in infancy and childhood. The too common practice of combining alteratives and cathartics does well where the case is not immediately urgent; but a diuresis which will *often* prove critical, and always be followed by the very best results, may be promoted almost at once by a purgative, composed of senna and salts, followed by frequently repeated doses of nitrate of potassa, which I conceive to be the most simple as well as the most efficient means that can be resorted to.

In health and disease the kidneys are carrying on an active eliminatory process, and the skilful physician will avail himself of it in treating all diseases, particularly those numerous and varied febrile affections of children, during the two or three first years of their lives.

Every practitioner of experience who may chance to read this imperfect article, will have his thoughts turned back upon some little patient which caused the deepest solicitude, while suffering from a tardy dentition. They will remember that while the little sufferer lay in a half comatose state, turning its head from side to side, they learned with infinite anxiety that the patient had not passed urine for the last twelve or twenty-four hours. A few hours more, and a crisis has come. The alterative treatment tells by frequent, dark discharges, that the patient is under its influence. The kidneys feel its power, and respond by copious discharges of urine, when the little sufferer is, though but a few hours before, on the verge of a fatal coma, free from danger.

The object of this communication is to tell the profession, that in my opinion, this moment of intense concern and point of imminent danger may be avoided by early and repeated stimulation of the kidneys with nitrate of potassa combined, where the state of the bowels will admit, with Rochelle salts. I would not be understood to recommend the preclusion of all other treatment. Mucilages and sedatives are important, and, indeed, must never be dispensed with; but potassa is the hobby upon which I hope some member of the profession will mount, who has a less tardy pen than mine, and give me through your valuable journal, the results of his experience.—[*N. H. Journal of Medicine.*

A Case of Puncture of the Stomach, with Protrusion for six hours. Reported by Charles William Ashby, M. D., of Culpepper C. H., Va.

A negro boy, 6 years old, the property of Mr. R. B., fell upon a pair of sheep shears, which he had in his hand, whilst running down a hill. The instrument penetrated the stomach obliquely from above, just grazing the left side of the sternum and edges of the ribs, making a flap-like orifice in the integuments.

I was called in consultation by my friend, Dr. P. C. Slaughter, and found nearly the whole stomach protruded, and discharging its contents through an aperture about three-quarters of an inch in length.

Aware of the controversy which has long existed among able surgeons, on either side, as to the propriety of stitching the stomach or bowels, the everted edges and gaping appearance of the wound in the stomach made it necessary, I thought, that a stitch should be taken. To avoid irritation, as much as possible, with the finest needle and silk I ventured to take a single stitch through the middle of the wound.

Before I saw the case, Dr. S. had made some efforts to restore the organ to its natural position, but it did not occur to me at the time that I should have any serious difficulty in replacing it, at least after enlarging the orifice a little. But such was the unruly nature of the boy—his violent screaming and resistance, the nausea and vomiting which constantly attended the handling of the stomach—that notwithstanding I enlarged the orifice several times to a considerable extent, our best

efforts not only failed to restore the organ, but it seemed to
protrude the more.

At this juncture, fearing the irritation resulting from further
efforts, I suggested the use of chloroform, notwithstanding the
necessary delay of having to send several miles for it. Whilst
under its influence, I found it necessary again to enlarge the
aperture slightly, and then had no farther difficulty, although
the boy vomited as freely as before from handling the organ.

The wound of the integument was rather ragged in its appearance, and of course a little bruised by our efforts.

The wound of the stomach was brought directly opposite
the tegumentary wound, and gently retained within its verge.
A single stitch, patent lint, with cold water and a bandage,
completed the dressing.

The patient was placed on his side, absolute rest was enjoined, and soon afterwards a large dose of opium was administered.

From the time of the accident until the completion of the
dressing six hours intervened, and yet the boy retained his
strength most remarkably.

Under the influence of the opium our patient rested well the
first night.

2d day. This morning the pulse is a little excited, and face
flushed—vs. to make a decided impression ; and this was repeated twice during the day, and opium after each bleeding—
absolute diet enjoined—but the boy desires no food.

3d. The wound had a healthy appearance, but tenderness of
the abdomen and tympanitis greatly increased our fears as to
the result. The pulse feeble and quick ; the bowels not moved
since the accident.

Turpentine enema and a succession of blisters were ordered,
and after the bowels were moved the opium was resumed.

4th. Our patient evidently improved, tympanitis and tenderness diminished, pulse more quiet, countenance and general
aspect of things more encouraging—takes a little hot water tea
this morning, for the first time—gum water and opium continued.

5th. The wound not healed by the first intention—has a dark
spot immediately over the wound of the stomach, and is discharging a very offensive sanious matter. A soft poultice, and
the same prescription continued.

6th. The ligature came out this morning. The same prescription continued. From this date the boy gradually recovered, without any particular change in the treatment.

Remarks.—1st It has occurred to me, that possibly it would
have been better for me to have restored the stomach, at least
partially, before the stitch was taken, as I ran the risk of break-

ing out the ligature by the subsequent efforts at reduction ; and
I am sure that the accumulation of gas, though some escaped
with an audible sound several times, did not increase the difficulty.

2d.   This case was admirably adapted to the use of chloroform, and illustrates most happily its incalculable value, when
used with discrimination.

3d.   As your journal is eminently practical in its character,
for the benefit of the younger members of the profession, it may
not be amiss to allude briefly to what I conceive to be a most
important principle in our profession, viz : that an *inflamed or
diseased organ must have rest.*   In this case, the stomach, instinctively sensible of its wounded and disabled condition, refused most emphatically, for four days, to receive any nourishment—not even gum water—and but very little of anything for
about ten days, notwithstanding the entreaties of master and
friends, contrary to our orders.

An inflamed eye instinctively excludes the light from itself,
so that the physician who interrogates nature intelligently, at
once gets the idea of confining his patient to a dark room, and
thus putting the organ entirely to rest.   When the lungs are
inflamed the patient breathes as much as possible by the abdominal muscles, and lymph is thrown out, gluing the organ to the
side, doubtless to prevent motion and friction as much as possible.   The same thing is true of inflamed bowels ; and because
some constipation, the result of this principle, exists, I have known
great error—and I may say even death—to result from goard-
ing and stimulating the organ with drastic purgatives.

This principle of rest is susceptible of very extensive application in practice; and any inflammation can be cured, I believe,
to which it can be applied.

The immortal Physic, always true to the laws of nature, recognized this principle in the treatment of coxalgia and other
diseases of the joints.   In conformity to this important law of
the animal economy, in the above case, we gave opium freely,
to prevent nervous and vascular reaction; and by thus adding in
keeping the wounded organ in a profound state of repose, it contributed, it is believed, no little to the favorable result.

[*Stethoscope.*

Observations on Pustule Maligne.. By C. Trenerry, M. R. C.
S. E., L. A. C., Assistant physician to the Civil Hospital,
Gibraltar.

It appears that Christoba Martinez, aged sixty, a Portuguese
by birth, presented himself as an out patient of this hospital on

the 21st of October, 1850, suffering from the pustule maligne ; he stated that he had been navigating on board a vessel laden with wool and salted bullocks' hides from Larachè.

On the 14th of the following month, Manuel Fernandez, aged sixty, a relative of the above, was admitted with a similar disease; he said he was a fisherman, and had not been near any wool or hides.

Francisco Lapena, aged forty-eight, a Spaniard, and Francisco Docarmen, aged sixty-eight, a Portuguese, both mariners on board a Portuguese vessel laden with hides and gum, were similarly affected.

Jose Pedro, aged fifteen, a Portuguese, had not been near any vessel, wool, or hides for fifteen days, but notwithstanding became affected with the disease, as did also Juan Bayestero, who had not been near the source of contagion for five days.

Juan Catania, aged thirteen, said he was standing on the wharf one Sunday afternoon, when he experienced a slight itching of the right upper eyelid, and the following morning the characteristic pustule showed itself.

On the 2nd of March, 1851, Lorenzo Pau, aged twenty-two, became affected, after being engaged in weighing salted hides on board a vessle that came from Tunis.

The disease was characterized in the above patients experiencing a slight itching in some part of the face, followed by a small pimple having a dark depressed centre, surrounded by several almost imperceptible phlyctinea, from which oozed an ichorous fluid ; the glands of the neck on the affected side, but more especially the parotid, became enlarged and indurated ; the head, face, neck, and upper part of the thorax were afterwards frightfully swollen and disfigured, the tumefaction having a peculiarly tense and elastic feel ; the respiration was laborious, and attended with a singular croaking sound whilst the voice was of a disagreeable guttural nature.

Two of the cases terminated fatally a few hours after admission ; the one with symptoms of suffocation, and the other of apoplexy ; the rest had a very protracted recovery, but more particularly the first case, whose life was compromised on different occasions by extensive suppuration and sloughs having formed on the left side of the face and neck, attended with frequent alarming attacks of hæmorrhage, so much so, that on one occasion my assistants was suddenly called for by Drs. Merry and Cortes, (who had the chief care of the patient at his own residence,) and it became a question whether the carotid artery should not be ligatured ; the poor fellow was spared the operation, and recovered after nearly four months suffering.

The treatment consisted in an immediate and free application

of the actual cautery to the affected spot, and afterwards the
diacetate-of-lead lotion, which were sure to arrest the disorder
if applied within twenty-four hours from its appearance ; the
bowels were cleared out by an aperient ; and other symptoms,
such as fever, suppuration, and sloughing, were treated on general principles.

The disease is generally considered contagious, and to depend upon carbuncles, or some peculiar virus existing in the
hides at the time the animal is slaughtered, which remains permanent, and whatever preparation the hides or wool undergo, it cannot be destroyed ; therefore whether sitting on a hair-
bottomed chair, lying on a woolen or hair mattrass, carrying a
hair trunk, or wearing a woollen garment made with the affected
material, disposes us to the dreadful malady ; an opinion that is
certainly not borne out by my experience ; for it must have
been observed how few became affected out of the numerous individuals that were necessarily engaged in those vessels having
the hides and wool ; besides, the immunity experienced by the
medical men and relatives in attendance on those affected, carries some weight in favor of its non-contagious nature; but as
additional proofs, I may mention that Drs. Merry, Cortes, and
myself, have unavoidably had our fingers frequently covered
with the blood and matter issuing from the sloughs that formed ;
further, I have inoculated some kittens with matter taken fresh
from some of the above subjects without the slighest ill effects
ensuing.

I am, therefore, inclined to suspect that insects are generated
at same particular period, or under some peculiar condition of
the animal, and lodge in the hide or wool, from whence they
are apt to escape and seek a nidus in the skin of any other animal, which in its turn becomes affected after a short time with
the poison secreted *sui generis* of this insect.—[*London Lancet.*

Chloroform in painful Micturtion.

We condense from the Journal des Con. Medico-Chir. the
following case, by Wm. Guisard :

My son, three years of age, affected with painful phymosis,
would not attempt micturition nor defication, through a dread of
the excessive pain which these acts produced. On the 8th July
last, the patient whilst under the influence of chloroform, taken
preparatory to the operation for phymosis, passed water and
feces remarkably freely. Twenty-four hours after, the patient
not having urinated, chlorform was again administered, and
was again followed by the same result as at first. At this time
the child was not entirely insensible, for he knew when the
water was passing, and said it gave him no pain.

𝔐𝔦𝔰𝔠𝔢𝔩𝔩𝔞𝔫𝔶.

MOBILE, (Alabama,) Nov. 1st, 1851.

Sir :—At the last annual meeting of the "American Medical Association," I was appointed Chairman of a Committee, to report at its next session, on the "*Endemic Prevalence of Tetanus.*" The subject is a novel one, its solution difficult of attainment and not easily controlled by any individual effort.

Permit me therefore to solicit your assistance, to the extent of your information, either from personal experience or inquiry, embracing the immediate circuit under your professional supervision. My object is not to tax you with long or elaborate replies, but simply, where admissible, to furnish affirmative or negative answers.

Your attention to the following queries, and answers seriatim, forwarded by mail to my address, on or before the 15th day of January, 1852, will not only serve the special object of the Association, but particularly oblige,   Very Respectfully,
                                                Your Ob't. Serv't.,   A. LOPEZ.

1st. Are there any physical causes, in or about your locality, productive of Endemic Disease, and if so, what form does such disease assume ?

2nd. Have changes by clearing of lands, change of culture, or any other circumstances, been the cause of such Endemic ?

3rd. Has Tetanus been of frequent occurrence, and if so, does it hold an analagous or independent origin ?

4th. Does it follow the laws which govern other climatic Endemics, in sufficient number, and simultaneous prevalence to warrant the belief of its identical origin ?

5th. What form of Tetanus have you most commonly met with ?

6th. The proportion of Traumatic to Idiopathic ?

7th. Have meteorological variations governed the production and character of the disease ?

8th. The average number of deaths from Tetanus ?

9th. Have adults or children been most liable to its attack ?

10th. What sex ?

11th. Proportion of whites to negroes ?

12th. Duration of disease previous to fatality ?

13th. Interval between cause and developements ?

14th. Does *Trismus Nascentium* ever observe an Epidemic or Endemic character ?

15th. Do you consider it Traumatic or Idiopathic ?

16th. Are negro or white children most liable to it ?

17th. Your belief as to its origin ?

18th. Proportion of deaths to cures ?

19th. Have you found any form of treatment more successful than another, in either Tetanus or Trismus Nascentium ?

AMERICAN MEDICAL ASSOCIATION.

Committee on the Radical Cure of Reducible Hernia.

To the Members of the Medical Profession throughout the United States :

The undersigned are a Committee of the American Medical Association to report on *" the radical cure of reducible hernia."* They are desirous of obtaining from their professional brethren any information that is calculated to throw light on this important and interesting subject.

They therefore take the liberty of proposing the following questions. An answer to any or all of them, or any facts connected with the branch of Surgery on which they are directed to report, would be gratefully received.

1st. Have you been in the practice of treating reducible hernia with a view to its radical cure ?

2nd. Have you ever performed any surgical operation for this purpose ?

3rd. If so, please to describe the operation and the mode of performing it.

4th. What proportion of cases, of all in which you have operated, has been cured ?

5th. Have any alarming or fatal effects, in any instance, been caused by the operation ?

6th. If so, please to describe them.

As the Report must be made at the Annual Meeting of the Association, to be held in Richmond, Va., in May next, it is desirable that the answers to the above questions should be forwarded to any one of the committee on or before March 1st, 1852.

> GEO. HAYWARD,
> J. MASON WARREN, } *Committe.*
> S. PARKMAN,

Boston, November 26, 1851.

ʼSTATE SOCIETY.

The annual meeting of the " Medical Society of the State of Georgia," will commence in Augusta on the *second Wednesday* in April. As we anticipate a session of unusual interest, it is hoped the members of the Association will come up from all parts of the State in their full strength. The presence of the Faculty, generally, is specially invited, and will be warmly welcomed.

> C. B. NOTTINGHAM, Rec'g. Sec'y.

Macon, 12th, January, 1852.

Female Medical College of Pennsylvania.—It appears that this *interesting* institution has recently held its first commencement : " An efficient orchester was in attendance and discoursed excellent music. The exercises were commenced with prayer by the Rev. Dr. Brainerd, after which Prof. T. S. Langshore, delivered an interesting address to the Graduates.   The degree of "Doctor of Medicine" was then conferred by Wm. J. Muller, President of the College, upon eight ladies, who had terminated their regular course of instruction, in these words :—" Ladies, after a careful and thorough examination, on the part of our Board, you have been found fully qualified to become practitioners in the healing art of Medicine and Surgery.   In the name and on behalf of the corporators of the Female Medical College of Pennsylvania, I present you a Diploma, signed by the President and Faculty, conferring upon you the degree of Doctor of Medicine, with all the honors, rights and privileges appertaining thereunto." The thesis were upon " Wounds," " Neuralgia," " Electricity," " Anemia," " Diagnosis," " True Physician," " Chlorosis," and ". Influence of the nervous system on the functions of Respiration and Nutrition."

Kinesipathy.—A new system of medical practice has been introduced into Europe, and it may naturally be expected that it will be imported, and sooner or later practised among us.   It would not be strange were it to supersede and take the place of homœopathy, to which it is assimilated in other points besides a common lack of science or reason.   It certainly is superior on the score of economy—for though the doses to be taken in the former are infinitesimal and therefore portable and cheap, in the latter no doses at all are required, and all the mysterious movements and " shakings" are to be accomplished on the sick body itself!   The originator of this improved system seems to have been a Swedish fencing master by the name of Ling, who is represented, in the Edinburgh Monthly Journal, to have been an universal genius.   He was successively a graduate in theology, a volunteer in the Danish navy, a fencing master (in spite of gout in his arm,) a lecturer on old Norse poetry, history and mythology, a professor of fencing and gymnastics, a student of anatomy, physiology and other sciences, a writer of poetry, and, withal, "a man of high moral tone, pious, sincere and honest," and died in 1839 with the honors of knighthood upon him.   His qualifications are therefore unquestionable !   All that Ling himself appears to have really accomplished, and probably all that he claimed at first, was set forth in a work published by him, and may be considered as merely an improvement in the practice of gymnastics and calisthenics.   Upon this has been engrafted the system of quackery alluded to above.   M. Roth, M. D., of London, who comes before us clothed with Ling's mantle, has sent out an octavo of 300 pages, devoted to the treatment of disease by "movements," alias Kinesipathy. His interpretation of the term is as follows :

. " By the word 'movement,' in a medical and hygienic sense, is to be understood every change of position and difference of form, determined by time and amount, in the whole body, or in any part of it, and which may be produced by the organism itself, or by any animate or inanimate mechanical agent."

In accordance with this definition, there are a great variety of movements—quite as many as there are dilutions and potencies in the homœopathic system—and each and all possess great power over the human body, as is rendered plain by another quotation :

"Whatever exists in our body, either as a part of it or as a foreign substance, must at a certain moment have a definite shape; therefore every change of the space in one part necessarily produces a corresponding one in the surrounding tissues—a change that is thence propagated to the most remote parts of the body, and which depends, with respect to its form, upon the amount of the alteration produced by the first movement."

Lest any one should still be in the dark, however, respecting what kinesipathy really is, we copy the full definition of one of the movements and its effects. It is called the

" *Chopping Movement.*—Chopping consists in alternative short blows, produced by the external sides of both the operator's hands. Choppings are principally used on the posterior surface of the trunk, chest, and also on the limbs. If it is desirable that the succession produced by this movement shall be less and softer, then the chopping is done with the external edges of the two little fingers, while the other fingers are spread apart, but not kept spasmodically fast, so that they act also by striking upon the little finger.

" Chopping may be confined to one part only, or may be exercised on a larger surface, by constantly moving the position of the hands. The chopping is called a ' longitudinal' one, if the hands are moved in the longitudinal direction of the trunk or of the limb ; and a 'transversed' one, if the blows are executed across the limbs.

" *Effect.*—Choppings produce generally a venous absorption in the capillary texture, not only of the external skin and the tendinous expansions, but also, if more strongly used, in the muscles and bones ; in imperfectly paralyzed muscles they excite the innervation both of the motory and sensitive fibres. If directed on the lower extremities, on the soles, they act very well in hæmorrhoidal complaints, headache, &c. On the chest or along the spine, there are efficacious specific movements in certain complaints of the chest, partly by their direct influence on the muscles of the chest, partly by the tremulous, passive vibration communicated to the lungs."

Then there is the " shaking movement," the "rising-up movement," the "letting-down movement," "transversal chopping," " vibration," &c. &c., which we have not room to describe. These " movements" are all claimed as a remedy in acute as well as chronic diseases. In gonorrhœa, even, cases are brought forward to show their great efficacy. Can quackery and imposture "further go ?" It does really seem as though we might hope that "things will come right at last," when such a multitude of absurdities and inconsistencies are countenanced and supported by those who break away from, or who never have entered, the ranks of legitimate and scientific practice.—[*Med. and Surgical Journal.*

Discovery of the Male Acarus Scabiei.—One of M. Cazenave's pupils, M. Lanquetin, has just found the male acarus scabiei upon the hand of a patient affected with the itch. It seems that this acarus had long been sought for in vain, and some works on skin diseases do not even mention its existence. As this parasite is very small, being less than half the size of the female, it had hitherto escaped detection.
[*L'Union Medicale. Med. News.*

Substitution of Iodated Oil for Cod-liver Oil.—M. Champouillon gave to the Acad. Méd. of Paris the following results of his experiments :—

102 phthisical patients were treated with cod-liver oil. Of these, 51 were in the first stage, of which 21 were cured; 37 were in the second stage, of which 9 were cured, 3 died; 14 were in the third stage, of which 6 were cured, 4 died.

75 other phthisical cases were treated with iodated oil. In none of these did any amelioration take place; in many the disease was aggravated.—[*Ibid.*

Medical College of Constantinople.—This school consists of two departments. The first comprises the study of the Turkish, Arabic and French languages, Geography, History, Cosmography and Mathematics. The second that of Medicine proper. Prof. of Botany, Zoology and Surgical clinic, M. Caratheodori; Chemistry and Pharmacy, M. Colleja; Physics, M. Basilidés; Anatomy, M. Warthbichler; Physiology, M. Gaspard; Materia Medica and Therapeutics, M. Archigènes; General Pathology and Hygiene, M. Mavrogeni; Minor Surgery, M. Steysan-Bey; Principles and Practice of Medicine, M. Fauval; Medical Clinic, M. Rigler; Medical Jurisprudence, M. Servican; Midwifery for the male department, M. Zohrab; Ditto for female do. Mehmed Effendi.

The number of students in the school is 444. In the course of the year, 11,000 persons were vaccinated there, 640 patients were treated in the clinics, and more than 160 operations were performed, about 11,000 patients presented themselves at the gratuitous consultations.
[*Journal des Con. Medico-Chir.*

Preparatory Medical Schools.—We perceive that our Charleston neighbors have organized two of these institutions upon quite a respectable footing, and that they are to go into operation in the ensuing spring. One of them is styled the "Charleston Preparatory Medical School," and the other "The Charleston Summer Medical Institute." We wish them both success.

A System of Operative Surgery : based upon the Practice of Surgeons in the United States : and comprising a bibliographical index and historical record of many of their operations, during a period of 200 *years.* By HENRY H. SMITH, M. D., Surgeon to the St. Joseph's Hospital; Assistant Lecturer on Demonstrative Surgery in the University of Pennsylvania; Lecturer on the Principles and Practice of Surgery in the Philadelphia Medical Institute, &c. Illustrated by numerous steel plates. Philadelphia: Lippincott, Grambo & Co. 1852.

The publication of the above title page alone would be sufficient to create in the mind of every American practitioner a desire to procure the work. Its intrinsic merits will secure it a place in the library of all who feel interested in Surgery. It was some time ago announced that a translation of the beautiful work of Bernard and Huette upon Operative Surgery was in preparation, but Dr. Smith has anticipated its issue by a very faithful reproduction of all the valuable peculiarities of the French work and by the addition of a very considerable amount of American matter, well calculated to make it, to us at least, the most desirable work upon the subject in our language. We were indeed much in need of a work to which we might look for the achievements of American surgery impartially and systematically set forth ; and we have every reason to think, judging from the specimen before us, that Dr. Smith will accomplish this object creditably. Errors of omission will doubtless be found in the Bibliographical Index, which may be corrected in a subsequent edition, or in the forthcoming volumes. The very bungling manner in which American views and doings were thrown into the poor translation of Velpeau's great work on Surgery, could not and did not satisfy the profession in this country.

Dr. Smith having already published an excellent work upon Minor Surgery, the present publication will comprehend—1st. General duties and Elementary operations; 2d. Operations on the Head and Face ; 3d. Operations on the Neck and Trunk ; 4th. Operations on the Genito-Urinary organs ; and 5th. Operations on the Extremities. The volume before us contains the two first parts, and the remainder will be issued as early as practicable. This, with Dr. Smith's former work, will constitute a whole which cannot fail to place the profession in our country under deep obligations to the distinguished author.

————

We are indebted to Publishers for several valuable works, which will be noticed in our next.

SOUTHERN
MEDICAL AND SURGICAL JOURNAL.

| Vol. 8.] | NEW SERIES.—MARCH, 1852. | [No. 3. |

PART FIRST.

Original Communications.

•

ARTICLE VII.

Epidemic Dysentery, as it prevailed in a portion of Floyd County, Ga., in the Autumn of 1851. *By* WM. C. BRANDON, *M. D., of Hermitage, Ga.*

In view of the fact, that ours is a progressive science, and that its whole history is made up of an accumulation of isolated facts and brief records, I am induced to ask a small space in the "Journal," that I may register upon its pages a short account of an epidemic as it occurred during the past autumn. I do not propose to offer any thing new, either in pathology or therapeutics. But as the present is greatly dependent upon the past, for the present state of medical science, for the historical accounts of epidemics, the opinions entertained as to their pathology, the remedies employed in them, &c., so the future may look back to the present period in the world's history with as much interest, for faithful and authentic records in medicine, as we now do to the past. This article of itself, I am aware, may be of little worth, but when taken in connexion with other accounts of this, or even different diseases, it may not be altogether without its value; and more especially, when we remember the fact that scarcely any disease appearing epidemically at different periods, possesses exactly the same features at each occurrence of the epidemic. At one time it may be very malignant and intractable, and upon a future occurrence be mild and readily amenable, to treatment. During the past year, two original articles on Dysentery have appeared in this Journal—one from the pen of Dr. H. F. Campbell, of Augusta, Ga., in the September number, another in the December number, from Dr. Weatherby, of Palmetto. I presume the disease (or rather the epidemic) treated of by those gentlemen, to be the same as that of which I propose to speak, bearing, perhaps, some modifications. The disease is said to have prevailed to a greater or less extent in several of the Southern States during the past summer and autumn. But as I can not say with positive certainty, that such is the fact, I shall confine my remarks to a personal knowledge of the extent of the disease; for my design is to record fact only.

The disease made its appearance in this and the adjacent counties, both in this State and Alabama, in the early summer months. It did not show itself at or near the same time in all places. Frequently it would prevail in a particular place or neighborhood for two months or more; while another point not five miles distant, would be wholly exempt, but in its turn become extensively infected, while the disease would be disappearing, or entirely arrested where it previously existed. It fell to my lot to see but very few cases during the first four months of its prevalence. The cases I did see presented nothing of particular interest, above that of ordinary sporadic dysentery, in this section of the country; and had not the disease shown itself to a considerable extent in other and various parts of the country, I should have considered them nothing more than sporadic cases. It was not until October, that the disease made its appearance to any great extent within the bounds of my practice. Although the disease had been migrating (so to speak) from place to place for four months, and frequently under a very formidable character, yet about this time (October) the type of the disease was somewhat changed, and unlike most epidemics, it became more malignant just previous to its disappearance. The disease now assumed a strictly typhoid type: this was a peculiarity which attended every case which came under my observation, whether the attack was mild or more formidable. So similar to occasional cases of typhoid fever were these symptoms, that it was, I learn, even by some physicians, pronounced typhoid fever; an error (if I may be allowed thus to express myself,) which might easily have been avoided, by a little attention as to what portion of the alimentary canal was bearing the onus of the disease.

In the greater number of cases, the attack came on without premonitory symptoms of any duration. The first warning the patients generally had, was severe griping pain, and sudden call to stool; the result of which was, the discharge of a small portion of blood, or blood and mucus, and occasionally of mucus alone. The frequency of dejections, or calls thereto, depended generally upon the character of the attack. In the worst cases, they were as often as every ten or fifteen minutes, for the space of an hour or two; then succeeded by an hour, perhaps, of rest to the patient, with entire freedom from pain, to be followed again by severe tormina and imperious tenesmus. The color of the blood discharged was variable; sometimes it was dark or venous, generally, however, it was of a bright arterial hue. In the more formidable cases the discharges presented a spumy appearance. I believe that no case recovered where this symptom was very persistent. There was one symptom which almost invariably attended every case; that was, the entire absence of fecal matter in the evacuations, even where the patient was attacked having the stomach and bowels in an ordinary state of repletion. And in many cases, it was with difficulty that a feculent dejection could be procured by cathartics, such as were thought advisable to be employed in the disease. In this respect, the disease differed from that form which prevailed in the summer, as reported by the gentlemen above referred to, at least in some instances. One of them speaks of serous or diarrhœal discharges, the other of feculent passages. In no single instance did I observe serous evacuations in any stage of the disease, and very seldom fecal matter until a change for the better. In one case, which proved fatal, for thirty-six hours prior to death the discharges were mixed with, and sometimes appeared to consist entirely of pus, giving out an exceedingly offensive odour.

Nausea, retching, and vomiting were present in the majority of instances. In the milder attacks, nausea was absent in a degree. The matter ejected consisted generally of the liquid which had been taken into the stomach, sometimes of a little tenacious mucus. In connexion with the excruciating pain, almost invariably referable to some portion of the colon, there was tenderness under pressure at some point along the bowels. This, however, was by no means an invariable symptom; for even in some very severe cases it was wanting to some extent. Very little tenderness was felt, in the early period of the disease in any case. The pain and tenderness under pressure was occasionally felt along the whole tract of the colon: and in fact, in some severe attacks the whole bowels with the stomach gave the same response; especially in cases attended by retching and vomiting. Tympanitis was not present in every case, but more frequent in young, than adult subjects. The febrile symptoms were of a low grade. The pulse ranged from a hundred to a hundred and forty, depending upon the character of the attack. It was always feeble, sometimes so feeble and thready as scarcely to be counted, even in adults of ordinary constitution. The skin was dry and usually cool, except over the bowels, where frequently there was pungent heat of the surface; ordinarily the extremities were cold and could be restored to normal temperature with difficulty.

The tongue at the onset of the disease was moist, and presented a dark appearance, as if deeply stained. This dusky appearance soon seemed to extend (if possible) below the epithelium itself. Unless the attack was a mild one, the tongue gradually became dry and of a heavy dark brown color, in some of the worst cases even black, along the back part. This organ was frequently cracked, or dotted with small superficial ulcers.

In the greater number of my patients the appetite was but little impaired, except during the period when they were labouring under nausea. The thirst usually was very considerable, ordinarily the urine was scanty and high coloured. In some instances, in children, it presented a chylous or milky appearance. The body of the patient as well as the discharges from the bowels exhaled a strikingly cadaverous and sickening odour. The breath possessed the same character.

One striking feature in the disease was, the almost entire

unimpairment of the mind. Even in the most formidable cases I observed very little mental depression, or low delerium, symptoms so common in diseases of adynamic character.

In but very few of the cases which I was called to attend, did it fall to me to make the first prescription. Some had been under the care of other physicians, but the greater number had been subjected to some domestic treatment, such as castor-oil, epsom salts, some of those death-dealing patent pills, "spirits and white sugar burnt with lightwood splinters with a little mutton tallow in it, and some black root tea;" often too, to the great detriment of the patient. In view of the feeble state of the pulse and coolness of the surface, I saw no case in which I deemed the lancet admissible. Cups were used in some instances along the course of the colon, but without the least discoverable advantage. ·

If I had reason to believe the bowels were loaded with fecal matter, my first object was to relieve them of this. My usual prescription was, an oz. of castor-oil with from 1 to 2 drs. oil of turpentine, for an adult ; diminished in proportion to the age of younger subjects. Often this dose had to be repeated, sometimes twice, before a fecal dejection could be procured.

The turpentine was left out in some instances, and my opinion is, with disadvantage to the patient. I used no saline cathartics, for in every instance where they had been used prior to my visit to the patient, I believe they had acted injuriously, especially where the stomach and small bowels were implicated to any great extent. The injurious effect may have resulted from the large quantity it was requisite to employ in order to get an operation; probably if they had been used in a diminished quantity and at proper intervals the effect might have been beneficial. After treating a few cases and seeing the tardiness with which cathartics acted, I was induced to commence at the outset with mercurials ; even where it was necessary to use cathartics. In connexion with the oil and turpentine, I administered 12 grs. calomel or 15 grs. blue mass, in divided doses; within 24 hours. Even that amount of the mercurial seemed to add but little force to the cathartic, it sometimes requiring two doses of the oil and turpentine with the mercurial conjoined, to produce one or two fecal discharges, and these were often small.

The mercurial was not given with a view to its cathartic effect, but as an alterative. It may at first view seem to the reader, rather heterodox that a mercurial should be used in what we term alterative doses, and for the purpose of obtaining its constitutional effects, while at the same time, cathartics are administered. But after seeing the slowness with which purgatives acted, I thought it possible that the mercury might make some impression upon the system before it would be carried off by them, and at least, it would but act favorably as an adjuvent to them. Where the stomach and small bowels gave evidence of considerable irritation the purgatives were withheld; however, in the greater number of cases, the patients had used them sufficiently before I was called. After having used the cathartics, and finding that they had been used sufficiently, my next object was to re-establish the· deficient, or rather, suppressed secretions, for it appeared that few, if any were in a natural state. To accomplish this I used from 2 to 4 grs. of calomel every four hours, or blue pill 5 grs. every six hours, combining opium to the amount of 2 to 4 grs. or its equivalent in morphine or laudanum, owing to the degree of pain, every twenty-four hours. The only perceptible effect of the opiates was the anodyne. And to me, it was a singular fact that but very few of my patients showed any signs of narcotism or stupor from these doses. Where they were kept up for several days and then diminished, no headache followed, as is frequently the case. And in speaking of the symptoms of the disease, I should have mentioned that headache was scarcely ever present. In some of the cases, where the mercurial did not make its impression early, which it seldom did, I combined ipecacuanha from $\frac{1}{8}$ to $\frac{1}{4}$ gr. with each dose of the mercurial. The nausea I believe, was not increased by the ipecac, even in cases where this symptom was already present. This combination, that is, the calomel and ipecac, appeared to exert a greater curative influence than any other prescription I employed. Where the calls to stool were very frequent, the acetate of lead was combined occasionally with other remedies. In some cases I employed emolient anodyne, and astringent enemata. Occasionally they showed decidedly beneficial effects, while in other cases no alteration was made in the condition of the patient

from their use. For several days after I commenced treating
this disease, it was my practice to employ blistering over the
most tender points and frequently over a considerable portion
of the abdomen. In view of the character of the disease, it
seemed to me a decidedly appropriate treatment; but to my disappointment, (I am of the opinion,) they exerted little or no influence over a large majority of the cases in which they were used.
From this opinion, I was induced to dispense with them, unless
in cases where the stomach was irritable. In comparing the
results of cases where blisters were, and were not used, other
things being equal, the difference was not considerable. Notwithstanding such are the conclusions which my observation
has induced, if a similar disease was again to come under my
care, I should resort to vesication with the expectation of
benefit, until facts proved the reverse.

Warm fomentations and gently stimulating rubefacients,
I found to be of service. If their therapeutic effect was not
great, they were decidedly soothing and agreeable to the patient. Where vesicatories were used serum collected in them,
but slowly and scantily, and they soon became dry and crusty,
unless some stimulating ungent was pretty freely applied. I
generally applied the mercurial ointment with the object of affecting the system.

The tepid bath was freely used in the cases of young subjects; the mustard foot-bath with adults. Where the vital
powers were considerably depressed, and this was generally
the case, I administered wine at intervals in small quantities.
I should have given quinine, believing the disese to be of malarious origin, but from the fact that the worst cases which came
under my care had been treated with quinine, with other remedies, as I was informed by the friends of the patients.

This was the general plan of treatment I pursued, modifying
it according to the age, constitution, condition, &c., of the
patient. As every practitioner is aware, though a general
plan of treatment may be pursued, it must frequently be altered
somewhat, according to circumstances. I lost no single case
where I succeeded in making any visible mercurial impression.
To do this, it was generally exceedingly difficult and in some
cases failed altogether. Some patients recovered without evi-

dences of ptyalism. I think my most successful treatment was, the mercurial and ipecac combined. And should it ever be my lot to meet with such a disease again, I should place my chief reliance upon these remedies, in connexion with wine and opium. Some of the milder cases were treated almost entirely with opium.

The result of my course of treatment was any thing but flattering. The proportion of cases which proved fatal was about 25 per cent. And shocking as this may appear, it was greater success than was obtained by some who treated the same disease. The mortality in all the cases which I knew any thing of—those treated by myself, those under the care of other physicians, and those not treated at all, except by domestic prescriptions, was about 37 per cent. The condition of many of the patients was unfavorable to proper treatment, being deprived of the comforts of life, and of proper nurses. The worst cases which fell into my care had been under treatment by others, and two-fifths of those I lost, were of this number. I do not make this remark as intimating that they had been improperly treated, for they doubtless had not, so far as the physicians were concerned.

During my short experience in the practice of medicine I have met with no disease possessing half the malignancy of the one under consideration. No age or sex was exempt. The child of two years and the matron of eighty-four were alike the subjects of the disease. The majority of the patients were below the age of puberty.

Dr. Campbell, in his article before referred to, remarks it as a singular fact, that negroes were not attacked by the disease, as it occurred to him. My observation was the same at a distance of two hundred miles from where Dr. C.'s cases were located, and at a different season of the year. While the disease was prevailing, I heard of one case in the person af a negro child, in the neighborhood of my practice. It was fortunate that some class of persons was exempt where the disease prevailed so malignantly. In some instances, from the very beginning of the attack, it seemed that death had marked his victim, and the disease progressed to a dissolution of the patient in despite of any remedial measures which could be adopted.

Fortunately this form of the disease was of short duration. It prevailed so malignantly but for the space of about six weeks, when the heavy rains and frosts, between the 15th and 25th of November, seemed suddenly to arrest the disease entirely. The rains and severe frosts may not have had any influence upon the disease, but I attributed its arrest to them. They may, however, have been coincident occurrences. The section where the disease thus prevailed was situated on a large creek, (the Armuchee,) and its tributaries—a region formerly considered malarious, and until within the last two or three years the location of autumnal fevers to a considerable extent. Doubtless the disease was of malarious origin. But it will require one more skilled in etiology than I am, to say why this malaria, or epidemic constitution of the atmosphere, as Sydenham terms it, did not produce remittent or intermittent fever, instead of a malignant typhoid dysentery. Was there some change in the constituents of this malaria, or could there have been a different state of susceptibility in the system of the subject, that determined the character of the disease? Was it the same idiosyncracy in the negro, which so often seems to exempt him from autumnal fevers, that preserved him in this disease ?

I might have extended these remark to double the length ; in fact, I might have given the history of all, or a certain number of cases in detail. But I deemed it more prudent to give · a general account of the disease, treatment, &c., rather than pursue a different plan, probably to the exclusion of more interesting and important matter from the pages of the Journal. And lest such should be the case, I have endeavored to be as concise as possible.

ARTICLE VIII.

Extracts from the Records of the Physicians' Society for Medical Observation, of Greene and adjoining Counties, Georgia. By D. C. O'Keeffe, M. D., Secretary.

January 12th, 1852. *Thrush in Children.*—Dr. B. F. Rea read a paper whose object was to lay before the Society some views of the pathology and treatment of a malady which presents itself, perhaps, as frequently to the practitioner as any other, yet is regarded by many as a disease of no great importance in a practical point of view, and even too lightly noticed in works on infantile disease.

"Thrush is readily recognized by the small curd-like deposit upon the epithelium of the lips and upper surface of the tongue, in children at the breast. It is at first of a milk-white or pearly hue, but occasionally assumes a yellowish color, sometimes covering the upper and under surfaces of the tongue, inside of the cheeks, gums and pharynx; and some authors—among whom are Armstrong, Marley, Gardien—assert that it extends quite through the stomach and intestinal canal to the anus. Having frequently met with thrush, and being interested in diseases of this class, I have, for some years, studied it attentively, and do not believe it is ever attached to the mucous membrane of the stomach and intestinal canal, although small portions of the aphthous (?) deposit may, and doubtless do, often escape into the stomach and bowels. The deposit is always found more firmly attached to the epithelium of the lips, tongue, &c.; and as the latter organ is so abundantly supplied with papillæ, which, with the epithelium, seem to afford the best soil for its growth, we here find it more firmly attached than any where else. Again: we know that the epithelium which covers the mucous membrane of the lips, tongue, cavity of the mouth, pharynx and œsophagus, extends only to the cardiac orifice of the stomach—the mucous membrane of which, as well as that of the intestinal canal, being covered with a coating or varnish of mucous matter, not adapted to the attachment and growth of the aphthous vegetations. Some of the best authorities consider it a diphtheritic inflammation, and describe it under the heads of pultaceous and pseudo-membranous inflammation. From this I dissent. Thrush cannot be a diphtheritic inflammation, for diphtheritis (from the Greek, diphthera) means a form of inflammation in which a false membrane is formed, and characterized by an exudation of fibrinous or albuminous matter, in the form of a pellicle *upon* the surface of the membrane, *underneath* the epithelium. Now we can have no diphtheritis without inflammation, and the exudation is *underneath* the epithelium; whereas, we may have *Thrush* without inflammation, and the deposit is *upon*, not *under*, the epithelium. Moreover, if thrush were an exudation, caused by inflammation, we would certainly sometimes see it become organized, which I have never seen ; nor have I seen the unusual redness and increased heat of the mouth which are stated by some authors to precede attacks of the disease.

I do not consider inflammation even necessary to the causation of thrush ; and although the deposit may often be upon an inflamed mucous membrane, yet I look upon it as a mere coincidence, and not as cause and effect. I believe, however, that if the deposit be allowed to remain undisturbed, it may excite inflammation in the epithelium, and by contiguous sympathy the mucous membrane underneath may become inflamed. The term aphthæ, which is sometimes applied to thrush, is incorrect ; for the very word itself leads to the idea that there is inflammation—which is true of aphthous affections, but not of thrush. Both may exist simultaneously, as I have myself seen ; but they are far from being one and the same disease—one being a vesicular affection, the other a *genuine parasitic deposit ;* and this constitutes the true pathology (if you will allow the expression) of Thrush.

The disease under consideration may sometimes occur without any general disorder of the constitution ; but more frequently we find general symptoms present themselves.

The diarrhœa which is often present, and which indicates disorder of the digestive organs, bears generally a direct relation to the extent and severity of the disease. There is usually an abundant formation of acid, as indicated by the green evacuations, which are so acrid in aggravated forms of the malady as to produce redness of the anus and nates ; and hence some suppose that the disease has extended through the alimentary canal. Sometimes there is vomiting of greenish acid matter.

Prof. Wood says: "Children prematurely born, or brought up by the hand, or nursed by unhealthy women, are more liable to be affected than others. In fact, whatever tends to impair the health and vigour of the infant, to induce acidity of the stomach, or other gastric and intestinal disorder, disposes to its occurrence. Yet it often occurs under apparently the most favorable circumstances, and in healthy, well fed children."

I shall proceed, as briefly as possible, to give the outlines of treatment I have found most successful, without, however, entering into particulars. As the disease is purely local, yet as the constitution sometimes, though secondarily, suffers, we must, when indicated, use a constitutional as well as a local treatment. I look upon topical applications as forming the most important part of the cure in most cases; and indeed in the milder forms, nothing more is needed. Borax, with sugar or honey; and alum combined with some vegetable astringent, I have found to answer only in mild cases, and doing little if any good, even when persevered in, in the severer forms of the malady. In such cases, my course is to apply some alkaline lotion prètty freely for a few days, and about the best is a solution of carb. potash (℥i. to ℥i. f. water); after this I use a solution of nitrate of silver, in the proportion of six, eight, and sometimes even more, grains to the ounce of water.

This is generally about all the local treatment that is required. A solution of bichlord. mercury, as recommended by the German physician, Eisenmann, may be very useful, but I have not used it. When there is diarrhœa, hydrg. c. creta, or the chalk alone, will be found very beneficial. If the diarrhœa is attended with flatulence and acid eructations, and greenish curdy stools, rhubarb combined with sup. carb. soda, in the proportion of 4 or 6 grs. of the former to 6 or 8 grs. of the latter, and given in some carminative infusion, *pro re natâ*, (a prescription peculiar to myself in such cases,) answers better than any thing I have used. After this, astringents must be resorted to, and I have found the mineral astringents best. Of these, a solution of nitrate of iron is to be preferred. I have used this for several years. It is much more astringent and efficient than a solution of chloride of iron, and not in the least caustic, and when given in doses of 8–10, or even more, drops, three times a day, or oftener if necessary, it diminishes the irritability of the weakened and relaxed mucous membrane of the stomach and bowels.

We must not, however, lose sight of alkalies, both topically and internally, whenever the indications call for their use. I always avoid any compound into which sugar enters, either as a local application, or as an internal remedy; for the sugar is converted into acid, which favors the increase of the malady.

We may often premise our treatment with an emetic, which sometimes has a very beneficial effect."

The opinions expressed by Dr. Rea, in the foregoing essay, were at variance with the views of some of the members of the Society; but, on account of the intense cold, it was received without any discussion.

Strangulated Hernia.—Dr. J. E. Walker reported a case of Strangulated Hernia which occurred in the person of a young man, J. L——, aged about twenty-two. "He was a laborer in one of our manufactories, of spare but muscular form and temperate habits. First saw him at 3 o'clock, P. M., of the 14th December ult., and found him in the most intense agony of pain, which he referred to the region of the umbilicus. Upon investigation, I elicited the following:

He has been the subject of a small oblique Inguinal Hernia of the right side, from a boy, but as he had suffered little inconvenience from it, he had never before made it known even to the members of his own family. He states that the tumor has never entirely disappeared since he first noticed it, which, as will he seen, is one of its chief points of interest. On the morning of the day above stated, his bowels became relaxed, and after straining at stool, he discovered that the hernia had descended much lower than usual, and that the tumor was much larger, which, however, did not create pain until after a second evacuation. He now felt as if a cord were being drawn tightly between the testicle and navel, giving rise to excruciating pain, and causing an entire inability to return the hernia. On examining the tumor, which was small, I found it so tender that the patient could not bear the slightest pressure—the greatest pain being at the seat of stricture. So great was the suffering, that the gentlest manipulations produced violent muscular agitation, amounting almost to convulsions. He had vomited freely before I saw him, and continued retching severely, and occasionally ejecting a thick yellowish matter, with some bile, but no fecal matter that I could discover—the whole surface was cold and of a purplish hue.

In this state of things I determined to apply fomentations to the tumor, with cloths wrung out of water as hot as could be borne, and also bloodletting was attempted but failed, in consequence of the coldness of the surface and smallness of the veins. After having used the warm applications for thirty minutes, I made an unsuccessful attempt to replace the hernia. I ordered the fomentations continued while I went to my office for medicine; and after my return, finding the patient a little more quiet, with a warmer surface, I attempted again to bleed him, but succeeded in extracting only a few ounces of blood.

I now determined to try the effects of Tart. Emetic, of which I gave him one-fourth of a grain at short intervals. The second dose having produced slight vomiting, and knowing the danger of my case being made worse by the straining of emesis, I guarded the tumor with the palm of my hand, to prevent a further descent until the vomiting should cease, at which moment I used the Taxis, and was much gratified to find that I could reduce the tumor to less than half its original size, but it could not be entirely returned. The pain was now mitigated, but not relieved. Farther interference being deemed improper for the present, I administered half a grain of Morphine and left him, with a promise to return at 7 o'clock. Dr. H. H. King, to whom I am under many obligations for his valuable suggestions and assistance, saw the case with me at the hour appointed. We found the patient about as I had left him, except that he was more composed and had less arterial excitement. He had just vomited, but without affecting the tumor. At the suggestion of Dr. King, he was placed in the warm hip-bath, and while in it, another attempt was made to bleed him. Although the V. S. was not as successful as we desired, the patient, partly from loss of blood and partly from the influence of the bath, was fast approaching syncope; while in that state he was placed in bed with the hips elevated, and Dr. King was requested to try the "Taxis," which he did for some minutes, with great pain to the patient and little effect on the tumor. I made another attempt with no better success.

The patient insisted that it was now as far reduced as it had been for years; was free from pain, except when the tumor was handled, and that in that condition, he suffered no inconvenience whatever. Accordingly, we agreed to give him half a grain of morphine and leave him for the night. On the morn-

ing of the 19th I saw my patient, and to my gratification found
the tumor had entirely disappeared, without his consciousness.
He had fallen asleep soon after we left him on the night previous, had rested well all night, and awoke in the morning to
the pleasant reality of finding his hernia gone and himself free
from pain. He was directed to keep his bed for a few days,
and to have a suitable instrument for retaining his bowels in
their natural cavity. I saw him in the afternoon of the same
day, and found him with some fever and tongue furred. Directed him to take half an ounce of castor oil, which acted
kindly; next day he walked about the house, and in a very
short time was attending to his ordinary business."

Case of Uterine Polypus, by Dr. H. H. King.—On the 19th
day of Feb., 1851, I was called to see a negro woman who had
been suffering for six months or more with a "misery," as she
termed it, in the lower part of the abdomen. I supposed the
pain was seated in the uterus, from the fact that she had not
been "regular" for some months, and as she told me she
thought it was about time for the catamenia to appear. I prescribed a cathartic and warm hip-bath, which relieved her for
a short time, although her catamenia did not appear. In the
early part of the spring I saw her again, when she told me she
thought she was laboring under prolapsus uteri. I made a digital examination, and instead of a prolapsus, I found a tumor
about the size of a hen's egg, which I partly succeeded in removing with caustics, not having a suitable instrument to operate with. On the 8th of July I saw her again. She told me,
when I arrived, that she had suffered all the pains of childbirth,
and, to use her own expression, "her body had come from her."
Being dissatisfied with the digital examination I had made, I
found, on occular inspection, that a polypous tumor, weighing
three pounds, had been extruded. Before removing it, I requested my friend, Dr. Walker, to see the case with me. After
examining the tumor and satisfying ourselves of its nature and
the manner of removing it, we proceeded to take it away,
which we did by ligating the pedicle as high up as we could,
and cutting it through with the knife. I endeavored to procure an instrument for the removal of the attachment, but

failed in doing so.   After several weeks, the ligature and a portion of the pedicle came away, and her general health improved
very much.   I do not look upon the case as cured, on account
of the great disposition of such tumors to form again, and from
not having a suitable instrument to remove the attachment.
This tumor has been deposited in the Museum of the Medical
College of Georgia.

Dr. Rea wished to know the nature of the polypus in question, and on being informed that it was of a fibrous character,
urged an objection to Dr. King's opinion that fibrous polypi
are prone to return; he (Dr. R.) thought such tumors seldom
returned.

Dr. O'Keeffe said that fibrous polypi of the uterus, as a general rule, do not reproduce themselves, unless they assume a
malignant character, as they sometimes do; but that fibrous
polypi, in other parts of the body, may grow again.

Pneumonia treated with Veratrum Viride.—Dr. R. S. Cal-
loway referred to three cases of pneumonia, well marked and
violent at their commencement, which he had brought to a favorable termination by the use of the American Hellebore.
They were treated for four or five days with the usual remedies: v. s. cal. diaphoretics, expectorants and blisters, without
any mitigation of their symptoms; indeed every thing seemed
to portend unfavorably when he commenced the use of the veratrum viride, and in a day or two, the condition of the patients
ceased to be dangerous, and their convalescence was rapid.
Dr. C. uses a saturated tincture of his own make, in the dose
of 12 gtt. every two hours until a decided effect on the system
is manifested by nausea and a diminution in the frequency of
the pulse; he then suspends its use for ten or twelve hours,
after which, he repeats it as before, and so on as long as the
symptoms require it.   In connection with the veratrum viride,
Dr. C. uses an anodyne expectorant occasionally, and aperients to keep the bowels in a laxative condition.

Dr. Rea gave his experience with the American Hellebore
as favorable to the good effects already attributed to it ; and
added that, in his opinion, its sedative properties were owing
to the nausea it induced, in the same way that ipecac. and tart.
antimony are sedative.

Dr. O'Keeffe added his testimony in favor of the report just made by Dr. Callaway, respecting the very beneficial effects of the veratrum viride in reducing the heart's action, and asserted that he had rather be deprived of all other sedative agents than the one under consideration. He did not believe that its great controling power over the circulation was entirely owing to its nauseating effects: he thought the remedy had a direct sedative influence over the heart and arteries through the medium of the nervous system, for he had seen the hellebore reduce the frequency of the pulse without any nausea or vomiting.

Dr. Jas. F. Foster made allusions to some interesting cases of midwifery which had come under his observation. One was a woman who had had nine children, intermitted child-bearing for nine years, during which she suffered from leucorrhœa several times—took "some medicine," and conceived again after nine years intermission. Another case was a woman he had attended and delivered of a full grown child without her having any knowledge of her pregnancy. She had borne no children for a few years, lived on good terms with her husband, in respectable society, and had no reason whatever to falsify.

Urethral inflammation in the female.—Dr. D. C. O'Keeffe read a report of a case of urethral inflammation in the female, supposed to be caused by the continued use of the catheter for two or three weeks. The subject was a woman of feeble constitution and lymphatic temperament. Six months previous to my seeing her, she was delivered of a full grown child after a somewhat tedious labor. After delivery the bladder was evacuated for two or three weeks in succession by the catheter, owing to a temporary paralysis of that organ. From this time dates the commencement of the state I shall presently describe. Her recovery from child-bed was slow and satisfactory, with the exception that she suffered very much from ardor urinæ and after urinating discharged some blood *guttatim*. For this she took various diuretic preparations with but little, if any, benefit to her sufferings. During this time she was under the care of the gentleman who attended her in confinement, and came under my care in the above condition.

Prescribed the tripple syrup of buchu, uva ursi, and pareira brava, lunar caustic injections into the urethra, and leeches to vulva and perineum. Of these but the first was used, owing to the patient's own objections, and the ext. belladonna was recommended as a substitute, which latter proved of no benefit. While under the use of the above diuretic syrup, she was entirely relieved from ardor urinæ and hematuria, but on discontinuing it, the ardor would return and continue a few days and be followed by the hematuria. She continued this remedy for four months without any suffering while taking it, but on its discontinuance, the same result would ensue that did at first.

Seeing no prospect of permanent benefit from the syrup, she at length consented to use the lunar caustic, to which she objected solely through fear of its severity. A solution of lunar caustic $\frac{1}{2}$ gr. to 1 oz. was injected into the urethra, but three times with a glass syringe, and no return of the disease has been experienced since. The pain in urinating, was quite severe after the use of the caustic, but it soon subsided and returned no more. She used none of the syrup after the first application of the caustic.

REMARKS. In this case we see exemplified the error of not yielding immediate and implicit obedience to the physician's prescription; for to her own reluctance to use the caustic may be fairly attributed her long and needless suffering. The present and beneficial effects of local applications of nit. silver to affections of the mucous membranes are also illustrated in the case before us, as well as the inutility of treating such affections with constitutional remedies. And from it, I would also draw the practical inference, that the promiscuous treatment of gonorrhœa in the female, by means of vaginal injections, is incorrect and indefinite, inasmuch as the vagina, the urethra or the cavity of the uterine neck may be each respectively the seat of the gonorrhœal inflammation; hence the use of the speculum is indispensable to a correct diagnosis, and consequently to a correct mode of treatment.

The cause of the urethral inflammation in the case just reported was attributed by the patient and friends to the long continued use of the catheter, and I think, in all probability, with good reason, as the patient and husband were altogether above suspicion in a moral point of view.   There was an error of omission, perhaps, in her management in childbed (as stated by herself and husband,) which consisted in suffering the bladder to become so distended before resorting to catheterism that it became entirely paralysed temporarily, thereby prolonging the necessity for the use of the catheter.   So that the whole difficulty might have been prevented had her attending physician obviated by the intervention of art, the supervention of the condition that rendered necessary the long continued use of the catheter.

In bringing these remarks to a close, I would wish to call the attention of the Society to the abnormal effects of cod liver oil on this patient, which she took, the year following the date of the above notes, for general debility.   She lost in weight, but gained in density of the muscular system.

ARTICLE IX.

Medical Statistics of the last Georgia Census.   By JOHN S. WILSON, M. D., of Muscogee county, Georgia.

There are some facts revealed by the last Census in Georgia, of such a striking character, that they cannot fail to engage the attention of the medical profession; and I have therefore compiled the following table (which has cost me much labor) for the benefit of the readers of the Journal.   The facts alluded to above, and which will be disclosed by the table, are these— viz: 1st. That the Middle Counties of Georgia are less salubrious than the Southern ones, contrary to the common opinion. 2nd. That Georgia, taken as a whole, stands unrivalled in salubrity, giving less than twelve deaths in one thousand persons.   3rd. The table will present some striking facts in connexion with the health of different counties, which are sufficiently remarkable to engage the attention of all who wish to find a healthy location.   I have divided the State into three parts—Northern, Southern and Middle—giving the total population of each county, and the number of deaths during the year 1850, together with the proportion of deaths in each Division, &c.—as follows:

Northern Counties.	Population.	Deaths.	Northern Counties.	Population.	Deaths.
Cass,	13,300	105	Brought up,	120,619	860
Chatooga,	6,815	79	Gwinnett,	11,257	110
Cherokee,	12,800	81	Habersham,	8,895	17
Cobb,	13,743	24	Hall,	8,713	69
Dade,	3,682	30	Jackson,	9,768	91
De Kalb,	14,328	118	Lumpkin,	8,954	46
Elbert,	12,959	143	Madison,	5,603	68
Floyd,	8,205	49	Murray,	14,433	67
Forsyth,	8,850	39	Paulding,	7,039	66
Franklin,	11,513	96	Rabun,	2,448	12
Gilmer,	8,440	54	Union,	7,234	64
Gordon,	5,984	42	Walker,	13,109	139
Carried up,	120,619	860		218,072	1609

A fraction over 7 deaths in 1000 persons. Least mortality in Cobb, which gives the remarkably small mortality of $1\frac{3}{4}$ or near that in 1000 persons.

Middle Counties.	Population.	Deaths.	Middle Counties.	Population.	Deaths.
Baldwin,	8,148	77	Brought up,	208,299	2550
Bibb,	12,699	177	Lincoln,	5,998	94
Burke,	16,100	326	Meriwether,	16,476	210
Butts,	6,488	55	Monroe,	16,985	210
Campbell,	7,232	62	Morgan,	10,744	216
Carroll,	9,357	70	Newton,	13,296	95
Clark,	11,119	149	Oglethorpe,	12,259	175
Columbia,	11,961	86	Pike,	14,305	150
Coweta,	13,635	218	Putnam,	10,794	160
Crawford,	8,984	118	Richmond,	16,246	291
Fayette,	8,709	99	Talbot,	16,534	208
Greene,	13,068	242	Taliaferro,	5,146	88
Hancock,	11,578	128	Troup,	16,879	148
Harris,	14,721	149	Twiggs,	8,179	107
Heard,	6,923	41	Upson,	9,424	74
Henry,	14,726	157	Walton,	10,821	135
Jasper,	11,486	180	Warren,	12,425	138
Jones,	10,224	85	Washington,	11,766	159
Jefferson,	9,131	131	Wilkes,	12,107	193
Carried up,	208,299	2550		426,673	5401

Nearly $12\frac{1}{2}$ deaths in 1000 persons. Healthiest county, Heard—next, Carroll, Jones, Fayette and Newton. Greatest mortality in Burke.

Southern Counties.	Population.	Deaths.	Southern Counties.	Population.	Deaths.
Appling,	2,949	27	Brought up,	127,066	1649
Baker,	8,120	126	Lowndes,	8,351	64
Bryan,	3,424	63	Macon,	7,052	00
Bullock,	4,300	28	Marion,	10,280	72
Camden,	6,319	61	McIntosh,	6,028	111
Chatham,	23,900	385	Montgomery,	2,154	22
Decatur,	8,262	92	Muscogee,	18,578	187
Dooly,	8,361	110	Pulaski,	6,627	87
Early,	7,246	55	Randolph,	12,868	130
Effingham,	3,864	68	Scriven,	6,847	32
Emanuel,	4,577	25	Stewart,	16,027	156
Glynn,	4,933	106	Sumpter,	10,322	140
Houston,	16,450	201	Tattnall,	3,227	10
Irwin,	3,334	15	Telfair,	3,026	9
Laurens,	6,442	54	Thomas,	10,103	125
Lee,	6,659	117	Ware,	3,888	18
Liberty,	7,926	116	Wayne,	1,499	10
			Wilkinson,	8,214	87
Carried up,	127,066	1649		262,154	2909

About 11½ deaths to 1000 persons. Healthiest county, Macon, no death—three next, Telfair, Tattnall and Scriven.

Whole population, 905,999. Number of deaths, 9,920—not quite 11 deaths to 1000 persons.

ARTICLE X.

Cold Water in Puerperal Convulsions. By G. W. Booth, M. D., of Carrollville, Mississippi.

In the year 1848, I was called early one morning to see Mrs. E. W., wife of P. W. On my arrival, I was informed that she had been in labour for several hours. She was about 18 years of age, short stature, and of ruddy appearance. This was her first pregnancy, and I was informed by the old midwife who was in attendance that the labour appeared to progress favorably till a short time before I was called in. The patient's friends had discovered some convulsive twitchings about her face which alarmed them, and I was consequently summoned.

The waters had been discharged sometime before I saw her. On examination, I found the head at the inferior strait presenting naturally, and the soft parts in a favorable condition. The

pains appeared to be effective.   Soon after I had made an examination, the muscular twitchings about the face deepened
into the most terrific general convulsions I have ever witnessed.   She was delivered in a few minutes after the accession of
the convulsions, of a fine healthy girl, of average size.   I was
in hopes, after this event, that some mitigation, at least, would
take place in the symptoms.   In this, however, I was disappointed, as the convulsions continued to recur as before.   She
remained perfectly unconscious, from the first severe paroxysm,
throughout the course of the disease.   I put into vigorous play
all the usual remedies for this formidable disease, but without
influencing it materially.   I continued this treatment till late
in the evening.   I now despaired of the patient's life, and announced the fact to her husband and friends.   As a dernier
resort, I determined to try the effect of cold water, applied by
pouring it freely over the whole system.   To carry this treatment into effect, I had her taken from the bed and laid on the
floor, with a quilt under her and a sheet thrown over her body.
I then, from a large pitcher, poured water, fresh from a well,
over her, from head to feet, for several minutes.   After the
application of the water, I had dry clothes put on the patient,
and she was replaced in bed.   In the course of half an hour
after this she awoke from the stupor, which had existed since
morning, perfectly rational, and had no return of convulsions
after the water had been used.   She now had no recollection
of anything that had taken place since the first convulsion, and
appeared to be surprised to learn that her child was born.

There was inability to pass of her urine, and I drew off a
large quantity with a catheter—the state of her bladder having
been unattended to in the earlier part of her labour.   I used
the instrument but once, as she was able afterwards to evacuate the bladder without its aid.   She had a fine "getting-up,"
and was as well in a few days as is common after the most
favorable labours.

Mrs. W. has borne two children since, without any untoward
circumstance attending either labours.

PART II.

Eclectic Department

Some Remarks on the recent Discovery, that the Chief motive
Power of the Blood is in the Lungs and not in the Heart,
and its application to useful Purposes. By SAMUEL A.
CARTWRIGHT, M. D., of New Orleans, late of Natchez.

I have elsewhere detailed the experiments proving, by ocular demonstration, in the vivisection of alligators, made in this city, that the chief motive power of the blood is in the lungs, and not in the heart.   Animation was restored by artificial respiration, after the animal experimented on had been perfectly dead to all appearances for about an hour.   Organic as well as animal life had been destroyed by tying the trachea. It is a remarkable fact that tying the trachea is the only means by which that amimal can be expeditiously killed.   They will live for days after decapitation, or immersed in water, but speedily die when the trachea is tied.   After life had been, to all appearances, completely extinguished, the heart, lungs and abdominal viscera were exposed to view by a careful dissection.   The inflating process was then commenced.   The blood, at length, was seen to move from the vessels of the lungs to the quiescent heart—thus proving that the primum mobile and chief motive power of the blood are in the lungs and not in the heart.   Dr. Dowler, who performed the vivisection, supposed that atmospheric air imparted to the globules of the blood a self-locomotory.   According, however, to the theory of Mrs. Willard, of Troy, to test which some of the experiments were made, it is the caloric evolved in the transformation of venous into arterial blood that gives the motion.   Be this as it may, the important discovery that the primum mobile of the blood and its chief motive power are in the lungs, rests not on theory, but on ocular demonstration, repeated again and again.   Mr. Crawford, long ago, attempted to explain the phenomena of animal heat by supposing that the caloric, generated in the lungs by respiration, was conveyed through the arterial system in a latent state to all parts of the body, and was there given out in the form of sensible heat.   The foundation of this theory was the greater capacity of arterial than venous blood, for caloric.   His premises were denied by Davy and the most of his co-temporaries—but subsequent observations have proved them to be correct in the main.   Mrs. Willard's theory of the motive powers of the blood rests upon the same basis as that of Mr. Crawford's doctrine of calorification—the different capacity of arterial and venous blood for caloric.   The theory itself is not the subject under consideration, but only in its main proposition, that the chief motive power of the blood is in the lungs, and not in the heart. Whatever be thought of the theory itself, it has the high merit of having announced a most important truth, which is proved by ocular demonstration, and will stand as an important discovery, whether the reasoning that led to it be correct or not.

I propose to make some remarks on the application of this important American discovery to useful and practical purposes. Lord Bacon truly says: "For of all the signs of philosophies none are more certain and noble than those taken from their fruits. For fruits and the discoveries of works are as the vouchers and securities of the truth of philosophies." "As it is in religion that faith be manifested by works, philosophy should be judged by its fruits, and held as vain if it prove barren."—(*Nov. Org., Sect.* iv. 73.) The discovery that the chief motive power of the blood is in the lungs, and not in the heart as Harvey supposed, I propose to show will not prove barren, but rich in useful fruits—"the vouchers and securities for its truth." Lest, however, some errors which have crept into physiology, may prevent any portion of those physcians, who are not too old or full of prejudice to receive a new idea conflicting with their former opinions, from seeing and believing in the discovery, it may not be amiss to surround it with some of the highest authorities in medicine, each holding a light so closely to it, as to convince the sceptical that it rests on the rock of the latest revealed truths in science, and not, as they might gratuitously suppose, on idle speculations behind the times.

Among the authorities, Sir Benjamin Brodie stands foremost and closest, he having, many years ago, come very near stumbling on the discovery. He killed a cat; i. e. paralyzed the action of the heart and lungs, with the poison called *woòrara*, and then by dint of artificial respiration, kept up for two hours and a half, brought the animal to life. He saw so far into the mystery of the motive power of the blood, as to ascertain that the heart's action depended upon the action of the lungs; and hence the experiment with the cat was to see whether life might not be preserved by artificial respiration until the effect of the poison on the nervous system had time to wear away. Sir Benjamin's idea was good, and true as far as it went, but it did not reach the main truth of the discovery first announced in Troy, and subsequently demonstrated in New Orleans. Although he brought the cat to life, he had no suspicion that the chief motive power of the blood was in the lungs, and that the heart performed a subordinate part in giving it momentum. His experiment, however, went far enough to prove, that Bichat

and some other physiologists, in supposing that the blood continued, for a time, to circulate through the lungs by the action
of the heart after respiration ceased, only becoming unaërated
after the lungs ceased to act, fell into a great error, which for
many years misled investigation from the true path of inquiry.

Dr. Kay, however, deserves much credit for correcting the
error, which he has done by proving, that as soon as respiration stops, the blood begins to stagnate in the pulmonary
capillaries, because it ceases to be transformed from venous
to arterial. In the language of the new philosophy, because
its motive power is taken away by the cessation of the process
of arterialization, therefore it stagnates. Dr. Kay ascertained
the fact, but he could not divine the cause. His researches do
not go far enough to detract from the merits of the discovery,
but they furnish sufficient light to show that it rests upon scientific truth.

Baron Cuvier, the highest authority in natural philosophy,
brings the light of that science in support of the new doctrine,
that the chief motive power of the blood is in the respiratory
organs. His great work, called "Animal Kingdom," revised
by Latreille, article Reptilia, says—" The blood derives its heat
and the fibre its susceptibility of nervous irritation from respiration." Not only that, but his other great work—" Le-
cons d'Anatomie comparée," abounds with proof of the intimate
relation of muscular motion and nervous influences, with respiration as their source and spring. Speaking of animals, he
says, "Chacune de ses classes jouit de la faculté de se mouvoir
précisément dans le degré qui correspond à la quantité de la
respiration."—(*Vol. I.* p. 52.) The blood could not derive
heat from respiration without deriving more or less power of
motion; because caloric is not inoperative. Those who object to the truths of natural philosophy as authority in medicine, forget that the former is the root of the latter. Hence
objections, drawn from medical theories, should have no weight
when brought against the truths of the mother science.

Harvey discovered the course of the circulation of the blood,
but he did not discover the chief power that moved it. His
discovery was incomplete, as it erroneously placed it in the
heart instead of the lungs. In consequence of this radical error,
the science of medicine has not been as much enriched by the
discovery of the circulation as was anticipated, as it only served
to lead the blind into a dazzling and uncertain light—whereas
the discovery that the chief motive power of the blood is located in the lungs, and not in the heart as was erroneously supposed, has opened a rich field for improvement in physiology,
pathology, and in the more successful methods of treatment in

disease. Before Dr. Bassi, charged, by the scientific congress
lately held at Genoa, to explain the reason why silk worms fed
on indigo leaves have a blue color imparted to the membranes
between the parietes of the air-tubes, can give a satisfactory
explanation of that phenomenon ; and before Prof. Bryan, of
Philadelphia, can interpret the experiments he is now making
on papilios, they will have to look into the anatomy and physiology of those insects, brought into the light furnished by the discovery locating the motive power of the blood in the lungs.
The dorsal vessel, called the heart, according to Cuvier, has no
muscularity, although these insects have upwards of four thousand muscles.   M. Lyonet counted in the caterpillar, called
the cassus lignéperda, 4041 distinct muscles.   The heart has
but one artery, and that artery no branches.   The muscles
have no blood-vessels distributed to them, nor is there any cellular membrane between the layers of their fasciculi, being
parallel and without attachment except at their origin and insertion—resembling hairs tied at their two ends.   There are
no veins, but more nerves than in the human body, viz : 47 pair
in the papilios.   Every part of the insect is pervaded by tracheal branches penetrating to the extremeties of every appendage of the body ; yet in the interstices between the tracheal
vessels the nutritive juices, which the experimenters found
colored in those worms fed on indigo leaves, are carried by
some unknown agency to all parts of the body—no doubt by
the same spring or locomotive power which in man is the primum mobile of the blood.

But it is not so much in explaining mysteries in entomology
that the discovery is valuable, but in leading the way to important improvements in therapeutics and other practical and
useful sciences.   Thus before roses can be planted on the pallid
cheek, it is important to know in what way healthy red blood
can be soonest made, warmed, depurated and kept in motion.
Before the " young idea can be taught to shoot." *with vigor,*
it is all-important that a current of red healthy blood be distributed to the brain—the organ of thought.   The same important agent, red healthy blood, is absolutely necessary to give
tone, vigor and symmetry to the body, and to prevent it from
falling an untimely prey to consumption and other ills.   But it
is not so generally known, that red healthy blood is just as
necessary for the full developement and integrity of the moral faculties as the intellectual ; and under this aspect, the discovery of its motive powers has strong claims to the attention
of theologians.   Church history bears witness, that *" the stony
ground "* where the seed of christian truth takes no deep root,
is the very ground trod by a people whose blood is vitiated by

idleness, filth, impure air and unwholesome diet.   Instance, the indolent Hindoos and other inhabitants of populous Asia, breathing the impure air of crowded hovels without sufficient food or clothing.   Instance, the idle eaters of ant eggs and caterpillars, overspreading Africa, and the denizens of the cellars of London. Education, therefore, in its broadest sense, physical, moral, religious and intellectual, is essentially and indissolubly connected with red healthy blood.   Hence, when Mrs. Willard indicated one of the chief ways, by which red healthy blood could be made at will, and that every child could be taught to make it for itself, she was not, as it was supposed, out of her province, as the head of a renowned institution of learning, but standing on the broad platform of her profession, and directing the building of a permanent basis for it to rest upon throughout all time. In forming that basis, she naturally looked into the science of physiology for certain materials in regard to the motive powers of the blood ; and not finding them there, after going as far as Harvey went, she brought that science back to natural philosophy, the parent from which it sprung, which receiving new strength and increase therefrom, readily conducted her to the hiding place of the materials she was seeking—a golden fleece, more valuable than that of fable.   If some medical men gainsayed her for overturning things on the altar of Harvey, it was because they had not reflected that the empire of science, so long encroached on by empiricism, calls for enlargement, and that America, like Rome, needs a Minerva.   Surely the almshouse, the hospital and the sick room, is too small an empire for the numerous votaries of the comprehensive science of medicine—a science, like the Crystal Palace, embracing almost everything worthy to behold in its study, but narrowed down in its practical exercise to a few common-place duties, associating it in the public mind with nothing but nauseous drugs, making it the terror of the people, and in too many instances driving them from its advantages until the fear of death is upon them. So much knowledge, with a field too small to call a tithe of it into requisition, requires the extension of the practical sphere of its operations, and that sphere will need enlargement until it embraces in its practical boundaries, not only therapeutics, hygiene, &c., but the art, long sought after by the ancients, of making the old younger, children healthy, men vigorous, and women pretty.   This art has always been imperfect ; its basis or starting point—a knowledge of the motive powers of the blood and the ways and means of making red healthy blood at will—having been unknown.   While the erroneous hypothesis of Harvey prevailed, that the heart, whose action is not under the will, was the primum mobile and chief motive power of the circulating fluids, instead of the lungs, which are under the will, there was no known way, except through the slow and uncertain process of diet, change of climate, exercise, or a course of medicine, by which the vitiated, cold, impoverished circulating fluids could be reached, depurated, or rendered red, warm and healthy. Body, mind and morals had to suffer all the effects of deteriorated humors as a necessary evil—the direct road to purify the blood through the respiratory organs being unknown, from incorrect theories of the power that moved it and the location of that power.

The true doctrine on this subject was no sooner promulgated, than I reduced it to practice, and have made it tell well as a valuable adjuvant in the treatment of many diseases, particularly those of a chronic kind, and the cold, phlegmatic ailments so common among females in hot climates. Some complaints, especially acute inflammations, require repose of the respiratory organs, absolute rest and a spare diet ; while the great mass of chronic and congestive disorders are greatly benefited by their activity. Thus in pleurisy, the curative process of nature prevents full respiration by piercing the side with pain whenever the ribs are expanded ; because the motive power of the blood being in the lungs, full breathing would aggravate a complaint consisting in too much heat and momentum. On the other hand, the cold, congestive and torpid affections require increased activity of the lungs to heat, redden, and vivify the circulating fluids. Full breathing in the open air and sun light is beneficial to children of infirm constitutions, and applicable to most of the diseases and infirmities peculiar to females, greatly assisting other necessary remedies, as malaxation, friction, inunction, bathing, &c., to improve the complexion, to prevent the hair from falling out, and the teeth from decay.

There has been a fearful increase of consumption and female complaints, and a large field opened for dentists, since the old-fashioned spinning wheel, called the big wheel, has been laid aside. In ancient times the women ground at the mill—that is, turned a horizontal stone with an upright staff for a handle, requiring them to stand up and to use both hands. Two women grinding at the mill, standing opposite to each other, was one of the best species of exercise to expand the lungs and to depurate the blood, without giving coarseness to the muscular system and no doubt greatly contributed to the health, grace and classic beauty for which the ancient women were so renowned. The discovery of the motive power of the blood, and the location of that power, will be a good antidote against the folies of Bloomerism, enticing women to assume indiscriminately the avocations of men. Most of these avocations would make them coarse, rough and masculine in appearance, like the weather-beaten female peasantry of Europe. The discovery is valuable as a key to find those species of exercise, which do not give coarseness, deformity and masculineness to the general muscular system and its tegumentary covering, but softness, symmetry, agility and grace, united with health, as the wheel and the mill-stone formerly gave. A substitute for the last-mentioned exercises is yet a desideratum. Mrs. Willard's substitute of early rising and running backward and forward before an open window, moving the arms and expanding the chest, is a very good one, but is defective in not being associated with some visible object of utility, and consequently somewhat difficult in being generally practised to a sufficient extent. The inventor of some species of play or kind of work, requiring similar movements, would be entitled to the thanks of the community. It could be improved by being performed in the morning sunshine, as sunlight is particularly beneficial to youth in strengthening their constitutions.

It was a rule in Egypt to bestow divinity and consecration upon the inventor of any useful remedy or thing ; and as instinct oftener than reason led to discoveries, the Egyptian deities were mostly in the form of reptiles and other animals of the brute creation. But if America, like Egypt, Greece and Rome, is to have mythological divinities, I am sure that none will object to their coming in the form and likeness of woman. Hence I have no apology to make to the profession, of which I am a humble member, for giving in my adhesion to an important practical truth in science, first announced by an American lady, long famous for her erudition and intelligence, and for the number of our country's fair daughters who have been refined and polished by her hands.—[*Boston Med. Journal.*

Report of three Cases in which Lactation was reproduced by the application of the Child to the Breast. By ARIEL BALLOU, M. D. (Read to the Rhode Island Medical Society.)

CASE I. In the autumn of 1836, Mrs. J. G., aged between thirty and forty years, of sanguine temperament, robust constitution, and the mother of several children, was confined. The presentation was natural, and no unusual circumstances attended her delivery. Subsequently she suffered from an attack of phlegmasia dolens in both of the lower extremities, attended with high febrile action, and, as is usual in such cases, extreme suffering. The secretion of milk ceasing early in the disease, the child was removed to a wet nurse, with whom it remained three or four months, during which time there was no return of milk. In the spring of 1837, the family being about to move a short distance from the village, where they could enjoy a better air and a more unrestricted exercise, the mother was anxious to take her infant with her, but did not like to deprive it of the advantages of the breast during the then coming warm season. I advised the mother to take her child and apply it to the breasts in the same manner she would do if she had a flow of milk, assuring her it was my confident opinion that in two or three weeks she would have milk, and a sufficient quantity, at least her usual supply.

She did so, and in about two weeks the secretion of milk was reproduced. She continued to nurse her child for more than a year, producing her accustomed quantity of milk.

Case II. Mrs. N. D., aged about twenty-five years, was confined in December, 1841. Nothing worthy of note transpired during her confinement and recovery. In April following her child weaned itself, in consequence of a sore mouth. Her milk soon entirely disappeared. In July following I was called to see her child, which was suffering from an attack of cholera infantum. Having lost several children about that time from this disease, I expressed my regret that the child was deprived of the benefits of the breast, adding, that in my opinion its chances of recovery were diminished in consequence.

The mother was informed of the course I had advised in other cases where it was desirable to reproduce the secretion, and of the results. On my visit the succeeding day, she informed me that she had applied the child to the breast, and that it nursed and seemed pleased and more quiet; but she was not aware that any milk was obtained or that she had any for it. I advised her to persevere in the application of the child to the breasts, which she did, and the child recovered, and in the course of a week or ten days obtained a full supply of nutriment from the breasts.

The mother continued to nurse for months with as full and perfect a secretion of milk as though no interruption in the secretion had occurred.

The following case I report as having an important practical bearing on the treatment and disposal of a class of cases which occur in our community at the present day, to cure which or otherwise dispose of satisfactorily to the physician, is often found difficult.

Case III. Mrs. O. H. H., aged about twenty-one years, of feeble constitution and nervo-lymphatic temperament, was confined in July, 1847. Previous to her accouchment she was troubled with chronic aphtha, red canker, or with that condition

of the system which is well known as "sore mouth attendant
on pregnancy and lactation." Nothing unusual occurred at
the time of delivery. No considerable loss of blood was sustained. As in similar cases, there was a remission of diarrhœa
and sore mouth for a few days after accouchment, giving rise to
a hope that, being relieved from the condition of pregnancy, she
would recover the powers of digestion and the assimilation of
nutriment, so as to enable the system to sustain the calls upon it
consequent to lactation. But in the course of ten or twelve
days after accouchment the sore mouth and diarrhœa returned
with increased violence, producing great debility. The secretion of milk was copious. Her pulse 120; the tongue flabby;
there were frequent copious dejections of yellowish water, the
face and extremities bloated, &c. Fearing the worst results
for my patient, I advised the immediate removal of the child
from the breasts of the mother to those of a wet nurse, at the
same time informing the parents that on the recovery of the
mother she could at pleasure reapply the child to the breasts
and have a full supply of milk, and be enabled to perform all the
duties and functions of a mother for an indefinite period of time.
The child was given in charge of a wet nurse, the milk gradually
disappeared, and the patient recovered under the use of tonic
remedies and a generous diet. Between two and three months
after this the mother called on me, having the appearance of
restored health, and inquired if she might now take her child
home with a hope of realizing my former assurances that she
would be able to reproduce her milk. I assured her there was
no doubt in relation to such a result, and her ability for the future
to nurse her child. She took the child, applied it to the breasts,
and in the course of two weeks had a good supply of milk.

I met her some nine months after, when she informed me
she was happy in the enjoyment of good health, and, to use
her words, she "had as good a breast of milk as if she had never
dried it up."—[*American Jour. of Med. Sci.*

---

*Retro-Pharyngeal Abscess, its Medical History and Treatment,
&c.,* By CHARLES M. ALLEN, M. D., Resident Surgeon of
the New York Hospital.

[A reprint from the *New York Journal of Medicine,* of an
article with the above title, deserves *condensation* for our
readers.]

Position of Abscess. Between the posterior wall of the
pharynx and the cervical vertebræ.

Acute Abscess, Predisposing Causes. Same as predispose
to the formation of abscess in other parts of the body; may be

the result of hereditary scrofulous taint, of the poison of syphilis, of long-continued habits of intemperance, of difficult dentition in children, of scarlatina, variola, &c. &c.

Exciting Causes. Exposure to cold, followed by inflammation of the pharynx itself, which, terminating in suppuration, deposits the pus betwee n the pharyngeal fascia, and the muscles lying upon it ; or inflammation of the lymphatic glands behind the pharynx, where these glands are found to exist, or by a foreign body, as a fish bone, passing through the posterior wall of the pharynx and forming the nucleus of abscess, or by retrocession of erysipelas, stricture of œsophagus, rheumatism, &c.

Chronic Abscess. Predisposing causes of the same character as in the acute form of the disease.

Exciting Causes. Caries or tubercular disease of the cervical vertebræ, progressing nearly in the same manner as psoas abscess.

Symptoms of Acute Form. Local uneasiness, stiffness in the back of the neck, chilliness, succeeded by febrile excitement ; though fever is not an invariable attendant, the chiliness being continuous. In young children convulsions are sometimes present, often œdematous swelling of the anterior and lateral portions of the neck ; as the disease advances soreness of throat is increased, and a sensation of a foreign body arrested at the base of the tongue is experienced; respiration difficult, voice nasal, cool perspiration about the head, pulse *always* quick and very frequent, though sometimes full and forcible. In children the dyspnœa often produces convulsions, which speedily terminate in death.

Attempts to swallow or to lie down increase the dyspnœa, and the somnolency or coma when present. The tongue is spasmodically thrust out when the patient is requested to show it, and returned with considerable difficulty, though it is often protruded from the mouth without the ability to return it.

The internal surface of the mouth and throat is congested with swelling of the tonsils and epiglottis, and an ovoid tumor may be felt by the finger pushing against the posterior wall of the pharynx, and in some instances, separating the alæ of the thyroid cartilage of the larynx. If death results, it is caused by asphyxia, or by spontaneous opening of the tumor, its contents deluging the air-passages.

Symptoms of the Chronic Abscess, are usually symptomatic of some constitutional disease, mostly traceable to hereditary taint. Pain in the back of the neck increased by moving the head, and often most severe in the after part of the day. As the disease advances, these symptoms become more marked, resulting in complete closure of the jaws. In such cases, the cavity of the abscess is liable to follow a more extended route, terminating sometimes in the mediastinal space, or again between the deep lateral fascia of the neck.

After (sometimes a long period of time) the dyspnœa, dysphagia, &c., appear as in the acute variety, but often attended with a low typhoid form of fever, which terminates in death unless promptly and skillfully treated.

For want of space we pass over the diagnosis, prognosis, and pathology of the disease, as presented by Dr. Allin, and proceed to state the treatment, which is divided into surgical and medical.

Surgical Treatment.   Make a free opening into the cavity of the abscess, as follows: suppoit the head of the patient firmly, pass the forefinger of the left hand into the mouth, raise the velum palati, and press the point of the finger against the tumor; then open with a common scalpel or bistoury, the blade being covered with sticking-plaster, to within half an inch of its extremity.   The incision should be free, at first, to avoid the necessity of repeating the operation.

Medical Treatment.   Apply emollient and soothing poultices, fomentations, &c., to the neck; after the discharge has ceased the local application of an astringent gargle, as follows :—

>   ℞. Bi-boratis sodæ ℨij;
>   Tinct. myrrhæ f℥j;
>   Syr. simplicis f℥ss;
>   Aqua puræ f℥vjss;
>   Misce.

The condition of the general system may need tonics, and even stimulants, but it is not usual to administer, where the appetite is good, and the patient's strength may be sustained by a generous system of nourishment.

The pamphlet contains, in addition to what has already been stated, a statistical table of fifty-eight cases.

[*New Jersey Med. Reporter.*

On some of the Causes of Pericarditis.   By Dr. JOHN TAYLOR.

In this communication, which appeared in the "Medico-Chirurgical Transactions," vol. xxviii. p. 453, the main object of the author is to determine what are the principal causes of pericarditis, and to ascertain their frequency, both absolutely and relatively to each other.

He does not profess to investigate all the causes of pericarditis. He has first inquired what were the causes actually observed in all the examples of the disease which have fallen un-

der his notice ; in the next place, he has investigated more in
dètail, their frequency, both absolutely and relatively to each
other, as well as some other of the circumstances connected
with each of the causes so observed ; lastly, he has examined,
incidentally, the influence of the same causes in producing inflammation of other internal organs, both in connection with,
and independently of, pericarditis.

The cases of acute and severe pericarditis examined are 35
in number.   Of these nineteen occurred in the progress of acute
rheumatism ; ten in connection with Bright's disease of the
kidneys ; three others may have had Bright's disease, but if not,
the cause is unknown ; one occurred with malformation of the
heart and consequent cyanosis ; two were produced by the extension of inflammation from a neighboring texture,—in one
from the liver and diaphragm, and in one from the left pleura.

These severe cases of pericarditis may again be conveniently
subdivided into two smaller groups.

1. Those occurring in persons previously in good health, or
in the course of an acute disease ; and 2nd. Those occurring in
persons in bad health or in the progress of some chronic disease.
A remarkable and important difference will be found in these
two divisions, in relation to the causes of the disease.   Of 29
cases examined, with a view to this difference, sixteen belong
to the first, and thirteen to the second, of the two divisions just
described.   Of the cases in the first class all were complicated
with acute rheumatism, and none of them, so far as is known,
with Bright's disease.   Of the cases in the second class, only
one was complicated with acute rheumatism ; whereas fully two
thirds were known to be associated with Bright's disease, and
all of them may have been.

The two great causes of pericarditis, therefore, appear to
have been acute rheumatism, and Bright's disease of the kidneys.   The author next enters into some considerations intended to show that these two diseases owe their power of inducing
pericarditis to the same ultimate cause, viz : an alteration in
the composition of the blood ; but he does not attempt to determine, whether the alteration in the blood be essentially the same
in relation to the production of pericarditis, in the two diseases
referred to.   If it be assumed that the pericarditis, which was
associated with cyanosis, likewise depended upon the state of
the blood in that disease, it will then appear that only two *generic* causes of the inflammation of the heart were observed in
thirty-five cases under consideration, viz : a morbid condition
of the blood, and extension of inflammation from a neighboring
texture.

The author next examines the cases of adhesion of the pericardium, and of white spots upon it, with references to the causes of the inflammation producing them ; and he arrives at the conclusion, that in every case in which any information is given upon the subject, there had previously been either acute rheumatism, or pleurisy, or there was found actually existing, either Bright's disease, or some other disease of the kidneys.

The two chief causes of acute pericarditis which were thus observed, viz : acute rheumatism, and Bright's disease of the kidneys, are next examined with more detail.

1. *Of Acute Rheumatism as a cause of Inflammation in the Heart.* The frequency of acute rheumatism, as an observed cause of pericarditis, has been already stated ; it was observed in two-thirds of all the cases of the latter disease.

Of seventy-five cases of acute rheumatism, treated by the author in University College Hospital, thirty-seven, about one-half, had, morbus cordis of some kind or degree ; the rest had probably none.

Among these seventy-five cases of rheumatism, there occurred six of acute pericarditis of considerable severity, besides two very slight cases. The proportion of the former, therefore was one in twelve and a half cases. In the same seventy-five cases of rheumatism, there were thirty two cases of valvular disease of the heart, either old or recent, besides two known to be recent. There was, therefore, one case of valvular disease in about every two cases of rheumatism.

The author next compares these results with those of various writers upon the same subject, and from this comparison he concludes—

1. That acute inflammation of the heart has occurred less frequently, as a complication of acute rheumatism, in his experience, than it has been believed to occur in the experience of those writers whose opinions seem to have been most generally adopted by the profession.

2. That the frequency of inflammation of the heart, even in his cases, has been such as abundantly to show the great influence of acute rheumatism in its production.

An attempt is next made to ascertain the real amount, and the causes of the difference between the observations of the author and those of the writers referred to. The result, as it respects most of these writers, may be briefly stated to be,—

1st. *Of Pericarditis.* In those instances in which such data have been given as enable us to compare similar cases, the results are very nearly the same. In various instances, however, no comparison can be fairly made, either from the want of figures, from the mixing together of cases of endocarditis, and of pericarditis, or from a great difference in the age of the subjects.

With respect to *Endocarditis*, the discrepancy is much greater than in the case of pericarditis, and one of the chief causes of
the difference appears to the author to be, that most writers
have given the proportion of cases of valvular disease in acute
rheumatism in such a manner as implies (when it is not directly
stated) that they were all cases of acute disease—omitting,
therefore, to distinguish the proportion of them which were of
older date.

The proportion of cases of valvular disease of all dates observed by the author is nearly the same as that observed by the
chief writers referred to ; but he attempts to show,—

1st. That the greater number of these are examples of old
valvular disease.

2nd. That, at all events, in most cases it is very difficult to
distinguish when the disease is recent and when old ; and, 3rd.
That, as far as he has been able to ascertain, acute endocarditis
is less frequent than acute pericarditis in rheumatism.

The frequency of morbis cordis in chronic rheumatism is
next inquired into, and compared with that in acute rheumatism
and from this inquiry it appears, 1st. That the total number
of cases of morbis cordis, old and recent, is nearly the same in
the two kinds of rheumatism. 2nd. That acute inflammation
of the pericardium and of the endocardium is much more common in cases of acute than of chronic rheumatism.

The frequency of other internal inflammations in the course
of acute rheumatism is next examined, and compared with that
of inflammation of the heart, and the result is that the last mentioned inflammation exceeds every other in the frequency of its
occurrence.

The next subject of examination is—the circumstances which
favor the occurrence of inflammation of the heart in the progress
of acute rheumatism.

1st. *Metastasis.* Metastasis of the rheumatism did not occur in any one of the cases observed ; hence it is inferred that
this is not the ordinary nor even a frequent mode in which rheumatism produces cardiac inflammation. It does not, however,
follow from these facts that metastasis never takes place, and
it is attempted to be shown that its occasional occurrence is
both consistent with theory and established by observation.

In this part of the paper the author refers—1. To some cases
of rheumatism in which the inflammation of the heart appeared
before that of the joints. 2. To some cases of what has been
termed "rheumatic fever without arthritis," *i. e.*, cases presenting all the symptoms of acute rheumatism except the affection
of the articulations. 3. To one of his own cases in which he
thinks it probable that there have been acute rheumatism, and

in which there was pericarditis, but no affection of the joints throughout.

2nd. *Form of the Rheumatism.* Adopting the divisions of rheumatism given in the treatise of Dr. Macleod, we find that all the cases of rheumatic pericarditis occurred in connection with the *fibrous* as distinguished from the *capsular* form of rheumatism. In estimating the influence of this circumstance, however, it is neceasary to remember that the fibrous variety of rheumatism is much more common than the capsular.

3rd. *Intensity of the Rheumatism.* From the cases examined, it appears to result that the violence and fatality of rheumatic pericarditis, are generally greater in the cases in which the accompanying rheumatism is very acute than in those in which it is sub-acute. Whether pericarditis be more frequent in the more severe than in the less severe form of rheumatism, the author's cases do not enable him with confidence to determine. As far as they go, however, they are opposed to such a view, for three-fourths of the examples of rheumatic pericarditis occurred in subacute rheumatism.

4th. *Stage of the Rheumatism.* In more than half the cases of rheumatic pericarditis, the affection of the heart appeared on or before the fourth day of the disease. With one exception, the pericarditis did not appear sooner in those cases in which it was very severe than in those in which it was much less severe.

5th. *Influence of Repeated Attacks of Rheumatism.* In the cases examined, pericarditis was found to be both more frequent and more severe in the first than in subsequent attacks of rheumatism.

6th. *Previous diseases of the Heart.* Ten out of fifteen patients had no previous disease of the heart, and among these were found all the most severe cases of pericarditis.

7th. *Age.* Of fifteen patients, nine, or about two-thirds, were only twenty years of age or under; five were between twenty and twenty-six; and one was about ferty.

8th. *Sex.* Of fifteen patients, nine were males and six were females. It is necessary, however, to remember that rheumatism is more common among men than women.

9th. *Influence of Venesection.* Twelve of the patients had not been bled before the pericarditis appeared; the remaining three were bled, one eleven days, one five days, and one three days, before the pericarditis supervened.

Mode in which Rheumatism produces Pericarditis. Upon this question the author adopts the following hypothesis as consistent with all the facts he is acquainted with:—

The cause of acute rheumatism is probably the presence of

some morbid matter in the blood, which has an especial affinity
for the fibrous and fibro-serous tissues of the body, and which,
by fixing itself in one or more of these, induces various local
inflammations.   The similarity of the structures implicated, is
probably the reason why rheumatic pericarditis or endocarditis often occurs at the same time with or succeeds to rheumatic
inflammation in the joints, just as rheumatic inflamation in one
joint occurs with or succeeds to that in another ; and the heart
is more frequently (?) and more severely affected in severe cases of acute rheumatism, for the same reason that more joints
are affected and more severely affected, and also that more fever
is present in such cases ; which reason may not improbably be
a greater abundance of the materies morbi in the blood.

II.   *Of Bright's Disease of the Kidneys as a Cause of Inflammation in the Heart.*   We have already seen that of thirty-five
cases of pericarditis, Bright's disease was the only assignable
cause of the inflammation in thirteen, or more than one-third.
It remains to institute the corresponding and complementary
inquiry, into the frequency of pericarditis and endocarditis in
Bright's disease.

1.   In the bodies of fifty patients, who had either died of
Bright's disease or who were ascertained to have this disease
in an advanced stage, acute pericarditis was found in 5, or in
1 out of 10. and acute endocarditis in 4, or in 1 out of 12.

2.   On the other hand, in 142 bodies, in which the kidneys
were not affected with any appreciable disease, acute pericarditis was found in 4, or in 1 out of 35, and acute endocarditis in
2, or in 1 out of 71.

Pericarditis and endocarditis, therefore, being four times more
frequent in fatal cases of Bright's disease, than in fatal cases
without renal disease, it seems clearly to follow that the influence of Bright's disease in producing these inflammations is
unquestionable and great.

III.   The frequency of other internal inflammations in fatal
cases of renal disease, is next examined and compared with
their frequency in fatal cases without renal disease.   From this
comparison it appears,—

1.   That the proportionate number of acute internal inflammations, exclusive of those of the heart, is twice as great in the
series of cases with renal disease, as in that without such disease;
the numbers being respectively ninety-six and forty-two per
cent.

2.   That the proportion of patients, likewise, among whom
these inflammations were distributed, is greater in the former
than in the latter series of cases ; the numbers being respectively sixty and thirty-six per cent.

Hence we may safely infer, that Bright's disease has a great tendency to produce other internal inflammations besides those of the heart.

IV. A further examination of the same facts shows, that the relative frequency of various internal inflammations, is different in fatal cases of Bright's disease and of other diseases, taken indiscriminately.

The following are the various inflammations inquired into, arranged in the order of their frequency, as they were calculated to be due to renal disease, or to the causes operating in other fatal diseases.

1. *Inflammations due to renal disease.* Cerebritis, pneumonia pleuritis, pericarditis, endocarditis, meningitis, peritonitis. 2. *Inflammations independent of renal disease.* Pleuritis, pneumonia, peritonitis, meningitis, cerebritis, pericarditis, endocarditis.

V. From a comparison of the numbers given in this paper, we may calculate the tendency to produce various internal inflammations of the causes operating in fatal cases of Bright's disease as compared with those present in cases without renal disease. If we use the term Bright's disease, to represent all the causes operating in fatal cases of Bright's disease, and then compare these with the causes in operation in fatal cases without any renal disease, we shall find that Bright's disease produces:—1. *Endocarditis*, almost 5 times as often as all other causes put together; 2. *Cerebritis*, fully $3\frac{1}{2}$ times as often; 3. *Pericarditis*, fully $2\frac{1}{2}$ times as often; 4. *Pneumonia*, just 5 times as often; 5. *Pleuritis*, just $\frac{3}{4}$ times as often; 6. *Meningitis*, 3 times less frequently; 7. *Peritonitis*, 100 times less frequently. The author next inquires into the comparative efficacy of acute rheumatism and of Bright's disease, in producing pericarditis and other internal inflammations.

In comparing these two affections, we meet with some difficulty, arising from the fact that one of them is an acute disease and is seldom fatal, whereas the other is chronic and generally fatal. It appears to the author that the best mode of avoiding this difficulty is, to compare fatal cases of Bright's disease with ordinary cases of acute rheumatism. If the object were to ascertain the proportion of cases, in which traces of previously existing inflammation were found, this method would be objectionable, because the one disease having run a much longer course than the other, it would have had much more time to produce any inflammation which it had the power to produce; but, if cases of actually existing inflammation alone be counted, then the objection does not exist, and the result should not be far from the truth.

Of seventy-five cases of acute rheumatism, eight, or one in nine and a half, were complicated with pericarditis acuta. Of fifty fatal cases of Bright's disease, five were complicated with pericarditis acuta—or one in ten.

Hence, Bright's disease in the advanced stage, and acute rheumatism, appear to have caused acute pericarditis in an equal proportion of cases.

An examination of twenty cases of old adhesion of the pericardium, however, shows, what the considerations stated above might have led us to anticipate, that old adhesions of the pericardium have been produced twice as often by Bright's disease, as by previous attacks of acute rheumatism.

From considerations which could not readily be made intelligible in this abstract, the inference is next drawn, that acute rheumatism has a greater tendency to produce pericarditis than has Bright's disease in its earlier stages, and consequently that the tendency of Bright's disease to induce pericarditis, and probably also other internal inflammations, increases in proportion as the affection of the kidney is more advanced.

The conclusion thus arrived at is quite in accordance with the *modus operandi* of Bright's disease in producing local inflammations, which has been assumed in an earlier part of the paper; for, if this effect of renal disease depend upon a morbid condition of the blood, arising from the excessive accumulation of urea, we should expect the effect to increase in proportion as the structure and the functions of the kidneys, and the consequent composition of the blood, deviate more from the healthy condition.

In conclusion, some remarks are made upon the probable occurrence of pericarditis in other blood diseases, besides those observed by the author.

Likewise some observations on the importance of the constitutional or predisposing causes of inflammation, as distinguished from the exciting causes.—[*Abridgment from Braithwaite's Retrospect.*

Cases of Synovial Articular Inflammation of the Knee, treated successfully with Urate of Ammonia.* By W. E. Horner, M. D., Prof. of Anatomy in the University of Pennsylvania, Senior Surgeon of the St. Joseph's Hospital, etc.

The liniment of ammonia is so well known in the treatment of chronic articular affections, that its character may be consi-

---

* This paper was originally read before the Academy of Natural Sciences, on Tuesday December 9th, 1851, though now published by preference in a Medical Journal.

dered as settled; but my attention has been only lately called
to the still higher powers of urate of ammonia, an article which
though sufficiently offensive to the olfactories, has a strong compensating quality in the efficiency of its action. My first observation in regard to it was the result of having accidentally been
called to a poor woman who was in a state of unremitted and
excruciating suffering, day and night, but especially during
the latter period, *from* a chronic inflammation of the knee joint,
attended with considerable swelling and tenderness, and some
degree of redness. I made to it the ordinary applications of
cold fomentations, and evaporating lotions, enjoined rest, attended to her diet and the state of her bowels, and gave opiates
at night in the shape of Dover's powder. After ten or twelve
days of attendance, in which no progress was made to a cure,
I was much gratified on a visit to find that the pain had ceased
suddenly, and that the preceding night had been spent in great
ease. The strong expression of satisfaction on my part, led to
a communication from her, with many apologies for herself,
that, finding the disease so little abated, she had been tempted
to try the remedy of a simple friend, who had been remarkably
improved by it in a similar attack. This remedy was a poultice
made of human urine, thickened with potter's clay, and put on
as warm as one could bear it; and to be repeated when it got dry.
She declared to me, that this rather indelicate application had
relieved her of all pain in a few hours. The fact of relief was
incontestible; the question was in regard to the remedial agency
of the article employed, and I therefore determined to make
some experiments on the value of ammonia in combination
with fine argillacious earth.

Having a similar case shortly afterwards, in the St. Joseph's
Hospital, I tried in it a solution of muriate of ammonia formed
into a poultice. No very distinct or satisfactory result followed,
and it was discontinued. Having the idea still in my mind,
and wishing to be satisfied about it, but reluctant to employ the
article resorted to by the poor woman, I determined to find my
urate of ammonia in some other form of an easy kind, and for
that reason adopted the guano, which has so large a proportion
of phosphate of lime, urea and of urate of ammonia in it. A
female patient, aged 34 years, Mrs. C——, from Tamaqua
in this State, who had for more than a year labored under inflammation of the right knee, was put under my charge at the
St. Joseph's Hospital, Oct. 8th, 1851. She had been well attended to by Dr. Scherner, who had conducted her through the
most acute period of her complaint. The joint had suppurated,
and she came to town with a small fistulous orifice on the inner
side of the knee, through which a probe could be easily passed

between the tibia and os femoris. From this there came daily a spoonful or more of matter, when a plug was withdrawn from the orifice. She still suffered great pain at night, the part was tender, and was in continual uneasiness, and she had some slight fever in the afternoon. Here was exactly the case to try the efficacy of urate of ammonia, as naturally formed in animals. I accordingly obtained some guano, and had it made into a hot poultice with clay. The joint was kept enveloped in the poultice with frequent changes, for nearly the remainder of the month, at the end of which time a very marked improvement had taken place in the amount of pain, and also in the degree of swelling; and the purulent discharge had almost ceased.

The application produced a very copious vesication of the knee, and it had to be weakened to reduce the caustic qualities. Having conducted this treatment as far as seemed necessary, the skin was permitted to heal. Some little pain recurring afterwards, she was blistered for it; that getting well, the emplastrum calefaciens was applied, and the leg was also kept supported by an extending hand on the ankle, and a counter-extending one on the thigh, their action being sustained by a splint on the outside of the limb. At the end of six weeks, November 25th, she has left the hospital without pain or uneasiness in the knee. The joint is in a state of false anchylosis, and straight. I have covered the knee with emplastrum adhesivum, and secured it in that position with strong paste board splints, moulded to the knee; and have recommended her to keep it so for two or three months, until all danger of secondary suppuration be removed. Probably at the end of this time the judicious use of frictions and of Stromeyer's screw splint, may impart some flexion to the limb.

The Hospital record sheet shows the following details of dates, which may be inserted in this place:

Oct. 9. Poultice of guano, (*urate of ammonia*) and potter's clay, equal parts.

Oct. 10. Poultice has blistered. It was discontinued, and simple cerate applied.

Oct. 11. Patient has less pain; soreness of knee reduced, and not so much swelling. A poultice with one-third of the urate of ammonia, and two-thirds potter's clay.

Oct. 13. Vesication.

Oct. 14. Quantity of urate reduced to one-fourth of poultice. Treatment continued pretty much in this state to near the end of the month. Vesication by Emplast. Cantharid. about this, but omitted on record.

Oct. 28. She was permitted to eat as she pleased.

Nov. 5. Emplastrum calefaciens.

Nov. 12. Discontinue emplastrum calefaciens, and re-apply the urate of ammonia as on 14th October.

While this case was in progress,-another occured in a boy who had the knee joint opened by a cut of half an inch or so in length. Synovial inflammation followed, with the ordinary symptoms. Its usual acute-period was passed through, under the depletory antiphlogistic treatment, and with evaporating lotions to the part. The disposition to fall into the chronic state, attended with tumefaction was relieved by five days use of the same argillacious, uro-ammoniacal poultice.

The Ward sheet exhibits the following entries in regard to this case : Patient, Timothy Roach, aged nineteen years, admitted September 23d, a day or two after accident. Knee painful and stiff, somewhat swollen. Rest and fomentations of warm water directed on that day. Also loss of ten ounces of blood from arm.

Sept. 24. Local bleeding by scarified cupping. Fomentatations continued.

Oct. 4. Warm fomentations to this date; in the mean time an evident articular effusion has occurred into the synovial membrane of the knee. A blister plaster 4 inches by 4, was then applied.

Oct. 6. Blister plaster 2 X 3 inches.

Oct. 7. The patient so much relieved from pain as to be permitted to leave his bed and promenade with a crutch.

Oct. 9. Some aching and temefaction indicated a persistence of articular irritation. The poultice of urate of ammonia (guano) one-fourth, potter's clay three-fourths, was then applied hot, with frequent renewals to the 14th of October, at which time all the symptoms were relieved. The patient was discharged cured on the 15th.

The above cases are reported much in outline. I shall continue, as opportunity offers, to test the value of the above remedy, and also compare its results with other remedies. It appears to me to have some special qualities, which are of a highly beneficial kind in the affections alluded to. It is so active a revulsive when applied strong, that I have no doubt of their being many cases of serous inflammation in which it may be usefully resorted to. I would here suggest a trial in puerperal peritonitis and in pleurisy. I see no objection except the odour.

The poultice of guano and clay dries very quickly, so that it is better to shield it with oiled silk or India rubber cloth. The clay I look upon as simply a vehicle, but it may also have some physiological action from its physical properties in regard to moisture.

The analysis of the best guano, by the chemist, presents the following constituents, which are mentioned here for facility of reference. The proportions will vary according to their atmospheric exposure and to the degree of adulteration in trade. As it is an expensive article for agricultural purposes, it has become common to reduce its chemical relations by the addition of common earthy substances:

Uric acid, thirty per cent.
Uric acid with ammonia.
Carbonate of ammonia.
Muriate, oxalate, and phosphate of ammonia.
Free ammonia.
Phosphate of soda.
Phosphate of lime.
Sulphate of potash and soda, and oxalate of lime.

It is the large quantity of ammonia in it which makes it so active a stimulant to vegetable growth, and so disagreeable to the smell. It, however, is not so intolerable medically, as assafetida, an article which we have but litte hesitation in prescribing.—[*Medical Examiner.*

On the Pathology of some Affections of the Ear which induce Cerebral Disease. By Mr. TOYNBEE.

Mr. Toynbee has presented a memoir to the Royal Medico-Chirurgical Society, in which he has endeavored to specify the diseases of the ear which are liable to extend to the brain, as well as to show that each division of the internal aural apparatus has its particular division of the encephalon to which it communicates disease. He states, for instance, that—1. Affections of the external meatus and mastoid cells produce disease in the lateral sinus and cerebellum. 2. Affections of the tympanic cavity produce disease in the cerebrum. 3. Affections of the vestibule and cochlea produce disease in the medulla oblongata. In speaking of the external meatus, its intimate relations with the lateral sinus and cerebellum are pointed out; the affection most frequently producing disease in these parts is shown to be catarrhal inflammation of its dermoid layer, one of the numerous diseases which have hitherto been classed together under the term otorrhœa. This affection of the external meatus is fully described; and it is shown that it is found to endure during many years, without the presence of pain, or any other symptom calculated to apprise the surgeon of the presence of a formidable disease, while the bone may be becoming slowly carious, and portions of the dura mater and cerebellum disorganized. In the second division of the paper, the tympanic cavity is described to be the part of the ear from which disease is most frequently propagated to the brain. This circumstance is accounted for, firstly, by the great liability of the mucous membrane of the tympanum to undergo pathological changes; and, secondly, by the existence of very intimate relations between this membrane and the dura mater. The affection of the tympanum which most frequently produces disease in the cerebrum is chronic catarrhal inflammation of the mucous membrane, an affection thus far only known as an otorrhœa. The four changes in the dura mater and cerebrum produced by the affections of the tympanum are—

1. Inflammation of the dura mater, and its separation from the surface of the petrous bone by serum.

2. Ulceration of the dura mater, and its complete detachment from the petrous bone.

3. An abscess in the substance of the cerebrum.

4. Undefined suppuration of the substance of the cerebrum.

From a careful examination of cases, it appears that chronic catarrhal inflammation of the mucous membrane of the tympanum may exist as many as twenty or more years, without the production of any disease beyond it, or at least, without the existence of symptoms by means of which the presence of such disease can be diagnosed; nevertheless, in the great majority of cases vital structures become sensibly affected in a much shorter period. In a third section of the paper the author devotes some space to the consideration of the labyrinth, and it is shown that purulent matter in the vestibule or cochlea sometimes causes disease of the auditory nerve, which is transmitted to the medulla oblongata, producing suppurative inflammation of the meninges, and death, without the presence of any caries of the bone. In the course of this paper the author shows the necessity of abolishing the use of the term otorrhœa, and of using in its place the names of the several diseases, eight in number, of which a discharge from the ear is one of the symptoms. In conclusion, the facts which he is desirous of impressing upon the minds of medical men are, that the bone, dura mater, and substance of the brain may be slowly undergoing disorganization, without the presence of any other symptoms calculated to reveal to the medical man the existence of formidable disease than the presence of a discharge from the external auditory meatus; and that, consequently, no person suffering from catarrhal inflammation of the dermoid layer of the meatus, the membrana tympani, or of the mucous membrane of the tympanum, can be assured that disease is not being prolonged to the temporal bone, the brain, and its membranes; and that any ordinary exciting cause, as an attack of fever or

influenza, a blow on the head, &c., may not induce the appearance of acute symptoms, which, as a general rule, are speedily
fatal.—[*Medical Times.*

Anti-Syphilitic Agents, to replace Mercury.

In the *Comptes Rendus des Sceances de l'Acad, des Sciences*
for the 3d of November, 1851, we find a *note* on this subject by
M. Edouard Robin, followed by experimental researches, by
Dr. Vicente.

M. Robin, reflecting on the fact that the mercurials, used in
the cure of Syphilis, did not probably exert any peculiar action
on the system, but removed the disease by entering the circulation and destroying the venereal virus, was led to the belief,
that other substances, besides those which had been employed
hitherto, might be found, which would exert the same power
over the poison.

All the anti-syphilitic remedies at present known, belong,
according to M. Robin, to the class of anti-septic substances;
and pertaining to the same class, two compounds appeared to
him eminently worthy of trial in this disease—these are the
bi-chromate of potash and the sesqui-chloride of iron.

Accordingly he invited a very experienced practitioner, M.
Vicente, to study experimentally the action of the bi-chromate
of potash. and the results at which he arrived were very favorable.   We insert the *resume* of the observations of M. Vicente:

"1. The bi-chromate of potash is undoubtedly an anti-syphilitic agent, and acts with more energy and rapidity than the
mercurial preparations.

"2. In the three cases in which I have administered this
new therapeutical agent, the patients have experienced no
inconvenience, except perhaps some nausea at the commencement, particularly when they neglected to drink water after
the pill, in order to prevent the slight local irritation; but with
this precaution, and the addition of opium, as a corrective, the
stomach soon tolerated the bi-chromate of potash, which, being
completely soluble in water, may be administered in a draught
or pill; taken after a meal the pills have never caused either
nausea or vomiting.

"3. The bi-chromate of potash being soluble, its absorption
into the system is complete and almost instantaneous; hence
the rapidity of its therapeutical action, even in doses of a quarter of a grain.

"4. The bi-chromate of potash does not appear to be anti-
plastic in its action like mercury; it did not cause salivation,
diarrhœa, or any particular phenomena.

" 5. Consequently, if these facts be confirmed by subsequent experiment, this agent will advantageously replace the mercurial preparations."—[*Transylvania Med. Journ.*   P.

Report of a fatal *Case of Tetanus following the ligature of Hæmorrhoids.* By JAMES BOLTON, M. D. (Read before the Medical Society of Virginia, at its October meeting.)

M. C., colored female æt. 35—married; has suffered intensely from piles since the birth of her first child fifteen years since.

Oct. 6. A mass of about the size of a hen's egg protrudes from the anus, and separates the nates.

Operation —The patient was fully anæsthetized. The mass was so vascular that merely sponging with cold water caused the loss of about half a pint of blood in a few minutes.

It was divided by sulci into three tumors. A needle was passed through the base of each, carrying a double ligature, which was tied on both sides of the tumor.

In forty-eight hours nearly the who'e had sloughed off. Chlorine wash was applied to correct the fœtor and to promote healthy action.

On the fourth day a moderate dose of sulphur and bitartrate of potash was ordered to remove constipation caused by opium used to allay the pain which was produced by the ligatures.

About three or four times the quantity ordered was given, and produced violent hypercatharsis. This was not checked until it had lasted several days, owing to neglect of directions.

On the 11th day the patient felt remarkably well until night, when she suffered from cramps of the hams.

On the 12th day there were symptoms of decided tetanus. Ordered morphiæ sulph. gr. ss.; quinine di-sulph. gr. x. every second hour. Chloroform to be used as often as necessary to subdue spasm. Directions not attended to until night.

Observing some fœtor from the anus, applied injection of strong solution of nitrate of silver.

13th day. Spasms continue when free from the influence of chloroform. Some tendency to sink. Inability to swallow. Directed mercurial inunction extensively. After relaxing the patient completely by chloroform, passed a stomach tube and injected morphiæ sulph. gr. i.; quinine sulphate ʒi. and brandy ℥ss. Only one spasm occurred after this, but the patient continued to sink, and died without a struggle in about four hours. A post-mortem examination was not permitted.

REMARKS.—Up to the time that hypercatharsis was produced,

the patient was doing very well.   Pain had ceased and the appetite and spirits were good.   From that time pain returned,
accompanied by physical and mental depression.   It is therefore highly probable that the irritation of the part, together
with general exhaustion, which no doubt caused the tetanus,
was really due to the improper administration of medicine to
the patient, already in a critical condition from the operation.
[*Stethoscope.*

Strychnine and Turpentine in the treatment of Cholera By J.
    Howes, M. D., Resident Physician of the Commercial Hos-
    pital, Cincinnati.

From the last of April to the middle of June, there were ten
cases of cholera in the Commercial Hospital, nine of which died
under the treatment usually adopted in such cases.   These cases
were mostly far advanced, as indeed, are neatly all those brought
to the Hospital.
    The success following this treatment was so small, that I con-
cluded none could be much less, and therefore considered every
case of cholera a legitimate subject for experiment; and as it
devolved on me, in the absence of the attending physician, to
prescribe for all patients who came into the wards over which
I, as resident physician, had charge, I tried the effect of several
different remedies upon persons attacked with cholera, and finally settled upon the following:

    ℞.   Strychnia,   gr. ss.
        Spts. Turpentine ʒii.
        Mucilage,   ʒviii. M.

Dose, table-spoonful, to be given every half hour, until the
discharges have ceased, and perfect reaction is secured.
    This treatment, with the consent of the attending physician,
has been made use of in the last twenty-five cases of cholera
which we have had in the hospital.   Of these cases, ten were
in a state of perfect collapse; twelve had a perceptible pulse,
but otherwise manifesting all the phenomena of collapse; and
three had a warm dry skin, and a pulse of nearly natural fullness, with vomiting, purging, and cramps, the discharges presenting the appearance of rice water.
    Of these twenty-five cases, three did not react at all, four died
of consecutive fever, and eighteen recovered.
    In some of the worst cases, we repeated the dose every fifteen
minutes instead of half hour.   One of the most desperate took
three and a half pints of the mixture, in forty-eight hours, and

reco'vered. None of them manifested any of the poisonous effects of strychnia.* We made as much use of external applications in our first cases, as in the last. Frictions of all kinds we always found to exhaust very much those patients who were in, or approaching very nearly, collapse. In a few cases we have made use of sinapisms or blisters.—[*Western Lancet.*

Extract of Beefs' Blood in the treatment of Anæmia. By Dr. VON MAUTHNER, of Vienna. Translated from the French by H. A. JOHNSON, A. B., Interne to Illinois Gen. Hospital.

Dr. Von Mauthner, Director of the Hospital, St. Amne, of Vienna, has employed for some time the extract of Beef's Blood in the protracted Anæmias of children. According to this distinguished practitioner a large number of diseases are caused by an Anæmic state, rather than is generally believed, by irritation, and ought, therefore to be treated by other than antiphlogistic means. Unfortunately, science has furnished, as yet but few remedies, capable of combatting successfully Asthenic diseases, having their point of departure in the constitution of the blood.

M. Von M. has employed with success the Ammonio Chloride of Iron in the treatment of children, presenting periodical symptoms of congestion, without any appreciable organic cause, and in debility attending intermittants, but he has become convinced that there are Anæmic conditions in which the patients do not bear the use of any of the preparations of Iron, and it is in such states that the Extract renders the most efficient service.

The extract is prepared in the following manner: Blood, fresh from the animal is thrown in a filter, and the residue evaporated to complete dryness. It is administered in the form of powder, or dissolved in water, in quantities of from grs. 10 to ℨi. per day. Under the continued use of this means the patients improve very much in appearance and gain rapidly in strength. This result ought to astonish no one when it is considered that the extract supplies just those substances which are wanting in the blood of these little sufferers, viz: the hæmatine and the fibrine.

According to Dr. Von Mauthner, this preperation is especially adapted to the following Anæmic morbid conditions:—
1st. Anæmia succeeding chronic diarrhœa of children of a cer-

---

* Since the above was written, we have had a patient to whom was administered one and a half pints of the above mixture, in sixteen hours, which produced quite severe tetanic spasms, which were relieved in a few moments by chloroform, and the patient is convalescing.

tain age. It is on the contrary of but very little use in very young subjects and in such as have just been taken from the breast. 2d. Anæmia after Typhus. The author who is perfectly convinced of the advantages which it offers in this case, assures us that it may be administered without any danger of fatiguing the digestive organs. 3d. Anæmia which follows severe pneumonia, when the lungs are not as yet restored to their normal state, and the patient is troubled with cough and fever ; but it is to be remarked that the remedy is not equally beneficial in tuberculosis. 4th. Anæmia succeeding wasting suppuration, and scrofulous ulcers. 5th. Anæmia after serous accumulations produced by scarlatina. In this condition of the system it seems to surpass all other remedies in use, since, contrary to the effect which has been observed of other tonics, it produces no irritation of the kidneys, a result often leading to hæmaturia and albumenuria and constituting a new disease.

This remedy, so simple in its use, and costing only the labor of preparing it, merits, as it seems to us, the attention of practitioners, especially for the poorer classes, among whom Anæmic effections are unfortunately so common.—*Annales, Med. de la Flandre Ocid.*—[*North-western Med. and Sur. Jour.*

On the Reunion of Wounds of the Spinal Cord, with Restoration of its lost Functions. By M. Brown-Sequard.

During the last three years, M. Brown-Sequard has made a considerable number of experiments, with the view of determining the degree of reparative power which exists in the Spinal Cord ; the results of which are very remarkable. The following is one of the most striking :—The spinal cord of a pigeon was *entirely divided* between the 5th and 6th dorsal vertebræ ; and the operation was followed by complete paralysis of the posterior part of the body, as regarded sensibility and voluntary movement. At the end of three months, voluntary movements began to show themselves, in the midst of reflex actions ; and sensibility also reappeared. These powers gradually augmented ; and six months after the operation, the bird could stand for some minutes, but fell if it attempted to walk. In the course of the seventh month it began to walk, but unsteadily, helping itself by its wings. By the end of the eighth month, it could walk, slowly without support ; but if it attempted to walk fast, it fell over, unless it supported itself by its wings. Twelve months after the operation, it could run ; and when the account of the case was drawn up, fifteen months after the section had been made, its progression seemed in all respects normal, save that a certain degree of stiffness remained in its gait.

In several Guinea-pigs, in which the section had only been made through one-half of the spinal cord, an incomplete return of voluntary power was observed within seven or eight months after the operation. In the case of one Guinea-pig, which had been subjected to this operation a year before, and in which sensibility appeared to have been completely restored, and voluntary movement less completely, a careful examination was made of the injured part. It was found that the section had traversed both the posterior columns, as well as the anterior and lateral columns, and a portion of the grey substance on the right side; all of which parts exhibited a sort of contraction, the continuity of the divided parts being re-established by a whitish cicatrix. On examining the substance of this cicatrix, it was found to be in great part made up of fibres of areolar tissue, the direction of which was transverse or oblique; but these were crossed by great numbers of nerve-fibres running in a longitudinal direction, which exhibited a double contour, and were uninterruptedly continous through the whole extent of the cicatrix. Amongst these were scattered some ganglionic corpuscles. A like reproduction of nerve-fibres in the cicatrix of the spinal cord, has been substantiated by M. Brown-Sequard in two other cases.—[*Gazette Médicale. Brit. and For. Med. Chir. Rev.*

On Kiestein. By Dr. Veit.

In consequence of the discrepancy of opinion which prevails among observers as to the value to be attached to the appearance of the urine termed Kiestein, as diagnostic of pregnancy, Dr. Veit has, during a year and a half, been conducting a series of experiments at the Halle Lying-in Institution. He has examined for this purpose the urine of 10 men, of 4 non-pregnant females, and of 48 women in various stages of pregnancy. He comes to the same conclusion as Höfle (*Chemie und Mickroskop am Kramkenbette*) and, recently, Lehmann, viz., that the so-called pellicle of Kiestein is no peculiar matter at all, and is not of the slightest value as a sign of pregnancy. In urine of both non-pregnant and pregnant women, pellicles are formed containing vibriones, and frequently the triple phosphate; the chief difference between the respective urines being, that in that of pregnant women, alkaline, and in that of non-pregnant women, acid, reaction more frequently manifests itself. This may, in some measure, depend upon the greater concentration of the urine in pregnancy, and the larger proportion of mucus mixed as a consequence of the changes induced in the condition of the mucous membrane of the bladder by the passive hyperæmia of that organ during pregnancy. Persons partaking of a more nitrogenous diet than did the poor pregnant women whose urine was examined, might furnish different results in this respect.—[*Zeitsch. jur Geburt. Brit. Amer. Journal.*

On the Induction of Premature Labour.

At a late meeting of the Edinburgh Obstetrical Society, Dr. Moir made a statement of the mode of inducing premature labour, which was introduced by the late Dr. Hamilton. The plan consisted in gently dilating the os uteri with the finger or a catheter, and separating the membranes from the cervix without rupturing them. When labour came on it proceeded as in the natural way, and the probability of the life of the child being saved was much increased by avoiding a premature rupture of the membranes. When this proceeding failed to induce labour, Dr. Moir was in the habit of passing a catheter along the posterior surface of the uterus, between it and the membranes, and by means of the stillet, puncturing the latter high up. By these means he had succeeded in every case but one.

Dr. Simpson is in the habit of inducing premature labour by dilating the os with sponge tents; and he considers this a more certain as well as a more safe mode than any other. Like Dr. Hamilton's plan, it had the advantage of not rupturing the membranes. It had also, in Dr. Simpson's opinion, other advantages. He has tried Dr. Kiwisch's plan of injecting a continuous stream of tepid water against the os uteri in one case with success.—[*Edinburg Monthly Journal.*

On the Effect of Pressure above the Pubis in Uterine Hæmorrhage. By EDWARD WILLIAMS, M. D., Resident Physician to the South-Eastern Lying-in Hospital, Dublin.

I was lately called to a case of uterine hæmorrhage, occurring after labour, and after the expulsion of the placenta. When I arrived I found the patient bandaged tightly; vinegar applications, also, had been used externally to the genitals; the pulse in both wrists was scarcely perceptible, and she appeared a good deal prostrated. The flooding had been arrested by the above means, at least partially. I applied pressure with the hand above the pubis, and instantly, not more than thirty seconds or a minute, it produced a magical effect on the pulse, which became bounding and strong, as if the heart had been stimulated to increased action. Theorise as you may, I leave this to learned physiologists; I merely state the practical results—viz., increased action of the arterial system and arrest of the flooding.

It may be said, all this is nothing new; all this is stated in books

on midwifery.   I am aware of this, and claim nothing original ;
but I believe that practical observations may strengthen and
confirm the views of theorists and authors, and thus continued
observation of many may do service to the talented few.

[*London Lancet.*

*On the Detection of Mercury in the Body of a Person Dying of
Mercurial Cachexy.*   By M. Gorup-Besanez.

That quicksilver is one of the metals capable of absorption
into the economy is a well-known fact, detected as it has been
by various chemists, not only in the blood, but in the secretions
of various organs, and especially the saliva, and in the structure
of the organs themselves.   But as to the mode of its distribution
the duration of its presence in the various organs, and whether
it is found in all or certain tissues only, are points yet to be investigated.   Dr. Gorup-Besanez relates the result of a recent
investigation of the body of a woman, who was long (twenty
five years) laboriously engaged in silvering looking-glasses, but
who, from the convulsive tremors that were induced, had been
obliged to desist from her occupation for a year prior to death.

The somewhat colapsed brain did not entirely fill the skull,
and the dura mater was of a reddish-blue from venous congestion.   The consistency of the brain was firmer than usual.   The
lungs were hepatized, loaded with dark-coloured blood, and non-
crepitant.

The chemical results obtained by following the processes of
Fresenius and Babo were as follows.   The lungs and heart
gave no traces of mercury ; a very small quantity was detected in the liver, and none in the bile.   A doubtful precipitate
was thrown down upon the gold plate by the brain, while the
spinal column presented no traces.   That any remains at all
should be found after a year is remarkable, and is confirmatory
of other facts, proving how long certain metals, *e. g.* antimony,
may be retained in the economy.   That the liver was the only
organ in which it could then be detected, confirms the doctrine
that metalic poisonous substances are longest found in that organ.—[*Buchner's Report.   Brit. and For. Med. Chir. Review.*

*On the distribution of the Blood-vessels in the Mucous Mem-
brane of the Stomach.*   By Henry Frey.

The distribution of the blood-vessels in the gastric mucous
membrane has an interesting relation to its double function ; for
the vessels of the surface, which are those most concerned in
absorption, are veins, and have a large diameter; whilst those

of the deeper portions of the membrane, which are subservient to secretion, are arteries, which form very delicate net-works around the gastric follicles. [*Henle and Pfeufer's Zeitschrift. Ibid.*

Meadow Sweet in Dropsy. By M. Tessier.

From experiments made by M. T., in certain cases of dropsy, he believes that spiræa ulmaria or meadow-sweet possesses diuretic properties; that it is also slightly astringent and tonic; that it is agreeable to the taste, and produces no disturbance of the stomach or of the nervous system; and that all parts of the plant seemed to possess the same properties. After all known diuretics had been used in vain in a case of ascites, connected with intestinal irritation, M. T. ordered a quart of the decoction of the meadow-sweet to be taken daily. From the third day, the patient passed much more urine than before. At the end of 16 days, the medicine was suspended, and the urine became àt once scanty; it was resumed, and continued six weeks; and the dropsy was removed without occasioning any debility. In a young woman affected with heart disease, it produced abundant diuresis, without lowering the circulation like digitalis.—[*Bull. de Therap. Northern Lancet.*

Sulphuric Acid in Diarrhœa.

The British medical periodicals contain additional testimony in favor of the diluted sulphuric acid in diarrhœa and affections approximating to cholera. The success obtained by some is represented as very striking. All concur, however, in repudiating this remedy in cases presenting dysenteric characters. It is most useful in passive diarrhœa or those forms of the disease in which there is not much excitement. The doses recommended vary according to circumstances, but are usually quite large. One formula suggested consists of $\frac{1}{2}$ oz. of the dil. sulph. acid (of the dispensatories) in $7\frac{1}{2}$ oz. water—of which 1 oz. may be given every two hcurs, or oftener, if rejected by the stomach. For children, it may be made palatable by sweetening.

Prurigo of the Genital and Anal Regions.

Various remedies are from time to time recommended in the journals for this disagreeable and obstinate affection. The

London Lancet, for December 15th, gives an application of M. Tournié's, as having been used with much success. "The affected spot is to be rubbed twice a day with calomel ointment, (one to two drachms of calomel to ounce of axunge,) and, after each application, dredged with a powder, consisting of four parts of starch to one of powdered camphor." We have used a great variety of applications, for the relief of this unmanageable affection, and have derived most advantage from a cerate made of calomel (3 i,) in Goulard's cerate (3 i.)—[*Medical Examiner.*

Sesquicarbonate of Ammonia in Lepra and Psoriasis.

M. Cazenave, so well known as a very successful dermatologist, has just published experiments tending to show that sesquicarbonate of ammonia may advantageously be used as a succedaneum of arsenical preparations, in lepra and psoriasis. The salt is mixed in the following proportions :—Half a drachm of sesquicarbonate of ammonia ; diaphoretic syrup, seven ounces ; take from one to three table-spoonfuls per diem. The physiological effects are very slight, but in the space of about a week the scales begin to fall off; those which succeed are thinner, the patches which give them support gradually fall in, the redness fades after a longer or shorter time, and a lasting cure generally ensues. If Diarrhœa, lassitude, cephalalgia, quick pulse, and rapid alterations of heat and cold, were to occur, as was the case with two or three patients, the remedy should be suspended.—[*London Lancet.*

New mode of Disguising the Taste of Cod-Liver Oil.

Dr. Routh exhibited to the Medical Society of London, a specimen of "Sardine flavoured oil," prepared by digesting a number of sardine fishes, as sent over from Italy, in some cod-liver oil. After a month or so, the oil acquired the tase and smell of the sardines, and was very pleasant to take ; spread over a piece of hot toast, it formed really quite a luxury. The bottle was handed round, and seemed to give general satisfaction.—[*Medical Times.*

Umbilical Superfœtation.

M. Danyau read (Nov. 18th) to the Academy of Medicine of Paris, a report on a case by Dr. Sulikowski, of a girl born in 1833, who had at birth a remarkably large abdomen, which increased in size till the age of ten years. During this period her health was greatly impaired, and she suffered much from abdominal pains and other symptoms. In 1843, a rupture took place at the umbilicus, and from twelve to fourteen pounds of serous liquid escaped; the tumor was notably diminished; through the opening left in the parietes a substance could be perceived, fleshy, resisting, red, and studded with teeth and hair. Several years afterwards the tumour was successfully removed by operation, and was found to contain a deformed male fœtus.—[*Medical News.*

On the Abortive Treatment of Gonorrhœa by Chloroform.
By M. VENOT.

M. Venot, of Bordeaux, states, as the result of a twelve-month's experience, that injections of chloroform, though of little avail in confirmed gonorrhœa, are possessed of a complete abortive efficacy, if employed during the first week.—[*Bull. de Thérap. Brit. and For. Med. Chir. Rev.*

𝔐𝔦𝔰𝔠𝔢𝔩𝔩𝔞𝔫𝔶.

Religious Monomania ; Self-mutilation.—(Under the care of Mr. Lloyd.)—We desire to call our readers' attention to a patient admitted a few days ago, under the care of Mr. Lloyd. The case is one of a very painful character, and falls as much under the cognizance of the psycologist as the surgeon : the former will therein find a new example of religious monomania with destructive tendencies, and the latter an instance of self-mutilation, somewhat startling in a purely surgical point of view.

It appears that the patient is a well-conducted servant girl, twenty-three years of age ; she has light hair and complexion, and has been in service for the last nine months with a widow lady at Islington, where she never showed any signs of mental aberration. Her father was a bricklayer, who died from a severe cold caught in a well; her mother and sister are alive ; and it would seem that no distinct signs of insanity have been known to exist in the family. The patient herself states very clearly that she was very happy in her situation, that she went to church every Sunday, and that she was in the enjoyment of good health. The catamenia have always been regular, and no uneasiness in respect of menstruation was ever experienced.

On the morning of the 7th of November, the mistress had left the kitchen but a short time when her attention was attracted to a very strong ammoniacal smell about the house. She inquired from the servant whom she had just left below stairs, whether some linen was burning, and receiving no answer, she proceeded into the kitchen, where she found the girl before the fire with her left arm thrust into it. The mistress, who was naturally very much alarmed, soon became aware that the hand had been completely severed from the arm, and was lying on the fire; and when anxiously inquiring for the cause of this frightful scene, the girl exclaimed that she had cut off her hand with the carving knife, and that God had told her to do so. When remonstrated with touching this sad mutilation, she seized a steel skewer, and attempted to destroy her own eyes by thrusting its point into them.

A surgeon, who had hurriedly been sent for, was soon upon the spot; and whilst he was endeavouring to take from the fire the severed hand which was lying upon it, the unfortunate creature rushed forward, and thrust her right and only remaining hand into the fire. By this last and desperate act she inflicted a severe burn upon the forearm and hand. She was finally conveyed to the hospital, a sad victim to a sudden and unexpected monomaniac attack.

On examination, it was found that the left hand had been severed from the arm as cleanly as a saw could have done it, the only difference from an ordinary amputation being, that no soft parts had been left for covering the lower ends of the radius and ulna, which latter were quite exposed, with small fragments of cartilage still half attached, the whole being somewhat obscured by charring. It would appear that the bleeding was inconsiderable, and as no actual hæmorrhage had to be stopped, it may be surmised that the actual charring to which the stump was exposed soon after the mutilation may have acted as the actual cautery. The left forearm was somewhat swollen, and on the right side the hand and forearm were found to be severely burnt, the action of the fire having penetrated to the cellular tissue. The poor girl was keeping her eyes closed, and when the lids were separated it was found that the skewer had principally wounded the conjunctive and sclerotic, between the lower eyelid, the external canthus, and the globe; there was much infiltration between the tunics, but the iris was untouched in either eye.

The patient seems to be strictly *mono*-maniac, as she gives very apposite and satisfactory answers respecting her age, state of health, family, and various other circumstances. When questioned, however, as to the unfortunate mutiliation she has inflicted upon herself, she invariably answers that God told her to do it. When closely pressed as to how she knew that she ought to commit such an act she appears wrapped in her monomania, and merely answers, " God knows."

On the second day there was some purulent discharge from the eyes; the stump, which had been simply dressed, and the right arm, which had been wrapped up in cotton wool, were rather painful; the bowels had been twice moved and the patient had been tranquil, composed, and even inclined to sleep. When interrogated she does not seem displeased at being disturbed, and gives short and clear answers to the questions put to her; she does not cry out or mutter, but now and then moves the upper extremities slowly in different directions and finally raises them above her head. The breathing is slow and regular, the carotids beat somewhat faintly and heavily, and when a certain pressure is made upon one of these vessels, the patient utters no complaint, nor do any cerebral phenomena become apparent.

Although the poor girl has been very quiet since admission, she is watched with great vigilance, as she might suddenly be seized with a fresh monomaniacal and destructive fit. Mr. Lloyd ordered some calomel ; and purposes, when the patient has been watched for a few days, to endeavor to render the stump a serviceable one. We shall watch the progress of this case with painful interest, and acquaint our readers with its subsequent features —[*London Lancet.*

The Microscope as a means of Diagnosis.—One occasionally hears the question asked—"Have you any faith in the microscope ?"—and asked, too, in such a spirit as to convey the answer in the question. This expression of doubt as to the value of this inestimable instrument, has in a great measure arisen from confounding the statement of the facts observed with the conclusions drawn from them by the observer. A microscope, such as can now be had for a very reasonable sum, cannot err. It may not be able to reveal all that is essential to minute structure, but it cannot add anything of itself to that which is placed beneath it for examination. The microscope is to the eyes of ordinary observers what a pair of spectacles is to the eyes of the short-sighted. Both individuals are enabled to see that which is invisible to the unassisted vision. It is when the observer begins to interpret, that error commences, and it is to him, and not to his instrument, that the question as to faith applies. Well, then, does it become those who seek to make use of the microscope—and who can now-a-days do well without it ?—to endeavor to render themselves competent interpreters of what they see, and until the accomplishment is obtained, to confine themselves to a description of facts.—[*London Lancet.*

A new Quackery.—In Naumberg a man named Mahner is preaching the necessity of a new regeneration, not in the spiritual but physical sense. He warns a sickly race that it must return to the lost state of "primitive health," or *Urgesundheit,* as the means of more fully enjoying life and attaining a patriarchal old age. It is to be secured by a diet of bread and water, going barefoot, and letting the hair and beard grow ; in short, making a nearer approach to man's original state in costume than the decencies or prejudices of modern society will altogether permit.—[*London Lancet.*

Amputation of the entire Lower Jaw, with disarticulation of both Condyles.—The January number of the New York Journal of Medicine contains the details of the above operation, as performed by Professor Carnochan. The result was completely successful, and adds another to the many brilliant achievements of American Surgery.

Fluid Extract of Ergot. By Joseph Laidley, of Richmond, Va. "It is prepared by treating fresh and good ergot in powder first with

ether, allowing the latter to *evaporate spontaneously*, thus securing all
the oil—then with alcohol, and lastly with water; the last two liquids
are evaporated below 212° until the fluid measures one-third as many
fluid ounces as the ergot employed weighed in troy ounces; sufficient
sugar is added to preserve it, and the oil is then thoroughly incorporated, and sufficient water added to render it of such strength that
one fluid drachm (one teaspoonful) will represent 40 grains, or about
two doses of ergot.

"Prepared as above, fluid extract of ergot is in the form of a concentrated syrup, possessing the advantages of being pleasant to take,
of being always ready for use, thus avoiding the delay sometimes
attendant upon administering a medicine where delay is so hazardous as in labour. The smallness of the dose is another recommendation in its favor. The writer believes that it will keep unchanged
for a long time. Some in his possession, after having been kept for
about two months in a moderately warm situation, is entirely unchanged. Some of this preparation was furnished to Dr. C. S. Mills,
of this city, who tested it in a case of labour about the middle of November. He informs the writer that it proved entirely satisfactory;
its action was almost immediate, and produced no nausea."

[Stethoscope.

Medical Institutions at Lima.—Lima, the population of which is
about 85,000, has a medical school, where a great many efficient
professors are appointed. The students are eighty in number, and
are admitted in the four hospitals of the city. The Santa Ana Hospital is exclusively devoted to women, and has 700 beds; that of St.
Andrew is for men only, and numbers 400 beds; the third is a military hospital, and the fourth an institution for incurable patients, with
80 beds. The latter hospital contains principally black people and
mulattoes, affected with local chronic diseases, especially lepra and
ulcers of a frightful description. In the other hospitals fever and
dysentery are the most common diseases, particularly among the
poor. Small-pox destroys a great many patients, as also elephantiasis. In the winter bronchial affections are somewhat common, owing
to the dampness of the climate.—[*L'Union Méd. London Lancet.*

Statistics of the Medical Profession in Paris and Russia.—On the
1st of January, 1849, there were 1389 doctors of medicine in Paris,
being 53 less than in 1847; and now, in 1851, the number is reduced
to 1351, being a still further diminution of 38. During the last two
years 65 have died, while, during the two former years, only 56 died,
and still fewer during the prior periods. In 1843–7, the mean annual
mortality was 1 in 75; in 1848–9, 1 in 50; and in 1850–1, 1 in 42.
There have emigrated 86, of whom 12 have repaired to California.
Towards following up the vacancies, 113 new doctors have been
made during the last two years.

Officiers de Santé have, however, increased from 156 in 1849, to
178 in 1851, and the *pharmaciens* from 363 to 381. *Sage femmes*

have diminished from 480 in 1847, to 385 in 1849, and 350 in 1851.
—*Révue Medico-Chirurgicale.*

According to the official lists, published Jan. 1851, there were, in the entire Russian empire, 7957 doctors possessing the right to practice, 552 veterinary surgeons, and 132 oculists, dentists, and others possessing restricted rights of practice.   There were also 714 *pharmaciens* having authority to sell medicines, viz: 77 in the two capitals, 150 in the governmental towns, and 487 in other parts.   Siberia and the oriental governments of the empire only possess 19 civil practitioners; and the insufficiency of this number has given rise to the establishment of a medical school at the university of Kazan.   In the course of the year 1850, there were treated 737,442 patients in the hospitals, of whom 609,564 are returned as cured, and 91,545 as dead, *i. e.* a mortality of 1 in 13.—*L'Union Médicale.*—[*Brit. and For. Med. Chir. Rev.*

Professor Henderson's Conversion to Homœopathy.—During the discussion which followed the motion of Mr. Syme, in reference to the exclusion of homœopaths from membership of the Society, and which was carried unanimously, Dr. Simpson related a very capital story, which will doubtless amuse our readers.   Some eight or ten years ago, an old schoolmate of Dr. S., who was a homœopathic druggist in Liverpool, presented to him a small, but very beautifully painted box of homœopathic medicines.   Dr. S. put it to a very natural use—he gave it as a plaything to his eldest son, then a child.   The youngster, full of mischief, oftimes uncorked the tiny vials, and pouring the contents into a heap, would re-fill them from the general mass. It thus happened that the globules belonging to the different bottles were more or less thoroughly mixed together, and then new and strange compounds were produced.   It also sometimes happened, that when the child, wearied of his performance, others engaged in the innocent amusement of re-filling the bottles from the general heap. A professional brother calling one day on Dr. S., who was not at home, saw this pretty box and pocketed it.   Weeks elapsed ere the two friends met, when Dr. S. was informed by him that he had been trying to practice homœopathically, and that he had seen some wonderful effects and *cures* from the drugs contained in that precious little box!   At this interview Dr. S. did not disclose to his friend the important fact that the globules he had been using were elaborately commixed; he was reluctant, cruel man! to spoil, at once, so good a joke.   In the progress of time, the physician became more and more a homœopathist, and then it became too serious a matter to joke about, when he actually published a list of supposed homœopathic cures.

[*New York Med. Times.*

Death of Priessnitz.—Priessnitz, the celebrated founder of hydropathy, died at Graefenberg on the 26th of November, at the age 52. In the morning of that day, Priessnitz was up and stirring at an early hour, but complained of the cold, and had wood brought in to make a large fire.   His friends had for some time believed him to be suffer-

ing from dropsy of the chest, and at their earnest entreaty he consented to take a little medicine, exclaiming all the while, "It is of no use."
He would see no physician, but remained to the last true to his profession. About four o'clock in the forenoon of the 26th he asked to
be carried to bed, and upon being laid down he expired.—[*London
Medical Gazette.*

BIBLIOGRAPHICAL.

Carpenter's Elements of Physiology—new edition.

We have to acknowledge the receipt, from the publishers, Messrs.
Blanchard & Lea, Philadelphia, of a new edition of Carpenter's
Elements of Physiology.

This, and other kindred works of the author are so well known in
this country, and so highly esteemed, that it is unnecessary to say
anything in commendation of them. It is proper to observe, however, that the present is not a mere re-print of former editions, but
has been carefully revised and subjected to material alterations :
several of the chapters have been re-written and made to conform
more nearly to ascertained facts in relation to the subjects of which
they treat. As a diligent compiler and as a successful cultivator of
the branch of science to which he has devoted himself, Dr. Carpenter occupies a distinguised position.

It is refreshing to note, that this and some other re-prints of English medical books have recently slipped through the press without
being saddled with an American editor. We trust that we have seen
the end of the shallow system of quackery in authorship which has
made us the laughing stock of Europe. Hereafter, it is to be hoped
we are to have English books, unmutilated by omissions and unde-
faced by notes and interlineations.   M....r.

*Lectures on Materia Medica and Therapeutics, delivered in the College
of Physicians and Surgeons of the University of New York.* By
JOHN B. BECK, M. D., late Professor of Materia Medica and Medical Jurisprudence ; prepared for the press by his friend, C. R.
GILMAN, M. D., Professor of Obstetrics, etc., in the College of
Physicians and Surgeons, N. York. Samuel and William Wood,
publishers, 261 Pearl-st., New York. 1851. 1 vol. 8vo. pp. 581.

We learn, from the editor's preface, that the lectures which compose this work were prepared for publication by the late Prof. B.,
with the exception of a few which were revised by Prof. Gilman.
This gentleman has also added notices of some subjects which Dr. B.
had not included in his course. Although the work cannot justly

claim any very high degree of merit, we think it a good digest of the present state of knowledge on the subjects of which it treats. It is handsomely printed, as indeed are all the medical books issued by the Messrs. Wood.   G.

The Elements of Materia Medica and Therapeutics. By JONATHAN PEREIRA, M. D., F. R. S. and L. S. Third American edition, enlarged and improved by the author. Including notices of most of the medicinal substances in use in the civilized world, and forming an Encyclopœdia of Materia Medica. Edited by JOSEPH CARSON, M. D., Professor of Materia Medica and Pharmacy in the University of Pennsylvania ; Fellow of the College of Physicians of Philadelphia, etc. Vol. 1st. Philad. Blanchard & Lea. 1852. pp. 838.

We are pleased to see that Messrs. Blanchard & Lea are engaged in publishing another edition of this valuable work. The first volume is before us, printed in handsome style, and containing all the " recent discoveries in Natural History, Chemistry, Physiology and Practical Medicine, relating to the Materia Medica. It is unnecessary to say anything in commendation of this work, as it is universally admitted to be the most comprehensive treatise on the subject in our language. We presume that there will be no delay in the publication of the second volume.   G.

Manual of Diseases of the Skin, from the French of MM. Cazenave and Schedel, with notes and additions. By THOMAS H. BURGESS, M. D., Surgeon to the Blenheim Street Dispensary for diseases of the skin, &c. Second American from the last French edition, with additional notes by H. D. BULKLEY, M. D , Physician of the New York Hospital ; Fellow of the College of Physicians and Surgeons, New York, Lecturer on Diseases of the Skin, &c., &c. New York : Published by Samuel and William Wood, 261 Pearl-street. 1852. 1 vol. 8vo. pp. 348.

This work is so well known and so highly appreciated that it is unnecessary to do more than to call attention to the fact that a new and enlarged edition is now offered to the profession. We think it the best manual extant, and should have a place in the library of every physician.   G.

The Pocket Formulary and Synopsis of the British and Foreign Pharmacopœias, comprising standard and approved Formulæ for the preparations and compounds employed in medical practice. By HENRY BEASLEY. First American from the last London edition, corrected, improved and enlarged. Philadelphia : Lindsay and Blackiston. 1852. 1 vol. 12mo. pp. 443.

This work has been favorably received in England, and has reached a third edition. It appears to be carefully prepared, and was probably called for by the profession in that country. We have now several Formularies, quite enough for all useful purposes ; but to those who have none of these, this work may prove convenient.

G.

Essays on Life, Sleep, Pain, &c. By S. H. DICKSON, M. D., Professor of Institutes and Practice of Medicine in the Medical College of the State of South Carolina, &c. Philadelphia : Blanchard & Lea. 1852.

We regret not having room to notice at some length this very creditable little work. It treats of subjects of general interest and in the distinguished author's happiest style.

An Analytical Compendium of the various branches of Medical Science, for the use and examination of Students. By JOHN NEITH, M. D., &c , &c., and F. G. SMITH, M. D., &c., &c. Second edition, revised and improved. Philad. Blanchard & Lea. 1852.

An excellent work for students who are preparing themselves for the ordeal of the " Green Room "—and may be consulted advantageously by practitioners who have allowed themselves to grow " rusty " in reference to first principles.

A Chapter on the Climate of the Isthmus of Panama, and its effects on Health. By C. D. GRISWOLD, M. D., recently one of the Surgeons of P. R. R. Co., New York. Dewitt & Davenport. 1852.

A pamphlet that ought to be procured by those who are going to California by way of the Isthmus.

Logic, in its relations to Medical Science: an address delivered before the Starling Medical College at its third Annual Announcement. By EDWARD THOMPSON, M. D., D. D., &c., President.

A very logical and readable production.

(Circular.)

PARIS, Jan. 12th, 1852.

At a recent meeting of American physicians in Paris, an association was established whose object is the promotion of Medical Science.

This association, essentially national, is progressing under the most favorable auspices. It is intended to be *permanent* in its nature, and is designated the " *American Medical Society in Paris.*"

Notwithstanding the vast advantages afforded by the French metropolis for the study of medical and surgical science, we feel ourselves isolated from our national medical literature, and, therefore, confident-ly appeal to the conductors of American journals and periodicals. We do this with the less hesitation, feeling assured that it will be not only a medium of improvement to ourselves, but a means of a more general diffusion and just appreciation of American literature.

By order of the Society.

A. J. SEMMES, M. D., *Corresponding Secretary.*

NOTICE.

The fifth annual meeting of the American Medical Association will be held at Richmond, Va., on Tuesday, May 4th, 1852.

All secretaries of societies, and of other bodies entitled to represen-tation in this association, are requested to forward to the undersigned correct lists of their respective delegations as soon as they may be appointed.

The following is an exstract from Art. II. of the constitution :

" Each local society shall have the privilege of sending to the association one delegate for every ten of its regular resident members, and one for every addi-tional fraction of more than half of this number. The faculty of every regular-ly constituted medical college or chartered school of medicine, shall have the privilege of sending two delegates. The professional staff of every chartered or municipal hospital containing a hundred inmates or more, shall have the privilege of sending two delegates; and every other permanently organized medical institution of good standing shall have the privilege of sending one delegate."

The medical press of the United States is respectfully requested to copy.

P. CLAIBORNE GOOCH,
One of the Secretaries, Bank-st., Richmond, Va.

State Medical Society.—The annual meeting of the " Medical So-ciety of the State of Georgia," will commence in Augusta on the *second Wednesday* in April. As we anticipate a session of unusual interest, it is hoped the members of the Association will come up from all parts of the State in their full strength. The presence of the Faculty, generally, is specially invited, and will be warmly welcomed.

C. B. NOTTINGHAM, Rec'g Sec'y.

Macon, 12th January, 1852.

SOUTHERN
MEDICAL AND SURGICAL JOURNAL.

| Vol. 8.] | NEW SERIES.—APRIL, 1852. | [No. 4. |

PART FIRST.

Original Communications.

ARTICLE XI.

Cases treated with Veratrum Viride. By Dr. D. C. O'KEEFFE. (Reported by J. S. CLEMENTS, of Penfield, Ga.)

The notes of the subjoined cases have been kindly furnished me by my friend and preceptor, Dr. O'Keeffe. In view of what has been said, in this Journal, on the remedial properties of the American Hellebore, by Dr. Norwood, and the erudite exposition of its botanical characters, by Prof. C. T. Quintard, I shall not embarrass the subject with preliminary remarks, but enter forthwith into the subject.

CASE I. Nov. 3, 1851.—Mrs. ——, aged 21, was delivered of her first child one week ago ; progressed satisfactorily until above date. Condition at that time : Skin hot and dry ; tongue furred, white on centre, red at tip and edges ; mouth dry and lips crusted ; slight headache ; pain in back and bowels—least pressure on abdomen causes pain ; pulse 115, small and hard ; dysuria for last twenty-four hours ; has had two stools during same period from castor oil and spts. turpentine she had taken. *Diagnosis*—Incipient puerperal fever. *Prescription :* Pepper poultice to abdomen, warm cloths to vulva, spts. nitre in parsley tea every two hours, until dysuria is relieved.

5 o'clock, P. M. Has urinated tolerably freely since morning, less pain in bowels, pulse 120 ; other symptoms the same.

Prescription : Eight drops tinct. veratrum viride every three hours until pulse is reduced.

8th—9 o'clock, À. M. Took but two doses of the veratrum viride, before nausea was induced, and lasted two to three hours. Simultaneously with the induction of nausea, perspiration set in, the pulse was lessened in frequency, and continued so all night. Present condition—Pulse 100, skin cool, tongue less red, feels but little pain and sleeps better, except during existence of the nausea, than she had done in several nights. Took a dose of oil and turpentine at 1 o'clock this morning, which has not operated yet; feels nausea occasionally.

9 o'clock, P. M. One stool; feels better, nausea occasionally all day; pulse 85; has taken none of the veratrum viride since last night. Ordered, 10 gtt. tr. veratrum viride every three hours, till nausea occurs, if fever returns. Has passed urine tolerably freely to-day.

8th. Has had no fever of consequence since last date, and therefore needed no medical attention.

REMARKS.—This case would, in all probability, have terminated in puerperal fever; of which it presented the essential characters, but for the timely administration of the hellebore. The febrile action could not have been owing to the dysuria and consequent distention of the bladder, for after these symptoms were relieved, the pulse numbered 120; neither could it be fairly attributed to want of action from the bowels, for they had been moved twice the day the first note was taken. She had had her " milk fever " three or four days before the date first noted, and got on well during the interim ; the lochial discharge was normal, and the untoward features were attributed by the family to " a cold she had taken." It is reasonable, therefore, to infer that it would have run its course, as a case of puerperal fever, had not the potent agency of the veratrum viride curtailed its progress. This is the first recorded case of puerperal fever treated by the American hellebore, and the sanguine expectations of its worthy pioneer, Dr. Norwood, have been fully answered.

CASE II. Nov. 8th, 1851.—Eliza, a negro woman, aged 25,

strong and vigorous constitution, was taken with pneumonia
of right lung on the 4th; was seen and treated by Dr. A. A.
Bell until the 8th, after the usual manner.   Calomel, tart. antimony, ipecac, Dov. powder and blisters, constituted the treatment.   He had used the tinct. of veratrum viride freely for
two days, without producing any perceptible effect whatever,
in addition to the remedies above enumerated.   The patient's
condition at above date was as follows: Skin warm and moist,
from ipecac and tart. antimony she had been taking freely all
day; pulse 120–130, small, compressible under influence of
tartar-emetic; bowels disposed to looseness, and tender to the
touch.   At 5 o'clock, P. M., she took 10 gtt. tinct. veratrum
viride to control the circulation, which had not been influenced
in the least by the calomel and tartar-emetic which she had
been taking for twenty-four hours.

7 o'clock, P. M.   Pulse the same; still perspiring—15 gtt.
veratrum viride.   8 o'clock, P. M.   Nausea and profuse perspiration; griping in bowels, which was followed by a copious
watery operation; pulse 110—took 60 gtt. tinct. opii. to check
bowels.   9 o'clock, P. M.   Nausea and perspiration the same,
bowels easy, feels drowsy, pulse 100, intermittent.   12 o'clock
at night.   Nausea and perspiration, pulse 100, not intermittent—
took 10 gtt. veratrum viride.

9th—10 o'clock, A. M.   One operation since last note, followed by 30 gtt. tr. opii; still perspires; skin cool; pulse 100,
not intermittent; no pain; feels drowsy.   Ordered, 10 gtt.
veratrum viride every three hours while the pulse numbers
100—should it fall before that, to be given less frequently.
Convalescence commenced at above date.

REMARKS.—This case Dr. O'Keeffe saw in consultation with
Dr. Bell, who had judiciously treated it with the usual remedies.
He had even given the hellebore a fair and impartial trial for
two successive days; but it failed—signally failed.   The present case was the second in which the incomparable remedy,
hellebore, failed in Dr. B.'s hands to produce any effect whatever, and he was on the eve of condemning it as an insignificant
puff, when a different preparation proved to him satisfactorily
that his was an inferior article—was inert.   Should this disap-

pointment happen to others, they would do well to pause, and consider the reliability and intelligence of their druggist. Dr. B. obtained his tinct. of veratrum viride from his druggist, while the preparation that fulfilled its mission—told the heart's arteries "so fast shalt thou beat and no faster," was prepared by a physician, in his own office, in the proportion of two ounces to the pint of alcohol.

It is difficult to say, with unerring certainty, what agency the veratrum had in bringing on a favorable crisis in this case, or how it would have terminated under the usual treatment. She took the first dose of hellebore at 5 o'clock, P. M., the tongue being moist and skin warm, but moist also; notwithstanding these favorable effects from the calomel and tart. emetic, the pulse was not reduced any. Two doses of the hellebore accomplished what several doses of the tart. antimony had failed to do. A crisis might have taken place without the veratrum, and its occurrence, after its exhibition, may have been a coincidence instead of an effect; but from the infallible certainty with which it reduces the action of the heart and arteries, I think it not unreasonable to attribute the favorable change, in the present case, to its potency..

CASE III. Mr. B., aged 45, complained of cold chills and acute pain in left side on 12th of November. Poultices, baths, diaphoretics and expectorants, failing to relieve him, he was bled next day 20 oz., the pulse being 100, full and strong. The v. s. and perspiration that followed relieved the pleuritic pain, partially, for a time, but it returned next day with some severity. A blister was applied to the affected side, which removed the pain; took 15 grs. of calomel, twice, in divided doses, which produced three dark operations. During this time, the tongue was covered on the middle with a whitish fur, natural at edges; the mouth dry, clammy, and exceedingly unpleasant, required cleansing frequently in the day; the pulse during the whole time 90–100.

8th day of illness. Skin hot, harsh and dry; tongue furred, clammy and sticking to roof of mouth; taste unnatural, very feeble and extremely restless; pain no where, pulse 90 to 100, variable, feeble and hard. Took several doses of diaphoretic pre-

parations, until altering the condition of the skin, which was so
hot and dry that he said he felt like he should "burn up." At
10½ o'clock, A. M., took 10 gtt. veratrum viride, the pulse being 100. At 11 o'clock, the skin was warmer and disposed to
become moist; pulse stronger and more frequent, 114; no
nausea. 1 o'clock, P. M. Skin moist, generally; large drops
of sweat on face, drowsy, no nausea; pulse 114. 3 o'clock.
Vomited considerable quantities of bilious matter several times.
After he had vomited twice, skin became cool and dry, and
the pulse fell to 100; and after he had vomited two or three
times more, the pulse fell to 80, was small and weak.
5 o'clock. The vomiting having continued, and feeling griping
pain in lower bowels, he took two tea-spoonfuls of paregoric,
which checked the vomiting and griping. Expectoration, of
which there was little or none before nausea, became profuse
after it, and relieved the lungs very much. He took no more
of the hellebore, and his pulse fell to 60, and continued so for
several days, when convalescence commenced, and progressed
satisfactorily to recovery.

REMARKS.—Here is a case in which the usual diaphoretic
remedies had been used freely and faithfully, without effecting
the desired result; whereas 10 gtt. of the veratrum acted like
a charm. The hellebore was not given in this instance to
diminish the frequency of the pulse—for that was not at all
imperative—but to act simply as a diaphoretic, and to remove
the great heat of which the patient complained so much.
It is proper to note that, before nausea set in, and after taking
the veratrum, the temperature of the surface was heightened,
and the pulse accelerated from 100 to 114 in the minute—a
result that ensued only in the present instance.

Without further notice of this case, which was considered
one of typhus fever, I propose to give, in detail, the notes of the
case of pneumonia in which the hellebore was administered as
a principal remedy during the whole progress of the disease.

CASE IV. Nov. 23d, 1851, 9 o'clock, P. M. A negro girl,
aged 20, of strong constitution, in seventh month of pregnancy,
felt pain (slight) for the first time, in her left side, this morning,

but attended to her usual duties until three hours before she
was prescribed for.   Condition: acute pain in her left side;
cough hard, painful and frequent; skin hot and dry; tongue
clean; pulse 120, and strong.   *Diagnosis*—Pleuro-pneumonia.

Prescription: Venesection 1 quart; poultice to left side,
and 10 gtt. tinct. veratrum viride.   12 o'clock.   The same;
15 gtt. veratrum viride.   3 o'clock, A. M.   The same ; 20 gtt.
veratrum viride.

24th, second day, 7 o'clock, A. M.   Skin a little cool, vomited some since last note, perspired some during nausea; other
symptoms the same—23 gtt. veratrum viride.   8 o'clock, A. M.
Nausea and vomiting several times, skin natural, pain almost
relieved; pulse 80, small and weak; deathly sick—Ginger
tea to relieve nausea, and poultice to chest.   6 o'clock, P. M.
Took the veratrum every three hours since last note; skin
warm and dry; one stool; pain in side returned; pulse 112—
15 gtt. veratrum viride.   8 o'clock.   Vomited three times;
skin moist; pain in side the same; pulse 80.   ℞. Calomel, Dov.
powder, *aa* 5 grs. ; ipecac, 3 grs. ; to be taken at once—cups
over seat of pain, and poultice.

25th—9 o'clock, A. M.   One stool; emesis several times in
night; skin harsh and dry, but natural in temperature; cough
hard and painful; pulse 120—15 gtt. veratrum viride every
three hours, poultice to chest, and expectorant to relieve cough.
7 o'clock, P. M.   Took three 15 gtt. doses of the hellebore,
after the last of which she vomited three times; no stool; skin
cool; pulse 80; respiration rapid, 50 in the minute.   11 o'clock,
P. M.   Took no medicine since last note; respiration rapid,
embarrassed and difficult; skin cool, but harsh and dry; very
restless, pulse 120, hard and constricted—15 gtt. veratrum
viride in 50 gtt. tr. opii., to produce sleep.

26th—1½ o'clock, A. M.   Took since last note 15 gtt. veratrum viride: respiration and pulse the same; skin warm and
moist, is in a copious perspiration; no nausea—20 gtt. veratrum.   8 o'clock, A. M.   Respiration and pulse the same;
skin dry and warm; no stool; pulse 120—20 gtt. veratrum
viride.   9 o'clock, A. M.   Was sitting up when last note was
made, which perhaps accelerated the pulse somewhat; skin a
little moist and warm; pulse 100, lessened 20 beats without

any nausea or vomiting; " felt worms creeping up her throat," attended with a flow of saliva and a desire to heave. (Complained of this sensation of worms in the throat since she has been taking the hellebore, and the same feeling was described by another patient who was taking the veratrum at the same time.) 15 gtt. veratrum viride every three hours, and intermediately a powder of calomel, Dover's powder and ipecac; blister to left side. 7½ o'clock, P. M. Took the above; no stool: after second dose of veratrum, vomited freely; skin warm; perspired none; blister well drawn; cough loose; pulse 90—continued veratrum every three hours, and gave injection to relieve bowels.

27th—9 o'clock, A. M. Two stools; emesis several times; cough very troublesome, causing vomiting; respiration very rapid, 50–60; pulse 100—15 gtt. veratrum viride, and same powders intermediately; blister dressed.

28th—8 o'clock, A. M. Followed prescription: two stools; constant nausea and vomiting; cough hacking and toublesome; tongue slightly furred; respiration same; pulse 100—continued hellebore and powders. Night visit: No improvement; felt labor pains since last note. *Prescription:* Discontinued hellebore; blisters to legs and right side; quinine, Dov. powder and ipecac, every three hours, and tart. antimony alternately.

29th—9 o'clock, A. M. Miscarried: pulse very frequent; getting worse—same treatment continued; brandy and quinine if pulse should sink. Night visit: Dead.

REMARKS.—This case of pneumonia tested the hellebore to its utmost capacity, and brings home to our mind the very reasonable conviction that it will not prove infallible in the treatment of pneumonia. On reviewing these notes, it will be seen that the heart and arteries seldom failed to respond to the sedative influence of the veratrum, while the respiration was not affected by it in the least: it was a singular phenomenon to observe the respiration as frequent as 50 or 60, the skin cool and moist and the pulse 80. Hence, in this case, at least, it did control the circulation, but did not affect the respiration or inflammation. There is every reason to believe that the pneumonic inflammation received no check whatever, notwithstanding the circumstance that the patient was kept fully and constantly under the influence of the hellebore. But it is a question of reasonable doubt, whether any course of treatment would have averted the inevitable doom that awaited this patient in view of her advanced state of pregnancy. It is the duty of physicians who submit this agent to the test of clinical experience, to watch carefully its effects, and report them for the benefit of the profession: the remedy is in a state of probation preparatory to its admittance into the sanctum of practice, ·and nothing should be withheld that may add to its value or detract from its merits. In view of the severity and well marked character of the diseases in which it is most likely to be used, its effects can be early determined, either as positive or negative: it will control the bounding pulse, or it will not; there is no half-way ground—no room for speculative propensities. In a type of typhoid fever, in which pulmonic symptoms predominated, Dr. O'K. assures us it had the happiest effects in curtailing the duration of the fever and expediting convalescence. But in cases in which inflammation of the intestinal mucous membrane exist, its exhibition may prove somewhat questionable. It may be said, that as far as the cases go, the claims of the American hellebore to a potent remedy are founded on no fictitious representations: they rest on the indisputable facts of rigid experience; and we have little doubt that when it shall have passed through an extensive trial, the conviction of its importance will become universal, and in the language of Dr. Norwood, a new era in the treatment of disease will be the consequence.

ARTICLE XII.

A Case of Tetanus—successfully treated. By W. W. Havis, M. D., of Houston County, Georgia.

Through the kind solicitations of my professional brethren, I am induced to give the details of a case of Traumatic Tetanus, which came under my care in January last; and if, by reporting in a concise and unvarnished style the features of the disease and the means used for its arrest, I contribute a mite (by data) in elucidating the same, I will realize an ample re-compense for my labor.

January 11th—5 o'clock, P. M., I was summoned to the bed-side of a negro man, æt. 28, of athletic form and robust constitution. On the 20th of December, he exposed himself, in a state of nudity, to the cold, which was severe, and from this congelation of his feet supervened. I saw him on the 28th: his feet were healing kindly; had been no constitutional excitement whatever; removed the lost phalanges of 2d and 3d toes of left foot.

Jan. 3d. Toes nearly healed. Boy walking about the yard without inconvenience, deemed farther attention unnecessary.

Jan. 8th. Exposed bare feet to the frost.

Jan. 11th. Found him resting upon occiput and nates; teeth separate ½ inch; articulates with hissing; face awfully disfigured; muscles of trunk, neck and face perfectly rigid; spasmodic twitching of diaphragm; extremities unaffected; tongue coated white; pulse 100, feeble; skin dry and hot; feet swollen, perfectly tense, very painful; severe paroxysms, at intervals of fifteen minutes, with aggravation of every symptom. Duration two minutes, pulse unchanged, articulation impracticable, excrutiating pain at scrobiculus cordis, bowels not evacuated since 8th. Placed him in warm bath; elm cataplasm to feet, sinapism to abdomen, emp. lyttæ from occiput to sacrum. Comp. ext. colo. and calomel *aa* grs. iij., followed by oleum ricini and ol. terebinth; pulv. Doveri, grs. x. every three hours.

Jan. 12th—11 o'clock, A. M. Bowels unmoved; pulse 98; volume sine force; paroxysms unaltered; tongue dry, and brown; viscid, frothy saliva exudes through teeth; dysphagia; skin hot and dry; feet very painful; teeth clenched during paroxysm; fine vesication upon spine. Ordered, ung. hyd. rubbed upon vesicated surfaces, enema of solution chloride sodium, opium cataplasms to feet, and mustard to abdomen; pulv. Dov. continued.

13th—11 o'clock, A. M. Pulse 88, tongue foul, paroxysm *in statu quo*, spasm reduced by attempting deglutition, small stool, pain in feet unabated, saliva profuse and ill-conditioned. Ordered, calomel grs. v., pulv. jalap grs. xx., followed by enemata of chloride sodium; cataplasms; alc. ext. cannabis indicus, grs. iss. every half hour.

14th—11 o'clock, A. M. Bowels moved, and no essential change—continued hemp. 15th. Pain at epigastrium very poignant during clonic spasm, tongue foul, respiration accelerated, saliva profuse, pulse 91, bowels unmoved. Ordered, salt enema—hemp continued. 16th. Dysphagia terrible, paroxysms irregular, induced by effort of any kind; hiccough troublesome; three copious stools. Ordered, quinia grs. xx., opium gr. i., every three hours. 17th. Clonic spasms greatly aggravated, pulse 100, patient groans piteously, lachrymation profuse, eyes blood-shot, fearful dyspnœa, pain at scrobiculus cordis severe, extremities affected and opisthotonos complete; every symptom unpropitious. Ordered, tinct. veratrum viride gtt. xii. every two hours; poultice, &c. 18th. Pulse 50, paroxysms modified in severity and duration, exacerbation one minute, respiration more free, twitching of diaphragm during tonic spasm, not present, tongue dry, skin hot and dry, suppuration in feet established, and copious stools, stench intolerable, breath offensive. Ordered, pulv. Dov. xv. grs. every two hours, emp. lyttæ to nucha, charcoal cataplasm, imbued with tinct. opii., to feet; jalap xx. grs., calomel v. grs. 19th. Pulse 75, skin cool and moist, tongue cleaning, saliva losing fœtor and vicidity, deglutition improved, clonic spasm at intervals of an hour, duration ½ minute, two copious stools, pain in feet abating, swelling subsided, appetite capricious, (takes chicken broth, the first nutriment of any consequence since invasion of disease,) pain in epigastrium diminished. Cataplasms, pulv. Dov., &c., continued. 20th. Pulse 80, swallows without much inconvenience, clonic spasm not appeared since 1 o'clock A. M., two copious stools, excessive nausea and emesis, tongue nearly clean. Ordered, sinapism to epigastrium, pulv. Doveri grs. xv., pulv. zinjiber grs. ij., until nausea and vomiting is relieved, every three hours. 21st. Pulse 100, tongue clean, red and dry; nausea and vomiting quelled, prostration great, severe pain at hypogastrium, two stools, all blood, lbj. aa.; tonic rigidity of muscles unchanged. Ordered, enema acet. plumb. and tinct. opii., sinapism to hypogastrium, Dover's powder, continued. 6 o'clock, P. M. Two stools, blood and mucus; enema repeated, elm tea as potation, opium and tannin aa. grs. ij. 22d. Pulse 90, small; tongue moist, profuse diaphoresis, prostration great, one stool semifœcal. Ordered, brandy ℥iss. every three hours, charcoal and opium cataplasm to feet, opium grs iss. every four hours. 23d. Pulse 80, tongue moist, skin cool and moist, sleeps, one stool, fœcal, small; tonic spasm abating, feet doing well; amputated middle phalanges of 2d and 3d toes of left foot, and gave flap. Ordered, quinia grs. ij., opium grs. ss., brandy ℥ij. every four hours.

This treatment was persevered in until tonic rigidity of muscles was overcome; then the quinia and brandy prescribed until his wonted strength and health were restored. Tonic rigidity was not reduced until the lapse of twelve days after arrest of clonic spasm. From arrest of clonic spasm to the 23d of January, there was tonic rigidity, and at no time within the period could his head be raised one inch without elevating the body the same length. In using the terms clonic and tonic, I wish to be understood as not employing them to express perfect relaxation from violent contraction, but a medium ground: from violent exacerbation, to mild. The risus sardonicus was perfect during tonic spasm—the violence of the clonic so distorting the features as to banish anything like a risus. His respiration was always difficult during clonic spasm, but easy during tonic; sore when twitching of diaphragm perturbed it. He rested upon his nates and occiput all the time of his illness, except one day and night, and then opisthotonos was complete. The Indian hemp which I used, presented all the physical qualities of a fine article, but was certainly devoid the action ascribed to it by Dr. O'Shaughnesey. The quinia seemed entirely out of place, notwithstanding its merit as an alterative and sedative; it proved rather a conservative of the spasm than otherwise, and I cannot attribute such a sudden exacerbation of the disease to aught save the drug. The veratrum viride effected such sedation as to give unwonted potency to the Dover's powder, and it was for this I stopped it, feeling confident that I could continue the sedation as well with the Dover's powder as with the hellebore, and secure a more decided action upon the gastro-enteritic functions.

The case may, by skeptics, (for want of autopsical facts,)

be termed a mild one, a mere flash; because its action was not
substantiated by the patient's death. But, because some cases
prove fatal in a few hours, it is not proof that other cases are
not as severe, because they procrastinate their "dead set" a
day or two, or even eventuate in restoration to health. But,
"*quantum sufficit.*" I do not consider the case as one of the
most active, but as one of inveteracy, and requiring medical
aid. Further comment is unnecessary: let the case and its
treatment go for its worth, and I am content.

ARTICLE XIII.

A Case of Onanism, presenting great difficulty of Diagnosis.
By J. A. Long, M. D., of McMinn Co., East Tennessee.

On the 15th of October, 1851, I was called to R. M., a young
man, æt. 25 years, of rather delicate constitution, had suffered
from several attacks of chill and fever, and was of a family
predisposed to renal affections. I found him sitting up by the
fire, complaining of a dull, heavy, listless feeling, with a general
aching and numbness all through his system, and particularly
in his limbs, more referable to the bones than other parts of the
body. He was somewhat cold, or rather chilly, at times, but
nothing like a distinct chill had he suffered from the onset of
his disease. His pulse was somewhat accelerated and rather
weak; skin warm, and perspiring; bowels costive; tongue
pale, and covered with a white coat; feet and hands rather inclined to be cool, and said he felt as he generally did previous
to attacks of chill and fever, which I thought myself he was
about taking. From the inactive state of his liver and bowels,
I gave him one or two calomel purges, followed by quinine,
with some benefit for a short time only.

In about a week I was again called, and found him in a similar condition, only somewhat worse, particularly in his back
and lower extremities. Ordered, blue pill, followed by oil, and
quinine to be given as before, and continued for several days.

I was again called in about a week, and found all of his
symptoms much aggravated, particularly in his back, of which
he complained greatly on being moved. Numbness and aching

down his legs, and in fact all over his body; fugitive pains through the abdominal muscles, and with more or less constriction around the abdomen; great soreness on pressure along the spine, especially the lumbar and lower dorsal region; pulse 140 in the minute, skin warm and perspiring freely. I now changed my opinion as to the nature of his complaint, and thought I undoubtedly had a case of *spinal meningitis* to deal with.

Treatment.—Local depletion, followed by a blister along the whole of the tender portion of the spine; calomel, until a decided impression be made upon the system; low diet, &c. The effect of this course of treatment was only to ameliorate the symptoms, reduce the fever and pulse, and to allay or remove the excruciating pains of the spine. The pains of the back have become more dull and deep-seated, as if they were in the kidneys; great soreness along the lumbar muscles, particularly on pressure; perspiration still profuse, and has a disagreeable acid odour; still complains much of his extremities, aching in his bones, &c. He now presents unequivocal symptoms of rheumatism of the lumbar muscles, which, however, only last a short time, and are followed by deep-seated pains in the region of the kidneys, of a spasmodic character, severe and excruciating, shooting down in the direction of the *ureters* to the testicles, these latter organs being drawn up. He has become greatly emaciated, notwithstanding his appetite has been tolerably good, and he has been generally allowed a generous diet. His case remained stationary, under the form of *nephralgia,* for at least two months, without fever or any excitement of the arterial system. Throughout the whole of his illness he has been remarkably restless, irritable (especially at night) and slept but little. Opium was used, in large doses, to allay his suffering, with only temporary relief. The whole class of diuretics was used without advantage. He had the appearance of a man of at least 45 years of age: his face became shrivelled and wrinkled, his countenance was bad and anxious, he wore his cap pulled down over his eyes during the whole of his sickness, and frequently exclaimed, "what a fix—what a fix to be in! death is far preferable. Oh, I will die! oh, I will die!" &c. In this stage of the disease, all hopes on the part of the patient and his friends were lost, and, in fact, death seemed to be his inevitable doom, unless some speedy relief were afforded him. There was but slight alteration of the urine, either in color, quality or quantity; at times it was slightly *albuminous*. His bowels continued costive, and were only moved when oil was given or the syringe used.

One of my pupils, Dr. G. A. Long, on visiting the patient, was asked by him if he knew what —— *self-pollution* was, and what were its effects. This conversation, on being reported to me, immediately unriddled the mystery of the case—my suspicions were confirmed at my next visit by a full acknowledgement of the baneful practice. I now put him upon a more nourishing diet, and the free use of tonics, quinine and the various preparations of iron, and directed as much cheerfulness as possible on the part of the attendants. This course was persevered in until he could go about the yard, and was able to take the cold bath. He began to improve immediately, under the iron and quinine treatment, though slowly and gradually.

REMARKS.—I have been thus tedious in the particulars of this case, because I thought it would be instructive, especially to the junior readers of the Journal. As this is the first case of the kind I have met during a practice of eight years I naturally conclude it is of rare occurrence, especially in country practice, though occurring sufficiently often to deserve the attention of medical men. By way of excusing himself, this young man mentioned to me another, equally guilty with himself, who had abandoned the practice on account of a severe spell of *chronic rheumatism*, affecting nearly everp joint of his body, but especially his back and lower extremities. He was down some twelve months, and his case was spoken of as a very strange one. His appearance was that of my patient— downcast countenance, old look in the face, dejected spirits, &c. There is nothing a young man can be guilty of that will undermine and sap the foundation of his constitution sooner and more effectually than this abominable practice.

PART II.

Eclectic Department

Throat Diseases. By IRA WARREN, M. D.

FOLLICULITIS.—This disease made its appearance in this country, so far as is known, in 1830, and the attention of the profession was first drawn to it, as a *distinct disease*, in 1832. Some have supposed its origin to have had a hidden connection with the epidemic influenza, which spread over the civilized world in 1830; but this is only conjecture. In its early developments, it attracted notice chiefly by its visitations upon the throats of the clergy. Hence its popular name of " *clergyman's sore throat.*" It was soon found, however, to attack all classes of persons, whether engaged in any calling requiring a public exercise of the voice or otherwise. It was more noticed by public speakers and singers, by reason of the greater trouble it gave them.

The disease consists simply in a chronic inflammation of the mucous follicles or glands connected with the mucous membrane which lines the pharynx, larynx, trachea, &c. The office of these little glands is to secrete a fluid to lubricate the air-passages. When inflamed, it spreads an acrid, irritating fluid over surrounding parts, and excites an inflammation in them. This, if not arrested ends in ulceration; the expectoration becomes puriform and undistinguishable from that of consumption, and the patient dies with all the symptoms of phthisis. Indeed, before its nature was understood by the profession, it was thought the most fatal form of consumption, because it could be affected only to a very small degree, if at all, by medicines taken into the general system.

When disease lays hold of those follicles in the larynx which supply a fluid for lubricating the vocal cords, and the secretion conducted to those instruments of speech is acrid and irritating, the voice becomes hoarse; and when at length the ulceration reaches the vocal ligaments themselves, the voice suffers a gradual, and finally a total extinction. I have treated a large number suffering entire loss of voice, and am happy to say it has been restored in every instance.

The approach of this disease is often so gradual as hardly to attract notice—sometimes for months or even years giving no other evidence of its presence than the annoyance of something in the troat to be swallowed or hawked up, an increased secretion of mucus, and a sense of uneasiness and loss of power in the throat after public speaking, singing, or reading aloud. At length, upon the taking of a cold, the prevalence of an epidemic influenza, or of an unexplained tendency of disease to the air-passages and lungs, the throat of the patient suddenly becomes sore, its secretions increased and more viscid, the voice grows hoarse, the difficulty of speaking is aggravated, and what was only an annoyance, becomes an affliction, and a source of alarm and danger. The disorder clearly belongs to the family of consumption, and needs early attention.

It is amusing to reflect upon the theories which writers were in the habit of constructing, a few years since, to account for the throat affections among the clergy. It was attributed by some to speaking too often, by others to speaking too loud. One class of writers thought it arose from high, stiff neck-stocks; another, from a strain of voice on the Sabbath to which it was not accustomed on other days.

The cause of the disease lies deeper than any of these trifling things. So far as ministers are concerned, it may be expressed in two words—labor, anxiety.

The clerical order are placed just where they feel the force of the high pressure movements of the age. They are the only class of recognized instructers of adult men, and are obliged to make great exertions to meet the wants of their position. The trying circumstances in which they are often placed, too, in these exciting times, by questions which arise and threaten to rupture and destroy their parishes, weigh heavily on their spirits and greatly depress the vital powers. And when we add to this the fickle state of the public mind, and the shifting, fugitive character of a clergyman's dwelling-place, and the consequent liability to poverty and want to which himself and family are exposed, we have a list of depressing causes powerfully pre-disposing to any form of disease which may prevail. As we have said, however, it is not the clergy only, but all classes of people who are afflicted with this dangerous malady.

The long and rather awkward name which Dr. Green has given to this disease is, Follicular Disease of the Pharyngo-Laryngeal Membrane. I call it Folliculitis, or, as this term does not describe its seat, follicular laryngitis, or follicular pharyngitis, according to its position.

Through a general lack of acquaintance with this disease, it has been often confounded with bronchitis. But bronchitis is an inflammation of the mucous membrane which lines the bronchial tubes, and of course has no existence except *below* the bifurcation of the trachea. In strictness it is not a throat disease at all.

Folliculitis is also often mistaken for laryngitis. But this latter disease is an inflammation spread over the mucous membrane of the laryngeal cavity. Bronchitis and laryngitis affect *mucous membranes;* folliculitis, the *follicles* of these membranes. Each is a separate disease, and they are easily distinguished by one who understands them. They are often complicated and unite in one subject.

There is yet another form of these chronic diseases, with which many are afflicted. Inflammation sometimes begins behind and a little above the velum palati, in the posterior nares, or back passages to the nose. Thus seated, it generally passes under the name of *catarrh in the head.* It often creates a perpetual *desire to swallow*, and gives the feeling, as patients express it, " as if something were sticking in the upper part of the throat." When the inflammation is of long standing, and ulceration has taken place, puriform matter is secreted, and drops down into the throat, much to the annoyance and discomfort of the patient. Many times the sufferer can only breathe with the mouth open. Upon rising in the morning, a great effort is generally required to clear the head, and the extreme upper part of the throat. Even distressing retching and vomiting are sometimes induced by the effort to clear the back nasal passages. There is occasionally a feeling of great pressure and tightness across the upper part of the nose ; and the base of the brain sometimes suffers in such a way as to induce headache, vertigo and confusion. The smell is frequently destroyed, and sometimes the taste.

If the inflammation be in the pharynx or larynx, there is a similar sensation of something in the throat, but the desire is not so much to swallow it as to hawk it up.

Beside these chronic forms of disease, there are a number of acute inflammations which attack the air-passages, and run a rapid and very dangerous course. Croup is well known as one of them. There is another, which attacks the mucous membrane of the larynx and epiglottis, which reaches also the sub-mucous cellular tissues of these organs, and which often proves fatal in a few hours. The effusion of serum into the epiglottis, in consequence of a high state of inflammation of that cartilage, causes it to stand upright, so that it cannot cover and protect the opening to the larynx; and the lips of the glottis, distended by the same cause, approach each other, thus closing up gradually the passage to the wind-pipe, and threatening immediate suffocation. It was this disease of which Washington died, as we learn from the clear account of the *symptoms* given by his medical attendants, though they mistook the disorder for another, the profession not being then acquainted with it.

Treatment of Throat Diseases.—Fifteen years ago, these

disorders were thought to be incurable; and by all the appli-ances of medical art then known, they were so. But time has brought a successful method of treatment, as well as a clearer knowledge of their nature. The honor of first employing such treatment in this country belongs to Dr. Horace Green, Prof. of the Theory and Practice of Medicine in the New York Medical College. It had been previously used by Drs. Trous-séau and Belloc, of Paris; but this detracts nothing from Dr. Green's just honors, as he had no knowledge of their discovery —for such it was—until after he had done the same thing on this· Continent.

This treatment, as is generally known to the profession, con-sists in topical medication, or the applying of the remedy direct-ly to the diseased part. The medicinal agent, more extensively used than any other, is a strong solution of nitrate of silver. This substance is not, however, adapted to every case—other articles succeeding better in some few ·instances. Modern chemistry has given us a variety of articles, from which the skilful physician may select a substitute, should the nitrate of sllver fail. This article has, however, proved itself nearly a *specific* for inflammation of mucous membranes, acute or chronic not connected with a scrofulous or other taint of the system ; and where such taints exist, it will generally succeed, if proper constitutional remedies are used.

Instruments.—The instrument employed by most physicians is a piece of whalebone, bent at one end, to which is attached a small round piece of sponge. I formerly used this instrument myself, and am happy to know, that notwithstanding its de-fects, it was generally successful. Yet where the larynx has been highly inflamed, with a swollen and ulcerated condition of the epiglottis and lips of the glottis, I have found the singular powers of the argent. nitratis put at defiance by an irritation evidently produced by the sponge of the probang. Upon its introduction in such cases, the parts contract upon and cling to it, and suffer aggravated irritation, almost laceration, upon its withdrawal, however carefully effected.

A case of this sort occurred to me in the person of a gentleman of great moral and intellectual worth, a teacher of a classical school, to whom I was called in Plymouth county, in August, 1849. He was at the point of death from starvation, not having been able to swallow anything, not even water for a number of days. The epiglottis and lips of the glottis were much swollen and deeply ulcerated, and the whole pharyngo-laryngeal mem-brane involved in a high state of inflammation. The first two applications of the nitro-argentine solution, made to the isthmus of the fauces and pharynx on Saturday evening and Sunday, so far relieved him, that on Monday morning he drank, with a sense of unspeakable satisfaction, a tumbler of cold water. Before I could see him on Wednesday evening, however, he was again sinking, the full activity of the inflammation having returned ; and every subsequent attempt to introduce the sponge, and to carry it down to the seat of the disease, caused such irritation as to exhaust the patient. He sank and died, leaving a void in his neighborhood which it will be hard to fill. I feel confident that with the instrument I am about to introduce to the notice of the reader, I could have reached the seat of the disease with so little disturbance of the parts, as to have saved his life.

Such defects in the probang led me to contrive an instrument, which I call a *Laryngeal Shower Springe.* It is in the form of a syringe, the barrel and piston of which are of glass. To this is attached a small tube, made of silver or gold, long enough to reach and enter the throat, and bent like a probang, with a globe at the end, from a quarter to a third of an inch in diameter, pierced with very minute holes, which cover a zone around the centre, one third of an inch or more in breadth.

This silver globe I daily introduce into highly inflamed and ulcerated larynges, generally without any knowledge of its presence on the part of the patient, until the contained solution is discharged. A single injection throws a *very fine* stream through each of the holes in the globe, and thus all sides of the walls of the trachea are washed at once. Moreover, the smallness and smoothness of the bulb allows of its easy and painless passage through the rima glottidis, so as to bathe the walls of the trachea as low as the bifurcation, and even of the large bronchi. Physicians will understand the advantage of this in the case of ulcers low down in the trachea. They will see its advantage, too, in the case of croup in children, into whose larynges it is not easy to introduce the sponge.

The introduction of this instrument into the larynx is easy. Upon the approach of any foreign substance, the epiglottis instinctively drops down upon the entrance to the larynx, guarding it against improper intrusions. It has been found, however, that when the root of the tongue is firmly depressed, this cartilage cannot obey its instinct, but stands erect, its upper edge generally rising into view. Availing himself of this fact, the surgeon has only to depress the tongue with a spatula, bent at right angles, so that the hand holding it may drop below the chin, out of the way, and as the epiglottis rises to view, slip the ball of the instrument over its upper edge, and then, with a quick yet gentle motion, carry it *downward* and *forward* between the lips of the glottis, and the entrance is made. I have often admired the heroic faithfulness of this epiglottic sentinel, who, when overborne by superior force, stands bolt upright, and compels us to enter the sacred temple of speech, *directly over his head!*

This instrument I have used with great satisfaction. A considerable number of physicians, in different States, have procured and are now using it.

For bathing the upper part of the throat, I construct it with a *straight* tube, with holes over the outer portion of the globe, and extending to the centre. This washes instantaneously the fauces and pharynx, without throwing the solution back upon the tongue.

Inflammations in the back passages to the nose, have been almost entirely inaccessible by any reliable healing agent, and consequently incurable. The probang could only reach a short distance, and caused great suffering. I have had this syringe constructed with a short bend, and the globe pierced with a few fine holes at the upper end. Carrying this globe up behind the velum palati, with a single injection I wash both passages clear through. I have had the pleasure of curing a large number of bad cases, of several years' standing, to the surprise and delight of the patients.

Many of these throat affections are connected with functional disturbance of the liver and stomach. In such cases the inflammation of the throat generally refuses to yield until the hepatic and gastric troubles are corrected. Indeed, in a majority of cases, the topical applications need to be accompanied, for the above as well as for other reasons, by a constitutional and alterative treatment.

One word respecting the tonsils. They are chiefly " an aggregated mass of mucous follicles"; and in many follicular diseases they are found enlarged, inflamed, and sometimes indurated. In such cases they secrete a thin, unhealthy, irritating fluid which is spread over the throat, increasing and perpetuating its disease. Much of this secretion, too, finds its way into the stomach, and thence into the circulation; and I am not sure that many cases of scrofula are not engendered by the poison thus conveyed to the blood. At all events, the throat seldom gets well in such cases, until the tonsils are removed.

For the excision of these glands, I found the same lack of instruments, as for making topical applications to the throat. The only one which had any claims to regard, was the guillotine instrument, invented some years since by Caleb Eddy, Esq., of this city. It had, however, no facilities for drawing the tonsil forward. Generally, all that could be done with it was to *trim* the gland, which did little good, for it became again enlarged. I attached the bull-dog tenaculum to it, with which I have been able to draw the tonsil from between the pillars of the fauces, and cut it through the root,.so as effectually to prevent a second growth. As there were still some defects in this instrument, I have prepared an entirely original one, with which the extirpation of these glands is so easy and expeditious, and withal so little to be dreaded by the patient, as to leave, I think, little further to be desired in this line.

As bearing directly upon this subject, I will add, that about three years since, Dr. Chambers, of London, reasoned that if nitrate of silver have a specific influence over inflammations of mucous membranes, it would cure bronchial consumption, and perhaps other forms of that disease, if it could be got into the lungs. He accordingly made a powder of that article and lycopodium to be breathed into the lungs. His account of it was published in the London Lancet, and has appeared in this Journal.

In August, 1849, I prepared the same powder; and not only in the cure of bronchial consumption, but in the treatment of the *first* and *third* stages of the tubercular form of this disease, I obtain results from it which I can derive from no other article.

I also use lycopodium for preparing powders in the same way, with sulph. of copper, crystals of nitrate of mercury (sometimes useful in secondary syphilitic troubles of the throat,) iodide of potassium, &c.

For breathing powders of every kind, I have constructed a neat inhaler, which consists of a glass tube and a receiver—the latter being something like a tube vial, perforated with holes around the lower end. The powder is poured into the receiver, which is placed in the larger tube, and twirled between the thumb and finger while inhaling.

In the bronchial forms of consumption, the local disease is confined to the mucous membranes; and in the tubercular type, the deposite *begins* upon the same tissue. Breathing medicine directly into the lungs is therefore the rational mode of attacking the local disease. The time must soon come when this form of treatment will be universally adopted. The mode of applying it will doubtless be improved, and the articles employed be multiplied. But we are on the right track, and the period may not be distant when this fearful malady, taken in proper season, will be held as curable as chronic diseases of the stomach or liver.—[*Boston Medical and Surgical Journal.*

Cerevisia Fermentum.—On the use of Yeast in Putrid Sore Throat, &c. &c.

To the Editor of the Boston Medieal and Surgreal Journal:

Sir,—The gratifying effects of the use of yeast, and the very happy result, in a case of putrid sore throat, that I have just had under my charge, induce me to offer the following suggestions for publication in your excellent Journal.

The case alluded to was a boy 12 years old. For a week previous to my being called in, he had complained of common sore throat. He had had the usual domestic remedies applied, and among them a flannel bandage around the neck. He considered himself well on Monday, 11th inst., and imprudently took off the bandage, going out and exposing himself to the inclement weather. He was taken severely ill on Monday, with a high fever, headache, &c, and early on Tuesday morning I was sent for, and found him laboring under all the symptoms of malignant inflammation of the throat, accompanied by an eruption on the face and neck, of a dark-red color; face somewhat swelled; skin of face and neck exceedingly *rugous,* like the surface of the leaf of sage; tongue of a fresh meat color; rima glottidis tumefied and inflamed: epiglottis erect and almost immovable from tumefaction, and the whole mouth and fauces dry and harsh. There was considerable cough, but the tough ropy sputa could not be expelled. I applied the usual antiphlogistic treatment, except bloodletting. A sinapism on the throat enabled the patient to swallow his medicine. The usual course of such a disease went on regularly till Thursday morning, the eruption having extended over the whole body. On that morning, unequivocal symptoms of ulceration and typhoid showed themselves. The pulse was small, thready, feeble and quick; the mind wandering, with incessant murmuring; inability to articulate intelligibly; alternate severe pains in the head and abdomen; little sensibility in the throat; small white and grey spots throughout the mouth, tongue and fauces, and numerous petechiæ on the face and abdomen. I immediately ordered half a pint of fresh brewer's yeast, mixed with half a pint of water, with brown sugar sufficient to give it flavor, and to take a table-spoonful of the mixture every two hours, suspending all other remedies, except the gargle (made of borate of soda, honey and infusion of sage) and occasional sinapisms to the throat. Up to this time the fever and eruption had been regularly intermittent, coming on about 2 o'clock in the morning, and subsiding about 12 M., at which time the skin became quite smooth, and very slight signs of the eruption. On Friday morning, a great change had taken place. He had rested tolerably well during the night; his tongue and mouth were nearly relieved and clean; the fever and eruption were quite moderate, and passed off before 9 o'clock. On Saturday, still further improvement was manifested. He could eat with facility, and begged for food, which was allowed him freely. On Sunday morning, all symptoms of the disease had disappeared, except the swelled and sore lips, and edges and point of the tongue. On Monday, all he required to constitute him perfectly well was strength; but even in that respect he was not very unwell, for he got up, in the absence of his mother from his room, and went to the window; and when I saw him last, on Tuesday, he was about the house with the rest of the family. He continued to take the yeast until Monday evening.

I have been rather particular in relating the case, that it might be understood; though I fear some will think, from the the rapid recovery and my imperfect description, that it was not a very severe one. I have seen many cases, during my thirty years' practice, of putrid sore throat, scarlatina maligna,* or whatever else it may be called, but I have never seen a more threatening one than this, particularly on Thursday morning. Its happy termination I attribute entirely, under Providence, to the free use of the yeast. I had used this article ever since the Rev. Mr. Cartwright, of Louisiana, published his account of its successful employment in nervous fevers some thirty years ago. I prescribe it in the typhoid stage of all eruptive diseases, especially small-pox, and generally with the happiest effect.

And now, sir, to the object of this paper. Do we not sacrifice too much in our endeavors to *refine* our remedies? Nearly all our writers discourage the use of yeast, saying we can avail of its active principles in far more elegant and convenient forms. I do not believe this. Who, I beg leave to ask, who knows what the active principles of yeast are? We can analyze and obtain from it potash, carbonic acid, acetic acid, malic acid, lime, alcohol, extractive mucilage, saccharine matter, gluten, water. But can we say that these ingredients or principles, artificially combined, in part or in whole, individually or collectively, will make yeast? And will the article thus made have the same effect as the natural article or compound does? Who can say that the effect of an article like this is attributable to its generation of carbonic acid, or to its tonic power derived from the bitter principle, or to the stimulating principle of its alcohol? We all have used carbonic acid in

---

* This boy had scarlet fever (scarlatina simplex) very severely, six years ago, and was attended by myself.

the form of carbonated water, effervescing draughts, &c.; and stimulants in the form of ammonia, alcohol, wine, &c.; and tonics in the form of bark, quinia, &c.; but never have I seen the effects from all these equal to those of yeast. Who can say that in the process of analyzation some very active principle is not lost? I think yeast exerts a direct and most powerful influence upon the degenerated blood, restoring it speedily to a healthy condition. It seems to generate some active principle while in the stomach, which acts upon the blood and nervous system. Certainly its effects on the system, in diseases of a typhoid character, are entirely unlike those of any other remedy. In our endeavors to render our remedies more " elegant," and " convenient," therefore, by the extraction of active principles, we should be careful lest we sacrifice utility to nicety. We all know that even *quinia* is not in all cases a substitute for Peruvian bark, although this article approaches nearer to a perfect embodiment of the active principle of a natural product than any other. Quinia is not always bark, nor morphia opium. But in the case before us, for yeast, in my opinion, no substitute can be obtained, even by a combination of every one of its active principles artificially; for, as before observed, there seems to be an active principle in the original that cannot he found by analysis, and that is destroyed by it. This principle seems to me to resemble the principle of life.

In conclusion, I hope your professional readers will bear these suggestions in mind, and when they have a case suitable for it, give the article a trial, and the patient a chance to be benefited by it. It is proper to say that *brewer's yeast* is the article I always use. Distiller's, baker's and common family yeast, do not act so well; though either are very far better than none. When prepared as above, it is by no means disagreeable. With children, I generally call it porter sangaree, and they are not aware of the deception.

Yours,   GIDEON B. SMITH, M. D.,

Baltimore, Md., Jan. 22, 1852.

BALTIMORE, January 27th, 1852.

Dear Sir—I feel it to be my duty to place at your disposal the following statement of facts, at the earliest moment.

I had scarcely returned from mailing my article to you on the subject of the use of yeast in putrid sore throat [see above], when I was called to visit a family of four children. I found them all laboring under severe symptoms of scarlatina maligna. The mother informed me they had been for two or three days complaining of dryness and some soreness of the throat,

headache, nausea, and pain in the back and stomach; but on
Friday evening, 23d inst., three of them went to bed, viz:—
John, 13 years; Mary, 8 years; and Robert, 4 years of age:
Charles, aged 10 years, not in bed, but complaing greatly.
When I saw them, on Saturday morning, the eruption was
fully developed on the face and neck of the three first, of a
dark dull red color; the throat very sore; the tongue dry,
with a dark fur on the middle and back portion; grey spots on
the tonsils and fauces; great mental uneasiness; eyes quite
red, and great anxiety of countenance. In fact, all three had
strong symptoms of the worst form of scarlet fever. The
pulse was almost too quick to be counted, and heat of the skin
very high. The skin of all three had also assumed the peculiar *rugous* appearance described in my previous article. I
had come to the conclusion that brewer's yeast was an antidote to the specific poison of scarlet fever, and I immediately
ordered its free use in these cases, administering it also to
Charles, who was not yet in the eruptive stage. I ordered the
yeast to be mixed with an equal portion of water, and to be
well sweetened with *brown* sugar, each patient to take a table-
spoonful every two hours, unless it affected the bowels, in which
case the quantity to be reduced one half. I gave no other
medicine, and did nothing else except applying sinapisms to all
their throats to enable them to swallow. On Sunday morning
I found they had all passed a tolerably comfortable night.
Their tongues were all clean, moist, and of a healthy color;
throats slightly sore; the eruption extended over the whole
body, but evidently on the decline. Charles, who was one day
later in the various stages than the other three, was now on an
equality with them. On Monday morning all of them were
so well they begged hard to be allowed to leave their beds,
except Robert, the youngest. This morning, Tuesday, 27th,
I have pronounced them all *well*. Robert had been dreadfully
burned several months ago, by the bed being accidentally set
on fire while he was in it. All the burnt surface had been healed,
except a place as large as my hand on the lower part of the
abdomen. His long confinenent and debility from that accident
rendered his attack of the scarlet fever much to be dreaded;
but even in this case the disease had passed away. The fact
that this remedy acts as an antidote to the poison of scarlet
fever, seems to derive great support from the case of Charles,
who commenced taking it before the fever and eruption were
developed, and who, though one day later than the others in the
development of the disease, got well at the same time they did.
    Now here are four cases, three of which commenced on
Friday night, the other on Saturday night, all presenting the

worst form of the disease, and all well on Tuesday morning—three days and a half in three of them, and two days and a half in one of them; and no remedy whatever used except brewer's yeast and occasional sinapisms!

As stated in my former paper, I have long used this remedy in scarlet fever, measles, small pox, and all other eruptive febrile diseases, when they degenerated into the typhoid state—or collapse, as it is generally called I have never before administered it in the first or eruptive and febrile stage, in which, from its success in these cases, it would seem to be even more efficacious than when delayed till the collapse takes place. I know you will think me very enthusiastic on this subject, and too easily led away by a single success with a remedy ; but, when you consider the nature of the disease, its extreme danger when it assumes a virulent form, and the uncertainty of all remedies heretofore used ; and when you consider, also, the formidable character of the case first reported in my former paper, and also that of the four now presented, and the very happy and speedy termination of all of them, I feel assured you will excuse me for calling the attention of the profession to the subject in the most earnest terms. I have rather underrated than exaggerated a single symptom of any of the cases. When l commenced attending them, the parents immediately became hopeless of any one of them, as soon as they learned what the disease was. The parents of the four children had lost a son, a few years ago, of the same disease, and they declared all these children were much more severely attacked than he was. I therefore feel it my duty to lose no time in making these facts public.　　　　　　　　　Respectfully,

GIDEON B. SMITH, M. D.

Observations on Diseases of the Ear ; with practical Remarks on their varieties and Treatment. By THOS. BARRETT, Esq , M. R. C. S., L. S. A., &c., Surgeon to the Ear and Eye Infirmary, Bath.

Acute Myringitis, with perforation of Membrana Tympani.

CASE 1. The Rev. J. H——, aged forty-five, on the 2nd March, 1850, performed the burial service in a damp country churchyard, and in the same evening felt he had " taken cold." He was attacked during the night with great pain in the left side of the face, extending into the ear, which increased and was followed by difficulty of swallowing, and tenderness round the angle of the jaw, and over the mastoid process ; all which symptoms, as he had previously suffered from neuralgia and rheumatism, he attributed to these causes, and took for his relief large doses of quinine and opium.   The pains and discomfort continued to increase, and he began to experience deafness and confused sounds in the ear, with great irritation over the whole of the auricle, and extending far into the ear-passage.

This alarmed him, and on the 9th of March he consulted me. I found him then labouring under considerable pain, as before mentioned, penetrating deeply into the head, and increased by every effort to swallow or open the mouth wide.   He feels the carotid of that side beating loudly in the ear; has tinnitus; the noise, he says, at one time is like the scraping of a saw-mill— at another like the rushing of the wind.   He does not fancy he is very deaf, but I find the hearing distance is less than three inches.   I take this opportunity of mentioning that, with a view to ascertain and note carefully the variation in the bearing power of patients, whilst under treatment, I always employ a metronome for this purpose; its steady, distinct, and uniform beat is more to be depended upon, and therefore is a much better and surer test than the ticking of a watch as ordinarily used.

An examination of the ear showed the auricle in a state of phlegmonous inflammation, and the tragus and commencement of the ear-passages so swollen that no inspection could be made by the speculum.

The next day after free leeching over the mastoid process and in front of the auricle, and the application of warm fomentations and bran poultices, I was enabled to examine the condition of the ear-passage and membrana tympani.

The whole length of the canal was covered with a muco-purulent secretion.   On this being washed away with warm water, the canal was found tender to the touch, swollen, and very red.   The membrana tympani, from its excessive vascularity, was bright rose colour; the projection of the malleus could not be detected; its whole surface looked pulpy and villous.   The tonsils on both sides were enlarged and slightly ulcerated; the fauces generally relaxed; and no air could be passed through the Eustachian tube on the affected side, the effort to do so being attended with great pain.   There is a good deal of constitutional disturbance.   The appetite is bad, and the night sleepless.   Leeches in front of the meatus were again ordered, and counter-irritation to be freely kept up over the mastoid process.   A pill, composed of extract of hemlock and colchicum, and blue-bill, was directed to be taken three times a day.

March 13.—The pain and irritation in the ear, and difficulty of swallowing, had considerably lessened; there is otorrhœa.

The noises in the ear continue most distressing. He is now able to force air through the Eustachian tube; the otoscope detects the air as gurgling through a mucous fluid, and with a peculiar hissing sound indicative of a rupture of the membrane. The speculum shows the membrana tympani still deeply red, though darker in colour, with two distinct vesicles on its surface, though so swollen and pulpy that the exact situation of the perforation could not be detected. The hearing distance is not an inch; indeed, the deafness is nearly complete. The medicine, and counter-irritation over the mastoid process, were ordered to be continued.

16th.—the constitutional symptoms much improved; the pain and irritation in the ear and the adjacent parts are lessened; the noise he likens now to the lowing of cattle. The discharge is very profuse: no improvement in hearing.

The ear was washed out with warm water, and I found a polypus excrescence had shot out from the interior wall of the canal and completely filled up the passage. I removed it by means of Mr. Wilde's ingenious and very useful "snare," and found the membrana tympani of a pale pink colour, with very little remains of its former villous and pulpy appearance. The perforation could not be seen; it was of an irregular shape, and situated near the anterior and inferior portion of the membrane. The removal of the fungus extended the hearing distance at once to about four inches.

As the mouth was rather tender, the pills were discontinued, and the iodide of potassium in bitter infusion was directed to be taken three times a day. A fine point of nitrate of silver was applied very lightly to the edge of the perforation, and gentle syringing with a weak tannin solution ordered twice a day.

This patient continued improving under treatment, both in his general health and in the local malady. On the 15th April, I found the membrana tympani rather thick and studded with opaque spots; there is slight discharge; the hearing distance is about one foot; the tinnitus still continues. Counter-irritation behind the ear with tartrate-of-antimony ointment; the occasional pencilling of the membrane and auditory canal with a solution of nitrate of silver (5 grs. to 1 ounce); and the Bath waters, formed the local and constitutional treatment for another month. At the end of that time the general health was perfectly restored; the discharge had quite ceased; there is still some tinnitus, and occasionally loud crackings, on gaping or swallowing, are heard by him.

I may observe that this gentleman has suffered a long time from dysphonia clericorum; the throat is always more or less relaxed, and the Eustachian tube, I doubt not, partakes of the same irritation of the membrane. The perforation in the tympanal membrane is of an irregular shape, occupying about a fifth of the membrane, the remaining portion of which has now assumed a tolerably healthy appearance ; the auditory canal is dry, and without any secretion of cerumen. The hearing distance is about two feet.

I considered this a favorable case for the use of the hydrated cotton, as recommended by Mr. Yearsley, and to the value of which, in judiciously selected cases, and when applied with due care and tact, I have before borne my full testimony.

Its application increased directly the hearing distance to nearly three yards.

I instructed my patient in its application, and on his visiting me about three months afterwards, I found him still deriving the same comfort from its use, though he says he cannot always "hit upon" the exact point of the membrane to which it should be applied, and then it not only fails in giving relief, but generally produces pain and irritation. An examination of the membrana tympani at this time showed it opaque and slightly vascular, the perforation existing as before. There were no remains of any polypoid growths, and a healthy secretion of cerumen was being established.

Tympanitis ; Exfoliation of the Ossicula ; Periostitis and Caries of a portion of the Mastoid Process.

CASE 2. Miss S——, aged 37, first consulted me in 1849. She stated that she had had scarlet fever at the age of nine years, which was followed by discharge from the left ear, and subsequent deafness in both ears. Her recollection of symptoms at that early period is, of course, not very clear, but she thinks the right ear was first affected. She never remembers having discharge from this ear, but from the left the discharge has been present at intervals from that period until now. On the right side the hearing distance is only two inches ; on the left, four inches. The right membrana tympani is thick, opaque, and studded with pearly deposits, and very much collapsed ; air is easily pressed into the tympanal cavity, but from probably old fibrous adhesions, the shape of the membrane is but little influenced by it. The ear-passage is dry and scaly. The left membrana tympani shows a large perforation, occupying its inferior portion ; the lining membrane of the tympanum seen through it is of a dark red colour ; there is otorrhœa ; air is freely passed by the Eustachian tube through the aperture.

Although from the extent and long standing of the disease, I felt little confidence in any treatment being productive of much good, I advised the application of glycerine to the right ear,

and the hydrated cotton wool to the left. The glycerine certainly did much to improve the condition of the former, and
the wool that of the latter, for the hearing distance was increased so much in each ear as to enable her to hear tolerably
distinctly across a small room.

I frequently saw this lady during several months after this
date, and she always spoke in the strongest terms of the immense addition to her comfort this treatment had induced.
Not content, however, with this, in an evil moment she made
application to one of the advertising quacks, and received, by
post, a nostrum, with directions to apply it freely to each ear.
This I afterwards showed to an experienced chemist, who informed me that it was an etherial tincture of horse-radish.

On the evening of July 1, 1850, she first used this application to both ears. Early the following morning she was awoke
by pain in the left ear, which continued increasing during the
day, but as she was led to expect pain from the application, she
not only bore it patiently, but even applied the drops again at
bed-time. The pain now became excessive, and her sufferings
were such that at an early hour of the morning, I was requested to visit her. She then told me what she had done. She
was experiencing no inconvenience in the right ear, but in the
left ear and left side of the head, she described her sufferings as
agonizing.

I could make no internal examination of the ear; the
whole auricle was so inflamed and sensitive, that the least
touch was unbearable to her. Leeches and fomentation locally
with salines and anodynes, formed the treatment, and when on
July 5, five days after her misfortune, I was able more easily
to inspect the parts, it was indeed sad to see the ravages that
this attack of inflammation, acting on a part already much diseased, had produced. The meatus was filled with a profuse
and offensive purulent discharge; its removal, by the most
gentle syringing, showed the membrana tympani nearly entirely
destroyed, throwing open the tympanal cavity, the lining membrane of which is of a dark red colour, pulpy and granular,
and covered with purulent discharge; the power of hearing,
even by contact is quite lost.

It is unnecessary to follow this case, step by step, in its progress. The general health, never good, now began to suffer
considerably from the increased local irritation, and it was to
improve this, that the treatment was principally directed. She
was put under a course of very mild alteratives and bitter tonics, with the iodide of potassium; but in spite of the most judicious management and careful watching, the local disease fast
extended. Large polypoid growths sprung up from the lining

membrane of the tympanal cavity. The otorrhœa became profuse and most offensive, and it was soon apparent that in addition to the disease of the soft parts, the bony structure was
becoming involved; caries and exfoliation of the ossicula followed, and she began to experience great and continued pain
over the mastoid process, with slight swelling, redness and
soreness on pressure—Leeching and counter-irritation locally,
and the most steady perseverance in constitutional treatment,
failed, however, to arrest these symptoms, and the periosteum
itself quickly became involved in the inflammation; a free incision down to the bone allowed the escape of offensive matter,
followed afterwards by a considerable exfoliation of bone.
The wound healed, and the general health improved, but deafness, permanent and incurable, remained, the consequence of
her unfortunate error.

*Acute Myringitis from the introduction of a Foreign Body
into the Meatus.*

CASE 3.—Master O——, aged nine years, a scrofulous lad,
dropped, while at play, a glass bead into the right ear. Four
days after, he complained of ear-ache, for the relief of which,
laudanum and stimulating applications were freely used. On
the next day he first told his parents of the accident, and the
removal of the bead was ineffectually attempted by forcible
syringings, poking with forceps, bodkins, probes, &c. I first
saw him on the seventh day after the occurrence. An examination by the speculum showed the foreign body at the bottom
of the meatus, and it was removed without difficulty. He was
suffering great pain in the ear, extending over the side of the
head; he was feverish and excited. The auditory canal in its
whole length was dry and red; the membrana tympani was
exceedingly vascular, the vascularity being greatest nearest
the attachment of the malleus. Warm fomentations and saline
purgatives were then prescribed.

On the following day (November 14) the little patient was
so ill that I was requested to visit him at home. I found that
he had passed a night of great suffering from intense ear-ache.
His pulse was quick; tongue loaded; face flushed; the pain
extends over the whole head; he is slightly delirious, and his
sensibility to sound is so great that the slightest noise excites
and disturbs him. An examination of the ear showed great
redness and swelling of the auricle; great pain over the mastoid process, extending round the angle of the lower jaw; the
auditory canal was so swollen as not easily to admit of the introduction of the speculum; a sufficient examination, however,
could be made to show the dry, puffy, and vascular state of the

passage; the membrana tympani was of a bright-red colour, the vessels branching and uniting in all directions, so as to form a mass of red.   His sensibility to sound is not so acute—indeed he is rather deaf, and complains now of strange noises in the ear.

This was a case of acute myringitis, in which, from experience, I felt assured of the necessity of bringing the system quickly under the influence of mercury—a practice, in the early stages of myringitis, so strongly urged by Mr. Wilde, in his valuable communication on the subject, and to the importance of which I can well bear my testimony.   In addition, therefore, to the free fomentations, and the application of leeches round the meatus, I ordered one grain of calomel, with two of James's powder, every four hours, with low diet and saline purgatives.   The leeches gave temporary relief, but during the night the pain returned with increased violence.   In the morning I found the constitutional disturbance very great.   The pain in the ear was acute, and the cerebral irritation very alarming.   He is now quite deaf; the noises in the ear remain as before ; the tumefaction of the meatus, and the general vascularity of the membrana tympani still continue.   Leeches were again applied, and the calomel continued.

Nov. 16th.—Slept better; in less pain; the noises in the ear, he says, are like the squeaking of trumpets.   He cannot hear a loud-ticking watch when close to the ear; hears it when it touches the auricle or mastoid process.   The pulse is very quick, and the febrile excitement considerable.   The membrana tympani is still very red ; two or three ecchymosed spots are seen near the attachment of the malleus.   The auditory canal is swollen and dry, and has several distinct vesicles on its surface.

18th.—Gums very tender ; general symptoms much relieved; is free from pain; sleeps well ; bowels much purged.   He says he does not hear the trumpet-sound in the ear: it is now like the constant whistle of a railway engine.   Can hear at three inches from the ear.   The auditory canal has now no swelling ; it is paler and dry ; the vesicles have healed ; the membrana tympani is much less red—indeed, except over the attachment of the malleus, it has assumed a yellowish-brown colour; it looks dry and inelastic.   The calomel was discontinued, and three grains of mercury with chalk ordered every night ; counter-irritation with tartar-emetic ointment was directed to be used over the mastoid process.

21st.—Very slight tenderness of the gums ; the constitutional condition continues improving ; the hearing distance extends to six inches ; the membrana tympani shows a marked improve-

ment ; any vascularity is scarcely perceptible, except when
air is forced through the Eustachian tube, when vessels are
seen starting over its surface ; it still looks dry and muddy ;
there is no secretion in the auditory canal, which is very dry,
and covered with scales of exuded cuticle. The tinnitus continues. He was directed to continue the grey powder, and to
take three grains of iodide of potassium three times a day.
The tartar emetic ointment having been rubbed in incautious-
ly and too freely, the whole of the covering of the mastoid
process and back of the auricle is a mass of pustules, which are ·
exciting a good deal of general irritation, to relieve which a
poultice was ordered.

28th.—The little patient is considered by his friends to be
nearly well. He is stronger, sleeps well, except that he is tormented hy the irritation of the pustules behind the ear, which
are healing very slowly ; says he hears very well. I find,
however, on testing his hearing, that though greatly improved,
it is far from perfect ; he is a sharp, intelligent, and attentive lad,
and catches conversation quickly. The auditory canal is less
dry and scaly, and is secreting a small quantity of pale cerumen. The membrana tympani is regaining its transparency ;
its surface is smooth, has lost its granular appearance, and now
no longer shows any vascularity, even on pressing air into the
tympanum. He lost all sound in the ear for two days, when it
returned slightly, but has again left him. I directed the bro-
mide of potassium in infusion of cascarilla to be taken twice a
day, with generous diet and change of air, and the discontinuance of all local treatment.

From this time the symptoms all gradually improved ; the
membrana tympani acquired its natural colour and elasticity,
all tinnitus ceased, and the hearing power became perfectly restored. The auditory canal continued very dry for some
time ; the application of glycerine appeared to make up for the
deficiency of ceruminous secretion, but a healthy formation of
wax was at last fully established.

I need scarcely say that any attempt to treat ear disease
without a full and complete examination of the organ, must
always end in unsatisfactory results. The speculum which I
am in the habit of using, consists of a funnel-shaped tube, with
a polished interior ; the light of a wax taper is concentrated on
a small polished mirror, and is reflected by a double reflector
into the tube : the tube does not expand like Kramer's speculum ; indeed, there is so much bony matter and so little soft
parts in the auditory canal, that I have rarely found any advantage from a dilator.

This speculum, originally made by " Jordan, Manchester,"

and to be had at Weiss's, enables me distinctly and easily to
examine the condition of the membrana tympani, if present, or,
if destroyed, deeply into the tympanal cavity. I know objections have been made to artificial light as being likely to mis-
lead, and I admit that the sun's rays are to be preferred ; but
how seldom in this country can we avail ourselves of them I I
feel that diffused light will very rarely enable the practitioner
to gain anything like the opportunity of a certain examination
of the lower part of the ear passage, and in the absence of the
sun's rays, I know no speculum which gives such advantages
as the one I have described.—[*London Lancet.*

On the Vaccine Fluid as an Internal Remedy in Small Pox.
By Dr. Jose Alves Nogueira, of Porto-Algre, Brazil.

The great number of patients which I have lost from small
pox, during fifteen years of practice, both while in charge of
military hospitals, in which this disease is very prevalent, and
in private practice in the city, has led to the use of a variety
of remedies, none of which has produced such satisfactory
effects as the vaccine pus diluted in water and taken internally.
My first case was a negro, attacked with confluent small pox,
which in spite of all the ordinary antiphologistic remedies, increased in violence until it threatened the life of the patient.
At this time it occurred to me to make trial of the vaccine pus,
which being a preventive, it might possibly possess the power
of curing the disease ; on the same principle that belladonna, so
efficacious in the treatment of scarlet fever, is also a preserva-
tive against it. Experience alone will decide, and as my
patient was rapidly growing worse, I resolved to put it to the
test. Procuring a lamina of vaccine pus, of the purest quality, I
dissolved it in an ounce of water, and gave him a tablespoonful
in the morning. In the afternoon the fever had diminished, and
I gave him another dose. He passed the night comfortably,
and slept for the first time in three or four days ; he awoke with
some appetite, his face was much less swollen, and he could
open his eyes. I gave him the remainder of the remedy, and
he convalesced without farther treatment, except a dose of
castor oil.

Case 2d. Child three years of age, whose body was completely covered with variolous pustules, nearly united to each
other, especially on the face and extremities. It had an intense
fever, disturbed sleep, vomiting, difficult deglutition, diarrhœa
and delirum. Under the use of the ordinary remedies, the pustules had arrived at their greatest perfection, and at this
moment I resolved to administer the vaccine pus. Soon after

the first dose the little patient had a quiet sleep, the delirium ceased, the swelling diminished and it rapidly recovered.

Case 3d.   Was a child, thirteen years of age, robust, and of sanguine temperament; two cases of this disease, in the same family, had recently proved fatal.   When first called, I found the symptoms of small pox well developed. the pustules being so united that it was difficult to separate them; the mother and others of the family, terrified at the fatality of the disease, had abandoned their home, and although they had never been vaccinated, could not be induced to submit to this operation.*   My little patient was left in charge of two ladies, who, with commendable charity, offered to nurse her.   The disease ran an unusually violent course, the face appearing at one time to be a single pustule.   With the exception of mild sudorific infusions at first, I used no other remedy than the vacine pus, taken as before described, and with the most complete success; the disease not leaving that disfiguration of the skin which is usual after recovery.

In conclusion, I may remark, that before using the vaccine internally, I applied it externally in the usual way, but without the least result.   It is necessary that the pus be of the purest quality, taken from a healthy subject, before the period of suppuration, generally on the seventh or eighth day, while in a limpid state, and preserved on glass plates, or better, in glass tubes.   I am not aware that any specific remedy, for combating the morbid effects of this terrible disease, has been suggested; but the vaccine matter, so well known to the profession as a preventive, when taken internally, I have found to be the most powerful agent that can be used for its cure, and may be considered as the specific remedy.—[*N. Y. Jour. of Medicine.*

Observations on Nitrate of Silver Stains of the Conjunctiva. Case of absolute Blackness. By James Vose Solomon, M. R. C. S., Surgeon of the Birmingham Eye Infirmary.

The application of a solution of nitrate of silver, if long and injudiciously applied to the conjunctiva of the eye, produces a discoloration which is indelible.   The sclerotic conjunctiva becomes of a dusky brown, or of an olive color; the palpebral linings, more particularly of the lower lid, assume a brownish or

---

* It appears incredible that, notwithstanding the government of Brazil spends a great amount of money, annually, for vaccination, there die every year of small pox, upwards of a thousand persons; and still more incredible, that there are many families who will not be vaccinated, because they consider it entirely useless; this ignorance of the benefits of vaccination, however, exists principally in the interior.

livid hue, or as will be presently shown, become black ; the sulcus between the inferior lid and globe is more deeply dyed than the other parts. In the majority of cases the conjunctiva of the superior lid retains its natural color. In a few rare instances the salt becomes incorporated with ulcers of the cornea, forms a subchloride of silver, and perpetuates one or more black lines in their cicatrices.

A still more uncommon, and I believe hitherto unrecorded change of color consists in absolute blackness of the conjunctiva, an instance of which, the only one that has ever come under my notice, is probably of sufficient interest for publication in your journal.

Case.—A young woman, aged 29, came from a small town in Radnorshire to consult me for a dimness of vision.

Both corneæ were extensively covered by opacities, which were irregularly streaked with black lines. The caruncula lachrymalis and tarsal borders were of a jet-black color, giving the appearance, at a cursory glance, of soot or dirt settled on those parts. The palpebral conjunctivæ were smooth, and in color not quite so black as their margins. The sclerotic conjunctiva presented a deep olive color. I found on inquiry, that she had, at one time, suffered from strumous ophthalmia, for the cure of which a strong ointment and some drops had been prescribed and freely used. These applications had been continued for three or four months.

The black streaks which traversed the corneal opacities, and the olived sclerotic conjunctiva, decisively indicated the nature of the other discolorations.

There is a much greater susceptibility to these stains in some individuals than in others. They are more common to adults than children ; possibly because ophthalmic disease among the latter is for the most part either of the strumous or purulent kind in both of which the surface of the eye and its appendages are continually bathed in secretion.

If we excise a portion of discolored sclerotic conjunctiva, a white cicatrix is formed, indicating that the sclerotic maintains its natural color.

At present we are unacquainted with any means for removing the stains under consideration. Our obvious duty is to prevent their occurrence by vigilant attention and care. This may be accomplished by prescribing the preparations of nitrate of silver in short and intermitting courses, and by frequently noting the condition of the lining membrane of the inferior palpebra. In public ophthalmic practice, it would be well if the solution were not dispensed in larger quantities than two drachms at one time.

Since writing the above, a man 60 years of age, who has been all his life a martyr to rheumatism, has become my patient at the Eye Infirmary. The right globe is collapsed; the left eye retains some vision; it has been repeatedly inflamed; the iris is of a dull leaden color, and convex towards the cornea; the pupil is puckered, adherent to the lens, and filled within a third of its area by opaque lymph (artesia irridis imperfecta.) Near the centre of the cornea is a leucoma.

Fifteen or eighteen months ago, he for the first time consulted a surgeon, who prescribed caustic drops, which he has ever since applied. The conjunctiva of the inferior palpebral sinus is of a greenish black color. The inner surface of the superior lid has lost somewhat of its natural polish; a few black drops assume an arborescent shape near the superior punctum; a light brown and well defined narrow stripe extends along the concave aspect of its tarsal cartilage.

I have cited this case to show the impropriety of allowing patients to use the preparations of lunar caustic *ad libitum;* and as an interesting example of how well the superior lid escapes serious change of color, even in the worst and most neglected cases. It also illustrates the destructive character of uncontrolled rheumatic ophthalmia.—[*London Med. Times.*

Medical Properties of the Scullcap.   By C. H. CLEAVELAND, M. D., of Waterbury, Vermont.

DR. PARRISH. I have received from Ariel Hunton, M. D., of Hyde Park, in this State, a communication in regard to *his* experience in the use of the *scutellaria laterifolia*, and as it embodies some observations that may be of use to the profession, I am led to offer it through the medium of the columns of the *Reporter.*

He writes: "I have been in the habitual use of this article some fifteen years. When I recommended the use of the blue side-flowered scullcap to my patients, I was in the habit of informing them, especially nervous females, that I had a *new* remedy, reputed to possess excellent and active *nervine* properties, which I wished them to use according to directions, to mark the effects, and to inform me if it did not prove to be far superior to valerian, foreign or *domestic,* (many in this vicinity have, of late, become accustomed to use the root of the cypripedium under the name of American valerian.) After a trial, those who had used it informed me they considered it preferable as a nervine to anything they had previously used, for, after taking a cup of the infusion of this herb, they were insured a happy exemption from their former nervous pains.

" It is now nine years since I was called to a Miss C., in this vicinity, who was suffering from *convulsion of her limbs.* They would jerk for an hour at a time, with such force that the *jar* might be plainly felt on the floor of an adjoining room.   I had never previously seen a case of this character, and it, of course, was one of uncommon interest to me.   The paroxysms did not recur at stated periods, but there were as many as two in the twenty-four hours.   The patient had already taken a variety of medicines previous to my seeing her, but without any apparent benefit.   I ordered a pill of the extract of stramonium, of my own manufacture, of half the size of a kernel of wheat, once in six hours, and a strong infusion of scullcap, a large spoonful each hour.   Under this course of treatment, the patient shortly recovered, and has since been entirely exempt from any difficulty of the kind.

" *Case second* was a Miss of about twelve years of age, afflicted with chorea.   In this case I was called as counsel, and was requested to adopt and carry out any course I might prefer.

" As the *primæ viæ* had already been thoroughly cleansed by cathartics, the patient was at once put upon the use of the infusion of the scullcap, a large spoonful each hour, and a pill of the stramonium once in six hours, and, before the end of the second week, convalescence was fully established.

" *Case third* was also a young lady, of about fifteen years.   I was called to see this patient in January, 1851.   She was also suffering from chorea, and was continually in motion.   In this case I adopted the same course of treatment as in the former, but the pills of the extract were used but a few days, while the infusion was continued longer and until recovery, which occurred after a short time.   The father was of the opinion that the recovery was wholly attributable to the infusion of the scutellaria."

Dr. Hunton is of the opinion that the S. *galericulata* possesses medicinal properties similar, and of equal potency with the S. *laterifolia,* and would prefer to use it, as it is less disagreeable to the palate, but it is by no means as common in this vicinity, and we have both been accustomed to use the latter.   He also considers the *scutellariæ* as one of our most valuable vegetable tonics.—[*New Jersey Med. Reporter.*

Paracentesis in Acute Pleurisy.

In an article contained in the Medical Examiner, No. for Jan. 1852, entitled extracts from a lecture 'On the present position in Europe of some of the most interesting and important points of modern Surgery,' recently delivered as an Introductory Discourse, by Thomas D. Mutter, M. D., Professor of Surgery in Jefferson Medical College, Philadelphia, we observe the following notice of paracentesis in Pleurisy :

"*Pleurisy.*—An operation altogether novel in the disease for which it was practiced, has been introduced by Prof. Trousseau, of Paris, one of the most distinguished practitioners of that city of eminent medical men.   Prof. Trousseau told me that he has succeeded in relieving several patients who were almost in articulo mortis: and I have myself known it to accomplish the same end.   The operation is nothing more than the evacuation of the fluid in cases of *acute pleurisy.*   You are aware that the secretion is here often exceedingly rapid, and unless the lung be relieved, the patient must die of suffocation.   When, therefore, you find a patient thus situated, recollect that paracentesis thoracis, promptly performed, will probably afford immediate relief."

That the rapid *secretion* of the fluid contained in the pleural sac in *acute pleurisy, often* exposes the patient to death by suffocation, is a novel fact.   It is to be hoped that young practitioners who may discover the chest on one side to be filled with fluid, will not deem it necessary to perform the operation of paracentesis without a reasonable delay, notwithstanding this injunction to resort to the operation promptly, by so distinguished a surgeon.

Dr. Walshe, a pretty fair authority, says that in acute pleurisy, "Death is so rare a result of the disease when attacking individuals free from organic affections, that I have neither myself (and I have carefully attended to the point since my attention was first drawn to it, a year ago, by M. Louis) lost a patient from pure primary idiopathic pleurisy, with or without effusion, nor known of an occurrence of the kind in the practice of others."   We may commend this statement to those who might be induced by Dr. Mutter's recommendation to puncture the thorax, as the reviewer of Dr. Walshe's treatise in the American Journal of Med. Sciences does to the "consideration of those who regard the disease as demanding bleeding, blistering, mercurials, and the whole armament of antiphlogistics."

The operation of paracentesis in cases of *chronic* pleurisy, in which the absorbing property of the membrane has been greatly impared by the quantity of fibrinous exudation, and the degree of distension, has been proposed and practiced in this country within the past year, by a method simple and devoid of pain and danger.   We allude to the plan originated by Dr. Morrill,

Wyman, of Cambridge, Mass., which was communicated to the profession by Dr. H. I. Bowditch, of Boston. Dr. Bowditch's article on this subject was copied into this Journal, and may be found in vol. VI. We observe in the January No. of the American Journal of Med. Sciences, a report, by Dr. Bowditch, of several cases in which paracentesis with the small trochar attached to a suction apparatus was resorted to with marked advantage.

This procedure in the large accumulations of chronic pleurisy, certainly merits farther trial, but the proposition to tap the chest to remove the serum rapidly effused in cases of acute inflammation, is another matter, and, as it seems to us, should be protested against.—[*Buffalo Med. Journal.*

On the Nature and Causes of Genu Valgum, or Knock-Knee. By Professor BOCK.

The most common deformities of the knee-joint may be arranged under the four following heads.

1. Contraction of the knee (*contractura genu*) is the name given to the condition in which the knee is in a state of abnormal constant flexion, with considerable, little, or no power of motion in the joint.

2. Recurved knee (*genu recurvatum.*) Here the knee is in a state of superextension, and the popliteal space forms the apex of an angle pointing backwards.

3. Genu varum, or bow-leg: called by the Danish wheel-leg (*Hjulbenet.*)

4. Genu valgum, or knock-knee: in Danish, calf-knee (*Kalveknæet;*) in German, goat's leg (*Ziegenbein,*) X-leg (*X bein.*)

The name genu valgum is borrowed from an imperfect analogy with pes valgus. In the latter, the foot is thrown outwards. In genu valgum, it is not the knee, but the tibia which is pressed outwards; and the more correct denomination would, therefore, be tibia valga, if the analogy with the foot were preserved. The same is the case with genu varum.

Genu valgum has been but imperfectly described in surgical works. Prof. Bock has for some time been collecting materials for a more accurate knowledge of this deformity, and now publishes the results at which he has arrived.

Pathology.—In the normal condition, the knee-joint deviates from the long axis of the lower extremity, on account of the greater extension downwards and inwards of the inner condyle of the femur.

The thigh-bones hence converge downwards, especially in

females, in whom the pelvis is wider, and the neck of the thigh
bone is larger and directed more outward.   It is the unnatural
exaggeration of this condition to which the name of genu valgum
is given.   It might be supposed, that this affection is more frequent in the female sex : such, however, is not the case, for it
is far more rare in women and girls than in men and boys.
Both knees may be affected, but one is generally more so than
the other : and it is then almost always the right knee which
is the chief seat of the disease.   When one knee alone is affected, it is the right in about twice as many cases as the left.   The
origin and progress of the disease are gradual and almost imperceptible.

The knee forms the apex of a triangle, the other angles of
which are at the ankle and the great trochanter, so that the
base consists of the straight line which may be drawn between
these points.   The altitude of the triangle, or the perpendicular
line from the knee to its base, points out the greater or less
degree of the disease ; this may naturally be denoted by the
anomalous proportions of the angle at the knee, which, from
being very obtuse, becomes, in the more advanced stages, a
right or even a very acute angle.

On examining the knee, the following changes are found :—
On its anterior surface, the united large tendons of the extensor
muscles, and the ligamentum patellæ, are found much stretched ;
and the more so, in proportion as the knee is bent backward
as well as inward.   The patella is displaced outwards ; so that,
in a more advanced stage of the disease, it rests on the external edge of the knee, in front of the condyles of the femur and
tibia.   The knee loses its natural convexity forward, and becomes acute-angled on its anterior and outer edge ; and the
anterior part which lies more interiorly forms a plano-convex
region in front of the inner condyle.   On the outer surface of
the knee, or in the angular bend, we often find the tendon of the
biceps much stretched, as well as one or two portions of the
external ligaments extended into sharp strings.   The external
condyles, both of the femur and of the tibia, are small, and can
scarcely be felt in the more advanced stages of the disease.
When the curvature is very remarkable, there is a transverse
furrow in the skin on the exterior part of the knee.   The natural hollow of the ham is obliterated ; and the posterior surface
of the knee joint is more or less plano-convex.   The inner
surface of the knee forms the obtuse apex of the angle ; and
here the internal condyles of the femur and tibia are felt always
prominent, usually hypertrophied, and, in rachitic cases, enormously swelled.

The condition of the whole extremity is at the same time

changed. The thigh assumes an oblique direction downwards
and inwards, towards the opposite knee. The knee is directed inwards, against or behind the sound knee, and the shin-bone
assumes a direction downwards and outwards, so that the foot
is at a great distance from that on the sound side. As the disease advances, the direction of the foot is changed : but this
will be treated of under the head of complications. In children,
where the affection is of a truly paralytic nature, and has followed convulsions, there has been constantly observed a sinking of the temperature, as much as two degrees, in the diseased
limb. In grown persons, the author has not found this symptom. In consequence of the bending of the limb, the distance
from the pelvis to the sole of the foot is diminished ; the direction of the pelvis in walking consequently becomes oblique, so
that the anterior superior spine of the ilium may be found an
inch lower on the affected than on the sound side. This obliquity of the pelvis becomes gradually permanent,- so that it is
observed both during walking and standing. In cases where
the deformity has not yet reached a high degree, and in children, the limb can generally be brought back with the hands to
its natural position : but the tension is felt to increase in the
biceps femoris and external ligament of the knee-joint ; and,
when the force is removed, the limb instantly resumes the bent
position. In rachitic cases, not only the internal condyle of
the femur, but also, in a still higher degree, that of the tibia is
enlarged. The concavity inwards, which is naturally formed
by the tibia, is obliterated ; and, in the more advanced stages,
there may even be a pretty conspicuous convexity, so that the
whole extremity more resembles a bow curved inwards than an
angular bending. The knee-joint generally retains it mobility.
In the higher degrees of curvature, this is indeed somewhat
limited ; but either true or false anchyloses are seldom met
with as consequences of the affection of the knee which has
been described.

When both legs are curved, the right leg is always slightly
more bent than the other, and the apices are turned towards
each other. This has given rise to the German designation of
the disease—X-lex (*X-bein*).

In this affection, the patients halt in a peculiar manner. If
one bone only is affected, there is a lameness—(*a*) because one
extremity is too short ; (*b*) because the foot of the diseased limb
falls beyond the centre of gravity of the body ; (*c*) because
the affected knee, in walking, both hinders the free swinging
motion of the healthy knee, and is in its turn impeded by the
latter. Each of these causes has distinct results, which modify
both the direction of the limb and the lameness. When the

extremity is too short, there is a natural attempt to compensate
the defect ; and this is effected partly by the already mentioned
obliquity of the pelvis, and partly by the formation of a curve
in the healthy leg. In healthy individuals, who have for some
time had genu valgum, there will almost always be found a
slight but true contraction of the knee in the sound leg. But
in children, almost without exception, the other knee will become curved, either as genu varum or valgum. The outward
direction of the tibia and foot causes the peculiar up-and-down
lameness to become rotary and swinging, like mowing, and
this swinging is increased, to prevent the collision of the
knees during walking. In the more remarkable modification,
the body seeks to maintain its equilibrium ; and it attains this
object more completely than in many other forms of lameness
—*e. g.*, from congenital dislocation of the thigh. This is partly
affected by the position of the pelvis, and partly by a greater
degree of mobility in the lumbar vertebræ. The diseased leg
is generally sufficiently powerful, in persons affected with genu
valgum, to enable them to walk for some distance. Naum-
burg has compared their gait to that of ducks ; but this is scarcely correct. The gait is more swinging than waddling, as in
persons with rachitic distortion of the pelvis or double congenital dislocation of the hip-joint. The patient who has genu valgum
in one leg, endeavors, while standing, to preserve the centre of
gravity by moving the sound leg somewhat outward beyond its
natural position. Hence the points of support in the feet are
at a greater distance from each other, and the surface within
which the centre of gravity of the body can fall is greatly increased. Patients with double genu valgum usually, when
standing, support the knees against each other, so as to form
there a mediate resting point for the body, while the feet stand
out from each other.

   Complications and Secondary Deformities.—These are more
various in this than in any other deformity whatever. Where
the disease has commenced in youth, a curvature of the spinal
column will generally be produced by the obliquity of the pelvis and the lameness. The affected limb is not unfrequently
more or less atrophied. Anchylosis of the knee-joint rarely
occurs, unless some chronic disease have preceded or accompanied the deformity. Prof. Bock has, however, seen two
cases of anchylosed knock-knee in elderly persons; in these
the limb was also directed backwards. But it is the feet which
are especially influenced by the gait produced by genu valgum ;
and hence knock-kneed patients have, almost without exception,
some deformity or other of the feet. The patient may, in consequence of the abduction of the tibia, tread and walk on the

inner edge of the foot, which hence often becomes callous. Hence there is a disposition to flat-foot, which is the most frequent complication. But, almost as frequently, the genu valgum is complicated with club-foot ; and, as the shortness of the limb leads the patient instinctively to endeavor to touch the ground with the points of his toes, it is evident that these forms will be accompanied by a greater or less degree of talipes equinus. It has been hitherto impossible to determine the reason, why these secondary deformities of the feet should in some cases assume one form, and in others another. In certain peculiar cases, the deformity of the knee is secondary. A patient in Dieffenbach's ward had had, from childhood, *cyphosis accurvata* of the lumbar vertebræ ; in his youth varus had been developed in both feet, and, in his sixteenth year, he had become knock-kneed in both legs. Not uncommonly there is genu valgum on one side, and genu varum on the other, accompanied by the same, or by distinct deformities in the feet.

Causes.—There is no doubt that genu valgum may be congenital ; this is, however, a rare occurrence. The causes of the development of the affection in latter years are partly external, partly internal, but most frequently both are combined. The greater convergence of the thighs in women may be supposed to be a predisposing cause ; and Lessing says that this affection is more frequent in females than in males ; this is, however, incorrect, for the deformity is twenty times more frequent in the latter sex, than in the former. Scrofula and rickets may be considered as predisposing causes, especially the latter. It still more frequently produces genu varum, in which case the external condyles of the femur and tibia are most affected and enlarged, while a similar swelling of the internal condyles give rise to genu valgum.

Genu valgum may, as a general rule, be considered as a disease of a paralytic nature, and its most usual cause as a depressed state of innervation. Hence the commencement of the affection is limited to certain periods of life, in which the nervous centres undergo a more than ordinary degree of disturbance, connected with the state of development. Genu valgum is developed either during the first dentition or during puberty. This rule is so constant, that the only exceptions are the cases in which some local malady has given rise to the deformity : but these are comparatively very rare. In children, the disease has always, in the author's cases, arisen between the eighth month and the completion of the second year, and has always been preceded by difficult dentition, with fever, convulsions, violent hooping-cough, or, as in one case, acute exanthematic fever. This agrees with what has been stated by Heine, with regard to nine cases of knock-knee observed by him. The external causes, which may give rise to the affection at this age, and under the circumstances which have been mentioned, are, that the children *walk* too early, or too soon after a weakening illness, while they have not yet recovered strength, or that they are constantly carried on one arm, by which one knee is pressed inwards.

Among 221 cases of genu valgum, which the author has observed, 17 originated during the first dentition. In a few instances he has not been able to ascertain the period; but in almost all the rest, or about 200, the deformity commenced between the fifteenth and eighteenth years, or at the time of puberty. In all these cases there was an evident external cause for the deformity—the patient's position or occupation: but the limitation of the age referred to above, together with the fact that many following the same occupation, under apparently similar external circumstances, do not become deformed, seem to show that the external conditions are not sufficient to produce the disease, unless they meet with a corresponding disposition in the system of the individual, or rather in his development. We correctly consider the periods of dentition and of puberty as stages of development, in which the body is more obnoxious, than at any other period, to the hurtful operation of various extrinsic or intrinsic influences. That the deformity in question less frequently arises during dentition than during puberty, may be ascribed to the fact, that the influences above referred to, are more easily resisted by the system in the former than in the latter period.

This deformity is more frequent in smiths, joiners, bakers, and grocers. In 1846, there were in Copenhagen 644 smiths, among whom were:—

225 blacksmiths and anchorsmiths; of whom 42 had genu valgum in the right leg, 7 in both legs=19 per cent.

359 locksmiths; of whom 23 had genu valgum in the right leg, and 3 in both legs=7 per cent.

30 nailsmiths; of whom 17 had genu valgum in the right leg, and 5 in both legs=73 per cent.

There were thus, in all, 97 cases of the deformity among 644 smiths, making an average of 15 per cent.

The following are the immediate causes of the frequency of the deformity among smiths. Almost all smith's work necessitates the long maintenance of the same position, whether at the bellows, the anvil, or the vice; and, while standing in this position, they often have to use much force, which leads them to seek a firm and solid footing. The feet are hence removed from each other, either both sideways, or one—always the left—forwards. In both these positions, any powerful effort will tend to produce genu valgum; for a great part of the weight of the body will, under the powerful movements of the arm and upper part of the body, act on the knee like a pressure from above and below. In blowing bellows, a work in which apprentices are generally employed, they must often stand uninterruptedly at work for several hours. At the vice and anvil, the left foot is placed forwards, the right backwards and rotated outwards, so that the toes are turned to the side. In this position they often stand with the leg and foot unmoved for several hours, while the upper part of the body is subjected to constant and violent swinging, in order to use the file or hammer. The influence of the position on the knee will be easily seen by any one who will make a trial of it. Blacksmiths and anchor-smiths are besides constantly liable to have to bear heavy burdens. The fact that nailsmiths are most liable, in spite of their work being least laborious, is explained by the circumstance that they almost constantly use a kind of vice, which is fixed near the ground, and against which they all, without exception, place the inner surfaces of both knees, " because it is impossible for them to work in any other way."

Of 1340 journeymen carpenters, about 60, or 5 per cent., had genu valgum. It has been impossible to make very accurate observations on this class, as they endeavor to conceal the deformity as well as they can. It does not reach in them so high a degree as in smiths. Notwithstanding that the work of carpenters is less laborious than that of smiths, considerable exertion is required: most of the labour of carpenters, as sawing, planing, and polishing, requires the same positions as are here described in speaking of smiths. The author has also observed that carpenters carefully watch for this deformity, and endeavor to prevent its development. Many masters have told him that they have had to set free their apprentices, or, in the first year to caution them against habituating themselves to the posture which favors the commencement of the disease.

Of 334 journeymen bakers, 27 were knock-kneed ; 24 were affected in both knees, the right being generally more bent than the left. One individual had the curvature only in the right knee. In 16, deformity had not reached a very high degree. Notwithstanding that bakers seem to be affected with this malady more than the other classes above named, and several of them have some difficulty in walking, the deformity is not strongly developed. The disease does not arise from the position in which they stand while kneading dough ; for in the first years, when this malady is developed, the apprentices are

not employed at this labour.   But the deformity is produced by
standing at night at the board, often half asleep or contending
with sleep, seeking ·for rest in the most varied positions ; or
partly by carrying water or sacks of corn.   It is possible also
that the great changes of temperature in attending to the oven
may have some influence ; but the author considers the night
watching as the most essential cause, for the constant struggling
with sleep produces a relaxation of the muscles.   All the bakers
in whom he observed genu valgum, also had flat-foot ; and the
latter deformity, in several cases, had preceded that of the knees.

The generally received opinion, that grocer's apprentices
should be liable to genu valgum, from standing long, or from
shutting drawers with their knees, Prof. Bock has not found
supported by facts : for, among 2000 individuals of this class,
he has in vain sought for any examples of this deformity.   It is
said to have been more frequent formerly ; and what has most
surely contributed to its removal, is the reform in working
hours, it having been formerly the custom to keep the shop
open much later at night, and to open it earlier in the morning.

It hence results, that the general causes of this deformity are
certain positions and habits, where these are often repeated,
and especially at times when the body is more susceptible of
their influence than at others.   Other more accidental causes
are, allowing children to walk too early, carrying heavy burdens, ulcers on the inner border of the foot, a burn on the outer side of the knee, resection of the upper end of the tibia,
tuberculosis in the legs, caries, necrosis, rickets, syphilis, chronic
abscesses, inodular bodies, &c.

The knee-joint is properly speaking, a ginglymoid articulation, and its essential movements are merely flexion and extension ; but the hinge-like movements are not so absolutely
limited as in other analogous joints.   The knee possesses a
slight power of pronation and supination, but only when bent :
and this power is dependent on the rotation of the tibia on its
long axis, being limited, when the limb is extended, by the cru-
cical ligaments.   It is not connected with any peculiar apparatus,
as in the rotary movements of the radius and ulna, and may
properly be considered as a slight twisting, which becomes
possible on the tolerably flat upper surface of the tibia, when
the knee is in such a position that rotation is not prevented by
the extensor muscles.   The knee has hence no power of abduction or adduction ; and therefore the motions of this joint do
not help to explain a deformity, which is characterized as an
abduction of the tibia.   Its immediate cause must be sought for
in the parts which form, hold together, and strengthen the joint.

Although the part which these structures play in the produc-

tion of this deformity is for the most part passive, the biceps
femoris seems to be active in those positions in which genu
valgum is chiefly produced, and to exercise the greatest influence on the increase, if not on the origin, of the deformity.

Supposing that one of the external influences which have
been referred to should steadily act on the knee-joint, at a time
when either convulsive disease (first dentition) or an unequally
powerful development, perhaps in connexion with a rapid slen-
der growth (puberty), have weakened the nervous system;
then the parts on the inner side of the knee have no power of
opposing the pressure outwards. They are overstretched and
slackened; and thus the conditions arise for the commencement of genu valgum. The most important relaxation takes
place in the internal lateral ligament, which is lengthened and
thinned in its whole extent: in the more advanced stages, the
four tendons on the inner side of the knee are also lengthened.
On the other side of the knee, the tendon of the biceps, and
both the external lateral ligaments, as well as the posterior, are
strongly stretched.

When the deformity commences, the angle at which the biceps femoris acts constantly, becomes more and more favourable to its increase. This is, however, still more favoured by
the circumstance, that the weight of the body, which in the
normal state is uniformly diffused over the upper surface of the
tibia, is now transferred to the upper surface of the outer condyle of that bone. The inner condyle of the tibia, and that of
the femur to some extent, are atrophied even in cases which
are not of rachitic origin. This hypertrophy is greater, in
proportion to the youth, or small size of the patient at the time
when the deformity commenced. In rachitic cases, it sometimes attains an enormous degree. It is probable, also, that
the internal semilunar cartilage is somewhat atrophied.

Prognosis.—As genu valgum is a deformity which depends
rather on relaxation than on active contraction, the prognosis
in general may be considered as scarcely favourable. It is,
however, curable, when it comes under treatment in an early
stage, and, which is more important, when the circumstances
which have produced and kept it up can be removed. In your
children the knee can be brought with the hand into its normal
situation; and in these the prognosis is most frequently good,
when the necessary continued watching of the growth can be
maintained, and when the general condition of the child does
not give a tendency to the continuance of the disorder, or to
relapses. In young men, also, the deformity can be cured,
when there are as yet no consecutive changes. But, under
all circumstances, the removal of the deformity must not be

looked on as complete; for, even when the curvature is completely removed, it will still be necessary to employ fitting means to insure the result desired.

Treatment.—The treatment of genu valgum in young children, consists in mechanical means to keep the knee outwards, and this must be always supported by such general treatment as the constitution of the child may indicate. The most simple apparatus is a splint, either straight or convex outwards, reaching from the hip-joint over the outer ankle, and fastened at the ends with circular bands. This apparatus, however, hinders the child from walking, and therefore can only be used constantly at night; hence it can only be used in the more unimportant cases. It is preferable to make use of a steel spring, convex outwards, furnished at the height of the knee with a hinge, fastened at the hip to a bow which can be stretched round the pelvis; just over the outer ankle, the lower end of the spring passes into another bow, which can be fastened round the tibia. The spring is furnished on the outside, through its whole length, with buttons, on which are fastened small leather straps, four or six in number. These are brought round the legs; and on the inner side of the knee they glide between flat *pelottes*, which exert a pressure from within outwards, when the straps are stretched or buttoned. An apparatus of this kind may be worn for a long time, and its action gradually increased. It must be used for at least a year after the deformity is removed, and even then it must be gradually ascertained whether it can be left off.

The same apparatus, on a larger scale, and with greater strength of spring, can be used in grown persons. The patient can easily accustom himself to use it—indeed, he feels comfortable with it. In grown persons it will generally be an indication, before employing mechanical treatment, to divide the tendon of the biceps, or of the most stretched fibres of the lateral ligaments, but generally only of the posterior lateral ligament. The mechanical treatment, after tenotomy, may appear tedious; but the result will be more perfect; but without great perseverance on the part of the patient, and careful watching of the deformity for several years, the treatment of genu valgum will in general be ineffectual.—[*Bibliothek für Lægen and London Jour. of Med.*

Aphorisms on the Treatment of wounds and injuries of the Abdomen. By G. J. Guthrie, Esq., F. R. S.

1. A blow on the wall of the abdomen, from any solid substance, causing a severe bruise, often, if not always, gives rise to the absorption of muscular fibre, and the subsequent forma-

tion of a ventral herna. It is desirable, in all such injuries, to prevent or to subdue inflammation as soon as possible, in order to obviate the formation of matter between the layers of muscular fibres, which is a disagreeable, if not always a dangerous consequence. Severe blows or contusions from falls may rupture the hollow as well as the more solid or fixed viscera, causing death. A child just able to walk was placed under the author's care in the Westminster Hospital, having been tossed up into the air by its father with his right hand, and caught in its descent in the crutch formed by the thumb and fingers of the left, on the thumb of which it at last fell. The integuments seemed to be unhurt, the small intestine was ruptured and the child died. The author has seen all the viscera of the abdomen ruptured, at different times, from non-penetrating blows or wounds, the sufferers usually dying from hemorrhage.

2. When an *incised* wound is made through the wall of the abdomen, except perhaps in the linea alba, the parts, when vascular, are rarely found to unite in a permanent manner, so that a ventral hernia is the result. The knowledge of this fact, acquired during the war in Portugal and Spain, led Mr. Guthrie first to doubt the propriety of, and when confirmed by subsequent experience, to forbid the introduction of ligature, through muscles for the purpose of keeping in apposition parts which could not ultimately cohere.

In all simple wounds of the abdomen, of even a moderate extent, the edges of the wound should be brought together by means of a small needle and silk thread, precisely in the manner a tailor would fine-draw a hole in a coat, or a lady a cut in a cambric pocket-handkerchief, sticking plasters over it, no bandage. The *position* of the patient should be of the gentlest inclination of the body towards the wound, the limbs being bent so that the parts may press against each other. *Absolute* rest is no less to be observed, and steadfastly continued. In the position the patient is placed in he should remain. When Mr. Guthrie became an examiner of the Royal College of Surgeons, the practice of the older surgeons he found there was to purge such patients *vigorously*, in the same manner as they purged persons who had undergone the operation for hernia; against both of which practices he protested until they were condemned and reprobated—improvements the surgery of civil life owes, among many others, to her elder but less fortunate sister, the Amazonian of warfare.

The custom of directing a man to be bled forthwith, as well as purged, because he had been stabbed, was another and not less esteemed error, with the author's older colleagues, which experience did not sanction, and which he could not approve.

The abstraction of blood before reaction has begun, after the constitution has sustained a severe shock, delays it, as well as the commencement of the inflammatory stage necessary for the cure of the wound. The abstraction of blood is to be directed and regulated by the signs of reaction which have taken place, and by the augmenting intensity of the symptoms of inflammation which may follow. The quantity required is often large, although too much will do harm. Leeches are very beneficial, and the author has often applied from twenty to a hundred with the greatest advantage.

The *pulse* is by no means a guide to be relied upon, a small, low, and sometimes not even a hard pulse, being more strongly indicative of an overpowering state of inflammation than a quick and full pulse ; and much more depends on the fixed pain, the anxiety, and the general oppression, than on the apparent state of the circulation. Long before general and local bleedings cease to be of advantage, calomel and opium will render most important services, particularly the latter.

3. Penetrating wounds of the abdomen are frequently followed by an immediate protrusion of some portion of the contents of the cavity. When the omentum has protruded, it should be returned as gently as possible ; the finger should not follow, to ascertain its position ; it should be left free from strangulation within, but in contact with the cut edges of the peritonæum, to which it is desirable it should adhere, as they are not likely to unite one with the other. The external wound is then to be sewed up as the author has directed, and the stiches are *not* to be carried through all the intervening parts down to the peritonæum, as is directed by most, if not all, authors whose writing are of ancient and even of modern date.

4. When the opening through which the omentum and intestine, or both, have passed, seems too small to admit of their being returned, the latest writers on this subject recommend that a director should be introduced between the upper portion of the wound and the protruded part, upon which a blunt-ended bistoury is to be passed into the cavity as far as the enlargement of the wound seems to require, when they are to be withdrawn together ;—*from all which the author dissents.* The difficulty does not usually lie with the opening in the peritonæum, but with that in the aponeurotic or tendinous expansions, and it is this part only should be divided. A small cut in the peritonæum is not dangerous ; a larger one is, and should always, if possible, be avoided, for however indifferent a quarter of an inch, more or less, may be in a large wound, it is not so in a small one. The protruded parts should be gently cleansed with warm water, with which the fingers of the surgeon should be

wetted, and then returned, the mesentery first, then the intestine, and the omentum last.   At a later period, if the omentum
be found protruded, adherent, inflamed, in a state of suppuration
or gangrene, it should be left to itself, and treated in the most
simple manner.   A ligature should never be applied to it as
whole, although it may be applied to a bleeding vessel of any
part which has been cut, or which it may be necessary to remove.   It should not, however, be spread out in these cases, and
cut off, as is usually recommended, as it will gradually retract,
and be withdrawn into the cavity of the abdomen, if the patient
survive.   An omentum wounded in the first instance, is in the
best situation when placed just within and against the cut edges
of the peritonæum; it is never in a better under any circumstances, except when it adheres to them.

5. When an intestine is protruded, it is to be treated in a
similar manner, and the three great directions on this subject,
of modern surgeons, are to be *avoided:* do not therefore cut
the peritonæum, do not unnecessarily introduce your finger
into the cavity of the abdomen, and be most careful to avoid,
above all, the third direction, "that the patient is to be placed
in such a posture, that the intestines should *least* press against
the wound." On the contrary: relax every part, keep the
patient perfectly at rest, and if you can so manage, that the
intestine shall be steadily applied against the cut peritonæum,
without protruding between the edges, so as to be in the best
possible situation for adhesion.   The external wound should
be accurately closed by the continuous suture, supported by
adhesive plaster and a compress, and a proper bandage, if it can
be methodically applied.

6. When the intestine is wounded, as well as protruded, the
case is complicated; a mere puncture, or a very small cut, is
not to be dreaded, the bowel should be cleaned and returned,
and the excess of inflammation closely watched.   When the
wound in the bowel is larger, but is less than a third, or not
more than a quarter of an inch in length, it is less apt than
might be supposed to permit the extravasion of its contents in
consequence of the villous coat protruding through the opening
in the other tunics, the edges of which being in great part muscular, have separated from each other.   This eversion of the
lining membrane, so conspicuous in wounds, is not seen in ulcerations, the previous inflammation having solidified the parts.
Whenever then an opening in a bowel is not filled up by the
internal coat, the edges must be brought together by ligature.
A ligature placed around an intestine of a dog, cuts its way
through, into the cavity ; and if the animal should survive some
months, the part which had been injured will not be easily discovered.

When the wound in the intestine is small, and yet larger than it would be safe to leave to nature, a ligature should be applied firmly around the opening, which should be raised with a pair of forceps, so as to admit of its application. When the wound is larger, the edges should be brought together by the continuous suture in a parallel line. A common needle carrying a fine well-waxed silk-thread, is to be introduced about half a line from the peritonæal edge of the opening, and brought out at the corresponding point on the opposite side, a knot on the end of the thread preventing its slipping. The first stitch should be a line from the end of the wound, and the last should terminate with a knot at a similar distance. The stitches should not be tightened when made, but left loose until all are inserted, when they may be drawn close, one after the other, the cut edges being turned in by a probe, so that the peritonæal surfaces may be in contact under the stitches, the divided edges being turned into the cavity of the bowel. It has been advised not to pass the needle through the mucous coat, but only through the strong areolar tissue connecting it with the transverse muscular coat. It is apprehended that if this could be accurately done, which may be doubted, the ligature might not ulcerate its way through to the cavity of the bowel. It is therefore better to pass the needle through all the coats, until further observations shall have been made on man on this point.

When an incised wound in the intestines is not supposed to exceed a puncture in size, or is less than a third of an inch in length, no interference should take place: for the nature and extent of the injury cannot always be ascertained, without the committal of a greater mischief than the injury itself. When the wound in the external part is made by an instrument not larger than one-third, or from that to half an inch in width, no attempt to probe, or to meddle with the wound, for the purpose of examining the intestine, should be permitted. When the external wound is made by a somewhat broader and longer instrument, it does not necessarily follow that the intestine should be wounded to an equal extent; and unless it protrudes, or the contents of the bowel be discharged through the wound, in the first instance, the surgeon will not be warranted in enlarging the wound, to see what mischief has been done. For, although it may be argued that a wound four or more inches long has been proved to be oftentimes as little dangerous as a wound of one inch in length, most people would prefer having the smaller wound, unless it could be believed, from calculation, that the intestine was also injured to a considerable extent. Few surgeons, even then, would like to enlarge the wound, to ascertain the fact, unless some considerable bleeding, or a dis-

charge of fæcal matter, pointed out the necessity for such operation; when there would be reason for believing that the
patient would have a better chance of recovery after the application of a suture to the wounded artery, or bowel, than if it
were left to Nature.

If the first two or three hours have passed away, and the
pain, and the firm, not tympanitic swelling in the belly, as well
as discharge from the wound, indicate the commencement of
effusion from the bowel, or an extravasation of blood, an enlargement of the opening alone can save the life of the patient,
although the operation may probably be unsuccessful. It is
not, however, on that account, to be always laid aside, when
the state of the patient offers even a chance of success. The
external wound should be enlarged, the effused matter sponged
up with a soft, moist sponge, and the bowel or artery secured
by a suture. When a penetrating wound, which may have injured the intestine, has been closed by suture, and does not do
well, increasing symptoms of the inflammation of the abdominal cavity being accompanied by general tendernes of that part,
and a decided swelling underneath the wound, indicating effusion beneath, and apparently confined to it, the best chance for
life will be given by reopening the wound, and even augmenting it, if necessary, to such an extent, as will allow a ready.
evacuation of the contents of the bowel. It is a point in surgery
which a surgeon should contemplate in all its bearings. The
proceeding is simple, little dangerous, and, under such circumstances, can do no harm. Mr. Guthrie has seen instances in
which it has been done, and others in which it might have been
done, with some hope of its being beneficial; and he recommends it for the serious consideration of those who may hereafter have the management of such cases.

8. When the abdomen is penetrated, and considerable bleeding takes place, and continues, it becomes necessary to enlarge
the opening, and look for the wounded vessel. If the hemorrhage
should come from one of the mesenteric arteries, or the epigastric, two ligatures are to be applied on the injured part. If it
should be presumed that the enlargement of the wound and
the search for the wounded vessel is not likely to be effected
with advantage to the patient, the wound should be closed by
suture, and a compress laid over it. If the bleeding should
continue internally, and the wounded part become distended
and tense, the sutures may be in part removed to give relief.

If the belly should become very painful, tense, and manifestly
full after a punctured wound, and not tympanitic, the wound
should be enlarged to allow the evacuation of the blood, which
cannot, in such quanity, be absorbed. Extravasations of blood

of a determinate quantity are not found to be diffused all over the surface, and between the convolutions of the small intestines, provided the person has outlived the period of extravasion, and may be readily evacuated, provided the wound be sufficiently open. It may, when confined without an external opening, be absorbed, but it is more likely to give rise to suppurative inflammation, and the formation of matter, requiring with it to be discharged by an opening made for the purpose. Cases of extravasion, terminating in this manner, are very rare in our northern climate, where inflammation usually runs high in the first instance. That they do sometimes occur should not be forgotten, and that surgery should not be wanting to give its aid.

For the proper treatment of gunshot wounds of the belly the author refers to his work on "Injuries cf the Abdomen," where it is fully pointed out.—[*Lancet.*

On the necessity of administering a Stimulant in certain cases, previous to using Chloroform. By Dr. C. FLEMING.

The most important point in the information contained in Mr. Fleming's pamphlet we consider to be that of the administration of a stimulant before allowing the patient to inhale the chloroform, in cases, where, from extreme depression of the vital powers, it becomes a serious risk to attempt the induction of anæsthesia. He says:

"The first case of this kind in which it struck me that salutary anæsthetic effects might be secured, occurred in one of the constabulary force, a patient in Stevens' Hospital. He was the subject of disease of the knee-joint, advanced to a stage to demand amputation, and was in a state of such extreme exhaustion that the operation was not free from danger. It was most desirable to save him the shock and pain of it; and yet his condition appeared to militate against the use of chloroform, for which he was most anxious. It struck me that some dietetic stimulant might answer as a protective, and I gave him, about half an hour before the operation, some brandy beat up with the yolk of an egg. The chloroform was now administered in his ward, previous to his removal to the operation theatre; the limb was removed by Mr. Wilmot, and he was replaced in bed, without knowledge or pain throughout the whole proceeding, and in a condition not appreciably different from that which preceded it."

The idea of giving a stimulant as a protective against the injurious effects of anæsthetic agents, in cases of extreme exhaustation, appears, as far as we know, to be original with Mr.

Fleming, for we are not aware that the plan was before adopted. Simple as the suggestion may at first appear, we are of opin- ion that it is one of the most important practical points we have recently gained regarding the administration of chloro- form. We have known surgeons refuse to allow patients in a weak condition to be brought into an anæsthetic condition, preferring that they should suffer the torture of even a pro- longed and exquisitely painful operation to risking their lives by the action of chloroform; and we have to mourn over the fatal consequences we have heard recorded, from the employment of that agent, when much debility existed. If the precautionary measure of exhibiting a stimulant before the inhalation of-the chloroform had been known and adopted, we are certain that, upon the one hand, many sufferers might have been spared unnecessary pain, and, upon the other, a large number, if not most of those who fell victims to its agency, have been rescued from death; and this suggestion receives increased importance by reflection, for, in reality, it is in cases where vitality is low that anæsthesia would be most desirable, since, during that state of the system, the shock of an operation must be greatly lessened.—[*Dublin Quarterly Jour.*

Case of Inversion of the Vagina coming on during Labor. By. Dr. LAMBERT.

The patient was a laboring woman. During the last six months of her third pregnancy she suffered from prolapsus of the vagina whenever she was working at out-of door labor. The swelling thus produced attracted her attention, but did not alarm her, as it disappeared when she lay down in bed.

When labor came on, the tumor again appeared between the limbs. The midwife in attendance finding the labor tedious, and ignorant of the nature of the case, recommended the wo- man to make the most of her pains, and ordered her a vapor bath. The only apparent effect of this advice was the increase of the tumor to double its former size. When Dr. Lambert arrived, he found it projecting from the vulva, of the size of the two fists, of a blueish-red color, round, wrinkled, and of con- siderable consistence. At its lower extremity was an opening through which the finger could be introduced to the os uteri.

Dr. L. recommended rest in the horizontal posture, with the pelvis a little elevated, cold applications to be made to the tu- mor, and slight pressure applied to replace it during the inter- vals between the pains. After considerable delay the tumor was reduced, and the woman delivered with the forceps. She made a good recovery, and the swelling has never returned. [*Lond. Monthly Journ., from Revue Med. Chir.*

The Sympathy between the Uterus and Intestines.

Dr. Vandeen, a Dutch physician, has published in the *Presse Médicale Belge*, a few judicious observations respecting the sympathy which exists between the functions of the uterus and intestines at certain periods. He considers that the reaction of the uterus upon the bowels at the time of menstruation produces diarrhœa, as both the uterus and large intestine (the latter sympathetically) are at that period in a congested state, and their secretion therefore abundant. During gestation, however, a great deal of functional energy is transferred to the breasts and uterus, and thus constipation is a frequent symptom both during the development of the fœtus and for some time after parturition. The author looks upon these facts as brought to light for the first time by himself; we were, however, in reading his remarks, forcibly reminded of a paper read by Dr. Tilt before the Medical Society of London. In this communication, Dr. Tilt pointed out how frequently diarrhœa is a precursory symptom to menstruation, and the following passage of Dr. Vandeen's remarks shows how identical facts may be simultaneously observed in different countries. The Dutch physician, namely, says: "The sympathy between the uterus and the large intestine is rendered evident by the fact, (which to my knowledge has not been pointed out before,) that with most women the alvine dejections are much more frequent and loose when menstruation is about to set in."—[*London Lancet.*

On the Post-mortem Duration of the Ciliary Movements in the Human Subject. By M. Gosselin.

The body of a decapitated criminal having been conveyed to the Ecole Pratique, the ciliary movement was recognised on the mucous membrane of the trachea, of the nasal fossæ, and on that lining the maxillary, frontal, and sphenoidal sinuses, 8 hours after death. The movements were still distinguishable, especially on the mucous membrane of the trachea, 32 hours after death. The movement had ceased on the mucous membrane of the nasal fossæ and of the sinuses, 56 hours after death; but this was perhaps due to the free exposure of these parts to the air; for the vibration was still active on the mucous membrane of the trachea, where it was distinctly seen to the 168th hour after death, after which putrefaction came on, and the movement ceased. In another case of the same nature the ciliary movements were much less durable; and this seemed to be consequent upon the earlier supervention of putrefaction, brought about by a higher temperature, the thermometer having ranged from 46° to 54° in the first case, and having risen to 68° in the second.—[*Gaz. Médicale. Medico-Chir. Rev.*

On the Nerves of the Uterus. By M. Boulard.

The author states that his dissections were carried on without any knowledge of the 'Memoirs' of Dr. Robert Lee and Mr. Snow Beck; which he only consulted after the termination of his own inquiries. He states that these have led him, in all essential particulars, to concur with the latter anatomist; and he particularly affirms that the nerves do not augment during pregnancy. He has made two comparative preparations of the uterus of a girl of 12 years old, and of a woman who died near the end of pregnancy; and he affirms that there is no difference in the arrangement of their nerves, except that which arises from the closeness of the elements of the plexuses in the first case, and their separation in the second.—[*Ibid.*

On some of the Histological Characteristics of Malignant Growths. By Prof. Albers, of Bonn.

1. No form of growth other than the malignant consists so exclusively, even to the acquisition of a large size, in cell-formation, all non malignant ones containing a great abundance of fibre-formations. It may be objected that *epithelial* tumours consist of cells, and yet remain innocent. It is to be observed, however, that such tumours always remain small, and have not proved so generally innocent as the polypus and fibroid. Epithelial tumour, too, frequently relapses, and is sometimes as destructive as cancer itself. Among other innocent tumours, the *fatty* especially exhibit cells, but the regular fibrous network, which is also present, essentially distinguishes them from all malignant tumours.

2. In innocent growths the cells decrease with the duration of these, while in malignant ones they increase. At the commencement of the so-called tumours of the cellular tissue, among the predominant fibres, cells are to be seen, which at an older date are entirely absent; and the same is observed in polypus and fibroid. In malignant tumours a great number of fibres are found at first; but the longer the tumours exist and the larger they become, the more completely do such fibres diappear, leaving the cells as the sole histological element.

3. Certain peculiarities are observed in these cell-formations, among which may be mentioned the incomplete formation of the greater part of the cells, when the tumour is old and large, ⸱ and especially in the case of relapsing and secondary formations. The cells exhibit either a different form, an unequal size, or an irregular degree of development. The equal development of the structural elements of polypus, fibroid or fatty

tumour, furnishes an entirely different general impression from that derived from any kind of malignant tumour.

4. Besides the incompleteness and irregularity of the development of cells in malignant growths, they are found in these to undergo a rapid disintegration, examples of which, though more frequently met with in the older tumours, are not wanting in the younger ones, showing the retrograde changes which are taking place. The elements proving this, are granules, granular bodies, and granular cells; and these are to be found in a greater or less number in every cancerous tumour proportionate to its age. If on the other hand, we consider the regular and unchanged conditions of the cells in fatty tumours or polypus, in which scarcely any granular bodies or cells are found, it becomes certain that the duration of the life of a cell· is much longer in innocent than in malignant tumours.

5. Malignant tumours are remarkable for the rapidity of their cell growth. In a few days an entire lung may undergo tubercular transformation, or a cancerous tumour acquire double its size. A relapse may occur in five or six days, and a few days later may attain enormous dimensions. No innocent tumour comports itself thus.

6. In malignant swellings we always find a more abundant juice, which flows out on pressure, and contains some of the elements of the disease, as the cells, and the same fluid blastema is obtainable from tubercular lungs. When fluid is pressed out from a polypus, it contains no cells or fibres, or very few, while in that obtained from cancer there are numerous cells in every stage of development. It follows from this, that the textural connection in the malignant tumor is always looser, and the proportion of fluid blastema always larger, than in the innocent; and that these slightly connected elements are easily separable, and are incapable of the degree of development observed in the innocent, being, therefore, endowed with a shorter duration of life than these.

It results from the above observations, that there is less *vital energy and durability* in malignant growths, as is shown by the fewer stages of development they are capable of: and by the great disposition of the cells to terminate their life, and to pass into granular bodies and granule-cells This retrograde course explains the inordinate increase of cells, just as we see an immense reproductive power in animals placed low down in the scale. The lower its vital energy sinks, the more rapidly does the growth increase, so that the second or third relapse takes on a much larger and more rapid development than did the original tumor—a point well deserving the attention of the operator, lest, by his interference, he lowers the amount of vital energy, and hastens death more rapidly than it would have occurred had the case been left to nature. It is to this diminution of vital activity, that the peculiar softening of these tumors is due. In the softened mass are found the elements of the degenerated structure with incompletely formed pus globules ; and when the vital power is increased, and, as in tubercule, stationary condition of the disease produced, a more complete pus formation takes place.—[*Canstatt's Jahrb.* *Ibid.*

Miscellany.

A Singular Epidemic.—The history of Epidemics is one of the most interesting departments of Medical Literature. Whether studied by the medical philosopher, the philanthropist, or the theologian, it furnishes the most fertile themes for observation and speculation. It has in all ages been made the subject of special research by minds of the first order. And yet, what do we know of Epidemics ?—Nothing more than the dates of their occurrence and the extent of their ravages! We are still in total darkness in reference to their cause, and powerless in our attempts to arrest their progress! Facts upon facts have been diligently accumnlated from the Mosaic and Hippocratic eras to the present time, without yielding the data from which we may deduce one single law of practical utility to the physician! We should not, however, be discouraged, but continue to keep a record of their manifestations, until, piled like Ossa upon Pelion, they furnish us the knowledge we need.

Upon returning to our post about the 1st of October last, we were surprised at the frequent occurrence of sore fingers among our employers, and on inquiry found that they were equally common in the practice of other physicians, and had been so for several months. In some families nearly every inmate suffered more or less. Upon a large plantation in this vicinity they were so numerous as seriously to interfere with working the crop, and to lead to the suspicion that they were designedly induced in order to furnish an excuse for idleness. We learn from physicians residing at various points between this city and our northern frontier counties that they also saw a very unusual number of whitlows during the same period. The cases commenced in July, and continued to present themselves until the beginning of November. We are not informed whether such a state of things existed in the counties south of this.

The disease generally assumed some one or other of the forms of Paronychia or Whitlow—the majority of them being superficial, and

the smallest number affecting the theca of the tendons and the periosteum.   Although occurring spontaneously in most instances, the
slightest abrasion or irritation of the finger or hand would terminate
in suppuration more or less troublesome—Erysipelas complicated
some of the cases, and proved fatal in one of them here.

The season was one of the warmest and dryest ever known in Georgia.   The health of the city, and indeed of the whole State, is represented as having been unusually good.   The supervention of cold
weather put a stop to the sore fingers, and the writer has not seen one
since.

It may perhaps be deemed out of place to dignify so trivial a disease with the epithet " Epidemic," although its general prevalence
may really constitute it one.   Other slight affections are occasionally
seen occurring in this way.   We think we have seen the common
Furunculus prevail as an epidemic here several times.   The mere
fact that they are not often fatal is no reason for not classing them
with epidemics whenever their prevalence becomes general in a community.

Our object is now simply to add one more fact to the record; and
to ask our readers, if they have observed the same in other localities.

Medical College of Georgia.—The exercises of the annual Commencement in this institution took place on the 2d day of March,
when the Degree of Doctor of Medicine was conferred upon fifty
gentlemen.   A learned address was delivered to the Graduates, by
the Rev. W. G. Connor, and a most appropriate and felicitous Val-
edictory to his class-mates, by Dr. P. C. Winn.

The Dean of the Faculty reported to the Board of Trustees, that
there were in attendance upon the Course of Lectures just concluded
one hundred and fifty-eight students, of whom, there were from Georgia, 128—from Alabama, 19—from South Carolina, 14—from North
Carolina, 1—and from Tennessee, 1.

The following is a list of the Graduates:

FROM GEORGIA.

T. G. Andrews, - - - Thesis on Dysentery,
C. H. Bass, - - - - "   " Fœtal Brain,
E. T. Bell, - - - - "   " Pleurisy,
J. W. Barber, - - - "   " Intermittent Fever.
E. J. Berrie, - - - - "   " Croup,
J. W. Bowdoin, - - - "   " Lymphatics,

R. L. Cummins,	- - -	Thesis on Inflammation,
J. A. Carter, -	- - -	" " Uterine Cancer,
L. P. Dozier,	- - -	" " Erysipelas,
R. E. Fryer, -	- - -	" " Scurvy,
J. J. W. Glenn,	- - -	" " Cynanch. Trachialis,
R. A. Gowin,	- - -	" " Croup,
W. J. Holt, -	- - -	" " Rheumatism,
N. L. Hudson,	- - -	" " Gonorrhœa,
W. T. Jernigan,	- - -	" " Signs of Pregnancy,
F. M. Jones, -	- - -	" " Remittent Fever,
J. S. Lane, -	- - -	" " Colo-Rectitis,
T. G. Macon,	- - -	" " Typhoid Fever,
Elijah Mattax,	- - -	" " Typhoid Fever,
B. R. Rives, -	- - -	" " Professional skill,
William Rhodes,	- - -	" " Menstruation,
W. J. Reeves,	- - -	" " Intermittent Fever,
J. H. Ragan,	- - -	" " Pleurisy,
Robert Ragland,	- - -	" " Menstruation,
W. R. Ruffin,	- - -	" " Syphilis,
E. J. Setze, -	- - -	" " Gonorrhœa,
J. M. Saunders,	- - -	" " Typhoid Fever,
J. N. Smith, -	- - -	" " Typhoid Fever,
Lawrence Smith,	- - -	" " Intermittent Fever,
J. H. Trippe,	- - -	" " Pneumonia,
J. F. Trippe,	- - -	" " Delirium Tremens,
J. R. Tucker,	- - -	" " Scarlatina,
J. S. Wilson,	- - -	" " Gastritis,
W. H. Wilson,	- - -	" " Tetanus,
Jubal Watts, -	- - -	" " Gastritis,
B. A. Ware,	- - -	" " Concussion of Brain,
C. R. Walton,	- - -	" " Infantile Rem. fever,
Z. L. Watters,	- - -	" " Apoplexy,
W. T. Wilchar,	- - -	" " Inflammation,
J. W. Whitlock,	- - -	" " Sub. Nit. Bismuth.

FROM SOUTH CAROLINA.

J. A. Evins,	- - -	Thesis on Typhoid Fever,
R. J. Gilliland,	- - -	" " Scarlatina,
J. A. Glenn,	- - -	" " Cholera,
D. M. Laffitte,	- - -	" " Aneurism,
R. W. Quarles,	- - -	" " Functions of Liver,
R. M. D. Russel,	- - -	" " Cholera,
P. C. Wait,	- - -	" " Hepatitis.

FROM ALABAMA.

Alexander Donald,	- - -	Thesis on Electricity,
Christopher Montgomery,	-	" " Pleurisy,
P. C. Winn,	- - -	" " Spinal Irritation.

BIBLIOGRAPHICAL.

A complete Treatise on Midwifery ; or the Theory and Practice of Tokology ; including the diseases of Pregnancy, Labor and the Puerperal state. By ALF. A. L. M. VELPEAU, M. D. Translated from the French, by Charles D. Meigs, M. D., &c., &c. Fourth American, with the additions from the last French edition. By Wm. B. Page, M. D., &c., &c., with numerous illustrations. Philadelphia : Lindsay & Blakiston. 1852.

The work before us is one of three productions of Velpeau's pen, either of which would alone have made him distinguished among the medical authors of the age. His Surgical Anatomy, his Midwifery and his System of Surgery are all monuments of his erudition and sound practical sense. The profession in our country should feel grateful for the zeal manifested by the learned translators, in issuing this new and fine edition.

A Treatise on the Diseases of the Chest : being a course of Lectures delivered at the New York Hospital. By JOHN A. SWETT, M. D., &c., &c. New York : D. Appleton & Co. 1852.

The diseases of the chest have been for many years a favorite study with Dr. Swett, whose opportunities as physician to the New York Hospital and as an extensive practitioner in a community very much disposed to those affections, must entitle his deductions to great weight. As an original American work of merit, we cordially welcome it and wish it a favorable reception.

The Medical Student's Vade Mecum : A compendium of Anatomy, Physiology, Chemistry, Materia Medica and Pharmacy, Surgery, Obstetrics, Practice of Medicine, Diseases of the Skin, Poisons, &c., &c. By GEO. MENDENHALL, M. D., &c., &c. 3d Edition—Revised and greatly enlarged. With 224 Engravings. pp. 690. Philadelphia : Lindsay & Blakiston. 1852.

The nature and object of this work may be inferred from its title page. Lazy students, fond of the multum in parvo, will here find a capital work.

Discourses delivered by appointment, before the Cincinnati Medical Library Association. By DANIEL DRAKE, M. D. Cincinnati : Moore & Anderson. 1852.

The subject of the first of these discourses is "Early Physicians, Scenery and Society of Cincinnati," and that of the second is "The Origin and Influence of Medical Periodical Literature ; and the benefits of Public Medical Libraries." Like every thing from the pen of the distinguished writer, these discourses are full of interest, and will constitute a valuable contribution to the Medical History of the United States.

Outlines of the arteries : with short Descriptioms. Designed for the use of Medical Students. By JOHN NEILL, A.M., M.D., &c., &c., 2d edition. Philada. : Ed. Barrington & Geo. D. Haswell. 1852.

As a mere remembrancer of the general distribution of the arterial system, it may be useful. The plates are, however, very coarse.

Review of Materia Medica, for the use of Students. By JOHN B. BIDDLE, M. D., formerly Professor of Mat. Med. in the Franklin Med. College of Philadelphia, &c., &c. With illustrations. Philadelphia : Lindsay & Blakiston. 1852.

A very convenient and well gotten up manual, well aclculated to aid medical students.

Homœopathy : an examination of its doctrines and evidences. By WORTHINGTON HOOKER, M. D., author of "Physician and Patient," and "Medical Delusions." New York : Charles Scribner. 1851.

We have always believed that the best way to destroy quackery is to pay no attention to it. Physicians are never regarded by the community as *ex parte* witnesses, and their invectives therefore have no weight, save to enable the charlatan to cry "persecution." The work of Dr. Hooker, however, differs vastly from the ordinary tirades upon the subject. It is a calm and sensible appeal to the common sense of common intellects—of those who need the aid of others to enable them to see the truth, and to distinguish it from falsehood. The "Fiske Fund Prize" was awarded it by the Rhode Island Medical Society, and it will doubtless do much to open the eyes of the people.

Another Journal Discontinued.—The British American Medical and Physical Journal, published at Montreal, has been discontinued because subscribers would not pay up as punctually as the publisher was obliged to do. It is succeeded by the "Canada Medical Journal," edited by Drs. Macdonnell and David, to whom we cordially wish a successful career.

Death of Dr. Sidney A. Doane.—The ship-fever which has been prevailing to such an alarming extent among the emigrants daily arriving at New York, has numbered among its victims Dr. S. A. Doane, the distinguished physician at Quarantine on Staten Island. Dr. D. was the translator of a number of French medical works.

Medical Society of the State of Georgia.—We would remind our readers that this society will convene at Augtusta on the second Wednesday of the present month (April). · A large meeting is expected.

SOUTHERN
MEDICAL AND SURGICAL JOURNAL.

| Vol. 8.] | NEW SERIES.—MAY, 1852. | [No. 5. |

PART FIRST.

Original Communications.

ARTICLE XIV.

*Pathology : its relations to Physiology, as based upon Abnor-
mal Nutrition—being one of a series of Lectures upon
Physiological and Pathological Microscopy, delivered at the
Medical College of Georgia in February last.* By W. J.
BURNETT, M. D., of Boston.

The domain which we have just left, Physiology, is by no
means so widely separated from the one upon which we now
enter, Pathology, as might be supposed from the commonly
received doctrines of medical science. I do not make this remark, however, as applicable to anything but their material
expressions ; for the difference as to essential nature between
truly normal and abnormal phenomena, must, of course, be wide.
But in our conversation with the material world, either natural
or unnatural, we can learn about it only through the intervention of material forms. It is in this way that we have learned
all we truly know in physiology, and it is in this way that we
are now to inquire into Pathology, and if from the minute character of our inquiries, the expectation is raised that thereby
will be solved the mystery of the intimate nature of disease,
that expectation will certainly remain unfulfilled and disappointed. In a general way it may be said that pathology is but an
erring physiology. This expresses a great deal that is true of its
nature ; and although, perhaps, not the whole truth, it approxi-

mates so closely, that it will serve as the basis of our inquiries. Such a view is well calculated to remove from the mind many erroneous notions ; one of which, for instance, is that disease is a self-existing entity, which notion, if well entertained, cannot but impede our correct interpretation of its phenomena, for we shall be constantly struggling between a fancy and a fact. Then, again, the ideas which we have of health and disease must be relative, since we have no positive data by which the one can be determined in contradistinction to the other. Our idea of normal life must be extremely indefinite, and especially so when the steps of its transition to that which is abnormal, have not been well made out.

Another question, which arises at the outset, is—Does disease always have a material expression, and that, too, of a corresponding and invariable character ? A negative answer to this would be deemed by many as quite *unphysical,* not to say unscientific ; but in the present state of our knowledge, I must regard it as by far the one most correct, for we are to reason from what we know, and although analogy is of great service in such matters, yet we cannot be too careful of its use. We should very naturally say, that in virtue of the great fact constantly before us, viz., that vitality has its expression only in organization, which is tangible and capable of being analysed, so should we always have a tangible expression of any perversion of that vitality. This may be very scientific, but at present it is negatively so only, for there are many transitory morbid changes of the vital phenomena—many morbid conditions, known by the name of functional, which leave no traces in the matter or organ in which they occur, at least as far as we can now detect by the most careful research. Too high an estimate must not therefore be placed upon these intimate microscopical studies of pathological conditions and phenomena. In the first place, with all the material product at our command which we could ask, we must expect to know of disease only subjectively ; and in the second place, we must not be surprised to meet with many of the best expressed pathological phenomena holding apparently no corresponding material relations.

If these two points be well borne in mind, much error and confusion will be avoided.

But let us return to our original proposition : Pathology is only an erring physiology. We can understand from this why that the genesis and general laws of pathological cells should be the same precisely as those of physiology. And I make here this general statement founded upon a pretty widely extended observation—that, *both as to their genesis and general aspect, as cells, those which belong to abnormal, cannot be distinguished from those belonging to normal conditions of life.* The genetic and general relations of cells in physiology and pathology are therefore the same, but the bifurcating point in the road appears when we begin to inquire about the destiny of each. Physiological cells must always be considered *teleologically,* that is, as having relations with a future and determinate result, in the attaining of which, they fulfil their destiny ; with pathological cells, however, all these conditions are absent. They exist as cells in virtue of the previous existence of a formative material, which must have an organized expression of its forces. This expression is necessarily a cell, but there it ends, it sustains no higher and future relation for a definite result.

Abnormal cells, or rather cells produced under abnormal conditions of life, therefore, are not characterized by any type or true individuality. I know very well that some, such as those of pus, tubercle and cancer, have an uniformity of appearance quite remarkable, but I cannot regard this as having any teleological signification at all, but rather as due to a corresponding uniformity of condition of the abnormal plasma in which they are found. I do not think that this view at all disparages the scientific accuracy with which they should be described, for experience has shown us that this uniformity of abnormal plasma is so constant, that it may always be counted upon in our determination of its products. With these considerations, founded on fact, the distinctions between physiology and pathology as based upon cells, are therefore not only broad, but definite as far as they go. I may say, farther, that they are the only distinctions upon which we can at present insist ; remove them and I can perceive no reason why all our pathology should not at once be resolved into physiology. It may be asked if this resolution of the two into one is not desirable, as simplifying our ideas of organic life, both normal and abnormal ? I say *no*, even were it possible, for it immediately takes away from the phenomena of organic life their philosophy as manifested in their teleological bearing.

There is one other result which may well be deduced from the foregoing remarks: it is that all pathological products are necessarily *infra*-formations—they are below the standard of those of health, of which they may, or may not, take on some of the characteristics. Pathological formations may be divided into two kinds, only; viz: 1st, those which simulate the type of the healthy tissues, called *homeomorphous*, and 2d, those which have characteristics of their own, called *heteromorphous*. All abnormal products are necessarily one or the other of these kinds. It is true that the latter are most important in a practical point of view, on account of their peculiarity of life, widely separated as it is from that of normal forms. Such, for instance, are cancer, tubercle and pus. Under the former, on the other hand, are included all those forms of tissue which are abnormal, not so much because they are dissimilar from healthy forms, but because they want very much their definite character as active tissues towards a conservative, economical end in the economy. They are therefore less severe and more amenable to treatment; but still, in an histological point of view, they are not the less worthy of our consideration.

It is difficult to get hold of this subject unless we take it up in a particular manner. Pathological products, as material forms, are superventions in and upon the healthy parts. In a causative point of view, they are therefore referable to nutrition and its perversions. And 1 shall take up the subject in this light, even though there is necessarily a blending of physiological and pathological phenomena.

Two conditions mark the existence of the healthy living tissue—these are *decay* and *repair*; the former occurring because the tissue is living; the latter because to live it must preserve its physical identity.

This round of actions constituting the sum total of those making up the live adult tissue, have their foundation in a function which we term *nutrition*. A word to which in later days we have been inclined to give a more pregnant signification than in former times; and this, because it thus embraces in function, either directly or indirectly, the whole phenomena of animal life. Many have thought that the relations of reproduction, or the origin and rise of the new being, should be viewed as belonging to another category of actions. But they have allowed themselves to be deceived by the importance of these processes; for we have seen on a preceding page, that such phenomena are only *cellular,* and are therefore only those of nutrition seeking an individuality of expression.

Nutrition, then, being considered as the basis of physiological science, it will be my object to show that its *perversions* can be viewed as the foundation of our rational pathology.

But, that my meaning may be fully comprehended, I will run over briefly the leading features of this nutrition as a physiological function—a task which I have hitherto omitted, anticipating as I did, its consideration more properly in this connection. This is not a new, but it is a most important physiological truth, that the blood or its analogue is that from which all the conditions of nutrition arise. It therefore follows that in it we should clearly recognise the elements of all these different tissues. The blood-vessels form a series of channels permeating the tissues, and terminating as it were in a set of vessels, functionally different from either arteries or veins—the capillaries—which are the dispensers of the nutritive fluid to the tissues; and although they cannot be traced minutely into every tissue or part, yet their function on such tissues is always indirectly felt.

It is asked how these capillaries are the immediate agents of this nutritive function. It is by their transuding through their parietes into the parts through which they pass, the hyaline plasma of the blood, and which is immediately appropriated by the contiguous tissue, or transferred by endosmosis through granular or cell-structure, to those more distant. This hyaline blastema is structureless, but it contains within itself the elements of structure. It is entirely amorphous, but it possesses in a latent form all the individualities of the different tissues. After effusion, it may serve its function as a pure plasma, by bathing the tissue and filling the vacancies made by liquids passed away. But this, I think, is not common, and belongs almost exclusively to the sclerous tissues. It gener-

ally gives rise to more solid products. These are utricles
and cells with all their various metamorphoses. The primitive
utricle appears as the first material expression, and in tissues
of a purely utricular character, such as the muscular, the development does not extend beyond this point, but as such they
are appropriated. But in tissues having an *existing* cell-structure, these utricles pass on to cells, replacing those passing
away. I believe that this hyaline plasma, immediately upon its
effusion, and before the primitive utricles have appeared in it,
is, whatever be its locality, identical in character. The reason
why it has afterwards so many ultimate expressions or developments, appears to me due to another cause. It is that directly upon its transudation it receives in coming in contact
with a tissue, the impress or type of that tissue ; so that whatever the former may be, the plasma in serving any purpose
follows directly in train of the *idea* on which the tissue is expressed.

Let me illustrate this doctrine by referring, for example, to
the epithelial tissue. This, as we have already seen, is composed
of a layer of cells, situated upon, and attached to a basement
membrane. The cells thus attached, whatever be their function, are constantly passing away, and must be renewed. To
effect this last, a plasma is effused by the contiguous vessels ;
this, as soon as it comes in contact with this tissue, takes on its
epithelial type, and the primitive utricles developed in it, immediately pass on to that ulterior condition of epithelial cells.
Other examples might be cited to show in the same way this
beautiful *type-form* of tissue ; without which the continuity of
structure could not be maintained. The full appreciation of
this idea cannot be two strongly insisted upon, and I will again
express it in a laconic way : A liquid containing the elements
of structure, upon being brought in contact with a living solid,
is immediately impressed with the type-character of the latter,
and therefore must subserve its repair. It is not properly *a*
selective power of the tissue, but a *living act*, occurring because
the tissue has an individuality of its own which it can impart.

I wish that I could illustrate this by any reference to common
examples of animal life : but as it is one of those immaterial
acts in physiology, we can appreciate it only by the recognition of the fact.

I might, perhaps, liken it well to the act of fecundation, in which a spermatic particle, by simple contact with the ovum, impresses upon it the full type of the male parent ; and, to carry the comparison still farther, if the completeness of an individual can, in this way, be thus stamped upon an ovum ; so, in the same way in the act of nutrition, may the singleness of a tissue be stamped upon a hyaline plasma.

I regard the recognition and application of this *type-power of tissues*, as one of the happiest results of modern physiology, not only as illustrative of the higher tone of our present studies in this direction ; but also, as enabling us to grasp many of the hitherto hidden forms of function in this science.

On account of its value as the hidden spring of the various nutritions, let me still farther notice its character.

If it is asked what is this *type-power*, I should say that its nature can be best expressed by an imperfect metaphor. It is the *memory* of the immaterial idea on which a tissue is developed, still persistent during its material life. And to carry the metaphor still farther, this memory may be bright and active, or may be fast fading away, according to the age of the tissue.

The younger the tissue, the more full and complete is its individuality and type-power, and if it suffers a lesion in its very early life, this breach of continuity is thereby so thoroughly repaired, that its physical identity is preserved. This is the reason why in wounds with very young children, the healing of them leaves no cicatrix. The *type-power* extends fully and completely into the plasma effused for repair, and this repair therefore has all the character of true interstitial nutrition. As the individual advances in life, and passes into, or beyond its adult period, this type-power appears to die out, or at least to lose some of its strength. This is the reason why at that time lesions are not perfectly repaired ; the material not taking on the character of the contiguous tissue, and an adventitious product occurring in the place of the lost part. The same reason may be assigned for the fact, that tissues having suffered no lesion, sometimes atrophy, the plasma effused not being appropriated, but which, taking on a new character, may give rise to new and morbid forms.

I might enter more fully into the consideration of this most

interesting subject, and it would afford me much pleasure to
take up its illustration in some of the most delicate tissues in
both man and the lower animals. But at this time, I have
thought proper to sketch only its general character, and which
is to serve as the foundation of considerations of another character soon to follow.

It is quite necessary that we should be very familiar with
this great *high road* of physiology, in order that we may well
know where the *by-road* of pathology divides from it.

Thus far, we have seen that two conditions are necessary
for correct and healthy nutrition. These are : 1st, that the
plasma effused shall be healthy, and such as may be fit for appropriation, and 2nd, that the type-power of the tissue to be
nourished, shall be sufficient to make the appropriation. Such
being the requisites of the healthy nutritive process, the perversion or suspension of one or both of these conditions, gives
rise to what has been justly termed *abnormal* nutrition—a
state of the animal tissues, which we have good reason to believe is at the very foundation of pathology. To illustrate clearly this point, we will take up separately each division.

I. *Perversions of the character of the Plasma.*—There
appears to be a law of affinity, or congruity of action in tissues,
which must be regarded as a very powerful conservative of
their integrity. By this, I mean, that when the circulatory vessels do not contain the proper elements for the tissues, the
latter do not call for the effusion of their plasmatic liquids—or,
to impersonate the matter, as would, perhaps John Hunter, I
should say, that the tissues perceiving the incongruity of the
nutritive fluids, refuse to have them effused ; but still it often
happens that this inappropriate plasma is effused, and then, not
being at all reconcilable to the type of the tissue, yet possessing
a certain vitality of its own, and which perhaps is still further
urged on by the very fact of its being in contact with. a *living*
tissue, the course which it pursues is wayward and thus we
have heterogeneous pathological products. This perverted or
abnormal plasma varies much as to its capacity, but is always
below that of health. Its capacity is expressed in the character
of its products; when quite low, granular and low cell com-

pounds are the result.   Such, in fact, are *pus and tubercle* which appear to constitute the lowest expressions of a plasmatic formative power.   When of a higher character, it gives rise to the highest pathological products, which often seem to have a kind of individuality of form and function.   A good example of this is seen in *cancer*.

The heterogeneous products, then, of pus, tubercle and cancer, I have considered as due to perversions of plasma.   But, perhaps, the subject will come home more clearly to the mind, if I say that *inflammatory products* may be regarded as due to this same perversion of plasma.   I do not mean to say that such products can always be traced as the results of inflammation; but, as far as yet studied, there appears to be here a connection, at least, assuring us that when we shall know more of the matter, our most comprehensive idea of inflammation will include all the conditions under which heterogeneous products occur.   In touching, then, here upon the subject of inflammation, I shall not be considered as diverging from the main point of our discourse.

I do not pretend to define inflammation, because I think we have not yet sufficient data to convey to the mind a clear idea of its character; still, if I say that there appears to be coëxistent with it a want of healthy relation between the bloodvessels and the blood, I think I have stated pretty clearly all that which is really known about the matter; and even then, it is very far from being certain if their *absence of relation* is not the first known *effect*, instead of the *cause* of the inflammatory process.

It is therefore a waste of time to dwell upon that, the nature of which we have yet so feeble an appreciation of.   We must take the results as we find them, waiting for the ultimate cause until we have more data.   I have said that the first visible sign of inflammation is an absence of the healthy relation between the bloodvessels and their contents : this leads to a partial suspension of the function of both, and also that that function which does occur is of an abnormal character.

When the otherwise nutritive processes are very active, scarce any appropriation of this plasma takes place, and the products arising in it, viz: granules and corpuscles seem so

alien to healthy tissues, that they are expelled as foreign substances; such is *pus* in all its forms, and such, I think, there
is reason to believe, is tubercle also. When, however, the
process is less active in its character, the plasma is appropriated to a certain extent, but the tissues thus badly nourished
sink below their normal type, and when these conditions are
kept up for any length of time, they seem to take on a character of their own. This is often seen as one of the consequences of a previously acute inflammation of an organ, but
especially is it observed in indolent ulcers. It is thus that we
see that the long continued use of a perverted plasma, by a
tissue, serves to modify the type-power of the latter. And,
in speaking of the minute pathology of some organs, at a future
time, I shall have occasion to enter more fully into the peculiarities of these changes and their consequences.

It may be asked how the etiology of cancer can be considered as belonging to the perversions of the plasma. The reply to this, is, that although eminently a morbid product, it
differs widely from those of which we have just spoken, and
this, in possessing in a high degree, a life of its own. The
plasma in which it takes its origin has a capability not much
below that of health, but still has a character as different as the
results produced. Although passing on to the higher cell-
structure, its inferior character is betrayed by the objectless
nature of its termination; for these cells appear to be the *ultimate* result of a morbid action, rather than the material agents
through which a higher function is to be performed.

The cancerous structure, however high it may appear in an
anatomical point of view, is aimless and without function.

In speaking then of pus, tubercle and cancer, as the results
of a perverted plasma, heteromorphous products, I think I can
best express their mutual relations and dissimularities, if I use
a figure, and say that normal nutrition being considered the
great high road, those forms of abnormal nutrition producing
pus and tubercle would be considered as small roads diverging
from it at nearly right angles; whereas, that form producing
cancer would be considered as a much larger road, and diverging at a smaller angle; in fact, often afterwards running parallel with it. But all these diverging roads never get back upon

the main one, and therefore have a termination unlike any thing of true function.

In concluding this section, the relations which this perverted plasma holds to inflammation, may be thus briefly stated. We cannot conceive of this want of harmony between the action of the capillaries and the constituency of the blood, unless we suppose at the same time an existing cause. Now, as it is true, that the more we investigate minutely their conditions, the more do we find the inflammatory process co-existent, and, as in the instances of pus and granular forms, the relations of cause and effect can be directly traced, we have a right to infer that the same is true, even although their relations cannot be fully made out.

And so, on the whole, we seem to be justified in regarding inflammation, whatever is its nature, as a condition always preceding, and in all probability causing this perversion of the effused plasma, and therefore the immediate cause of pathological heterogenous products.

II. *Perversions of the type-power.*—We now enter upon the consideration of quite another class of phenomena. The vessels being healthy and the blood normal, they cannot be viewed as being in the same category as those of inflammation we have just considered. I have therefore thought proper to designate the results of such conditions as the *homogeneous non-inflammatory* products : in fact, they are forms, which, while they are really morbid, partake nevertheless of the type of the healthy tissue, as far as that condition will allow.

We have just seen how, when the type-power was good and the plasma bad, the dissimilar results were referable almost entirely to the plasma. We shall now see that where the inverse is true, the results produced have more an affinity with the tissue, than with the plasma. In one sense, it can scarcely be called a perversion of type-power, but rather a decrease or increase; but on the other hand, these words do not express the whole ; for, besides these variations of amount, there is involved a pathological principle not easily or readily expressed.

Suppose that, from some unknown cause, the type-power of an epithelial tissue in the body had become changed. The nor-

mal plasma is thrown out as usual, but it is not delicately and
nicely appropriated as in health; and although the tissue has
given it its impress, yet this is all, for the relations of size and
shape appear to be absent.   There therefore appears a new
form, which, while it bears the outward aspect of the healthy
tissue, is an abnormal product; it is, as it were, the representation of disease, under the garb of health.   This product is
epitheloid, but not *epithelial*.   Such, for instance is the so-called
cancer of the lip, the cancer of the antrum, &c., &c.

In the same category may be considered many, if not all, the
hypertrophies of tissues.   Where a product appears with the
general character of health, but with the profligacy of disease.

It is not difficult for us to understand how, in some of these
immense growths, a sufficient amount of plasma is supplied;
for it appears to be a law in the nutrition of tissues, that the
greater the demand the greater the supply; and, so when the
demand has once been made, even by a morbid product, it is
furnished and the whole may go on increasing, the vessels con-
forming to these changes exactly as though a healthy tissue
was experiencing a rapid normal growth.   But, if we thus have
products, from what, in one sense, may be called an increase
of type-power, constituting hypertrophy, there is quite a different class arising from a *decrease*, in fact a suspension of it, and
which ought in this connection be noticed.   I cannot say that
it is primitively of tissue-origin, but, at any rate, it seems to be
a dying out of the type-power; in fact, so thoroughly is this
the case, that the individuality is gone and nothing is appropriated; and in accordance with the law just mentioned, there
seems ultimately to be scarce any supply; and then the tissue
loses its physical identity and gradually recedes to its primitive
utricular condition.   This condition of things has generally
been considered in the light of an *atrophy*, but I have thought
that it merited a distinction, and have proposed for it the name
of *retrograde metamorphosis*.   Its leading characteristics may
be thus briefly stated.   Bichat's definition of life, as applied to
an individual, was, "the sum total of the functions by which
death is resisted."   Now, what applies to an individual, may
be taken as at least applicable to a tissue.   Its life consists in
the conservation of those two conditions by which its integrity

is maintained. ·These, I have already regarded as involved in
what is called nutrition; the balancing of decay and repair.
Now, whatever function a part may discharge, it is necessary
that it (the function,) should be kept up in order that the nutrition should continue normal; when, from either an unknown
cause, or from suspension of function, it ceases to have that
even changing vitality, then it seems to lose its type-power, and
the small quantity of effused plasma is feebly appropriated, the
vital cohesion of the tissue in part disappears; so that although
there is strictly no decomposition, yet the individuality of the
part is gone, and with it all those forces that elevated and sustained its character above that of the primitive elements. We
have, then, in place of the normal tissue, what is called a granular mass; and as such it cannot be called a special product, for
it is alike, whether it occurs in a muscular or a glandular organ.
It consists simply of oil and albumen, uniting in their usual
way. This point, however, will be touched upon at a future
time. I have said that this condition differs from *true atrophy ;*
for this last can scarcely be regarded as an abnormal state, it
being only a decrease of tissue-function, and which we see daily
exemplified in the muscular tissue. The same is true in an
inverse sense of *true hypertrophy ;* and which is *not,* as I have
before said, the cause of *homeomorphous products.* They are
both rather variations of nutrition, as to *quantity,* than as to
perversion.

Such is a rapid survey of some of the perversions of nutrition which lie at the foundation of many of our best views of
pathological changes. It may be asked, if under this head may
be included the causes of all pathological phenomena having
their expression in a material product? With our present
knowledge, I do not think that the question can be positively
answered. Nevertheless, I think I am safe in saying that the
tendency of the present enquiry is to show that in abnormal
nutrition is to be found the causes of all *organic* pathological
changes.

These considerations may perhaps serve as the ground-work
of our subject, it being now our task to look into the specific
character of its details. I shall therefore, take up first, the subject of hetero-morphous products, each in its proper character,

commencing with the lowest.   But before this, the phenomena
of inflamation as elucidated by the microscope should be considered, and this will serve a sa proper prologue for the next
lecture.

ARTICLE XV.

Report of Cases of Typhoid Fever and Typhoid Pneumonia,
treated principally with Veratrum Viride.   By W. J. SUM-
MER, M. D., of Lexington, S. C.

Since the publication of Dr. Norwood's articles on veratrum
viride, I have extensively employed it in the treatment of
Typhoid fever and Pneumonia, and with the most gratifying
success.   I would, therefore, most cordially adduce my experience in support of the remedy, as being at once safe and efficient.   Before I became acquainted with this valuable agent, I
regarded the treatment of a severe case of typhoid fever with
something like dread, as to its results, but now I am less concerned about my cases of this disease, than of other affections
generally deemed more trivial.   A brief notice of a few cases
treated with this remedy, will not, I hope, prove unacceptable
to the profession, and will, perhaps, induce others to make
trial of this valuable agent.

CASE I. Rebecca, aged 8, daughter of Mr. F.   I was called
to see her on the 5th Oct. last.   She had been suffering under
the premonitory symptoms of typhoid fever for four or five
days, and the disease was now fully formed.   There was headache ; hot, dry skin ; small and frequent pulse ; tongue coated
with a whitish fur, with tip and edges red and rather dry ;
loss of appetite, amounting to a disgust for food.   There was
tenderness of the abdomen in the right iliac region, pressure
over which produced the gurgling noise, so characteristic of
this affection—no diarrhœa.   I prescribed pil. hydrarg. gr. v.,
to be followed, if it did not act on the bowels, by castor oil.
Scarified cups were applied to the abdomen—pepper poultices
to be used subsequently.   After the bowels were cleared, neutral mixt with a minute quantity of tartar emetic.   (I had no
veratrum viride with me.)

Oct. 6th. Called and found my patient in pretty much the same condition : had two evacuations from the bowels, without taking oil; headache somewhat relieved ; abdomen still a little tender ; pulse 130. Discontinued previous treatment, and ordered tinct. verat. vir., to be given in doses of three drops every three hours, and if nausea, emesis, or a reduction of the pulse did not take place after giving three or four doses, to increase the dose one drop each time. Pepper mush to be kept constantly applied to the abdomen.

7th. Called eighteen hours afterwards. Patient had vomited once, a short time previous ; skin cool ; pulse reduced to 80 : the vomited matters consisted of a quantity of mucus and watery fluid. The dose of tinct. veratrum had been increased to six drops. Directed it to be given in doses of four drops every four hours. At my visit next day, the patient seemed entirely free from fever—pulse 72, soft and full. Bowels had acted twice since previous visit, dejections resembled what had been vomited. The dose was now reduced to three drops, repeated at intervals of three or four hours and continued for several days, for fear of a return of the fever, after which it was discontinued—the patient convalesced rapidly.

Case II. Henry, aged 10, brother to the above. Called 20th Oct. Found this patient with symptoms very much resembling the first, though more severe, particularly the headache. The parents had administered a dose of epsom salts, the bowels having been constipated. The salts, however, operated drastically, and diarrhœa was subsequently very obstinate. There was considerable tenderness in the right iliac region, and gurgling on pressure. Cups were applied to the temples and abdomen, followed by poultices to the latter; hyd. c. creta et pulv. Dover, in small doses, for the diarrhœa, and the patient at once put upon the use of tinct. veratrum, in small doses, gradually increased. Gum-water was the only article of drink or food allowed.

Oct. 21st. Patient complains less of headache ; pulse reduced from 130 to 84 ; has vomited once or twice without much nausea ; diarrhœa still persistent, yet the discharges are not so watery. Continue same prescription—the veratrum in slightly diminished quantity.

22d. Diarrhœa rather worse, there being frequent watery discharges, telling rapidly on the strengh of the patient; tongue dry and red, but the skin cool, and pulse only 70 ; no nausea. The family were averse to using the syringe, or I should have directed opiate enemeta ; as it was, I had recourse to acet. plumbi combined with pulv. Dover., a dose of which was given every two hours, veratrum to be continued in small doses.

23d. Patient is better to-day.   Bowels have acted but three or four times in the last twenty-four hours ; tongue less red and dry ; pulse still about 70, full and soft ; skin cool and moist, no tenderness of the abdomen, though it is still a little tympanitic. Continued same treatment.

24th. Better in all respects ; diarrhœa is sufficiently checked ; tongue is becoming moist and clean ; abdomen more natural ; pulse and skin about natural.   Discontinued my visits.   Next day the pulse showing a disposition to rise ; the father called on me again, and not being well enough to ride, I gave him some of the tinct. veratrum, of which he gave small doses for a few days, with the same happy results.   Recovery was slow, but steady and perfect.

Case III. A negro girl, aged 7, the property of Mr. H——, was called to her on the 6th Dec.   She had been ill for more than a weak previous, and the disease was now fully formed, and unusually severe.   The pulse was feeble and very frequent, amounting to 140 ; the tongue was quite dry and red ; the abdomen tender and very much distended ; diarrhœa, also, was present, there being from six to ten discharges daily of a watery fluid, resembling new cider.   She was more or less affected with delirium, particularly at night.   Scarified cups were applied to the abdomen, followed by poultices ; small doses of acet. plumbi with Dover's powder were given every two hours, and tinct. verat. vir., every four hours, commencing with three drops and increasing one drop at each dose until its ordinary effects were obtained.

7th. Patient has less fever this morning ; pulse 110 ; diarrhœa almost as bad as ever ; patient rested better through the night, though there was slight delirium.   Ordered in addition to the lead and Dover's powder, laudanum injections, and applied a large blister to the abdomen.   The veratrum to be continued in full doses.

8th. No fever to day; pulse 80, full and soft. Patient this morning passed about eight ounces of nearly pure blood from the bowels—blister drew well and the abdominal distention is diminished. Directed acetate lead and opium in large doses, to be repeated as often as could be well borne—veratrum to be continued in diminished doses.

9th. Patient is much better: no hemorrhage from the bowels nor watery stools; pulse 75 and natural; tongue is becoming moist and clean. Left off all medicine except veratrum, which was still to be given in very small doses.

13th. Saw this patient, and she seemed so much improved that I ceased visiting her—directed the owner to watch her for a day or two, and if she took fever again, to resume the use of veratrum and send for me.

16th. Was summoned in haste to this patient. She had, a few hours before, been attacked with severe pain in the lower part of the abdomen, which rapidly spread over its whole extent—the abdomen was so tender as not to bear the weight of the bed-clothes without pain. The pulse was a mere thread, and so frequent as scarcely to be counted; respiration short and hurried; stomach very irritable—in short, she had all the symptoms of peritonitis, and caused, undoubtedly, by perforation of the intestines, allowing the contents to escape into the cavity of the abdomen.

I attempted the administration of large doses of opium, hoping that under its influence, in connexion with perfect rest and the avoidance of all substances internally, which could in any way disturb the bowels, the system might be supported until adhesive inflammation might possibly unite the perforated intestine to the adjacent parts. But such was the irritability of the stomach, that nothing could be retained, and reluctantly I had to abandon the case as utterly hopeless. She died 18 hours after the commencement of the symptoms of peritoneal inflammation.

I regret exceedingly that I had not the privilege or time to make a post-mortem examination; yet I am confident that the disease was in the first place typhoid fever, and that the fatal termination was due to perforation of the intestines, followed by general peritonitis. Equally certain am I, also, that

had not perforation of the intestine occurred, this patient would
have recovered.

Case IV. Mr. S., aged 30, and of delicate constitution. I
was called to him on the 4th Jan. last—he had been in bed for
four or five days—I found him with the usual symptoms of
typhoid fever, in addition to which he had pain in the left side,
a distressing cough, and was expectorating the rust-coloured
sputa, as characteristic of pneumonia. On examining his chest,
I detected inflammation involving the lower half of the left
lung, and, seemingly, verging into the second stage, or that of
real hepatization. His tongue was covered with a whitish fur,
with tip and edges red and dry; bowels acted about twice a
day, without medicine; abdomen a little full, though nearly
natural; no appetite whatever. Pulse 128, and without much
strength; respiration hurried and laborious.

He was already much prostrated, so I contented myself with
the abstraction of a couple ounces of blood from the side by
cupping. I at once put him upon the use of tinct. veratrum
viride, in doses of eight drops every three hours, gradually increasing the dose until nausea, vomiting, or a reduction of the
pulse was induced. Not feeling satisfied to trust the life of
my patient to this remedy alone, (I had not used it in such
cases,) I desired to employ, in conjunction with it, an alterative
mercurial course, but no reasoning or persuasive power of
mine could induce him to give his consent. He had once been
under the specific influence of mercury, and now declared that
he would take no more of the subtle mineral.

5th. Patient seems in much the same condition, with the
exception of fever. On increasing the veratrum to twelve
drops, slight vomiting, without (as the patient said) nausea,
was produced, and the pulse came down to 90, at which I found
it. Has still some pain in the side, particularly on coughing;
expectoration free, and redder and less viscid than in sthenic
pneumonia. Applied a blister, 6 by 8 inches, over the inflamed
lung; directed veratrum to be given, in full doses, until the
pulse was reduced to 70, then diminished one half, and continued.

6th. Better to-day; veratrum is well borne, has reduced the
pulse to 68. Respiration slow and easy; cough less trouble-.

some, and expectorates freely; no pain; blister has drawn
well: tongue tremulous and pointed, but moister; bowels move
about twice daily; abdomen slightly distended. Veratrum to
be continued in doses sufficient to maintain the reduction of the
pulse, and along with it, small and frequent doses of the decoction of polygala senega.

7th. Patient still better; feels stronger since taking the seneka. Pulse rather below 70, and strong enough; respiration
good, though, of course, a little hurried. Continue same treatment.

9th. Patient still improving; has gained a little more
strength; takes light nourishment with some relish. Blister
is healing, and the solidified portion of lung is becoming permeable to air, though slowly; the cough is better, and expectoration diminished and more natural. Still to take small
doses of veratrum, and sulph. quinine grs. ij. thrice daily, as a
tonic.

11th. Called and found patient doing well in every respect,
except that his bowels were much too irritable, there having
been three or four watery discharges in the last twenty-four
hours. Prescribed a combination of acid. sulph. aromat. with
tinct. opii. in sufficient quantities to check the diarrhœa; the
tr. opium then to be continued, or omitted, as should be necessary; the acid to be taken freely as a tonic. The patient now
improved, and has recovered without farther treatment.

One or two remarks, and I have done. It will be seen that
I have not depended on veratrum viride alone, in the treatment of the cases in which I was employed, but have called
into requisition other agents of acknowledged therapeutic value, and, as I believe, with better effect than could be obtained
from its single action. At the same time, I am confident that
without the use of this extraordinary medicine, I should, within
the last few months, have lost many patients by typhoid fever
and pneumonia—indeed, since I have learned its valuable properties, I would not know how to dispense with it. About a
year ago I had a case of typhoid pneumonia, similar to the one
above stated, which, in spite of my best directed efforts, ran on
to a fatal termination. Had I, at that time, been acquainted
with the properties of this invaluable medicine, I have not a

doubt but I could have saved this patient. Something was wanted to control the excited circulation, which was beyond my reach. Although it is not the only medicine to be depended on, it is certainly the chief one. I have used the remedy in at least a dozen cases of pneumonia, after depletion, when that was indicated, and with a success beyond any thing I ever anticipated. With the exception of the case reported in this communication, (Case iii.,) I have not lost a case in which I have used the remedy. In a general way, I have not found the medicine act harshly or disagreeably,—it is true, it sometimes makes the patient deathly sick, but its unpleasant effects are easily obviated, and after the system is fully under its influence, its unpleasant effects usually soon pass off. It is applicable to many diseases, but is particularly suited to pneumonia. By reducing the circulation, it very materially lessens the amount of labour thrown upon the lungs, a circumstance greatly to be desired, when we remember that well established principle— an inflamed organ must have rest. I have found it to possess all the powers and properties ascribed to it by Dr. Norwood, yet I have usually found it necessary to continue it a day or two longer than he directs. I use the saturated tincture of the root.

ARTICLE XVI.

Remarks upon Mrs. Willard's Theory of the Motion of the Blood, and Dr. Cartwright's Experiments. By Wm. T. Grant, *M. D., of Culloden, Ga.*

We feel considerable embarrassment in writing an essay on a theory advocated by so celebrated a member of the Medical profession as Dr. Cartwright; but, as we are writing for information, we think we may dismiss this without more ado.

Dr. Cartwright establishes his theory of the motion of the blood, by ocular demonstration, in the form of experiments on the alligator. In reply to this, we would cite an animal, that belongs to the same class as the alligator, and also to the same order, by which we can prove the very opposite to that which he has so satisfactorily proved by his experiments on the alligator. The animal to which we refer, is the frog. It is a Physiological fact in natural history, that in the frog, the circulation is carried on, without any assistance from the air ; when the animal is in the dormant state. Now, as said above, the alligator and frog are animals, both of which belong to the class called Amphibia ; so then, everything being equal on this point, in these two animals, the argument deduced from experiments on the frog, performed by Naturalists long ago, serves us to counterbalance that drawn from experiments performed on the alligator by Dr. Cartwright, and as they are equal, it is necessary for the advocates of his theory to advance others in its support.

But, then, there are objections to his theory, some of which it is our object to bring forward ; and we will first lay down a premise, viz : if the theory be *true*, it is consistent with every anatomical and other truth with which it has any connection, and furthermore it harmonizes with every fact that is a fact, by which it is surrounded.

In the first place, then, " like causes will produce like effects," under any circumstances, at any time, and in any place. Now, to apply this to the point in question : it means, that as the motion of the blood is produced by the action of the air on the blood, under *certain* circumstances, it ought, *cæteris paribus*, to do the same in certain *other* circumstances. Or, in other words, if the air acting on the blood, which is the cause, produce the motion of that blood, which is the effect, under *certain* circumstances, then the same cause must produce the same effects under other circumstances. If then this cause produce this effect in a *living* man, ought not the blood to flow in the *dead* man, if artificial respiration keeps the air acting on the blood, from the moment that natural breathing ceases ? And cannot the system, in the same way, be made to perform all the functions natural to it, in the dead as well as the living man ; the warmth of the body be kept up ; the different organs secrete the juices peculiar to them—and indeed, everything that is not dependent on the will, be carried on as well after as before death ? This new theory would answer these questions in the affirmative, but it is useless to say that reason proves the fact, that such is not, cannot, and will not be the case. So then the theory is inconsistent here.

The second objection is axiomatic : if, in any case, the cause ceases to act, then the effect is no longer produced ; but, if the effect ceases, it does not follow that the cause must likewise cease.   Now, to apply : If the action of the air on the blood, the cause, ceases, then must the motion of the blood, the effect, also cease, which is not *always* true, as is proved by reference to several of the lower animals.   This latter opinion, was held as . Dr. Cartwright says, by Bichat.   So, then, the theory is inconsistent here.

The third objection may be embraced in the following words : " This theory mistakes the effect for the cause."   Now, to prove this.   " When the chest expands, the lungs follow, and consequently a vacuum is produced in their air-cells.   The air then rushes through the nose and mouth into the trachea and its branches, and fills the vacuum as fast as it is made.*   And when the chest is contracted, the air is expelled from the lungs.   This then is breathing.   Now, then, whatever causes this alternate contraction and expansion of the diaphragm and chest, must be the prime cause of breathing.   The blood does this, therefore it is the cause of breathing ; and we can prove that the blood does do it.   All the muscles are divided into two sets— the voluntary and involuntary ; the involuntary muscles act independent of the will ; and their action must have a cause, and this cause must be inherent, or dependent on something external to the muscle.   It cannot be inherent, for in that case, if one of these muscles be taken out of the body, it must move about in consequence of its inherent principle of action.   Therefore, it must depend upon something in connection with the muscle ; now then, when this is taken in connection with the fact that the power of the muscles is greatly exhausted by a copious depletion, it proves beyond a doubt that the blood produces the action of the involuntary muscles ; therefore, we come to the conclusion that respiration is the effect and not the cause of the motion of the blood.   It is not necessary to explain how the blood produces the action of these muscles, but it can be done in a few words : it acts as a vivifying and stimulating principle in all parts of the system and especially on the muscular fibre. So then the theory is inconsistent here.

* Cutter on Respiration.

As it seems that some of the profession are dissatisfied with the old explanation of the motion of the blood, and as new theories are advanced on almost every subject, we think it could not be considered presumption in us, if *we* were to advance a new theory; and we embrace this as being a good opportunity, more especially as it is on the very question that we have been discussing. Our theory of the motion of the blood is simply this: the motion of the blood is caused by galvanism, the heart, arteries, veins, and capillary vessels acting as a battery, one pole of which is situated in the heart, and the other in the capillaries. This is only our opinion, and as such we advance it in the form of a theory, hoping that those who have more advantages than we, may put it to the test and sift it well. We have reasons for entertaining this opinion, but think it unnecessary to give them to the public at present. We think with *this* theory of the motion of the blood, a great many things that are now considered as inexplicable, can be easily explained; the why and wherefore of the different secretions, &c., we think could be explained on this principle.

PART II.

Eclectic Department

On Healthy and Morbid Menstruation. By J. Henry Bennett, M. D., late Physician-Accoucheur to the Western General Dispensary, etc.

The Physiology of Menstruation; Dysmenorrhœa; Menorrhagia; Amenorrhœa.—The function of menstruation has been much elucidated during the last ten years by the labours of the numerous physiologists who have investigated the phenomena of generation, amongst whom stand prominent, Pouchet, Gendrin, Negrier, Barry, Wharton, Jones, Bishoff, Raciborski, &c. I would, however, more especially, refer to the elaborate work on "Spontaneous Ovulation," by M. Pouchet,[*] in which will be found a full and complete account of his own important researches, as also of those of nearly all the ancient and modern writers on the subject. To M. Pouchet, whose life appears to have been partly devoted to the study of this interesting and

---

[*] Théorie Positive de l'Ovulation Spontanée, par F. A. Pouchet, Professor of Zoology to the Museum of Natural History of Rouen, Paris: Baillière, 1847.

important physiological point, belongs the credit of having been one of the first to broach the doctrine of spontaneous ovulation as a law in the females of all mammiferæ, and also of having established this law in the most irrefutable manner by numerous experiments, and by a close and powerful analysis of all that had been done by his fellow-labourers in this field of observation.

The researces to which I refer prove, in the most satisfactory and conclusive manner, that menstruation is intimately connected with the evolution from the ovary of matured ova, which takes place periodically in the virgin as well as in the married female. In the human female the maturation and evolution of ova occur at frequent intervals, and are marked by the exudation from the uterine cavity of a greater or less quantity of blood. In the lower animals, the interval is generally longer, and the menstrual phenomena are less marked, consisting merely in congestion of the sexual organs, accompanied by the exudation of mucus, mingled with a few blood-corpuscles. But in both, the phenomenon is the same; in both, nature directs a tide of blood to the uterine organs, as the ova contained in the ovary arrive at maturity, in order that the uterus may be in a fit state to receive and nourish them should they be fecundated after their emission from the Graafian vesicle.

A decided physiological connexion exists between the different organs which constitute the sexual apparatus in the female —viz: the ovaries, the uterus, the external sexual parts, and the breasts. All are dormant as it were, until the advent of puberty, the great and essential characteristic of which is the developement of the Graafian vesicles or ova. Previously deeply imbedded in the tissue of the ovaries, small, and rudimentary, as puberty approaches, some of their number begin to enlarge, and gradually to approach the surface. The installation of puberty and the first menstrual show coincide, and are evidently connected with the arrival of one or more of these vesicles at the full period of development. A few red streaks formed by capillary vessels are first observed on the surface of the Graafian vesicles, which protrude from the surface of the ovaries. These capillaries gradually increase in number and intensity of colour, giving the membrane on which they ramify the appearance of being the seat of acute inflammation, until at last, in the centre of the vascularized surface, an opening shows itself, the result of a tear or rent, or of absorptive inflammation; the ovule is expelled, and having been grasped by the fringed extremity of the Fallopian tube, passes down its canal, to be lost, no doubt, in the uterus, if not fecundated.

According to M. Pouchet, the opening of the Graafian vesicle and the evolution of the ovule take place either at the epoch that menstruation ceases, or one or two days later. If this view be correct, the progressive vascularization of the proper membrane of the ovum or Graafian vesicle would coincide with, and to a certain extent occasion, the uterine congestion that precedes and accompanies menstruation ; as also the sympathetic irritation and swelling of the breasts which so frequently precede and accompany the menstrual flux.

I have qualified the above statement by the words " to a certain extent," because it appears to me that the uterus is not merely a passive organ, receiving and responding only to impressions originating in ovarian phenomena, but that it exercises a marked influence over their development. Thus we find that its diseases very frequently arrest and modify in various ways the function of menstruation, and also diminish and annihilate sexual feelings and appetites. We may therefore fairly presume that they exercise the same unfavorable influence over the maturation and evolution of the ova. In other words the attentive consideration of the reciprocal influence of the uterus and of the ovaries on each other in disease, must lead all impartial observers to the conclusion that in health they constitute one system of organs, the integrity of which in its component parts is necessary for the normal accomplishment of the functions of ovulation and menstruation.

The above, I am firmly convinced, is the only true and rational view that can be taken of the uterine system both in health and in disease. To attribute both the healthy and the morbid conditions of menstruation all but exclusively to ovarian influence, as has been done by some pathologists, is to take much too narrow a view of uterine pathology, and is as far from the truth as would be the negation of all ovarian influence on uterine phenomena. The ovaries, it is true, preside over the function of menstruation, as we have seen, but the uterus cannot certainly be considered a "mere reservoir" or bladder, destined only to receive and nourish the ovum after impregnation.

The more accurate knowledge which we now possess of the cause, seat, and mode of manifestation of the menstrual function, tends greatly to corroborate the view at which I have long arrived from clinical experience, respecting irregular or morbid menstruation, viz : that it is nearly always, when strongly marked and *inveterate*, the result of positive disease of some portion of the uterine system, and, generally speaking, of the uterus. That such is the case must be admitted as probable, when we consider that the function, although presided over by the ovaries, is accomplished by the uterus, which contains an extensive mucous surface. Those who have hitherto written professionally on menstruation are, however, so totally unaware

of this important fact, that their works, even the most recent,
are replete with cases the true nature of which they do not
even suspect—cases in which it is most evident to me that menstruation was modified by positive disease, but which they view
as physiological, or as the result of constitutional causes. In
the present essay, I shall endeavor to point out the data by
which mere physiological modifications in the menstrual function may be distinguished from modifications the result of
actual disease. Although a difficult task, I hope to be able to
accomplish it satisfactorily by bringing to bear on the question,
the facts respecting uterine disease which I have developed at
length in my work on Uterine Inflammation. I must first, however, be allowed to enter into a few details respecting the mode
of manifestation of the menstrual function in the normal state.

From what precedes, it is evident that the term menstruation ought in reality to be applied to the totality of the conditions that co-exist with the maturation and evolution of ovarian
vesicles. Until recently, however, the exudation of blood from
the uterine organs in the human female, the all but invariable
concomitant of this periodical function, having been alone observed, it has been to it only that the term menstruation has
been given. The necessary connexion between the ovarian
and uterine phenomena having only been discovered and established of late years, it is not surprising that the meaning of the
word menstruation should have been thus limited. Henceforth,
however, it will have to be taken theoretically in its more extended and truer sense, although, practically, we may still be
obliged to limit the term menstruation to the uterine element,
or the exudation of blood, as it is the ostensible indication and
evidence of the changes that are taking place in the ovaries.

It is now universally admitted that the menstrual secretion
takes place from the mucous membrane lining the uterine cavity. For one or two days before it commences, in the healthy
uterus, a tide of blood sets in towards the uterine organs ; and
if the cervix uteri is then brought into view, its mucous surface
is found greatly congested, and of a livid hue. When the secretion has commenced, the blood may be seen to ooze *guttatim* from the os uteri. After it has ceased, the tide of blood
gradually recedes, and in the course of one, two, or three days,
the uterus is restored to its normal condition, the cervix assuming its naturally pale, rosy hue. If the uterus is the seat of
disease, the flux to it begins earlier—often a week before.
After menstruation has ceased, there is also, in disease, a great
tendency to the perpetuation of the menstrual congestion, the
uterus frequently not appearing to have the power to expel the
menstrual blood.

Menstruation in the human female oscillates physologically between great extremes, or, in other words, it may vary to an extreme extent in its mode of manifestation, and yet these variations may be compatible with health, and with the perfect integrity of the uterine organs. Indeed, there is not a greater difference between the human female and the female of the lower mammiferæ, in which the menstrual function only shows its presence by a congested state of the genital organs and a slight mucous secretion, than there is between different females. Thus, for instance, in some, the menstrual flux only shows itself for a day or two, or even for a few hours, throughout life, and is very scanty ; whereas, in others, it lasts seven or eight days, and is always so profuse as to be all but hæmorrhagic.

The physiological variations of menstruation may be referred to its epoch of first manifestation, to its duration, to the quantity of blood lost, to the amount of pain experienced, and to the periodicity of its return.

The epoch at which menstruation first sets in, is very variable, but may be said to range between eleven and nineteen or twenty, the cases in which it occurs before or after these ages being rare. The medium age, in temperate climates, according to Raciborski, who deduced it from the analysis of a large number of cases, is about fourteen—a statement which my own experience completely corroborates. There are cases on record, in which menstruation has set in as early even as the third or fourth year, but they can merely be considered freaks of nature. Climate was formerly considered to exercise great influence over the epoch at which menstruation appears, but this influence appears to have been greatly exaggerated. So far from cold greatly retarding, and heat greatly accelerating, its appearance, it would appear, from the valuable researches of Dr. Roberton,* of Manchester, that the medium age is pretty nearly the same all over the world. Raciborski finds a difference in the medium age of the cases he investigated for the north and south of Fance, but that difference only amounts to a few months, and would require to be deduced from a larger number of persons, to be definitely accepted. Menstruation generally ceases between forty-five and fifty, but the menopause may occur much earlier or much later.

The duration of the menstrual flux, and the quantity of blood lost, vary very considerably in different females. The average duration may be said to be about four or five days, but many are only unwell two or three, and with many again, it lasts six or seven. When menstruation is of short duration, the loss of blood is generally scanty, whereas it is greater when it lasts

---

* Essays and Notes on the Physiology and Diseases of Women. 1851.

a long period; not only on account of its longer duration, but
also because it generally flows more freely. The influence of
climate in this respect also appears to have been much exaggerated. The fact of menstruation being constitutionally of
long duration and profuse, I have found to be a powerfuly predisposing cause of uterine inflammation, owing probably to the
intensity of the mollimen hæmorrhagicum, and to the length of
time during which it persists, during which the patient is exposed
to many perturbing causes. The intensity of the physiological congestion is evidenced by the fact, that for one, two, or
three days before and after menstruation these females often
have a slight white or leucorrhœal discharge, even when in perfect health.

With many females the first manifestation of the menses is
unaccompanied by pain. The menstrual flux makes its appearance with scarcely any previous admonition of its advent, and
continues to appear without pain or uneasiness; or if pain is
present, it is slight and limited to the first few hours. This is
the most favourable mode in which the menstrual function can
take place, and the one which affords the greatest guarantee of
future immunity from inflammatory disease. It is, however, by
no means the rule; with many women, the first advent and the
subsequent appearance of the menses, are attended, physiologically, throughout life, with great uterine pain. With some the
pain is limited to the first few hours, with others it exists for a
shorter or longer period before, and lasts throughout, the period.

The periodicity of menstruation also varies physiologically
to a great extent. I have found that four weeks or twenty-eight
days, the lunar month, is the most general term; but the periodical return of the menses may take place at any time between
the third and the fifth. Most authors allow even a greater
latitude; but I believe that the constant return of the menses
at an earlier or later period will nearly always be found, on a
careful inquiry, to be a pathological symptom, and to be connected with local disease.

From what precedes, it will be perceived that the physiological variations of menstruation—variations quite compatible
with health—are so numerous and so great, that it is impossible
to lay down any standard by which the integrity of the function can be generally tested. The above fact would much
diminish the importance of the changes that occur in the menstrual function in disease, as an element of diagnosis, were it
not that this irregularity is not observed, physiologically, in
each individual case. In other words, every female has *her
own individual standard*, to which she generally remains true
throughout her life, unles the uterine organs be the seat of dis-

ease, or the general health be deeply modified by some other cause. Once, therefore, we have ascertained the mode in which menstruation occurs in any particular female, at an epoch when it may be fairly presumed that she was in good uterine health, we, are authorized to surmise the presence of uterine or ovarian disease—and, generally speaking, the former—if any marked and permanent change takes place.

It is the ignorance of this important fact that has filled with errors, as I have already stated, all existing treatises on menstruation, at nearly every page of which are narrated, as physiological, cases which I at once recognise as most decidedly pathological. This circumstance, therefore, must greatly invalidate the value of the conclusions at which these authors have arrived, whether statistical or otherwise, with respect to the physiology of menstruation.—[*London Lancet.*

[To be Continued.]

On Irritable Uterus. By F. W. MACKENZIE, M. D.

The term Irritable Uterus is applied to a painful condition of the organ, not caused by displacement, inflammation, or appreciable organic disease. It is met with in various degrees of intensity, from slight uneasiness to excruciating suffering. Although apparently a simple lesion of innervation, it is found to be a very obstinate disorder.

The slighter forms of the disorder are characterized by pain in the uterine region, increased by standing or walking, and relieved by lying down. The pain radiates from the uterus to the groins, loins and hips. A sensation of bearing down is often complained of, and there is leucorrhœa or dysmenorrhœa. On examination, the uterus is found to be excessively sensitive to the touch, but not displaced, or sensibly diseased. The general health is generally feeble, the circulation languid, and the digestive organs are generally in a faulty condition. The patient will often be found to have suffered from severe mental affliction, or has undergone physical privation and fatigue, and that, as a consequence, spinal irritation and anæmia have resulted.

The more severe form of this disease has been very graphically described by Dr. Gooch. He remarks that a patient, suffering from irritable uterus, complains of pain in the lowest part of the abdomen along the brim of the pelvis, and often also in the loins. The pain is worse when she is up and taking exercise, and less when she is at rest in the horizontal posture. If the uterus is examined, it is found to be exquisitely tender. As soon as the finger reaches, and is pressed against, the uterus,

it gives exquisite pain ; this tenderness, however, varies, at different times, according to the degree of pain which has been
latterly experienced. The neck and body of the uterus feel
slightly swollen ; but this condition also exists in different degrees ; sometimes being sufficiently manifest, sometimes scarcely or not at all perceptible. Excepting, however, this tenderness, and the occasional swelling, or rather tension, the uterus
feels perfectly natural in structure. There is no evidence of
scirrhus in the neck ; the orifice is not misshapen, nor are its
edges indurated. The circulation is but little disturbed ; the
pulse is soft, and not much quicker than is natural, but it is
easily quickened by the slightest emotion. In a few instances,
however, there has been a greater and more permanent excitement of the general circulation. The degree in which the
health has been reduced has been different in different cases.
A patient who was originally delicate, who had suffered long,
and has used much depletory treatment, has been, as might
reasonably be expected, the most reduced. She has grown
thin, pale, weak, and nervous. Menstruation often continues
regular, but sometimes diminishes or ceases altogether. The
functions of the stomach and bowels are not more interrupted
than might be expected from the loss of air and exercise ; the
appetite is not good, and the bowels require aperients ; yet
nothing more surely occasions a paroxysm of pain than an active purgative. Such are the leading symptoms of this distressing complaint. To embody them in one view, let the reader
imagine to himself a young or middle-aged woman, somewhat
reduced in flesh and health, almost living on her sofa for
months or even years, suffering from a constant pain in the
uterus, which renders her unable to sit up, or to take exercise ;
the uterus, on examination, unchanged in structure, but exquisitely tender, even in the recumbent posture ; always in pain,
but more or less frequently subject to great aggravations.

With regard to the pathology of these cases, Dr. Gooch observes, that the causes, to which this disease has been attributed,
are generally considerable bodily exertion at times when the
uterus is in a susceptible state ; but he remarks, that the patients had previously manifested signs of a predisposition to it.
They were all sensitive in body and mind, and many of them
had previously been subject to painful menstruation. As to
its proximate nature, he is satisfied by stating that it consists
in a morbid condition of the uterine nerves, attended by pain,
and sometimes vascular fulness ; and he likens it to the irritable breast, the irritable testis, and the painful condition of the
joints which is sometimes met with in hysterical females. He
does not venture to explain its pathology any farther.

A consideration of the cases of this disease which have come under my notice, appears to me to justify the following conclusions :—

First. That, in the majority of instances, irritable uterus is rather a sympathetic than an idiopathic disease of that organ.

Secondly. That it is sympathetic of irritative disorder of various organs with which the uterus has intimate relations, the irritation of which is reflected, either partially or entirely, upon the uterine ganglia and nerves.

Thirdly. That whilst such reflected irritation is its immediate cause, it is remotely dependent upon a defective condition of the blood, which would appear to operate by producing a morbidly irritable state of the nervous system generally, and of the uterine ganglia and nerves in particular.

[These propositions are supported by the detail of nine well selected cases, upon which Dr. Mackenzie makes the following general observations:]

Upon a general review of the preceding cases, the first inference I would venture to draw from them is, that they are affirmative of the truth of the propositions which were advanced at the commencement of this paper. In all, the uterine affection appeared to be consecutive to, or sympathetic of, constitutional derangement or irritative disorder of other organs. In none could it be regarded as dependent upon idiopathic disease of the uterus ; and additional corroboration is derived from the fact, that it disappeared, in most instances, under the influence of treatment of a general rather than of a specific character.

Another inference which may be drawn from them is, that the influence of gastro-intestinal disorder and spinal irritation are very considerable in the causation of uterine derangements. In the majority of the cases reported, these co-existed, and would seem to have had a similarity of origin. In all, they were associated with anæmia, and had been preceded by much mental anxiety. How much, therefore, is due to each in the production of the uterine symptoms in these cases, it is impossible to say. Many circumstances, however, which have come to my knowledge, lead me to believe that derangements of the uterus, involving more particularly its nutritive and secretory functions, such as leucorrhœa and disorders of menstruation, have rather a gastro-intestinal origin when sympathetically induced; whilst those which affect more particularly its sensory functions, producing neuralgia and various irritable conditions, are, for the most part, connected with an irritable or morbid condition of the spinal cord.

But it is not contended, that hysteralgia is in all cases necessarily connected with spinal irritation, or gastro-intestinal disorder. I believe them to be very frequent causes, but I have met with instances in which it existed irrespectively of either. In gouty and rheumatic subjects, considerable uterine pain, more or less of a persistent character, is often met with, doubtless of a gouty or rheumatic nature; and I believe that severe irritation of any important organ or nerve may, under certain circumstances, be reflected upon the uterus, so as to give rise to very distressing symptoms.

[In further illustration of the pathology of these affections, the author has made the following analysis of thirty-seven cases, in which the uterus was in a morbidly irritable state, not in consequence of displacement or appreciable disease. In all there was marked pain and uneasiness in the region of the uterus, which varied in intensity in different instances, and in some had been of long continuance:]

1. UTERINE COMPLICATIONS were observed in the following proportions:—
In 3 there was no other uterine disease.
" 15 the pain was complicated with leucorrhœa.
" 7 " " leucorrhœa and dysmenorrhœa.
" 3 " " leucorrhœa and amenorrhœa.
" 1 " " leucorrhœa and menorrhagia.
" 4 " " leucorrhœa and irregular menstruation.
" 4 " " dysmenorrhœa alone.
" 2 " " menorrhagia.
" 1 " " fibrous enlargement of the neck of uterus.

2. ANTECEDENTS. The irritable state of the uterus had been preceded:—
In 4 cases, by weakening discharges, such as profuse hemorrhage, and protracted suckling.
" 5 " mental anxiety and distress.
" 8 " mental anxiety, with disorder of the digestive organs.
" 2 " sudden fright.
" 18 " disorder of the digestive organs.

3. CONCOMITANT AFFECTIONS:—
In 18 there was well-marked anæmia, with disorder of the stomach and digestive organs.
" 12 " anæmia, with spinal irritation.
" 3 " spinal irritation.
" 4 " great irritability of stomach and digestive organs.

[The facts contained in the foregoing analysis appear, to the author, to justify the following conclusions:]

First.—That, from the operation of the same causes, various and dissimilar uterine diseases may be occasioned. Thus the principal antecedent circumstances in these cases were, for the most part, the same, and yet very different disorders were the consequence. In some, there was simply a painful condition of the uterus; in others, this co-existed with leucorrhœa, amenorrhœa, dysmenorrhœa, menorrhagia, &c. The probable explanation of this is, that the operation of the different causes in question is primarily upon the nerves of the uterus, and that irregular actions, in regard to these, precede and give rise to those particular symptoms, which, in the aggregate, constitute disease as known by a given appellation.

Secondly.—That, all these lesions may arise from constitutional disorder, may be perpetuated by it, and in many instances will cease on its removal. In these cases the chief circumstances which had preceded were either of an enervating or depressing nature ; such as loss of blood, over-suckling, &c., or mental depression or uneasiness. The obvious effect of these would be to lower the tone of the nervous system generally, and to render it morbidly susceptible to impression. Thus it would happen in regard to the uterine ganglia and nerves, that they would be prone to irregular actions, and to participate readily in the morbid affections and conditions of other organs. If,.again, the impressions leading to such abnormal actions are received from or through the medium of the ganglionic system of the nerves, it is reasonable to suppose that the functions to which these are more immediately subservient, such as nutrition and secretion, would be more particularly disturbed, whilst those received from or through the medium of the cerebrospinal system would rather give rise to painful and uneasy feelings; and thus may arise the difference in the uterine derangement, which is consecutive to chylopoietic disorder and spinal irritation.—[*London Journal of Medicine.*

Some Practical Observations on Pelvic Abscesses. By FLEETwood CHURCHILL, M. D., Fellow of the King and Queen's College of Physicians, Ireland, &c., &c.

The peculiar disease, then, to which I would very briefly call your attention, is that phlegmonoid inflammation, which, by some, is termed pelvic abscess, and by others inflammation and abscess of the uterine appendages, according as the attempt is made to be more or less explicit. Of the nature of the disease, there is no difference of opinion among modern writers ; the older ones, indeed, regarded it as a metastasis of the milk, and termed it "milk abscess."

I have no doubt that the attack is much more common than is even yet believed, although the attention of the profession has been latterly a good deal directed to the subject by writers in Dublin, London, Edinburgh and France. Within two months this year, for example, I was called to three such cases.

We find this local inflammation occurring under very different circumstances, some of which we should hardly have anticipated.

1. It may occur, not only unconnected with parturition, but in unmarried persons at different ages, and independent of all the ordinary irritants of these organs. A case occurred in the person of one of the nurses at the Meath Hospital, a single woman, about 50 years of age, and without apparent cause. It exhibited the usual symptoms which I shall notice by and by, and ran the usual course, softening and opening into the rectum, after which the patient recovered.

2. I have seen several cases of the disease in married women who never had had children; in two instances it occurred within a few months of marriage; in both the tumefaction was considerable, but both terminated in resolution.

3. In some few cases, it occurs as a secondary complication of severe uterine irritation, apparently from the use of local irritants, the too frequent employment of the uterine sound, the introduction of the pronged pessary, &c.

4. I have seen the disease follow a smart attack of ephemeral fever several times; in one case it terminated in resolution after several weeks; in another in suppuration and evacuation by the rectum; and a third is at present under treatment.

5. It not unfrequently complicates or terminates an attack of simple hysteritis, of which several examples have come under my notice, terminating most generally in suppuration. One such case was the largest abscess of the kind I have ever seen, occupying about one-fourth of the abdomen; and in another, at present under my care, the tumor acquired the size of an orange, and after remaining stationary for some months, is now nearly resolved.

6. In certain epidemics of puerperal fever, inflammation of the uterine appendages appears as a special variety, with or without a corresponding affection of the uterus.

It is not unlikely that the disease may occur under other circumstances, but these have each and all come under my own observation, and I can therefore vouch for their accuracy.

With regard to the nature of the disease, as I have said, there is no difference of opinion, it is a phlegmonoid inflammation of these parts, but there is a distinction of some practical value as to the locality and the parts affected. In this respect all the cases I have seen may be divided into two classes :—

1. The first and largest exhibits a tumour just above the brim of the pelvis, and closely connected with it, fixed and immoveable, extending downwards internally outside the vagina, through the sides of which it can be felt.

2. In the second class the tumour is distinct from the pelvis, rounded, and quite moveable in every direction.

In the latter cases, the inflammation appears limited to the uterine appendages—*i. e.,* the ovary, broad ligament, and Fallopian tubes. In the former, the soft parts which line the anterior and lateral wall of the pelvis are also involved in addition to the uterine appendages; these are more properly named pelvic abscesses.

I may add, that although either side indifferently may be affected, I think the left side is more frequently the seat of the inflammation.

As to the causes of the disease, it is not easy to be very precise.

1. In certain cases, to which I have alluded, the abscess is undoubtedly the result of mechanical injury, and the cause is quite intelligible.

2. In others, again, there would appear to be a sort of metastasis of inflammation from the uterus, which in these cases occurs towards the termination of the uterine affection.

3. In a third class of cases, especially when the patient is unmarried, it seems more fairly attributable to cold than to any other cause; but what may be the influence which determines the attack to this region, it is quite impossible to say. In one of the cases, to which I have alluded, all the uterine functions had been some time quiescent.

4. Lastly, in puerperal epidemics, when the uterus is involved, we could hardly expect, that its appendages would escape; and accordingly we find that they generally share in the disease, though much more remarkably, in some epidemics than in others. In another place I have given statistics of the comparative frequency.

Now, with regard to the symptoms, I must beg you to bear in mind what I have said as to the two varieties of the local affection; the one involving the soft parts lining a portion of the pelvis, and the other limited to the ovary and its appendages, strictly speaking.

The disease may, and generally does, I think, commence by a febrile attack; but this is not always the case. There may be a rigor, followed by heat, or this may be entirely absent. Sooner or later the patient complains of pain or uneasiness in the lower part of the abdomen; but the amount of suffering varies a good deal, and pretty much in accordance with the amount of fever.

If we examine the abdomen carefully, we shall either find a tumor just above Poupart's ligament, of varying size and thickness, and firmly fixed to the pelvis, or a moveable tumor, rounded, firm, and elastic, lying above the pelvis in the abdomen.

In the former class of cases, a vaginal examination adds

nothing to our information, as the tumour is out of reach ; but in the latter, we can trace it extending more or less down into the pelvis, adding a lateral thickness, extremely tender on pressure. Generally speaking, the uterus is pushed a little to one side, is not tender on pressure, but moving it gives pain. In one or two cases I have seen the uterus fixed and nearly immoveable ; in one case only have I seen both sides affected. This occurred in a married woman, unconnected with delivery.

In the former class, also, in addition to the pain, tenderness, &c., the movements of the leg of that side are affected ; the patient cannot stretch it out straight without great pain, nor can she walk or stand up without bending forward.

In the latter cases the movements of the limb are quite un- affected. This distinction is, I think, of considerable practical value.

The tumour, I have said, varies in size ; it is, however, always tender, on pressure, and not less so as the disease ad- vances. When it attains a considerable size or is attended with much irritation, I have seen the bladder and rectum sym- pathetically affected ; the former more frequently so, giving rise to a frequent desire to evacuate their contents. In only one case have I had reason to believe that the tumor offered a mechanical impediment to the passage of the fæces.

These are the principal symptoms present in a simple case of pelvic abscess ; but they, as well as the course of the disease, will vary much according to the extent of the local affection, the amount of constitutional disturbance, and, in some degree, according to the circumstance under which the attack has oc- curred.

1. In some cases I have seen, the affection had a purely local character. There was the tumour tender, firm, moveable, or immoveable ; but the pulse was scarcely quickened from beginning to end ; the appetite but little affected ; the bowels regular, &c. The patient was confined to the sitting or recum- bent posture, and suffered pain locally, but that was all.

2. In other cases, the local suffering was very considerable and unceasing ; the pulse very quick, at least 120, with sweat- ing at night ; utter loss of appetite ; irregularity of bowels ; no sleep, and great emaciation.

3. Lastly, the cases which occur during an epidemic of puer- peral fever will present its general characters in addition to the local symptoms already mentioned.

With more or less of these symptoms, but with the local ones always, the disease runs its course not quickly ; often, on the contrary, very slowly, but with an uncertain duration in each case. I do not think I ever saw the tumour disappear or suppurate in less than a month ; and I have known it run on to three or four, as in two cases at present under my care.

The disease may terminate either by resolution or suppuration.

1. By resolution. I have seen repeated instances of this termination, both when the tumour is free and when it is attached to the pelvis, though more frequently in the former than in the latter, and much more frequently in those cases where there is but little constitutional irritation. In such cases, the tumour may increase to a certain degree with the symptoms I have described ; it then remains pretty stationary for a time, often a considerable time, after which it gradually and slowly subsides. It is worthy of notice, that if the patient be imprudent during this process, the morbid action in the tumor may be re-excited, and the case may terminate in another manner. In one of my cases the tumour had nearly disappeared when the lady's servant became suddenly insane, and so frightened her that the tumor enlarged, and all the symptoms re-appeared. The time occupied by the process of resolution is generally considerable. I have two cases under my care at this moment illustrative of this ; in one, the tumour, which was free, has all but disappeared, after nearly five months ; and in the other, the fixed tumour has considerably diminished after three months.

2. In the majority of cases, however, the tumour suppurates, softens, generally perceptibly, and after a process of absorption of the intervening tissues, terminates by the evacuation of the purulent matter ; this formation of matter being generally, though not always, marked by the occurrence of rigors. The channel, through which this takes place, varies a good deal.

1. In some cases it has been evacuated into the peritoneum, giving rise to peritonitis ; but this must, I think, be very rare —at least, in upwards of twenty cases which have come under my notice it never occurred. I recollect a case which ocurred to my friend the late Dr. Haughton, which now appears to me to have been a case of the kind. The poor woman had recovered badly from her confinement, and some time afterwards, when at the night-chair, she felt something give way, and peritonitis immediately followed.

2. Cases are on record in which the abscess opened into the bladder. If I mistake not, I saw one recently in one of the Journals ; but such cases I believe to be the most uncommon of all.

3. The tumour may soften at its lower part, and the matter may find its way through the coats of the vagina, and be discharged through that canal. I have seen several cases of this

termination, the results of which have been very favourable. It has been suggested that we should puncture the tumour in this situation, when the situation of the softening is suitable ; nor do I see any objection to the plan. I have, however, not found it necessary.

4. The most common situation, certainly, for a spontaneous opening, is into the rectum, and then the matter will be found discharged along with the stools. On this account, when the tumour is observed to become softer, and we have reason to suspect that matter is formed, the alvine evacuations should be carefully examined. Except when the matter escapes into the peritoneum, no degree of pain seems to accompany its evacuation. It often passes unobserved by the patient, and sometimes seems marked by a sense of relief in the tumour.

5. In a considerable proportion of cases, the tumour approaches the surface gradually, and engages the integuments, which become tense, fixed, and sometimes red and shining. The fluctuation can be felt, the intervening integument is absorbed, and the matter points, as it is called.

The extent of these abscesses superficially, is generally not much beyond the size of the tumour at an earlier period, but in some cases I have seen them very large ; in one case, scarcely less than one-fourth of the abdomen seemed involved. I do not think it would be wise to wait for such an extent of disease, but we ought to open it at an earlier period, and thereby save the patient much suffering.

The symptom which most surely indicates this mode of termination, or rather this locality, is the skin becoming fixed over the tumour, not rolling freely, but being adherent to it.

Diagnosis.—There can hardly be any difficulty in the diagnosis or pelvic abscesses which occur after delivery, and as part of a mere general puerperal affection ; the attention being directed to the uterine system, a careful local examination will detect the tumefaction, whether it be fixed or not. If it be situated deep in the pelvis, and scarcely appearing above the brim, still the pain down the leg, and the difficulty of extending the limb, will leave but little doubt.

Perhaps an equally careful examination might be equally successful in the unimpregnated condition ; but as the disease is not generally expected under such circumstances, a less minute investigation may, and often does, lead to a false conclusion. I have myself known a case of pelvic abscess pronounced to be a fibrous tumour by very competent authority.

Now, the pathognomonic symptoms are, the pain in the tumour and down the leg, the impossibility of standing quite upright, or extending the leg completely, and the tumour detected on external and internal examination.

1. From fibrous tumours it is distinguished by its comparatively quick growth, the amount of uneasiness, and the termination. The former increase very slowly, and insensibly give
rise to few or no symptoms, and, above all, are not common in
the uterine appendages.

2. In women of a certain age, the filling up more or less of
the pelvic cavity, might be supposed to result from cancerous
disposition; but here we have no general cancerous diathesis,
the uterus is always unaffected, and the occurrence of suppuration or resolution solves the difficulty.

3. That one variety of abscess which is unconfined resembles much ordinary ovarian enlargements, at first sight, but it
differs in this, at least according to my experience, that it never
occurs except in connexion with childbirth or miscarriage; and,
as a general rule, the growth is much more rapid in the cases
under consideration.

The affection, then, may be considered as well marked, and,
with care, not difficult of appreciation, but requiring special
care and attention when it occurs independent of parturition.

Prognosis.—For so serious an attack, involving such important organs, and liable to such various terminations, the prognosis is very favourable. I have seen more than twenty such
cases, and have never seen one in which any unpleasant result
occurred. Some fatal cases are on record, but they must be
very rare, and probably in consequence of secondary peritonitis.

The disease is, however, very tedious, and may reduce the
patient considerably, so that there may be some risk of the in-
cursion of other diseases, if the patient be predisposed thereto.

Treatment.—Whether the attack come on after delivery or
independent of it, if we see the patient during the acute stage,
it will be necessary to apply leeches over the tumour, to repeat
these, if required, in numbers according to the amount of irritation and the patient's strength and to follow them by constant
poulticing.

The bowels should be kept quite free, and I have found benefit from small and repeated doses of calomel or blue pill, but
not continued so long as to affect the gums.

The diet of the patient during this period must be low, and I
need hardly say that she must be confined to bed.

After we have somewhat subdued the acute inflammation,
we must still continue the poultices until suppuration is established; but if the pulse be quiet, we may allow a little better
diet, such as chicken-broth or beef-tea.

When we are satisfied that suppuration has taken place, that
matter is formed, then our anxiety is as to the place where it is
to be evacuated. If by the bladder or intestine, we can do

nothing but continue the poultices; but if, on a vaginal examination, we find the tumour soft and the intervening parietes thin, we are advised to make a puncture with a bistoury into the tumour, first ascertaining the presence of pus by an exploring needle. If we succeed, the after-treatment is simple; so long as purulent matter escapes, the poultice may be continued, and occasional pressure made upon the tumour, so as to empty it as much as possible.

But if the tumour enlarges above Poupart's ligament, involves the skin, and becomes soft, with a sense of fluctuation, it must be opened freely in this situation : and it will save the patient some suffering if we make an incision reasonably early. Sometimes a large amount of matter is discharged with great relief, sometimes only a small quantity, but the discharge will continue so long as suppuration goes on. When it ceases, the poultices may be omitted, and some dressing substituted if the wound remains open.

When once the abscess is opened, we may allow the patient a more generous diet, with wine, &c., and in many cases bark may be given with benefit.

But if the tumour shows a disposition to resolve itself, it will be advisable by degrees to leave off the poultices, and substitute cotton wool or flannel. In some cases, this process is hastened by a small blister applied occasionally, or by painting the part with strong tincture of iodine, and I have seen great benefit and improvement result from warm hip-baths twice or thrice a week.

Such, Mr. President, is the imperfect sketch I have ventured to lay before you. No one can be more sensible than I, that it needs an apology, and I trust it will be found in the fact, that it has been written in the midst of great anxiety and hurry, without time to refer to books, and from an earnest desire to show my willingness to co-operate with you in your noble efforts to advance the science of medicine and surgery.

[*Dublin Med. Press.*

On Epithelial Cancer. By G. MURRAY HUMPHRY, Esq., Surgeon to Addenbrooke's Hospital.

[We extract the subjoined remarks from a Course of Lectures delivered in the Medical School of Cambridge, and to which we have before been indebted for contributions. The author divides cancer into four varieties :—1. Epithelial cancer. 2. Schirrous and encephaloid. 3. Melanic cancer. 4. Alveolar or gelatiniform cancer. The first only is here spoken of.]

The epithelial cancer affects usually the skin or a mucous surface in the first instance. It differs from the other forms of cancer in being composed almost entirely of cells more or less flattened out, and closely resembling those of ordinary epithelium ; it does not present the malignant qualities in so marked a degree ; it is more tardy in its progress, sometimes remaining for months or years in a quiescent state, or growing very slowly ; it generally appears at some part of the skin or mucous membrane which has been exposed to a long-continued irritation, and its ravages are confined to the vicinity of that spot and to the adjacent absorbent glands ; that is to say, it does not often make its appearance in any other organ, being, in a greater measure than the other forms of cancer, a local affection, less associated with any particular diathesis, and much less likely to return after extirpation.

For these reasons some pathologists are inclined to exclude the epithelial species from the family of cancer ; mistaking, as it appears to me, differences in degree for differences in kind, inasmuch as the epithelial disease does really present all the leading features of cancer, though it may do so in a less decided and less active manner than the other members of the class. It is attended with the destruction of the original tissues whenever it occurs ; it possesses the quality of spreading from point to point, assimilating the adjacent tissues of every kind and in every direction, and reducing them all to one homogeneous structure ; it affects the neighboring absorbent glands, converting them also into a substance like the parent mass ; and it is prone to decay and ulceration ; moreover, it is unceasingly destructive ; it yields to no treatment, and pursues its relentless course till death puts a stop to its ravages.

Watch the progress of the disease when it affects the lip, by far its most frequent seat. It usually begins on the edge of the lower lip, a little to one side of the middle line, probably at the spot where the pipe is habitually rested. I have seen it in the middle of the lip, originating in one of those cracks which are often so troublesome in that situation, and in two or three cases have met with it in the upper lip ; in one of the latter it originated in the cicatrix of a wound inflicted several years previously. A slight thickening or wart-like elevation of the skin is generally the first symptom ; the cuticle is also thickened at the part, and, in course of time, becomes rubbed or scratched off, leaving the surface a little abraded or cracked, or superficially ulcerated. Upon this a succession of scabs are formed and detached, while an increasing lump is produced underneath them, and the ulceration proceeds deeper ; so that in the course of time a considerable ulcer is engendered with an indurated basis. an excavated, or deeply fissured, or warty surface covered with white dirty secretion, or perhaps with pale firm granulations, and having a sinuous, raised, everted margin. The discharge from these ulcers is thin and pale, like serum ; occasionally it is mixed with blood. They are not painful or tender, and the patients often think little of them. However they gradually increase, extending along the margin of the lip and towards the chin, the thickening and induration preceding, the ulceration following, till the whole lip and part of the cheek may be involved in the disease. Before such extensive ravages have been effected, the absorbent glands under the jaw are generally found to be enlarged and hard, the skin over them becomes adherent and inflamed, and ultimately giving way, an ulcer is formed which extends deeply, presents the usual can-cerous aspect, and leads to the like fatal termination. If a sec-tion be made through the ulcer in the lip, even in an early stage, its indurated basis is found to consist of a compact, opaque white, pearly substance, of uniform appearance, or speckled, it may be, with small yellowish spots, which are softer than the rest of the mass, and which are generally situated in greatest numbers near the ulcerated surface. In this substance all the natural tissues of the lip are blended and lost. Not only are the skin, the mucous membrane, and the labial glands transformed, or assimilated by the new structure, but the muscular fibres of the orbicularis as well as the areolar and fibrous tissues are traceable into the mass and are lost in it. When examined under the microscope, the new substance is found to be com-posed almost entirely of flattened cells, like those of epithelium, compressed together, and arranged in laminæ superimposed upon one another. Some of those which are newly formed or which are swollen by the imbibition of moisture, are round, oval, or fusiform, and present nearly the characters of the ordinary cancer cell. It is an interesting fact, first announced, I believe, by Mr. Paget, that the microscopical characters of the diseased absorbent glands correspond with those of the primary disease in the skin ; the glands, like the tissues of the lip, being conver-ted into masses of flattened and closely compressed scales, in-termixed with cells in various stages of transformation. This fact, taken in conjunction with the acknowledged success that attends the removal of epithelial cancer of the skin, makes us somewhat bold to extend our incisions for the purpose of ex-tirpating also the morbidly affected glands.

The disease is most commonly seen in elderly men, though middle aged and younger men are sometimes affected by it. The patient's health generally appears to be good till it be-comes impaired by the distress, discharge, and inability to masticate, occasioned by the extensive destruction of parts about the mouth. A complete and permanent cure in most instances follows the entire removal of the mass by the knife, which should be done at an early period ; before the absorbent glands are involved, if possible, because they are sure to enlarge and lead to the results just described when they have begun to participate in the disease. Occasionally we find this to be the case after the operation, although there was at the time no evidence of their being in a morbid condition. In three or four cases, after the removal of the mass from the lip, and when the cicatrix remained perfectly sound, I have known the disease spring up in the periosteum, make its way through the jaw, and destroy the patient. Even the complete excision of the portion of the jaw thus involved does not always save the patient.

In the cancer of the penis and of the scrotum the progress of the disease is very much the same as in the lip ; the ulcer originated in a pimple, a wart, or a little thickening of the skin, has the same foul or coarsely granulating surface, everted edge, and indurated base, goes on increasing with equal or even greater virulence, involves the inguinal glands, and destroys the patient in a shorter space of time than the corresponding affection of the lip. I have seen the disease at the anus, on the anus, on the extremities, the trunk, the face, and head, and believe it may attack the integuments at any part of the body. It presents very much the same characters, and runs the same course in whatever situation it occurs ; exhibiting the qualities of malignancy in a sufficiently marked manner, quite as strongly, indeed, as we could expect, considering that it is very generally the result of some local irritation.

Nevertheless, it must be admitted, and this is one of the most interesting features in their pathology, that these cutaneous growths vary a good deal in their malignancy;—so much as to constitute, it would seem, a very instructive link between simple hypertrophy and genuine cancer—between an ordinary wart and well-marked scirrhus, proving that these diseases must be studied in their relation to one another no less than in their points of difference, if we would attain a correct idea of their real nature. There is good reason to think that the neglect of this mode of considering the subject, together with the too great stress which is usually laid upon the distinctive features of cancer, has been the source of many narrow views, if not of much misconception, upon this very important class of disease. Any information upon this subject which the cutaneous growths may afford, is peculiarly valuable, because they are directly under our observation ; and if there be any rela-

tion between simple and malignant disease, we may expect to
find some evidence of it in them.

Now, there are numerous instances of warts occurring upon
the skin in elderly persons, respecting which we have a difficulty in deciding whether they be cancerous or not, and which
we are in the habit of extirpating, because we know that if they
are allowed to remain they will go on increasing, will in the
long run ulcerate, affect the adjacent glands, and terminate fatally.   For example, a healthy man, æt. 63, was in John's ward,
a year ago, with a broad, flat, warty growth on the right temple; it overhung the surrounding integuments, which was
purplish and a little pimply.   The surface of the growth was
covered by a soft, white secretion, and when this was washed
away it was seen to be granular and warty, with superficial
ulceration at places.   There was no induration about its base,
and no enlargement of the adjacent absorbent glands.   It had
commenced a year and a half previously.   About the nose was
several small pimply or warty elevations of the cutis, which
he said had existed for a longer time than that on the temple,
though the latter at its commencement resembled one of them.
I removed the growth, completely dissecting it away from the
temporal fascia, to which it was loosely connected by cellular
tissue.   After the wound had healed, there was a return of the
disease at one spot in the edge of the cicatrix, requiring a second
operation, which left him quite well.   A short time ago the
part was sound, and the warts on the nose remained unaltered.
A section of the mass showed it to be composed of pale, blunt,
thick fibres, parallel to one another, and at right angles to the
surface of the body, doubtless enlarged and elongated papillæ;
together with epithelial sheaths of papillæ.   This appearance
is often seen in cases of the like kind, and is probably the result
of a change analogous to that which causes the thickened striated condition of the intestinal muscular coat accompanying
cancer of the bowel.   The association of an actively increasing
warty growth with a number of others of similar appearance
which remain in a quiescent state is very common.   I remember a chimney-sweep, the subject of cancerous ulcer of the
scrotum, whose skin was covered in many parts of the body
with little warty elevations, attributed by him to the same
cause as the more malignant disease in the scrotum, viz., the
irritation of the soot.   They were in a quiescent state, and
hardly attracted attention.

[The author here narrates two cases of warty growths, both
of which ultimately caused death.   He then proceeds as follows:]

These warty growths, which exhibit the stubbornness, and

are apt to assume the destructiveness of malignant disease, are almost always met with in elderly persons. It is the best plan to extirpate them at once, where that can be done, and not to waste time in the anticipation of caustic and other remedies, which are more likely to excite than to repress the growth, and which often hasten the enlargement of the absorbent glands. I remember regretting that I had treated with nitrate of silver a warty growth of this kind on the labium, in a woman, æt. 60; for though the growth was without induration, presenting the appearance of a simple affection, and was diminished in size for a time, yet it subsequently advanced more rapidly, the inguinal glands participated in the disease, ulceration took place, and proceeded as in ordinary cancer, and the patient died.

Perhaps it may be stated, as a general rule in these and in other affections of a similar kind, that the degree in which the natural structure of the part is altered, will be found to be proportionate to the malignancy of the disease. Thus, where the change consists simply in an outgrowth of the papillæ, with a thickening of their epithelial coats, after the manner of the wart, there the mass is slow in its increase, slow to extend to the stratum of tissue under the skin, slow to ulcerate, slow to make any impression upon the absorbent glands, and may be removed with great prospect of a complete cure. Secondly, where the warty disposition is less manifest, the alteration of structure being attended rather with a destruction of the papillæ than their hypertrophy, and with the substitution of flattened cells, like those of epithelium, for the natural tissue of the cutis ; there the malignant qualities are more evidently displayed, the mass increases more quickly, extending beneath the skin, involving the subcutaneous areolar tissue, muscular fibres, and even the bones; it ulcerates at an earlier period, the absorbent glands are more quickly affected, and we are not quite so free from apprehension of a return after removal. Still the disease is generally local, unattended with any constitutional indisposition, and is not likely to appear in distant parts. In the third class of cases, which comprises the scirrhous or encephaloid cancer of the skin, the morbid elements have still less relation to those naturally existing, the tissues are replaced, not by epithelial, but by cancer cells, or nuclei—that is to say, the new products do not exhibit a tendency to liken themselves to any one of the components of the skin, but assume the form, and are endowed with the endogenous productive qualities of cancer-cells ; they breed others in their interior, instead of being themselves transformed into any kind of tissue. In these cases the disease commences, not with a wart, but with a tubercle, spreads quickly in all directions, ulcerates, attacks the absorbent glands, and is commonly associated, either as a primary or secondary affection, with cancer of some other organ ; its removal, therefore, is attended with comparatively little hope of a permanent cure.

The warty growths described by Mr. Cæsar Hawkins and others as cicatrices, more particularly in the cicatrices of burns, partake, I suppose, in a greater or less degree, of the nature of epithelial cancer, being, for the most part, intractable by ordinary means, and requiring extirpation for their cure. I have not happened to meet with any cases of this kind.

Epithelial cancer attacks mucous surfaces, no less than the skin ; sometimes commencing under the tongue, about the orifices of the salivary ducts, in the form of an indurated elevation of the membrane ; it extends upon the jaw, and the under surface of the tongue, as in the case of the woman from whom I lately removed the mental portion of the jaw, the anterior and under surface of the tongue, and the parts intervening between the two. The patient recovered, and has not at present (six months after the operation) suffered any relapse. In another woman the disease, commencing at the same spot, had involved the submental and submaxillary absorbent glands to too great an extent to admit of extirpation, and proved fatal within two years from its commencement. More commonly it attacks the tongue, beginning on one side, opposite the molar teeth, with a little thickening and induration of the part ; the papillæ being sometimes prominent, so as to give a warty appearance, ulceration soon follows, and extends into the substance of the organ. The pain or inconvenience attendant on the early stage of the disease not being great, we frequently do not see the patient till an excavated ulcer of considerable size has been formed, with a raised indurated base which extends probably to the side of the fauces, and involves the mucous membrane between the tongue and the jaw. The ulcer has a foul, grayish surface ; and the induration is caused, as in other cases of the like kind, by the infiltration of a new product in the structure of the organ, and its substitution for the natural tissue. Examined microscopically, this new product is found to consist of epithelial cells, compressed and matted together, perhaps concentrically arranged, or elongated, and showing some tendency to split into fibres. In the further progress of the disease the palate and lower jaw, and submaxillary glands become involved, the movements of the tongue and jaw are impeded, deglutition is difficult, the flow of saliva increased, the breath fetid, and the patient's condition is altogether very miserable during the short period of life which remains.

On the whole, there can be no doubt that, although it often

is excited by a local source of irritation, such as a decayed tooth or stump, the epithelial cancer of the mucous membrane of the tongue and mouth, is far more actively malignant in its progress than when it affects the skin.   Indeed, I think it exhibits in this situation as rapid and as determined destructiveness, with, perhaps, as great disposition to return after extirpation, as do the scirrhous and encephaloid cancers in other parts of the body ; though it is not so likely to affect distant organs.   Our hopes, therefore, of ultimate success from operative interference, are far less than in the treatment of the corresponding affection of the skin.   Nevertheless, we may give the patient the benefit of the chance, when there is a fair probability of our being able to remove the entire mass.—[*Provincial Med. and Surg. Journal.*

On Hysterical Affections of the Hip-joint.   By Mr. Coulson.

Mr. Coulson gives the following diagnostic signs of nervous, as contradistinguished from organic, disease of the hip-joint :—

In the nervous affection pain is felt from the commencement in the hip, and extends to the loins and down the thigh.   There is great nervous excitability and extreme sensitiveness in the part ; and the patient, from the first, is unable to walk.   Combined with this extreme suffering, the trochanter major retains its proper bearing to the spine of the ilium.   There is not the characteristic wasting of the glutæi muscles, and, consequently, no flattened appearance of the nates.   Pressure in these situations, when the bone approaches the surface, does not excite greater pain than elsewhere.   There are no involuntary startings during sleep.   On the contrary, the patient sleeps calmly through the night.   In true hip disease the reverse is the case, the sleep, if unaided by opium, is broken by sudden shooting pains and frightful dreams, or vague anticipations of coming pain.

Of the pathology of the disease Mr. Coulson admits that little is known.   The joint is healthy in structure.   He asks whether the spine is not in a morbidly excited state, and responds truly, or whether the brain is not itself perverted as to its functions, and the pain is not a delusion ?   His own opinion inclines the other way, and he looks to the sensorium as the organ chiefly affected.

With regard to the treatment, he remarks, that if it be mistaken for organic disease, the line of practice adopted on that supposition will be positively injurious.   The patient must be persuaded to leave her couch, and to take air.   The diet must

be plain and nutritious.   Among medicines, he prefers the vegetable tonics and antispasmodics—as valerian.   Copland has
found most benefit from turpentine internally by enema, but he
also associates various tonics and local sedatives.—[*London
Journal of Medicine.*

On the Position of the Limb in Diseases of the Hip-joint.   By
Holmes Coote, Esq., M. R. C. S.

Mr. Holmes Coote makes the following observations on the
difficulties attending the diagnosis of this affection :—There are
but few surgeons who have not experienced occasional difficulty
in forming an accurate opinion as to the character of the morbid changes which occur during life in chronic disease of the
hip-joint.   In the early stages there is frequently but little pain,
and children so affected, especially amongst the poorer classes,
are permitted to walk about and pursue their daily avocations,
without notice being taken of their lameness, until at last a fall
or some other accident excites more acute symptoms, and induces the parent to seek professional assistance.   The surgeon
finds the pelvis oblique ; the affected limb apparently elongated,
and slightly everted; he finds that in bending the thigh upon the
trunk, the whole pelvis moves with the femur ; pressure over the
hip-joint excites, perhaps, little pain ; there is flattening of the
buttock, and the trochanter major appears more sunken that
natural.   The history accompanying such a case is often as
follows :—The child was in perfect health, and able to run
about until about a week or two ago, when, in consequence of an
accident, it was thrown down upon the side.   Upon being taken
up, it was found to be lame and has been unable to walk ever
since.   The history of the case, and the position of the limb,
might lead to the belief that the head of the bone was dislocated
upon the thyroid foramen, especially amongst those who consider that inversion and not eversion of the foot, is the position
assumed by the inferior extremity in the earlier stages of hip-
disease.   I propose offering a few remarks upon the position of
the limb, granting that, as is commonly asserted, there may be
inversion and not eversion ; that there may exist a resemblance
to dislocation on the dorsum ilii, or to dislocation on the thyroid
foramen ; but denying that such varieties can ever be referred
to accident.
In the commencement of an inflammatory affection of the
hip-joint, the thigh is bent upon the body ; the whole limb is·
slightly everted and abducted ; the anterior superior spinous
process of the ilium of the affected side is either raised, when

the limb appears to be shortened, and the sound hip more sunken than the opposite, or it is depressed or thrown forwards, when the whole limb appears elongated, the knee being bent, and the toes touching the ground a short distance in front of the toes of the sound limb.

The elevation or the depression of the anterior superior spinous process of the ilium of the affected side depends upon whether the patient happens to have been forced to follow his occupation during the early stages of the disease, or whether he has been in circumstances which allowed him to rest when in pain or uneasiness. The spine of the ilium is generally sunk and thrown forwards, and the limb apparently elongated; that position being the one in which the diseased joint will be easiest, the patient standing upright. But if he be forced to walk about, the pelvis becomes oblique in the opposite direction, the spine of the ilium is raised, and the limb is apparently shortened. The patient, throwing as much as possible of the weight of the body upon the sound side, limps upon the extremities of the toes of the affected limb, the foot being extended that its tip may just touch the ground.

The flexion, eversion, and abduction of the limb constitute the position into which it would be naturally thrown by the combined action of the powerful muscles which surround the hip-joint. The synovial membrane is inflamed and tender, and unfit to bear pressure; the patient, therefore, instinctively endeavors to relax every muscle directly in contact with the joint. The psoas and iliacum, passing over the front of the synovial membrane and tightly pressing upon it where the limb is extended, flex and evert the thigh, the gluteus minimus will contribute to flex it; the pyriformis will abduct the limb; the gemelli and the two obturators, especially the obturator externus, will evert the limb; it is unscientific to refer the position of the limb to effusion of fluid into the synovial membrane; it is but rarely that we find the joint so distended, especially at the commencement of the disease, when eversion is the common symptom. It may be true, that if the joint be tightly distended by the artificial injection of fluid after death, the limb will assume the position above described. The attachments of the capsular ligament are in harmony with the sphere of action of the muscles which surround the joint. That the muscles which evert the limb may act with greater freedom, the fibrous capsule is unconnected with the posterior part of the neck of the femur; it forms there a ring not very unlike that which surrounds the head of the radius in the forearm. After a sudden fall, or a blow on the hip, the limb becomes at once everted, if the joint is bruised, long before sufficient time has passed for the capsule to become distended by fluid.

In course of time, as has been proved by innumerable *post-mortem* examinations, the disease produces thickening of the synovial membrane, absorption of the articular cartilage, and ulceration both of the head of the femur and of the acetabulum; the shortened neck of the femur slipping upwards and backwards in the enlarged acetabulum, approximates the fixed points of insertion of all those muscles which have everted the limb. They waste and become atrophied, being no longer in action, and the buttock appears much flatter than on the sound side. The gluteus medius and the adductor muscles then influence the position of the limb, their power being increased by the absorption of the neck of the femur. We may therefore say that, in the second stage of the disease, the limb passes from abduction to adduction; from eversion to inversion. Still flexed it is drawn across the sound thigh, the toe pointing downwards, when the position somewhat resembles that of a limb in dislocation upon the dorsum ilii.—[*Medical Times.*

On the Presence of Sugar in Pus. By George D. Gibb, M. D., L. R. C. S. I., Lecturer on the Institutes of Medicine, St. Lawrence School of Medicine of Montreal. Physician to the Montreal Dispensary.

In January, 1850, I opened a large abscess situated on the back below the right scapula, in a female aged 23, the subject of general external scrofula. The fluid withdrawn, was of a yellowish colour, spec : gr : 1028 ; inodorous, neutral, and of a creamy consistence. In the course of a chemical examination, I applied the different reagents for testing the presence of *sugar ;* when, to my surprise, I found that Moore's test, and Trommer's tests gave positive proof of the presence of a considerable quantity of that substance. Microscopical observation showed the usual characters of tuberculous matter, in the presence of cells filled with granular matter, free granules and fat globules, together with pus and lymph corpuscles. In February, this large abscess having become again filled, was opened, and exit given to a thick cream-like fluid of a dark drab colour. On examination for sugar, the results were again positive, and the microscope showed a larger number of pus corpuscles.

These experiments were not sufficient in themselves to prove that pus necessarily contained sugar ; and to test the subject further, other kinds of pus were examined with the following results :—

Pus from *Chronic fistula* in left breast of a female in which

Cyanuret of iron was found.   (This case was published in the
6th volume of the *British American Medical and Physical
Journal.*)   Moore's and Trommer's tests, quite satisfactory.
Pus from sac of an abscess over the *right malar bone* in a girl,
very fœtid : all the tests satisfactory.

Crude and softened Tubercles from left lung of a Phthisical
patient, aged 40.   Tests satisfactory, but sugar not large in
quantity.

Fatty liver, same case, that variety described by Louis ; su- .
gar found in *large* quantity by the usual tests.

Pus from a *Bubo.*   Tests satisfactory.

Large Mammary Abscess.   Healthy laudible pus, sugar in
small quantity, by Moore's and Trommer's tests.

These results conclusively prove, that sugar is one of the
normal constituents (so to speak) of pus, and it is to its presence
that the sweetish taste is due.

Dr. Mason Good, in the second volume of his Study of Medicine, in describing pus, says "It has a sweetish, mawkish taste
(apparently from its containing sugar,) very different from that
of most other secretions."

He appears to have been the first author who has supposed
its presence in this fluid.   Its presence may possibly be due to
the albumen found in pus, which, according to Dr. Wright, *
contains 58 to 83 per cent.   It has been shown elsewhere, that
sugar exists largely in the serum of the blood, † which contains
albumen principally, and also in the albumen of eggs. ‡   Pus
also contains fatty matters which may likewise account for its
presence.   In fact, the presence of either fat or albumen, both
being proximate principles, is a sufficient proof of its elaboration
from the body.

That fat may have some influence in the transformation, is
supported by the evidence afforded in the amount of sugar contained in the fatty liver examined, which was very large.   And
in some experiments performed on the livers of Birds, (which
will be described in a future number of this Journal) the amount
of sugar was found to be large in those containing much fat, as,
for example, in the liver of the goose.—[*Canada Med. Jour.*

---

*Cases of Delirium Tremens successfully treated by the admin-
istration of Chloroform.*   By STEPHEN H. PRATT, M. D.,
of Baltimore.

CASE I.   May 7th, 1850, I called to see E. B., laboring under
delirium tremens.

---

* Ranking's Abstract ; vol. 1, 1845.   † Bernard in *Archives Générales,* 1848.
‡ Gazette Medicale, 1849.

E. B. had, that day, been taken from the ——— Infirmary,. where he had been for the last seven days under judicious treatment for the above named disease. During the time (seven days) he had not slept any, as I had been, that morning, informed by the resident physician ; and his case was deemed almost hopeless. His friends became alarmed, and (very injudiciously,. I thought) removed him, and placed him under my care.

It was 1 o'clock, P. M.. when I saw him. He was very feeble, and much exhausted by disease and protracted wakefulness: His pulse was feeble and frequent. There was subsultus, muttering, great incoherence, with cold and clammy extremities.

Having been advised that he had been on a mixed opiate and stimulant treatment, at least a part of the time, and having had some success previously in the use of chloroform, I determined to use it now. Accordingly one drachm of chloroform, diluted with water, was exhibited. At 5 o'clock, P. M., another drachm was administered ; and at 9 still another, diluted as before. At 10' he fell asleep and slept till morning. At 8, in the morning, he waked and drank some gruel, after which he soon fell asleep and slept till noon.

He now waked with a good appetite, which he too freely indulged by partaking of soup. However, he was quite comfortable during the afternoon, and slept well through the night. Next morning he vomited two or three times freely. The emesis was not violent, and was easily controlled. From this time, paying strict attention to his diet, he rapidly convalesced.

During this sickness no medicine was exhibited but chloroform (not even aperients), and this but three times. On the fifth day, the patient left the house to attend to his affairs, and was soon in health.

CASE II. Was called to see J. H., June 4th, 1851, laboring under delirium tremens. Put him upon a mixed opiate and stimulant treatment through the day, and exhibited opium in full doses through the night. This was continued two days and nights, without benefit. Indeed the patient grew worse. The third morning I put him upon : R. Spts. sulph. ætheris. comp., tinct. valerianæ, ana ℥iss. ; to take ℥ii. every two or three hours, intermediately giving tinct. opil. At 8 P. M., gave a large opiate. At 10 P. M., gave tinct. opii. ℥j. At 12, repeated the dose ; and at 2, again repeated it. All this time the patient grew worse, and became " furiously delirious," frightening all the household.

Three men were appointed to prevent him from jumping out of the windows (several attemps at which he had made), or otherwise injuring himself. At times he was a match for them all. At length he grew weak, becoming more and more prostrated by his great exertions. The family became alarmed, and wished further advice. A consulting physician was called in. A hot stimulating pediluvium and an opio tartar emetic treatment was agreed upon.

I suggested chloroform internally, which was not wholly objected to, though not preferred by the consulting physician. Accordingly the former was tried, but unfortunately without success, the patient rapidly growing worse.

He was now beyond control, a raving maniac, a terror to all present. His pulse was feeble and frequent; so frequent it could not be counted with the existing tremor. His tongue was dry; there was also muttering, subsultus, and perfect incoherence, with cold and clammy extremities.

Under these circumstances, I determined to exhibit chloroform as a dernier resort. A tea-spoonful nearly, diluted with water, was administered. After one hour, the following was given: ℞. Spts. sulph. ætheris comp: tinct. valeriana, aa f ℨ ii., chloroform f ℨ i., at a draught.

(The compound spirit of sulphuric ether and tinct. valerian were added in order to obviate, if possible, the danger of fatal prostration.) Fifteen minutes after its exhibition, the patient fell asleep, and slept soundly three and a half hours. Meantime, perspiration ceased; his extremities became *warm;* his pulse grew *calmer, fuller* and *firmer.* He then awoke much refreshed and quite rational, and had a free, natural dejection.

Three tea-spoonsful of the mixture, ℞. Hoff.'s anodyn. and tinct. valeriana, with half a tea-spoonful of chloroform, were then exhibited. After this, he washed his hands and face, and bathed himself generally. In one hour, I exhibited f ℨ iv. of the mixture, with f ℨ i. of chloroform, and persuaded him to lie down. In a few minutes he was asleep, and slept comparatively soundly four hours, when he arose, went down stairs, and evacuated his bowels. In fifteen minutes he was again asleep, and slept three hours, when he walked and drank a tumbler of milk, took a dose of spts. sulph. ætheris comp. and tinct. valeriana; fifteen minutes afterwards he was asleep again, and continued sleeping through the night, rising, meantime, but once.

In the morning he rose, drank some milk and beef tea, and after evacuating his bowels again went to sleep. His pulse was now good; extremities warm, glowing; subsultus greatly diminished; delirium almost entirely wanting. He slept till about noon, and then waked still more tranquil. During the afternoon, he slept and waked alternately, and rested well the following night. His sleep was not comatose. When awake, he was wide awake, cheerful and lively. A day or two passed thus as he rapidly convalesced.   On the 9th, he was walking about the city a comparatively well man.   He has continued well since.

Such are the facts.   From a furious delirium, with subsultus, perfect incoherence, cold, clammy extremities, a feeble, fluttering, frequent pulse, costiveness, &c., by the tranquilizing and peculiar (shall I say specific ?) influence of chloroform, he was *rescued*, in a little more than an hour, and thrown into a condition the most favorable possible ; from which in a few days, he was restored to his usual health.   No emesis, or irritation of the bowels, occurred.   No cathartics were exhibited, yet gentle motions followed the administration of chloroform.

The methodus medendi of this wonderful agent, I will not here attempt to explain.   Facts are of more importance than inferences, and if, by this contribution, I add one to the *facts* already recorded, I shall be satisfied.—[*Amer. Jour. of Med. Science.*

The Skin as a Diagnostic of the General Health.   By Mr. Hunt.

The author commenced by observing that the subject naturally divided itself into two parts, viz:—1. The indications presented by the healthy skin. 2. Those presented by the skin in a state of disease.

Having alluded cursorily to the former, by pointing out some of the indications presented by changes in the condition of the skin as to smoothness or roughness, moisture or dryness, temperature and color.   Mr. Hunt proceeded to discuss the constitutional indications presented by the diseased skin, confining his remarks to a single topic, viz: the rapidity or slowness of development, which characterized respectively the various orders of cutaneous diseases, as arranged by Dr. Willan.   To explain this point more fully and forcibly, he placed the first seven orders of Willan in a new rotation, selecting two diseases as types of each order, by way of illustrating the subject, as follows :—

Orders.	*Types.*
1. Exanthemata	Urticaria. Erythema.
2. Bullæ	Erysipelas. Pompholyx.
3. Vesiculæ	Eczema. Herpes.
4. Pustulæ	Ecthyma. Impetigo.

5. Papulæ	{ Lichen. { Prurigo.
6. Squammæ	{ Lepra. { Pityriasis.
7. Tubercula	{ Acne. { Lupus.

The first three of these orders, viz: *Exanthemata, Bullæ,* and *Vesiculæ,* were described as comprising for the most part diseases of rapid evolution or development: the last three, viz: *Papulæ, Sqammæ,* and *Tuberculæ,* as containing diseases of slow development; the order *Pustulæ* taking an intermedite position in this respect. On this basis the author proposed to establish a theory, for the support of which he produced many curious facts relating to the artificial production of the various forms of skin disease, as well as facts connected with the development of spontaneous eruptions.

The theory consisted in regarding eruptions as defensive efforts of nature, tending either to prevent the absorption of poisons, or to eliminate them when absorbed ; those poisons or injurious agents which are most actively mischievous, being most rapidly eliminated or repelled : exciting the blush, (*Exanthema,*) the blister, (*Bulla,*) or the vesicle, (*Vesicula ;*) those which are less rapidly destructive, exerting a slow and feeble effort at elimination, as observable in the pimple, (*Papula*) the scales, (*Squamma,*) or the tubercle (*Tuberculum ;*) while those poisons which are of intermediate intensity of action originate the pustular form of eruption.

Taking seven diseases as so many types of these orders respectively, the author observed that their average duration when unchecked by treatment was strikingly illustrative of the truth of this theory of development. Thus—

Urticaria continues usually a few hours only.
Erysipelas - - - a few days.
Herpes - - - twice as long.
Ecthyma - - - a few weeks.
Lichen - - - as many months.
Lepra - - - as many years.
Lupus - - - for the whole life.

Each eruption showing the relative degree of intolerance of the poison manifested by the system, and thus becoming a signal of danger. Mr. Hunt contended that if this theory prove to be true, it might throw some light on the *prognosis,* the *pathology,* and the *therapeutics* of cutaneous disease ; assisting the prognosis by determining how long the disease might be expected to last ; the pathology, by pointing out the sudden cause of the disease, and its relative activity or destructive power ; the therapeutics, by sugesting long perseverance in one judicious plan of treatment in the diseases at the bottom of the list, and by indicating some error of treatment when the cure of those at the opposite end of the chain does not proceed at a rate corresponding with their natural rapidity of development.

These positions were illustrated by allusions to the action of external agents in the production of various eruptions, as well as to internal sources of cutaneous disease ; and among other important facts it was stated that, while the diseases included in the first four or five orders were producible by external agents, with a readiness diminishing from above downwards, it was impossible to establish the eruptions at the bottom of the list, (Lupus, Acne, Lepra, Psoriasis, &c.,) by any external application whatever.—[*London Medical Gazette.*

Application of the Nitrate of Silver to the Pharynx and Larynx in Hooping Cough. By Dr. E. WATSON.

I think that one great cause of the want of success hitherto experienced in the treatment of hooping-cough, has resulted from the prevalence of unsound ideas regarding its seat.   It is very generally treated with emetics and expectorants, with embrocations over the chest, or perhaps with leeches, as if it were some inflammatory *pectoral* affection.   No wonder that with such treatment the disease generally runs its course, and either wears out itself or the patient.

I think a much more correct theory of the disease is, that it is the product of a poison which exerts its first influence on the mucous lining of the pharynx and larynx, and on the sentient nerves—viz : branches of the superior laryngeal supplying these parts ; that in the next place the inferior laryngeal becomes excited, and partial spasm of the glottis follows.   It is a peculiarity of the action of this morbid poison, as of most morbid poisons acting on the nerves, that the symptoms caused by its presence are of a periodic or intermittent character. Hence it is that the disease commences with a periodic cough, differing in many respects from that which accompanies bronchitis ; hence arise the pains of the neck generally complained of by the patients, and hence, finally, the hoop, or back-draught, when the tendency to frequent spasms of the glottis has supervened.   In like manner the vomiting which generally accompanies the fits of hooping-cough, is caused by an extension of the morbid excitation to the branches of the pneumogastric nerve supplying the stomach.

Such are the symptoms which, in my opinion, are alone essential to a case of hooping-cough, and which of themselves constitute the disease. But whether this disease be or be not complicated with other affections, it ought to be treated *per se*, and not, as is too often the case, as if it were bronchitis or pneumonia, or some affection of the head or even of the stomach.

Entertaining these views, and being aware of the powerful influence of topical applications of solution of nitrate of silver, in allaying nervous irritability of the glottis, it occurred to me, about eighteen months ago, when hooping-cough was more than usually prevalent in this city and its neighborhood, to employ that remedy in the disease just named.   I therefore gave up all the usual treatment in the cases which I was attending at the time, and contented myself with confining my patients as much as possible to one apartment, well aired and properly heated, attending to the functions of the alimentery canal, and .touching the pharynx and larynx every second day with solution of caustic. Pursuing this treatment, I met with very considerable and unwonted success. My first cases, which occurred in summer, ceased to hoop in about ten days or a fortnight after the solution had begun to be applied; and of late, in our worst winter weather, I have treated several cases to a favorable *termination* in from two to six weeks.

In November last, I read to the Glasgow Medical Society a paper, detailing the results of this treatment, which induced several gentlemen to use the remedy proposed.   Most of them report favorably of their success, and I earnestly hope that a more general trial will soon be given to it, and that its true therapeutic value will be speedily recognized.—[*Lon. Lancet.*

Profuse Salivation and Sloughing, caused by three small doses of Mercury. By ROBERT HARPER, M. R. C. S., L. S. A., London.

W. W——, aged eleven years, a delicate boy, was attacked in the early part of last month (November,) with fever, and for which he was treated in the usual manner, namely, salines, antimonials, &c., followed by wine and other support, and under which he greatly improved.   The bowels, however, being in a torpid state, mild aperients, with mercury and chalk, were administered, when required.   Altogether only three doses of this mercurial were given, one of six grains on the 14th, a similar dose on the 17th, and four grains on the 20th; but most .profuse salivation followed, the salivary glands and features becoming swollen to an enormous size, the saliva flowing constantly away, and the breath having the fœtid mercurial odour. Port wine, arrowroot, good beef-tea, in fact all the support that could be got down, was given, and lotions employed to the mouth; but nothing would stop its fearful ravages: sloughing commenced in both checks, and rapidly extended through them; that on the right cheek was not larger that a shilling, but on the left side it extended from one-third across the lips backwards to the edge of the great masseter muscle, and from the malar bone to the lower edge of the inferior maxilla; it presented a frightful appearance, the whole of the teeth on that side 'being exposed. Everything that could suggest itself was done for the poor boy, but all was of no avail, and he died four days after the commencement of the sloughing.—[*London Lancet.*

Yeast Mixture in Petechial Typhus.

Dr. Jones (in Dublin Quarterly Jour. of Med.) speaks very highly of the stimulating and antiseptic properties of the following mixture in cases of typhus attended with petechiæ and other forms of passive hemorrhages:

R. Cerevisiæ fermenti, ℥x;
    Camphoræ, ℈ss;
    Ætheris nitrici, ℨiv.   ℥j to be taken every first, second or third hour. This removes the dark livid hue of the skin within a few hours; administered in cases of dysentery, attended with great fetor of the dejecta, it has speedily removed all odour, and at the same time rather counteracted the frequency of the discharges from the bowels.—[*Northern Lancet.*

Use of Diluted Pyroligneous Acid as a Gargle. By JOHN EVANS, M. D., Prof. of Obstetrics, &c. in Rush Medical College.

I have for several years been using diluted Pyroligneous Acid as a gargle in case of inflammation of the fauces and tonsils with better success than any other article that I have prescribed.

I put a teaspoonful of the Acid obtained from the shops into a wine glass of water and direct the patient to gargle the throat frequently with it.

In the sore throat caused by exposure, so common throughout the country, it generally relieves the soreness and stiffness felt in swallowing very promptly.

In chronic inflammation, with or without ulceration, of the throat, I have found it a very valuable remedy.

In the sore throat of Scarlatina it has generally afforded a very prompt amelioration of this symptom of the disease.

In several cases of habitual tonsilitis, by using this gargle

freely at the commencement of the disease, I have been able
to arrest the progress of the inflammation and secure a resolution.

Its use is not unpleasant; it is safe, even if used for hours
continuously, and has an additional advantage in removing the
fœtor of the breath.—[*North-Western Med. and Sur. Journal.*

Cannabis Indica as a substitute for Ergot.

Dr. Christison, of Edinburgh, considers Indian hemp (Cannabis Indica) to possess a remarkable power of increasing the
force of uterine contraction during labor. He reports, in the
August number of the *Edinburgh Journal of Medical Science*,
some cases in which it was given, with this view, at the Ma-
ternity Hospital of Edinburgh. As compared with the action
of ergot, that of Indian hemp presents the following points of
difference : First—While the effect of ergot does not come on
for some considerable time, that of hemp, if it is to appear, is
observed within two or three minutes.   Secondly—The action
of ergot is of a lasting character, that of hemp is confined to a
few pains shortly after its administration.   Thirdly—The action of hemp is moie energetic, and perhaps more certainly
induced, than that of ergot.—[*Med. Examiner.*

Miscellany.

Anonymous writers and Personalities.—Although fully appreciating the benefits of a free press, and of the multiplication of media
for the diffusion of knowledge and morality, we cannot refrain from
the expression of the profound regret with which we have observed,
especially during the last twelve months, certain periodicals ostensibly devoted to the cause of Medicine, allowing their pages to be
prostituted by anonymous writers to the grossest personalities and
misrepresentations, and occasionally containing even Editorials equally objectionable.   If licentiousness in secular newspapers be an evil
deeply lamented by all good men, how much more must it be desecra-
ted when found invading the sacred arena until now reserved exclusively for the efforts of minds in search of scientific truth and
usefulness !

We would not do injustice to the Medical Profession of our country,
by supposing that such Journals can ever secure or retain any countenance.   Yet their demoralising influence is incontestible, and can
only be arrested by an immediate withdrawal of patronage.

The whole Medical Profession of Georgia and some of its members in particular, the Medical Society and the Medical College, have been repeatedly and are still being made the subjects of most scurrilous anonymous communications to Medical Journals published at a distance, and in various quarters of the Union. The articles are not dated from any particular point, and bear different "*noms de guerre ;*" yet their style and general bearing show them to be all written by the same pen, and to have been indited in Georgia. Editors at a distance can surely have no good reason for not rejecting at once such miserable productions ; and we have been induced to make the above pointed allusion to articles bearing upon our own State, in the hope that their eyes may be opened to the plan by which they have been misled.

Medical Society of the State of Georgia.—We are indebted to the politeness of Dr. O'Keeffe, Recording Secretary, for the following abstract of the proceedings of the Medical Society of the State of Georgia.

This Society held its third annual session at Augusta on the 14th and 15th April, when quite a respectable number were in attendance. In the absence of the President, (Dr. R. D. Arnold, of Savannah,) the Society was called to order by Dr. A. Means, the 1st Vice-President. But little business had been transacted, however, when Dr. Arnold arrived and took the Chair. 44 new members were now admitted, which makes the whole number of members 152.

The election for officers to serve until the next annual meeting then took place, and resulted as follows:

President—A. MEANS, M. D., of Oxford, Newton Co.
1st V. President—H. F. CAMPBELL, M. D., of Augusta, Richmond Co.
2d V. President—C. T. QUINTARD, M. D., of Roswell, Cobb Co.
Rec'g Secretary—D. C. O'KEEFFE, M. D., of Penfield, Greene Co.
Cor'g Secretary—G. F. COOPER, M. D., of Perry, Houston Co.
Treasurer—R. C. BLACK, M. D., of Augusta, Richmond Co.

The President elect took the Chair, and in a few pertinent remarks returned thanks for the honor conferred upon him.

The following gentlemen were then elected Delegates to the approaching meeting of the American Medical Association in Richmond, Virginia.

Drs. H. F. Campbell, Juriah Harriss, J. D. Mackie, J. J. Robertson, C. B. Nottingham, L. C. Pynchon, R. C. Black, T. P. Janes, W. N. King, H. A. Ramsay, E. W. Alfriend, R. Campbell, A. C. Hart, E. Girardey, W. R. Ruffin.

On motion, it was Resolved that the President be authorized to fill any vacancy that may occur in the Delegation to the American Medical Association.

The South-Western Medical Society of Géorgia, the De Kalb Auxiliary Medical Society, and the Medical Society of Greene and adjoining counties were admitted as Auxiliaries.

On motion of Dr. Quintard, it was Resolved that Committees be appointed to furnish Essays upon such subjects as shall be designated by the Society.

On motion of Dr. H. F. Campbell, it was Resolved that the Standing Commitiees on the several branches of Medicine be abolished.

On motion of Dr. Dugas, it was Resolved that a committee of five be appointed, whose duty shall be to report upon the Contributions to Medical Knowledge by Physicians residing in Georgia during the year preceding. The Chair appointed Drs. L. A. Dugas, R. D. Arnold, G. F. Cooper, J. A. Eve, and H. Rossignol, this committee.

Dr. Robert Campbell, Chairman of the Committee on "Empirical Remedies," read an able Report, which was received and ordered to be printed.

Dr. G. F. Cooper read an interesting Report, prepared by Dr. Culler, upon "Health Statistics," based upon data obtained from the U. S. Census, which was ordered to be deposited in the archives of the Society, and for which the thanks of the Society were voted to Dr. Culler.

Able and interesting Reports were read by Drs. G. F. Cooper, C. T. Quintard, P. F. Eve, H. F. Campbell, and L. A. Dugas—all of which were received and ordered to be printed.

Dr. Juriah Harriss, of Augusta, was appointed to deliver the address at the next annual meeting of the Society, and Dr. W. Gaston Bulloch, of Savannah, the alternate. It was determined to hold the next annual meeting in Savannah, on the second Wednesday in April, 1853.

The thanks of the Society were voted to Dr. H. F. Campbell for his chaste Address, (a copy of which was requested for publication,) to the Committee of Arrangements, to the Faculty of the Medical College of Georgia, and to the officers of the past year.

On motion of Dr. Arnold, it was Resolved, to assess each member of the Society Two Dollars to defray the expenses of publication, &c.; and on motion of Dr. Cooper, it was also Resolved, that the Transactions of this Society, when published, be withheld from such members as may fail to remit their assessment to the Treasurer, Dr. R. C. Black, at Augusta.

The following resolutions were offered by Dr. Dugas, and adopted :

Resolved, That a Committee of three be appointed by the President for the purpose of proposing subjects for Essays to be presented at the next annual meeting. (Drs. L. A. Dugas, H. F. Campbell and L. D. Ford, were appointed.)

Resolved, That the President appoint Committees of one for each of the Essays above referred to, whenever he shall have been furnished with the subjects selected.

Resolved, That a Committee of two be appointed to superintend the publication of the Transactions of this Society, with authority to draw upon the Treasurer for the necessary funds. (Drs. I. P. Garvin and T. B. Phinizy were appointed.)

On Wednesday evening the Society partook of a fine collation prepared in one of the College Halls by the Faculty of this Institution. This entertainment, as well as the whole proceedings of the Society, were characterized by the warm-hearted cordiality and good feeling so peculiar to associations of men devoted to Science and to the cause of humanity.

. The National Institute of France, has recently awarded the following prizes :

"The prize of experimental physiology was given to M. Claude Bernard, for a paper on a new function of the liver in men and animals. M. Masson and M. Sucquet obtained prizes of 2000fr. each ; the first for his method of preserving vegetables, and the second for his disinfection of dissecting theatres. The Monthyon prizes for physic and surgery were awarded as follows : 2,500fr. to M. Jules Guerin, for the generalization of sub-cutaneous Tenotomy ; 2,000fr. to M. Huguier, for his researches into female maladies; 2,000fr. to MM. Briquet and Mignot, authors of a practical treatise on cholera ; 2,000fr. to M. Duchenn, of Boulogne, for his electro-physiological researches, applied to pathology and therapeutics ; 2,000fr. to M. Lucas, for his physiological and practical treatise on hereditary maladies ; 2,000fr. each to MM. Tabarie and Pravez, for the medical use of compressed air ; 2,000fr. to M. Gluge, for his pathological histology ; 1,500fr. to M. Gosselin, for his researches into the obliterations of spermatic channels ; 1,500fr. to M. Garriel, for his application of vulcanized caoutchouc to medicine and surgery ; 1,000fr. to M. Serres, for his researches respecting the phosphenes; and 1000fr. to M. Boinet, for his work on the treatment of chronic abscesses by injections of iodine."

Medical Colleges in the State of New York.—An application has been made to the Legislature of New York, for a charter for a seventh

Medical College, and an adverse report presented by the Committee to whom it was referred. Among other reasons assigned, is that of the inability of the existing Colleges to sustain themselves, as evinced by this indebtedness. The College of Physicians and Surgeons, owes $15,000; the Geneva College, $400; the New York University College, $47,000; and the Buffalo College, $3,300. We derive the above information from the New York Medical Gazette.

New Medical Periodicals.—A new feature in the periodical medical literature of our country, is the publication in New Orleans of " L'union Médicale " in the French language. A portion of the " Canada Medical Journal " is also published in French. This will doubtless enable many of our medical men to keep up their knowledge of that polite and useful tongue. We have received " The East Tennessee Record of Medicine and Surgery," edited by Frank A. Ramsey, A. M., M. D., Knoxville. It is to be issued in quarterly numbers of 100 pages each.

A New Method of Whitening Bones. By ELLERSLIE WALLACE, M. D., Demonstrator of Anatomy in Jefferson Medical College, Philadelphia.

To the Editors of the Medical Examiner.

Gentlemen,—During the past year, I have used sulphuric ether for the purpose of extracting the greasy matters from bones of which I have desired to make preparations, and have uniformly found it entirely satisfactory. I have used it for entire skeletons where they have been of value.

Twenty-five or thirty pounds of ether (which can be obtained for 18 cts. per lb.,) is enough for a skeleton, if the bones be closely packed in a proper case. After pouring the ether on them until they are entirely covered, they may be left for some hours, or a day; then removing them, they should be allowed to dry thoroughly. This process should be repeated as often as may be necessary.

Six immersions have been enough for a very greasy skeleton. It is prudent to wash the ether before using it, to remove free acid, and we may have the ether re-distilled after it is saturated with the oil. To morbid specimens, as of caries, &c., it is admirably adapted, as it removes the grease entirely, without injuring the delicate structure at all, which is not the case, as we all know, with any of the ordinary alkaline solutions.

Mortality of Children.—According to Quetelet, 22,472 children in every 100,000, die within 12 months after birth; and more than 2 in every 7 within the first 2 years. This may be true in Europe, but we think that, it is certainly not so in our country.

Tribute of Respect.—At the regular meeting of the Georgia Medical Society, held on the evening of March 4th, the Committee appointed for the purpose, reported the following Preamble and Resolutions, which met with unanimous adoption by the Society :

Since the last regular meeting of the Georgia Medical Society, our esteemed President, Dr. Cosmo P. Richardsone, has departed this life.   The many and various tributes to his worth as a citizen, which were poured in on all sides, the distinguished honors paid at the interment of his remains, truthfully attested the high estimation in which he was held by his fellow-townsmen.   While we rejoice that one of our number should have so faithfully fulfilled all the duties of his social position, as to have descended to his grave amidst the sorrow of a whole people, it becomes our duty to pay our tribute to him more exclusively as a member of our Society, and as an ornament to his Profession ; a Profession which we are pioud to consider as inferior to none in dignity of calling and humanity of purpose.

To a mind of great quickness of perception, he united a decision of character and action which rendered him ever prompt and energtic in ministering to the sick.   A large practice and the unbounded confidence of his immediate patients were the legitimate results of these qualities.   His intercourse with his Brother Physicians was marked with all the courtesy and liberality due to his own high sense of the requirements of a liberal Profession, whose standard he ever labored to elevate.   While he endeavored to do this he treated with the contempt of conscious superiority, those self-styled systems of medicine which are tried more as a royal road to money than to learning, and in the success of his own practice gave ample evidence that in following the lights which had been hung out by the experience of ages, he followed no " Will-of-the-Wisp."

It is therefore Resolved by the Georgia Medical Society, That in the death of Dr. Cosmo P. Richardsone, they have lost one who was endeared to them as a man by his kind and generous feelings ; one who from his large experience and great natural qualifications, and his high tone in all situations, in which he came in contact with his Brother Physicians, was an ornament to his Profession, and whose loss in the meridian of life and usefulness, they unaffectedly deplore as a most serious one to them.

Resolved, That this Society do most deeply sympathize with the Family of the deceased, and that a copy of these Resolutions be furnished them ; and that they also be published in the Daily Prints of the City, and in the Southern Medical and Surgical Journal of Augusta.

R. D. ARNOLD, Chairman Committee.

J. Ganahl, Secretary.

ERRATA.

Page 264, fourth line from bottom, for "live," read *life of the.*
" 265, sixth line from top, for "page," read *lecture.*
" 266, thirteenth line from bottom, for "type-form," read *type-power.*
" 269, fourteenth line from bottom, for "their," read *this.*
" 270, eighth line from bottom, for "dissimularities," read *dissimilarities.*
" 271, seventh line from top, for "existing," read *exciting.*
" 274, second line from top, for "inflamation," read *inflammation.*

SOUTHERN
MEDICAL AND SURGICAL JOURNAL.

| Vol. 8.] | NEW SERIES.—JUNE, 1852. | [No. 6. |

PART FIRST.

Original Communications.

ARTICLE XVII.

Remarks on Craniotomy, with a case. By Wm. Nephew King, M. D., of Roswell, Georgia.

Instrumental parturition has probably been practiced from the earliest times. Indeed, it is impossible to trace the history of many operations of obstetrical surgery to their origin or to say who were the originators of them.

The Cæsarian operation, for example, is of very great antiquity. Dr. Mansfield, in his work on the Antiquity of Gastrotomy and Hysterotomy, on the Living, informs us that in the Thalmud, Gastrotomy is mentioned under the article on Hereditary Rights, and re-asserts that in an earlier work called Mischuajoth, bearing date A. M. 140, this passage occurs—"in a twin-birth neither the first child, which by the section of the belly is brought into the world, nor the one coming after, can attain the rights of heirship or the priestly office." But even this great antiquity is lost in the still remoter period fixed by fabulous historians: thus, Jupiter snatched from the abdomen of the wretched Semele, his son, yet unborn, when the Goddess was killed by the thunder and lightning in which her divine lover was obliged to approach her. The Romans held that Æsculapius was delivered in the same way by Apollo. Virgil states that Lycus was born in the same manner. Pliny is, however, considered the first writer of authority on this point. Although the operation is of undoubted antiquity, yet it is not mentioned in the works of Hippocrates, Celsus, Paulus Ægineta, or Albucasis, and the earliest account of it in any medical work is said to have been published about the middle of the 14th century. In 1491 *Nicolai de Falconüs*, recorded a case; but Velpeau states that it was performed in 1424. Sprengel asserts that it was not performed upon the living subject before the year 1610, while many writers deny altogether that it was known to the ancients; among whom are Deleurye, Levret, Mauriceau and Mendel. In proof of its remote antiquity, Plenck, Dionis and Gardien refer to the thirty-fourth book of Pliny's Natural History.

Organikotocia or Instrumental Parturition was practiced by Hippocrates, and in his works are recommended all the obstetric instruments now in use; but of course imperfect in their construction, and some of them difficult of application. Thus, for a perforator, he used and recommended a small sword, and his forceps had teeth—he speaks of a blunt hook also.

The application of instruments in obstetrical practice, always requires delicacy and decision; the practitioner is often swayed by the opinions and prejudices of those around him—imperceptibly, it may be, but none the less certainly: in those operations which require a solution of continuity, not only the prejudice of ignorance, but religious faith often determines the character of the operation.

One instinctively shrinks from the destruction of a living infant, and is anxious to delay all action until death shall have supervened; and in every case requiring the operation of embryotomy, the accoucheur is glad to observe a *want of pulsation* at the *fontanels*—an *absence* of *motion* in the child—the shivering fits—the placid breasts and fœtor of the uterine discharges in the woman that are characteristic signs of the *death* of the fœtus, before proceeding.

These, although *signs of death*, are not *true diagnostics*; and many instances are recorded in which the operation has been performed and the child been born alive. This is readily accounted for when we remember the origin of the cerebral nerves, and the functions of which are not always destroyed.

In those cases in which the child is living, and where the brim
or outlet of the pelvis is so deformed as not to admit of a
delivery, the accoucheur has the choice of two formidable operations : in the one, the life of both mother and child *may* be
saved—in the other the child must be sacrificed.

That the child is often unwarrantably sacrificed, in this and
in other Protestant countries, no one can doubt, and indeed, we
understand that, in a medical society in our State, a gentleman
not long since, argued that the *destruction* of the *child* was
proper, in order to *avoid* the probable contingency of a *vesico-
vaginal fistula*.   In England, the preference given to Craniotomy, arose from an essay by Osborne ; but his deductions are
abundantly answered, exposed and ridiculed, by Dewees ; and
since the great success which has attended the Cæsarian section
Embryotomy has gone somewhat into disfavor.   Craniotomy,
says Ryan, is impracticable in cases of extreme deformity, and
from mature consideration of the history of the Cæsarean section, it is obvious that the extraction of the infant by Craniotomy is as fatal an operation to the mother, and there is often
much more injury inflicted on her than by timely removing the
infant through the abdomen.   "I would venture to predict,"
says he, " that Embryotomy will be nearly discarded in a few
years ;" and again, " the absence of a religious motive, is a
cause of the comparatively frequent performance of embryotomy in this empire—the necessity of its too frequent performance
in all Protestant countries, is almost exclusively founded on the
impracticability of delivery by the natural passage."   "I know
these are unpalatable assertions, but truth is great and will
prevail."   Tyler Smith, in his work on Parturition, says, "The
Catholic doctrine of the value of extreme unction, as regards
the mother, and the necessity of baptism to infant salvation ;
the different views on these points held by Protestants, are visi-
bly written in the precepts of practical midwifery, and taking
France and England as the types of the two great varieties of
practice, he presents us with the characteristics of each type.
Protestantism, always considers the social relations—always
preserves the mother, when the destruction of the infant will
secure that object.   It considers the child as already dead—
Catholicism, ' *au contraire*,' makes the life of the child practi-

cally of more importance.   The mother receives the sacrament of extreme unction, and being thus secured, her life is sacrificed and the child saved, if possible, that it may be spiritually washed with baptismal water."

The following is the division of Dr. Smith.

PROTESTANT PRACTICE GIVES THE DECIDED PREFERENCE TO THE LIFE OF THE MOTHER.	ROMAN CATHOLIC PRACTICE, LEANS TO THE LIFE OF THE INFANT.
This is seen	This is seen
In the partiality for Craniotomy.	In the favorable opinion entertained of the Cæsarian operation in Roman Catholic countries.
In the induction of premature labor.	
In the proposed separation of the placenta in placenta prævia.	In the high opinion in which the Sigaultian operation has been held.
In the dislike of the Cæsarian section, the Sigaultian operation, and the frequent use of the long forceps.	In the frequent use of the long forceps.
	In the great dislike to Craniotomy, and the induction of premature labor.

In our country, the attempt to save both mother and child, by Cæsarian section, is rapidly growing in favor, and very justly so, from the success which has attended the operation— but there is beyond question, too little attention given to the life of the fœtus.   Practitioners do not esteem the fœtus in utero as having sufficient claims upon their consideration, to authorize the jeopardizing the life of the mother ; though the risk, in which that life is placed, may be comparatively trivial.   In many instances, in which the interest of the mother and the offspring clash—as in the plan of detaching the placenta, and extracting it before the child, in placenta presentations, there is as much indifference shown to the life of the child, as in Craniotomy.   This "revived plan," of practice has been termed, "an excessive and unjustifiable application of the British rules ;" but it finds very many advocates among us, although it does not hesitate to sacrifice the life of the fœtus, for "an assumed but improved advantage to the mother."

We have thus briefly glanced at some points in obstetric practice, more for the purpose of suggesting reflections, than from any expectation or intention of deciding any disputed points of practice.   The case which we have to offer is one in which we were not called upon to question the propriety of our course. Indeed, we have thought, that had the case come under our care, at an earlier period of its progress, we would have been able to have effected the delivery without the use of instruments.   We should not have hesitated however—had there been signs of life in the fœtus, and such deformity as to have rendered delivery impossible by the natural way—to have made an attempt to save the lives of mother and offspring, by the Cæsarian section, after the manner we saw the operation performed, with great skill and perfect success, by M. Paul Dubois, in his wards in Paris, during the last season.

On the morning of the 13th December last, was called to Mrs. T., aged 18 years, first child, said to have been in labor 52 hours, her attendant "*une sage femme de la campagne.*"

The pains were during this time of short duration and at long intervals, of course very ineffectual. At the time we saw the case, there was considerable acceleration of the pulse, and the pains were severe, and had been so since the "waters," were discharged, some eight hours previous; as they were described to us, they must have been strong, vigorous, expulsive labor pains.

Upon making an examination per vaginam, found the external organs in a soft and relaxed state, and the head of the fœtus wedged very firmly within the pubic arch, the presentation was the "occipito sacrée secondaire" of the French. An attempt was made to introduce the forceps, but it was found impossible. Turning was out of the question, and now all that remained was to perform the operation of Craniotomy, which was accordingly accomplished in the manner recommended by M. Chailly of Paris—which may be found in his excellent work L'art des Accouchements. (See page, 582.)

The position there mentioned, viz. the Dorsal, is that usually selected by the obstetricians of continental Europe, while the left lateral is preferred in England. The left hand being greased, the fingers introduced into the vagina, and having them placed on the fontanel (or in the course of the sagital suture) the perforator was then introduced along the palmar surface of the hand—great care being taken to avoid wounding the soft parts of the mother, when by a rotary motion, the perforator was passed through the cranium, and the cerebral mass broken up. The perforator, now having been closed, was carefully withdrawn. In the case under consideration, the brain was removed, it not escaping, as is usually the case when uterine action is present. Slight traction was then made upon the fœtus, when it escaped without difficulty.

After the fœtus had been extracted, we perceived that the abdomen remained unusually distended, and on introducing the hand, another fœtus was discovered. By this time, the female was almost exhausted; we administered brandy and carb. ammon., which revived her—the pains came on, and the last fœtus, very diminutive in size, was expelled.

The case terminated very favorably; was attended with no hemorrhage. She was discharged on the 10th day after, and is now in the enjoyment of as fine health, as at any time prior to her accouchement.

Observations on the use of Veratrum Viride, By W. H. ROBERT, M. D., of Orion, Pike county, Alabama.

Although several articles have appeared in this journal, since Dr. Norwood's first communication, the importance of the subject must justify the present. I now propose to notice the use and effects of the Veratrum Viride, as observed in my practice.

Pneumonia.—It was in May, 1851, that I first used the article. I was called to a case of Pneumonia of the right lung, The patient was a man, 45 years of age, who had been suffering for a few days from general inflammatory symptoms, and was apparently relieved, when he suddenly took a chill, followed by high fever. I saw him 24 hours after the onset of the chill and found him laboring under confirmed Pneumonia. Difficult and hurried respiration, frequent coughing, severe pain in the right side, and *bloody* expectoration; pulse, 126 in the minute, full and hard. Without any hesitancy, I applied a very large blister to the affected side, and put him on the use of the tinct. veratrum viride, in doses of twenty drops every three hours, until it produced sufficient nausea to affect the pulse. I then reduced the dose to 15 or 10 drops, provided the latter dose controlled the action of the heart. On my next visit, I found the pulse reduced to 75 in the minute; respiration easy and natural, expectoration white and scanty, skin very much relaxed, and the surface cool. The blister had drawn well, and relieved the pain in the side. The medicine had produced very distressing sickness and vomiting during the first part of the night ; now it only produces sickness immediately after taking each dose. I pronounced the patient safe from that time, but directed the continuation of the medicine for some three or four days, in gradually reduced doses. At the end of that time, he complained of nothing but the medicine, nor had he since the first 24 hours after commencement of the medicine.

I would here take occasion to remark, that in pneumonia, I always apply a very large blister to the affected side, and sometimes cups. I find that very free vesication gives more relief in subduing the pain and calming the respiration than any other remedy. While the blister is doing this, the veratrum viride is producing its specific effect upon the heart.

Case 2, occurred in September last. The right lung was inflamed ; very similar in its onset to the first ; was treated in the same manner, and with precisely the same results—reducing the action of the heart in about 18 hours. In this case, the medicine produced its hiccough effect, which alarmed the patient very much.

Cases 3 and 4, occurred at the same house, in November last. One was a negro woman, six months advanced in pregnancy : she had been very sick for four days previous to my visit. The secretion from the left lung was so abundant as to threaten suffocation; expectoration could not clear the lung long enough to procure any rest—constant coughing, pulse 125 per minute, and very irritable. After applying the blister, I commenced the Veratrum Viride, in 20 drop doses. On my next visit, 24 hours after, I found the patient no better ; the system had not been affected by the medicine in the least ; the distress of the lung fully as great as the day before ; added to all this, she was now threatened with abortion. I immediately gave half teaspoonful of the tinct., and directed the 20 drop doses continued as before. As I lived but two miles off, I requested to be informed if abortion took place before morning. At 10 o'clock P. M., a messenger informed me that abortion had taken place. I sent word to continue the medicine.

On my visit next morning, I found such a decided relief of

the distressing symptoms, that I was truly afraid to express myself. The pulse had fallen to 70 ; respiration free, expectoration easy ; sputa (before very bloody) now scarcely tinged. I continued the medicine a few days longer, which sealed the convalescnce.

So confident was the master that the woman would die after the abortion, that he was not willing to bury the fœtus until he saw there was no probability of putting the mother with it, that time.

The other case (4th) was a young lady, sick (at the same time as the negress,) with double pneumonia, and who was relieved entirely in a few days, by the tinct. veratrum viride and extensive blistering.

Case 5, occurred in December, in a man, aged about 28 years. He had pneumonia of the left lung, blistering and the tinct. veratrum viride relieved him in a few days. He had no fever after the first day.

Case 6. From some peculiarity attending this case, I must give a more minute account of it than of the preceding :

The patient, (a ditcher by occupation,) contracted pleuro-pneumonia of the right side, early in January last. He had been bled and purged before I saw him, which was two days after the onset of the disease. I found him suffering intensely with pain, (which was confined to the posterior and inner parts of the right side of the chest,) and difficult respiration, and was unable to lie down or to cough. Pulse 115 per minute, and an intermission of every fourth pulsation. I cupped the side very freely over the seat of the pain; after which, I covered the part with a very large blister, I then put him on the use of the tinct. veratrum viride, in 20 drop doses, every three hours. On my next visit, I found that the blister had drawn very well, but with only partial relief to the distressing symptoms. Expectoration was however better established, and the matter expectorated, was a mixture of mucus and pure blood.

No perceptible effect of the medicine. I ordered the blister dressed with basilicon ointment, and continued the medicine as before. On my third visit, I found less pleuritis, but more pneumonia, which was gradually extending to the superior and anterior part of the lung. There was less pain, except in coughing; the secretion from the lung was not very copious, and when expectorated, appeared to be a lump of coagulated blood. The medicine had produced its specific effect in a very singular way : the pulsations at the wrist appeared to be only 40 to the minute; yet on a careful examination of the heart, I could detect an effort made by it to produce a contraction between each pulsation at the wrist ; but apparently too much depressed to perform its office *fully* more than 40 times to the minute ; added to this, the bowels had become very irritable, and the attendants were of the opinion that the tincture operated on the bowels. Not liking the depressed condition of the heart, and the irritable state of the bowels—yet not perfectly willing to suspend the use of the veratrum, I determined to persevere with it in combination with opiates, for at least 24 hours longer. The opiate controlled the bowels, but produced a good deal of stupor. The depression of the heart continued the same. I suspended the use of all remedies, only such as particular occasion would demand, such as opiates, &c., internally, and relied upon the effects of the blister. The pneumonia gradually advanced so as to affect the whole lung. I covered the whole anterior part of the right side of the chest with a blister ; on the drawing of this, the heart became regular in its action, but pulsating only sixty times per minute. This was some days after the entire suspension of the veratrum viride, and yet with active pneumonia all the time. Every mouthful of sputa was of the character last mentioned—that is, having the appearance of coagulated blood ; gradually, the respiration became easier, expectoration better, the case progressed on favourably, and recovery took place, without any increase whatever in the action of the heart. The last time I examined his pulse, I counted only 60 beats to the minute, and this when he was going about. This is the only case where I have ever entertained the least idea that the veratrum viride would purge, and this, too, the only case where the heart failed to react upon a suspension of this medicine after so short a trial.

CASE 7. Was under treatment at the same time as the preceding. It was a much milder case of pneumonia, but complicated with rheumatism of both knees : both complaints were relieved at the same time. I blistered the chest, and gave the tinct. veratrum viride for some four or five days, with the happiest result.

I have some 6 or 8 cases more on my note book, treated in precisely the same way, but I consider the above to be enough.

I have supplied some of my brother practitioners with a small quantity of the tincture for trial, and all are well pleased with it. In a conversation recently with Dr. A. S. Johnston of Troy, upon the effects of it in pneumonia, he made this answer to me—"I do not know how I have been treating Pneumonia, nor what I could do without it."

Cynanche Trachealis. I have used this remedy in one case of the above disease. I produced the specific of the medicine, on the child, and continued it so, for two days, but without any beneficial effect. The child died.

Typhoid fever. I have used it in five cases, and I cannot say that I derived any benefit from it, except in one of them. This was a relapse. The patient suffered no pain; there was some tympanitis of the bowels; the tongue was but slightly altered in colour or appearance; bowels were not relaxed; the pulse 125 to the minute, and rapidly increasing in frequency, and just such a case as I have in my practice denominated the nervous form of the disease. For two weeks, I had been using all such remedies as are commonly resorted to in cases of the kind, but without avail. As a last resort, I determined to try the effect of veratrum viride. I succeeded in twelve hours in producing its specific effect in a very powerful degree, attended with considerable prostration. I kept up the effect of the medicine eight days, and convalescence was fully established. I continued the remedy thus long in the above case, because experience had taught me, that a much shorter time would have no permanent effect, at least in typhoid fever.

In the other cases of typhoid fever, in which I used the remedy, I could produce its specific effect; but, as soon as I relaxed in giving the medicine, the disease would resume again its regular course.

In Mammary Abscess, I used the remedy in one case, with the happiest effect. The lady had been confined two weeks previous, and was taken with a very severe chill, which lasted half a day. I was called to her in the afternoon of the same day, and found her suffering very much with pain in the left breast, and in the axillary glands of the same side. There was some nausea and tenderness of the bowels, which were costive; pulse very rapid and irritable. She was purged freely, and warm poultices were applied to the breast; small portions of spts. of turpentine were administered internally. On my visit next morning, I found the patient no better; the breast more painful than yesterday, glands also very sore, pulse exceedingly rapid. I determined to try the effect of the veratrum viride in this case. I produced its specific effect in about ten hours: the prostration was so great as to alarm the friends of the lady, and I was sent for. On my arrival, I found reaction had taken place as much as I cared for it to do ; the pulse had come down to 70 per minute, the pain in the breast and glands had sensibly diminished. I did not give any more of the medicine ; she had no more fever, and escaped one of the most painful of diseases, mammary absess.

Some may imagine, that the cases of Pneumonia above detailed were slight, and not a fair test. In answer to this, I only say, that before the employment of quinine to the present extent, bilious fever always lasted from 7 to 13 days ; but who sees a case of bilious fever last that long now? Those who are prejudiced against the free use of Quinine, can best answer. I look upon the action of ver. vir. on the system, (at least in pneumonia,) as giving such a decided check to the disease, as to effectually prevent its progression to that severe type which it so commonly assumes, under any other mode of treatment.

I have to record only one fatal case of pneumonia occurring in my practice, since I have employed this remedy—and that case was a dear infant of my own, sixteen months old. In this case, the medicine produced violent vomiting and great prostration ; but I never could reduce the frequency of the action of the heart. The disease became chronic, and proved fatal in three months.

While practicing medicine in Middle Georgia, in 1844, '45, and '46, there occurred a very severe epidemic, (pneumonia,) producing great distress, in a large scope of country. I saw

fully the fatality attending it in the ordinary modes of treatment ; and I am perfectly satisfied that had this remedy been
used then, the result would have been far different.

In a few words, I will give the effects of the tinct. veratrum viride, as I have seen them. The first appreciable, is
its emetic effect : gradually, during the nausea and vomiting,
the pulse loses its fulness and frequency, very free diaphoresis comes on during the vomiting, and sometimes continues so
long as the medicine is kept up ; at other times, only when nausea exists ; this is accompanied generally with a cool state of
the surface. I have found that the depression of the pulse will
generally continue twelve or fifteen hours after the vomiting
is first produced, if no more medicine is given. I generally
reduce the doses from 25 drops down to such doses only, as
will produce nausea, not caring to produce any more vomiting
after the first time, unless the heart reacts too much under the
nauseating doses. In some cases, I have found the stomach so
susceptible to the presence of this medicine, that I have been compelled to disguise 8 drop doses in a draught of sweetened water.
For the first two or three days after taking the medicine, there
is a very free discharge of mucus from the fauces, afterwards
the whole buccal cavity becomes very dry. Hiccough is
sometimes a very distressing effect of its long continued use.

As I have said more than I intended in the first instance, I
will close with but a few more words. If I can induce some
physicians to listen to the appeal of Dr. Norwood, and give this
medicine a fair trial, I have no fears that they will reject it.
In conclusion, allow me through the medium of this valuable
journal, to present to Dr. Norwood my sincere thanks, for his
efforts to introduce properly to the profession this medicine ;
one which I now consider second to none. I do not claim for
Dr. Norwood the discovery of this medicine, but I do claim
for him, the discovery, in this medicine, of certain effects upon
the system which he ascribes to it, which he has fully proven
to belong to it, and which any one may observe who will use it.
The tincture I use, is made by digesting ½ lb. of the root in a
quart of alcohol.

ARTICLE XIX.

Cases demonstrating the utility of Electricity in the treatment of disease. By A. DONALD, M. D., of Alabama.

CASE I.   On the 27th day of September last, I was invited to see Mrs. G. C., a lady about 47 years of age.   She complained of severe pain in the ends of the fingers of her right hand—I examined them, and found them to be insensible to the touch and to cold, and of a deep purple hue, presenting over the back of the hand a shrivelled appearance, with some longitudinal depressions on the palmar surface of the fingers.   She was a lady of the sanguine temperament, with round, full features, blue eyes, light hair and small extremities, and when in health a florid complexion; but, at this time, she looked pale and manifested some slight agitation; there were also some purple spots over the palmar surface of her hand, about the size of a dime; the pulse at the wrist very small and somewhat irregular in its action; the pain at night prevented sleep; but little appetite for food; constipation, and occasionally very sick at the stomach.   Diagnosis: a tendency to mortification, or gangrena senilis, caused by obstructed circulation.   Having observed that the treatment generally resorted to, under such circumstances, had failed, I resolved to try Electricity, as I believed it to be, if *not vital force,* at least capable of *performing the office of the vital force.*   I at once began the use of this agent, with one of Dr. S. B. Smith's Torpedo-Electro-Magnetic Machines.   After putting the machine in operation, I made the first application, by placing the negative pole on the back of the neck, and the positive pole on the ends of her fingers; and finding that she gave no evidence of its power, I then placed one pole on each side of her fingers, and, as before, she gave no evidence of its presence.   I continued the application for half an hour, and still there was no impression made; I then ordered a basin of water, quite warm, placed her hand in the water and then put the positive pole in the basin, with the negative pole on the back of her neck.   After some ten minutes had elapsed, she experienced *very slight* sensations; but after continuing this application for one hour, the pulsations were more distinct, though only slight.   I then discontinued the application for that day, and ordered that the hand be kept continually warm and dry. This application was made for twelve days, in succession, and a perfect and complete cure was effected at the end of this time; the hand looked to be at least ten years younger than the other hand. I would remark that I occasionally applied it to the whole system in this case.

Case II. J. M. a highly respectable planter, of Butler county, Alabama, had been afflicted with chronic rheumatism, in both knees, for several years, and had tried nearly all the remedies generally resorted to in such cases. I determined to try electricity in this case: I did so, and in one month had the satisfaction of seeing him perfectly cured. In this case, I made the application by placing the negative pole on the sacrum, and the positive pole over the parts affected.

Case III. Mrs. B., of Lowndes county, Alabama, about 60 years of age, had been vaccinated in January, 1851, which occasioned high fever for several days, after which she found herself to be quite blind: she could not distinguish a man from a horse across the road. After being in this condition about seven months, she came to me for relief. Finding no structural change in her eyes, I concluded that the blindness depended upon debility of the optic nerve, and began the use of electricity, by applying the positive pole to the back of the neck, and the negative pole over the eyelids, (the eyes being closed,) as I only wanted its tonic effect. I continued the application from fifteen to twenty minutes, each day, for two weeks, at the end of which time she was so much improved that she could see how to take up a stitch in knitting.

Case IV. Jacob, a negro man, the property of Mr. J. M. Yeldell, of Butler county, Ala., had rheumatism in his left vastus externus muscle, and in his right ankle, which was very much swollen. I put him upon a long table, and began with electricity, by placing the negative pole on the sacrum, and the positive pole freely over the parts affected. The first application was continued one hour, for the purpose of producing a perfect reaction in the parts; the application was made about candle-light in the evening; the next morning I was astonished to find that the swelling in the ankle had entirely disappeared, and that there was no pain in the parts. I applied the poles again, as before, and have understood that he has been well ever since.

CASE V. Two years ago, I was seriously troubled with rheumatism in the whole of the deltoid muscle of the left shoulder, and tried many remedies, with only partial relief. My arm continued to be almost paralysed—I could not support any degree of weight, with my arm in the horizontal position. Finally, last spring, I had another attack, involving the right arm, in the same manner, and tried colchicum, guaiac., nitrate of potass., and various other remedies, without relief. I began to think that I should lose the use of both arms, and commenced the use of electricity, by applying the negative pole to the cervical region, and the positive pole over all the parts affected. In about ten days I was much improved. One *fact I observed in my own case*, was that, in a few moments after the application of electricity, the pain, however severe before the application, would be entirely relieved, and, in many instances, would not return again for twenty-four hours.

CASE VI. On one occasion, I was afflicted with dyspeptic head-ache, with nausea and vomiting; I used electricity, and in a moment (after taking one pole in each hand) the sickness at the stomach was entirely relieved, and the pain in the head disappeared as suddenly. I am satisfied, from repeated trials, that nothing in the materia medica will relieve vomiting so soon as electricity.

CASE VII. Mrs. C., after delivery and removal of the placenta, was threatened with dangerous uterine hæmorrhage. Electricity was employed in the following manner: the positive pole was placed upon the sacrum, and the negative pole (being properly insulated) was applied to the os uteri; in an instant the contraction was effected, and the hæmorrhage successfully arrested.

CASE VIII. Mr. G., had been afflicted for several years with a fistula in-ano. After syringing the parts with warm water, the negative pole was placed over the external orifice, and the positive pole over the sacrum; the applications were continued for thirty minutes, twice a day, (always after cleansing the parts,) and in ten days the cure was complete, and has continued so ever since. In this case, the opening was in the cellular tissue.

CASE IX. A lady about 45 years of age, had been afflicted with menorrhagia for seven years: she had taken a great deal of medicine during this time, with but partial relief. I had treated her myself with tonics, to improve her general health and with the secale cornutum, for its specific effect, without success. I finally had recourse to Electricity—I placed the positive pole over the sacrum, and the negative pole to the os uteri, and after daily application for two weeks, it was discontinued, and the lady is now entirely well.

CASE X. Miss H., aged about 22 years, had, from puberty, been afflicted with that most painful malady, dysmenorrhœa. She had been treated for it, under the presumption that it originated from a rheumatic condition of the uterus. I had used Dr. Dewees' famed remedy, " comp. tinct. of guaiacum," without success, and then proposed Dr. McIntosh's treatment of the bougie. This was objected to, and I then proposed Electricity, believing that the canal was subject to spasmodic constriction; for I found that this painful condition did not last more than *eight hours*, whereas, if it had been a permanent constriction, the pain would have continued throughout the *four or five days*. Having found by observation that the positive pole was expansive, and the negative contractive, and that one of the effects of electricity was to soothe pain, I began by placing the negative pole on the sacrum, and the positive pole to the os uteri, with a moderate power, for from 15 to 20 minutes each day, for two weeks. A complete cure.

CASE XI. A young man, aged about 23 years, had a gleet of about 12 months standing. When he came to me, he looked pale; his appetite was bad; it was evident from the history of the case, that debility existed, which had perhaps been induced by excessive sexual intercourse. Without doing any thing else, I advised electricity, which he used about 3 weeks, and was perfectly cured. In this case, I placed the negative pole on the end of the glans penis, and along the urethra, from the frænum backward, and the positive pole on the sacrum.

CASE XII. A young gentleman had been troubled with chronic gonorrhœa for about 12 months. I advised him to use Electricity—(he had used many other remedies)—he did so, for about one month, and the cure was completed. It was used, in this case, in the same manner as in the one of gleet.

CASE XIII. Miss L. C., of Butler county, Ala., about 17 years old, was affected with partial paralysis of the right side, from the time that she was six months old. At that time she had an attack of fever, which terminated in the affection above mentioned; she could not, by volition, control the action of her hands or feet; if she attempted to place her toes outward, they would be just as likely to turn inwardly; if she attempted to take hold of any thing, she could not grasp it at will. In this case, I also advised Electricity. I began, by applying the negative pole to the back of the neck, and the positive pole over the whole of the affected side, from the toes upward. I continued this application every night for two weeks, one hour each time. In this case, the improvement was beyond my most sanguine expectations. Miss C. can now use her foot sufficiently well to dance, and can grasp a dipper and take a drink of water, which she never could do before. I am now sanguine enough to believe, that if the treatment were continued, she would get well, or recover the use and fullness of the affected side completely.

[NOTE.—I am under promise to continue the case, and will report the result.]

I have seen a great many painful affections relieved, by the use of electricity—such as head-ache, tooth-ache, neuralgic pains about the face, neuralgia of the head, sciatica, &c., &c. In amenorrhœa, where it is caused evidently by a want of capillary circulation, electricity would be suggested to my mind as a most valuable remedy—for we have seen our Professor of Chemistry cause water to flow in a stream, through a tube, by running a current of electricity through the tube with the water, when previously this only went through by drops. We have also seen persons relieved of boils or furuncles in a few days, which had been very troublesome before.

We see in the Dublin Journal of Med. Science, May, 1849, that an obstinate case of hydrophobia was successfully cured by the use of Galvanism, applied by Dr. Rossi; also, in the same Journal, 1847, that it is announced that a case of poisoning by opium was successfully treated by the same agent. We have seen also, in the London Medical Gazette, that Archord, of Berlin, made an experiment upon himself, which, if true, is

worthy of notice: He placed a plate of Zinc in his mouth,
and a piece of silver in the anus, and having connected them
by a piece of copper wire, his bowels were immediately discharged of their contents.

We have seen that Professor Means, of the Medical College
of Georgia, (in the South. Med. and Surg. Journ., vol. 4, No. 3;
March, 1848,) says, "Under the generating power of a large
electro magnet and revolving armature, I have seen a case of
paralysis, of the muscles of the eye, cheek, lips, &c., entirely
relieved, after a few applications, of fifteen minutes each, *which
had resisted the ordinary treatment for several months previous.*"   And again, he says, page 150, "My esteemed colleague, in the Chair of Surgery, has kindly furnished me with
a case of spasmodic contraction of the flexor muscles of the
knee joint, which yielded to the *first* application of a moderate
magneto-electric current."

We have it stated by A. D. Bacon, M. D., of Massachusetts,
that he cured a case of tetanus, by the use of electro-magnetism.
Dr. Wilson Philip observes, " that in cases where there was a
failure in the secreting power of the liver, I have repeatedly
seen from Galvanism, the same effect on the biliary system,
which arises from calomel, a copious biliary discharge from
the bowels coming on a few hours after the employment of
Galvanism." (Sturgeon's Galvanism, p. 112.)

M. Martinet reports the case of a man aged 66 years, admitted into one of the clinical wards of Prof. Récamier.   For
a long time he had suffered from asthma, which, two days before his admission to the Hotel Dieu, was very much increased.
When the use of this agent (Galvanism) was begun, the asthmatic disorder was in full force ; but before the first essay was
over, the respiration was free.   Galvanism was continued
every second day, and at the end of twelve applications, the
patient was perfectly cured of his dyspnœa—he ran up a stair
of fifty steps, with a quickness and facility, and without being
at all oppressed.   (Dublin Quarterly Journal Med. Sci., May,
1847.)

ARTICLE XX.

Specific Cutaneous Eruption, produced by the internal use of Tartar Emetic. By John S. Wilson, M. D., of Air Mount, Ala. (formerly of Georgia.)

Case I. In November, 1851, J. H. was attacked with pneumonia of the upper lobe of the right lung. He was treated at first by venesection and an emetic of tart. ant. and ipecac ; the antimony was then continued, as a contra-stimulant, until the disease was subdued : it was given in doses of $\frac{1}{2}$ gr. every three hours, for about 12 days, and then in $\frac{1}{4}$ gr. doses, every four hours for three or four days longer. (The medicine was sometimes suspended during the night.) No symptoms of gastric or intestinal irritation occurred during its administration ; and the disease, though obstinate, progressed favorably under this treatment, aided by cups and blisters. But soon after convalescence was established, I was much surprised on finding the chest and abdomen thickly studded with the peculiar and characteristic pustular eruption of tartar emetic. The pustules were at first small, but they gradually enlarged and spread, extending themselves over the arms and forearms. They continued much longer than they usually do, when the tart. emetic is applied externally, and is discontinued after the crop of pustules have appeared. I did not learn that he had ever used the tart. emetic ointment, previous to his attack. The eruption was *so well marked* and characteristic, that I cannot entertain a doubt as to its nature, although I have seen but one similar case during several years' free use of the remedy.

Case II. In January last, I treated Mrs. L. for acute catarrh, with the tart. ant., giving it nearly in the same way as in the first case—the only exception being that the medicine was used but three or four days, when the subsidence of the disease rendered its continuance no longer necessary. This patient had used the tart. emetic ointment, to the spine, for a nervous affection, many months previously ; and in her case, the eruption was confined to that part : she was perfectly conscious of its nature, for she said that she experienced the very same feelings that she did when she applied it locally.

Remarks.—Authors mention an eruption on the mucous

membrane of the mouth and fauces, as an occasional effect of
the long-continued use of tart. emetic, and they may notice
this cutaneous eruption ; but I do not remember seeing any
thing of the kind in my reading, nor can I find any such, by
referring to the works at my command: but my opportunity
for consulting authors being limited, at this time, I may be
mistaken in supposing that they have not noticed it, and it
may be more common than I imagine. If it be common, it
may be made available in practice, as an evidence of saturation, by warning us not to persist in the antimonial, for fear of
bad consequences—if it be unusual, (as I suppose it is,) its occasional occurrence should still be borne in mind, lest we fall
into errors of diagnosis, by mistaking this eruption, for itch or
something else, as a practitioner of medicine did in one of the
above cases. Another interesting feature of these cases is
this: they add to the list of disagreeable effects sometimes resulting from the use of this truly valuable article. It is true
that the unpleasantness produced by the tart. emetic in the
above cases, is of small moment, when compared with the
"fatal effects," so strikingly described by Dr. Wm. M. Boling;
(vide his article in this Journal, Jan. 1852, taken from the Am.
Journ. Med. Sciences,) but still it *is* a disagreeable effect, and
it should make us cautious in using this medicine after the Ra-
sorian plan.

While on this subject, I would remark that I have never
ventured on the use of tart. emetic, in enormous doses, regardless of emesis or catharsis, as recommended by the Italian
school of contra-stimulant physicians: I give it in pneumonia,
in small doses, regulating these by the effects on the stomach
and bowels, as I would in any other disease. I have thus been
able to avoid, so far, the very bad effects mentioned by Dr.
Boling, but still, notwithstanding this cautious use of the remedy, I must confess that I have been in sight of the breakers;
and I think I have seen a few cases of inflammatory pneumonia, become complicated with intestinal irritation, and assume
a typhoid type, by the use of the antimony in the cautious manner above described. But in this I might have been mistaken,
as there was a prevailing tendency to adynamic fevers. While
I adduce these examples of the disagreeable effects of the

tart. ant , I must be allowed, in conclusion, to add my tributo to its merits, for I consider it superior to all other remedies in the treatment of pulmonic affections.

PART II.

Eclectic Department.

On Healthy and Morbid Menstruation. By J. Henry Bennett, M. D., late Physician-Accoucheur to the Western
General Dispensary, etc.

[Continued from Page 289.]

Dysmenorrhœa.—By the term dysmenorrhœa, is implied painful and difficult menstruation. Most females experience slight uterine and ovarian pains, accompanied by slight exter-nal tenderness in the hypogastric region, with or without aching pain in the back, for the first few hours previous to and after the advent of menstruation. When these feelings are not usual-ly experienced, they will often manifest themselves accidental-ly, as the result of over-fatigue or mental emotion, or without any appreciable cause. To such conditions, however, the ap-pellation of dysmenorrhœa cannot be applied ; it must be re-served for those cases in which a very considerable amount of pain is experienced, either invariably or by exception.

Dysmenorrhœa may exist—1stly, Permanently as a consti-tutional condition, or accidentally or temporarily in connexion with general morbid states. 2dly, It may be the result of the presence of uterine or ovarian disease, or of a contracted state of the cervical canal.

Constitutional Dysmenorrhœa.—This form of dysmenor-rhœa is often observed in the females whose uterus appears na-turally predisposed to congestion, and with whom menstruation is very abundant and is preceded and followed by a white leucor-rhœal discharge. It is met with also when this is not the case. It may be limited to the first day or two, or extend throughout the entire period. In such women the dysmenorrhœa is evi-dently functional, the result of the distention produced by the over-congestion, or of a peculiar susceptibility of the uterine innervation. The pain is by no means the same in intensity at every period, but varies according to hygienic and moral cir-cumstances. Under the influence of fatigue, excitement, or anxiety, and frequently without any appreciable cause, the dysmenorrhœa will become much more intense than usual, and last a much longer time. In some instances I have known it to exist every second period only. This form of dysmenor-rhœa may persist with varying intensity throughout the entire duration of the menstrual function, although occasionally it is modified or even removed by marriage, by parturition, or by the mere influence of time. Constitutional dysmenorrhœa can scarcely be considered a morbid condition, although verging on disease. It may be said to be characterized by its com-mencing with the menstrual function, by the entire and com-plete absence of all uterine symptoms in the interval of the monthly period, and by the general similarity of the menstrual epochs. Although one period may be, and often is, more pain-ful than another, on comparing menstruation during any two given periods of several months, the amount of pain suffered, and the mode of manifestation of the function, are found to be pretty nearly the same. If a permanent increase of pain oc-curs, it is a suspicious circumstance, as indicating the possible or even probable existence of some inflammatory condition of the cervix uteri, to which these females, as we have seen, are peculiarly liable, or of some morbid ovarian condition.

Accidental dysmenorrhœa.—Dysmenorrhœa may occur *ac-cidentally* in a female who usually menstruates without pain, as the result of over-excitement or fatigue, from exposure to cold, or as the result of some temporary disturbance in the general health. When this is the case, the dysmenorrhœa is probably occasioned by a disturbed or congestive state of uter-ine circulation, or by an exaggeration of the nervous suscepti-bility of the uterine organs. It is characterized by its merely temporary existence, and by the fact of its passing away with the cause that has produced it.

Inflammatory dysmenorrhœa.—Non-constitutional dysmen-orrhœa, however, according to my experience, is much more frequently the result of inflammatory disease of the uterine organs, and principally of the cervix, than, as is generally sup-posed, of functional derangement, or of nervous susceptibility. When menstruation, naturally easy, becomes permanently painful, or when, naturally but slightly painful, it becomes ex-tremely so, we are warranted in looking for local disease. Such a change *does not take place without a cause,* and that cause is, generally speaking, inflammation of the cervix or body of the uterus; dysmenorrhœa being one of the most prominent and most ordinary symptoms of that disease.

This fact applies to the virgin as well as to the married fe-male, and is of extreme importance, as affording a key to those extreme cases of dysmenorrhœa, accompanied sometimes by spinal irritation and hysterical epileptiform convulsions, which appear to resist every form of treatment, and are alike distressing to the patient, her friends, and her medical attendant. Since I have ascertained that such is the case, nearly all the instances of *extreme* dysmenorrhœa in the unmarried female that have come under my notice have proved to be of this description, and, however intractable before, have yielded as soon as a proper antiphlogistic treatment has been adopted.

The history of two patients formerly under my care, which I have elsewhere published, strongly illustrates these facts, and their importance. In the younger female, a young, unmarried lady, dysmenorrhœa from the first was the prominent symptom. She had always suffered *slightly* from painful menstruation, but not carried so far as to inconvenience her. About two years before I saw her, the dysmenorrhœa became much more intense, and at last so agonizing, as immediately to produce hysterical epileptiform convulsions, which ended in partial paralysis. In the other lady, who was thirty years of age, and the mother of a family, the uterine inflammation commenced six years before, with a laborious confinement. The most prominent symptom with her, also, was dysmenorrhœa, which increased rapidly, so as at last to bring on intense convulsions at every monthly period, and thus to occasion partial paralysis of the left side, as in the former case. Both these patients were considered to be merely suffering from hysteria, spinal irritation, and functional derangement of the uterus, and had been treated for several years, solely in accordance with these views; whereas, in reality, they were labouring under severe inflammatory ulceration of the uterine neck.

In these cases the dysmenorrhœa is a mere symptom of the inflammatory condition of the uterine organs, and is only to be removed by their restoration to a healthier state. Generally speaking, it is the neck of the uterus that is found to be the seat of the disease that occasions the dysmenorrhœa. The latter is nearly always very intense when the body of the uterus is affected. Sub-acute inflammation of the ovaries may also give rise to dysmenorrhœa, but I cannot agree with Dr. Tilt that it is a frequent cause. This difference of opinion is connected with that which exists between me and my esteemed friend respecting the frequency of sub-acute inflammation of the ovaries, inasmuch as I consider the symptoms which Dr. Tilt supposes to indicate the existence of such inflammation—pain and tenderness in the ovarian region—to be merely symptomatic of disease of the uterus or of its neck, in nineteen cases out of twenty in which they are observed.

We may connect with inflammatory dysmenorrhœa that form which has been described under the head of pseudo-mem-

branous, and which is characterized by the expulsion of shreds
and casts of plastic lymph from the cavity of the uterus. I
believe that the formation of these membranes coincides almost
invariably with the present or past existence of uterine inflammation.   In other words, I have found, in the great majority of
cases of this description that have come under my observation
that there has been at first inflammatory disease, although the
removal of this disease has not always freed the patient from the
liability to the formation of the pseudo-membranous casts.   It'
would appear as if habit alone sufficed in some instances to
perpetuate their formation, or at least their occasional formation
even after the removal of inflammation, once they have occurred under its influence.   M. Pouchet states that in all females,
even in virgins, a delicate decided membrane or cast is formed
in the cavity of the uterus at every menstruation, and is thrown
out about the tenth day.   If so, the deciduous pseudo-membranes of dysmenorrhœa may be considered as merely an exaggeration of a natural condition, but occurring, generally speaking, only under the influence of inflammatory disease.   The
expulsion of these psendo-membranous shreds is always preceded by an aggravation of the uterine pains, which are evidently
occasioned by the efforts of the uterus to get rid of the casts
formed in its cavity.   That the difficulty of expulsion is partly
the cause of the uterine tormina, is proved by the fact that I
have repeatedly relieved them by dilating the cervical canal in
the interval of menstruation, in females who continued to expel pseudo-membranes, and to suffer after the removal of all
uterine disease.

Inflammatory dysmenorrhœa may be said to be characterized
by the development of pain as a permanent menstrual condition, in a female previously free from it, or by the increase of
pain experienced constitutionally, but in a less marked degree.
In other words as pain during menstruation may exist constitutionally without local lesions, its value as a symptom of disease
can only be ascertained by comparing the past state of the patient with the present.   Generally speaking, there are other
uterine and general symptoms present *during the interval* of
menstruation which tend to assist the diagnosis. This, however
is not always the case.   I recently attended a young unmarried
lady, only twenty-one, who had suffered ever since the menses
appeared, at seventeen, from severe dysmenorrhœa.   The pain
was indeed so severe, that for the first five days she was always
obliged to keep her bed, writhing in agony, and for eight days
out of every lunar month she was confined to her room.   In
the interval she had not a uterine symptom, and beyond a certain amount of general languor and anœmia, which the mere

physical pain she had to go through at short intervals sufficiently explained, the general health did not appear to have much
suffered. Previous to my seeing her, she had been under constant medical treatment, and the total inefficacy of the remedial
means usually resorted to in such cases had been over and over
again tested. Under such circumstances, after treating her
without any result for sub-acute ovaritis, I considered myself
warranted in making an examination of the uterine organs,
being impressed with the idea that dysmenorrhœa of so severe
a character, and so rebellious to general treatment, must be
occasioned by some local morbid condition, and probably by
congenital contraction. To my surprise, I found the cervix
the seat of decided-inflammatory ulceration. I may also add
that the dysmenorrhœa has quite subsided under the influence
of the appropriate treatment of the local disease. This case,
however, is an exceptional one, from the entire absence of all
uterine symptoms in the interval of menstruation, and shows
the difficulties that occasionally surround the diagnosis of these
forms of uterine disease.

Physical dysmenorrhœa.—Dysmenorrhœa may also depend
as demonstrated by Dr. Mackintosh of Edinburgh, on a physical imperfection of the uterine neck, on contraction of the
os internum, of the canal which constitutes the cavity of the
cervix. This contraction may be either congenital, or the result of inflammation. The peculiar character of the dysmenorrhœa, when caused by congenital contraction, is the absence
of *any* uterine symptom during the interval of menstruation,
and intense agonizing pain for a few hours before the flow of
blood appears, either then disappearing, or lasting throughout
the period ; these pains commencing with menstruation in early
youth. If they are occasioned by inflammation, there are the
same symptoms at the time of menstruation, but there is not
the same immunity from uterine symptoms in the interval of
the catamenia.

The cause of the pain experienced under these circumstances is evident. The cavity of the non-pregnant healthy uterus
not containing more than about ten or eleven drops of fluid, as
soon as the catamenial secretion commences from the lining
membrane of the uterine cavity, unless the blood find a free exit
through the os internum and the cavity of the cervix, it distends
the uterus, and gives rise to great pain. The obstruction may
merely be at the os internum, spasmodically contracted ; in
which case, as soon as it has been overcome, the blood escapes
freely, and pain disappears. But if the os internum, is permanently contracted, or the contraction exists in the cervical canal, the pain may continue throughout the catamenial period.

A contracted state of the upper part of the cervical canal, or of the os internum, is not, I believe, an unfrequent complication of inflammation of the cervix, from the swelling and hypertrophy of the substance of the organ which it occasions. This remark, however, does not apply to the *inflamed region* of the cervical canal, which is uniformly dilated by the existence of inflammation.

I do not, however, think that Dr. Simpson's criticism of the existence of contraction of the os internum is entirely to be depended upon. Dr. Simpson believes, if I am right in my interpretation of his views, that unless the uterine sound pass without effort into the uterine cavity, there is contraction of the os internum. Now the careful examination with the sound of many hundred females has led me, as I have elsewhere explained, to a different conclusion. There evidently exists at the os internum a kind of muscular sphincter formed by a strong band of the circular muscular fibres of the cervix, and destined to close the uterus during the latter stages of pregnancy. Generally speaking, the sphincter, in the natural state, is sufficiently closed to prevent the uterine sound passing into the cavity of the uterus, unless a considerable amount of pressure be exercised. In nearly all the females I examine, in the interval of menstruation, the sound passes easily along the cervical cavity, but stops at the os internum ; and that when there is no reason whatever to suppose the existence of a morbid coarctation.

It appears to me, on the contrary, as I have elsewhere stated, that a free communication between the cervical and uterine cavities, allowing the *easy* introduction of the uterine sound, is generally an anomalous condition, indicating the existence of disease, unless observed soon after menstruation, when the os internum relaxes, or soon after parturition, when it has not yet had time to recover its normally contracted state. The principal morbid conditions in which I have observed a free communication between the two cavities, are inflammation and uterine tumours. If the inflammation which exists at the os uteri, and in the lower part of the cervical cavity, ascends as far as the os internum, it appears to release the muscular contractility of that region. The os internum is always open when the inflammation passes into the uterine cavity, and implicates its lining membrane. The same effect is also produced by the development of the uterine cavity, through the formation of tumours in the substance of the uterus, or from any other cause ; the os internum gradually opening as the uterus enlarges, probably by the same mechanism as in pregnancy. This is so generally the case, that the fact of the uterine sound penetrating easily through the os internum into an enlarged uterine cavity, may be considered a valuable symptom of the existence of such tumours, to add to those with which we are already acquainted.

Extreme dysmenorrhœa from congenital contraction of the cervical canal and os internum, independent of inflammation, is, I believe, of *rare occurrence.* This is a fortunate circumstance, as it is most embarrassing to treat, requiring an amount of interference with the uterine organs which it is very painful to have to propose to an unmarried female. Dilation of the contracted cervical canal is, however, sometimes the only means we have of remedying an amount of suffering at the catamenial period, so extreme as to render life nearly a burden, and as to re-act deeply on the general health.

A very strongly marked illustration of this fact occurred to me some time ago, in dispensary practice :—A young female, aged twenty-two, was sent to me by a medical practitioner in town, for dysmenorrhœa. It appeared that she had suffered in the most excruciating manner at every menstrual period, since the menses first appeared, at the age of eighteen. The pain always continued without intermission throughout the three days and nights that the catamenia lasted, and was of so severe a character that she never closed her eyes, and was confined to bed for the whole time. She had generally been under medical treatment, and the usual remedies had been repeatedly tried—anti-spasmodics, anodynes, sedatives, &c. Laterly she had been taking very large doses of opium without the slightest benefit. On inquiry, I found that after the menstruation ceased the pain gradually subsided, and that during the menstrual interval she was perfectly well, and was then *altogether* free from any uterine symptom. In appearance she was rather stout and healthy-looking. The hymen was intact, but dilatable, and I was thus enabled carefully to examine the neck of the uterus, which I found perfectly natural in size, colour, texture and density, and free from any tenderness. The cavity of the cervix, however, was evidently very narrow, not even admitting a very small-sized bougie. Thinking this might be the cause of the dysmenorrhœa, I at once decided on dilating it. This I effected to a considerable extent in the course of the three weeks which ensued before the next monthly period, by means of small sponge tents. I had not, however, dilated the os internum sufficiently to admit of the sound penetrating into the cavity of the uterus, and was consequently rather surprised to hear from the patient, after a week's absence, that not only had the catamenia been more abundant than usual, but that she had been entirely free from pain. The dilatation was continued irregularly, and as the next period was equally free from pain I ceased all treatment, although the os internum was still undilated; at least, it was only sufficiently open to admit of the entrance of the small extremity of the wax bougie.

The dysmenorrhœa which accompanies inflammation of the cervix, is evidently increased in some cases by the narrowing of the cervical canal, which the inflammation occasions, inasmuch as it may persist in a mitigated form after the inflammatory disease has subsided, and be readily removed by dilatation. The persistence of dysmenorrhœa from this cause after the removal of uterine inflammation, is not, however, of itself sufficient to necessitate or even to warrant dilatation of the cervical canal being resorted to, except in some special cases, until a few months have been allowed to elapse. After the removal of inflammatory disease of the uterus and of its cervix, a resolutive action is set up by nature,·which will often soften and relax the still swollen and indurated tissues, and thus open the cervical canal, and render mechanical dilatation unnecessary. It is therefore well to give the patient the benefit of this chance of recovery without further surgical treatment.

Whatever may be the cause of dysmenorrhœa, the mode in which the menstrual secretion takes place is modified by its existence: instead of a flow of bright blood, regular and continuous, although generally increasing by exercise and diminishing by rest, we have a dark, interrupted, clotted discharge. After severe uterine pains which may last many hours, and are often accompanied by tenderness and swelling in the ovarian regions, and pain in the back and down the thighs, more or less dark, clotted blood is thrown out. Its expulsion is generally followed by relief, and by a freer flow for a while, when it again diminishes, and the same ordeal again takes place. Sometimes the interruption will be complete for one, two, or three days, the pain subsiding with the menstrual flux, and returning when it again makes its appearance. The venous condition of the menstrual secretion shows plainly that, either from inflammation, congestion, or some other cause, the uterine circulation is defective, the blood stagnating in the vessels of the uterus, remaining in its cavity, and distending it after it has been secreted.

Treatment.—Constitutional dysmenorrhœa may be palliated in its attacks, but can seldom be removed by medical treatment. A great deal of subsequent uterine disease would, however, be spared to those young females who unfortunately present it, were mothers more generally aware that its existence constitutes throughout life a strong predisposition to uterine inflammation, and that they cannot take too great care of such of their daughters as suffer from it. For such young females the discipline of public schools may be said to be nearly always too severe, and often to lay the foundation for much future physical and mental misery. That this must be the case, will be easily understood when we reflect that the domestic treatment of this form of dysmenorrhœa consists principally in *rest* and *warmth*. Females who suffer habitually from dismenorrhœa, whatever their age, should remain quietly at home, taking care to preserve themselves from atmospheric vicissitudes during the first day or two of menstruation, which is the period during which the pain is mostly felt. A warm hip-bath will often be found useful. If the pains are very decided it is even best to confine the sufferer to bed, and to apply warm linseed poultices to the lower abdominal region, a valuable and simple mode of soothing pain.

In mere constitutional dysmenorrhœa, these simple means nearly always suffice to render the pain very bearable. If they do not produce relief, that fact alone constitutes a suspicious circumstance, and should induce the medical attendant to scrutinize narrowly the state of his patient, lest there should be some morbid or physical cause.

In severe dysmenorrhœa, connected with uterine disease, the only *efficacious* treatment is that of the cause of the disease which occasions the dysmenorrhœa. As time is required, however, we are often called upon even in these cases, to treat the dysmenorrhœa as a symptom ; and, warmth and rest failing, recourse must be had to medicinal agents. By far the most efficacious remedy with which I am acquainted, is the injection of laudanum, or any other preparation of opium, into the bowel. From fifteen to thirty minims of laudanum, mixed with a little warm water, should be injected into the rectum, and will generally exercise, if retained, as much influence in soothing the uterine pain as would double the quantity taken by the mouth. Moreover, the nausea and headache which opiates occasion are much less likely to be produced when they are thus administered. If the first opiate injection is not retained, a second, half an hour later, will generally be more successful. I have also found chloroform of great value in these cases. It may be inhaled or administered by the mouth in doses of from twenty to forty minims, mixed with mucilage, the yolk of an egg, or with camphor, which favours its suspension in water. I have given it by injection, but with less success, as it appears, generally speaking, to irritate the rectal mucous membrane, and is consequently not retained. When it is retained, the sedative effect is nearly always effectually produced. Although chloroform may thus often be resorted to with great benefit in dysmenorrhœa, I do not find that as much reliance can be placed in it as in opiates.

There are various other medicinal agents, principally anti-spasmodics and narcotics, which may be administered with benefit in dysmenorrhœa. We may mention more particularly the various ethers, and especially sulphuric ether, hyoscyamus, belladonna, musk, valerian and camphor. It must not, however, be forgotten that these remedies are mere temporary palliatives; that dysmenorrhœa, when constant and not constitutional, nearly invariably recognizes some physical cause—generally speaking, uterine or ovarian inflammation, and that it is this cause which we must find out, and remove, during the interval of menstruation.

-It is the fact of dysmenorrhœa being so frequently caused by inflammatory disease, that explains the success which often attends bloodletting, both general and local, and which has induced so many authors to recommend it, although unaware of the pathological state which it relieves. General bloodletting acts by revulsion; whilst local bloodletting directly relieves the congested and embarrassed abdominal circulation. I seldom, if ever, resort to general bleeding in dysmenorrhœa, because the relief which it gives is obtained at too great a sacrifice of the strength of the patient, and cannot, moreover, be depended upon. A few leeches applied to the groin, or, better still, to the neck of the uterus, when possible, if the discharge is scanty or temporarily arrested, is much more likely to mitigate the pain, and with less loss to the economy. Purgatives, which are frequently useful, act in the same way as leeches, by depleting the abdominal circulation. Some authors—amongst others, Dr. Gooch—have considered dysmenorrhœa to be frequently akin to rheumatism, and have recommended colchicum, guaiacum, and other medicines usually given in rheumatic affections. That the uterus may be the seat of such an affection, is undeniable; but I am persuaded that its frequency has been greatly exaggerated, as likewise that of irritable uterus. Indeed these two conditions may be said to have been, to a great extent, mere theoretical creations, destined to account for pathological conditions, the real nature and meaning of which has, until recently, been a mystery to the profession.

It will be seen, by what precedes, that dysmenorrhœa is by no means so simple a disease, or so easy to treat, as has been generally supposed, involving, as it often does, the question, whether or not local disease requiring local treatment may not exist as the real cause of the morbid state. If it resists all general treatment, it is probably the result of such disease, and the health and happiness of a young female are seriously endangered. Of course the medical practitioner has a duty to perform to his patient, before which all scruples must be made to succumb. I, however, here repeat, what I have so often said elsewhere, especially with reference to unmarried females, that nothing can warrant manual or surgical investigation and treatment, but months, or even years, of unsuccessful treatment, and the conviction with the latter, that unless they be resorted to, the case must be abandoned as hopeless. I would also repeat the advice given in my work on Uterine Inflammation, that a consultation should always be held first when the patient is unmarried, to decide the point, whether the examination of the uterine organs be warranted and necessary.

[*To be continued.*]

External Diuretics. By D. J. CAIN, M. D.

In reporting the three following cases, illustrative of the effects of external diuretics, I would remark that it must be obvious that the conditions in which they are indicated and would prove beneficial, are identical with those in which their internal exhibition would be resorted to. In cases of local or general dropsy, resulting from structural lesion of the heart, liver, mesenteric glands, peritoneum, etc , their effect can, as a matter of course, be but palliative.

The employment of diuretics *externally*, instead of *internally*, dates only a few years back. According to Dr. Christison, the idea of substituting the one for the other originated with a French physician, who reported several succesful cases from their use. But it would seem that the medical world did not adopt this mode of practice, for we hear nothing more of the subject until the appearance of Dr. Christison's paper in the Edinburgh Monthly Journ. of Med. Sci., of last November. With the contents of that communication, all present are doubtless familiar. So favourable was the opinion expressed by him, in reference to their action, that I determined to use them in that manner, in the first case of effusion that should present itself to me.

I was soon furnished an opportunity, by a patient who was admitted into the Marine Hospital, Jan. 28th, 1851, labouring under extensive inflammation of the medius finger of the right hand, with caries of all the phalanges, rendering amputation necessary. This was performed while he was in a state of complete anæsthesia from chloroform.

" While the healing process was going on, I perceived that his abdomen began to enlarge, and, on examination, fluctuation

was very evident. On inquiry into his antecedent history, I
learned that his general health had not been previously very
good ; he had been troubled with diarrhœa from childhood, but
he had had violent attacks, from time to time, during the last
five years, and his bowels were, at the time I speak of, much
disordered, the stools being more or less fluid and frequent, and
of a white or ash colour, denoting inactivity in the hepatic
organ.   He also told me that, about four years ago, he had a
hydropic collection in his abdomen for which he was treated in
Baltimore, and from which he recovered in about a month.   I
prescribed for him small doses of taraxacum, with a view to
its effect upon the liver, and cinchona with iron as a tonic.
The swelling increased to so great a degree, in the course of
two weeks, as to sensibly impede respiration.   I now began
the administration of watermelon seed tea, and continued it for
a few days, without any great increase in the quantity of urine.
It was still scanty and red.

"I then used the formula recommended by Dr. Christison,
viz : equal parts of the tinctures of digitalis, squill and soap of
which compound two drachms were rubbed upon the abdomen
three times daily.   In forty-eight hours, the effects were manifested by a considerable increase in the quantity passed.   By
the fourth day, I found him discharging between three and four
quarts, by measure, which reached nearly five quarts, by the
7th, when the whole dropsical collection had disappeared.

"After keeping up the action of the kidneys for two or three
days longer, the diuretic was discontinued, and the urine began
to diminish in quantity.

"It may be well to observe here, that, during the use of the
diuretic, I caused the patient to be restricted to about one pint
of fluid for the twenty-four hours—thus carrying out the plan
I have always followed in allowing the patient the smallest
quantity of drink, for the reason that, if the watery portion of
the blood is evacuated by diuretics, either alone or by cathartics,
and its place is not supplied by the introduction of water through
the stomach, the blood will become inspissated, and, in accordance with physical laws, an endosmotic movement will go on
from the rarer to the denser fluid : that is to say, the dropsical
effusion will permeate the tissues, enter the blood-vessels, (the
veins,) and will be carried into the circulation, where it will
dilute the blood.

"But, although the effused fluid had disappeared, the cause
was not removed, and, after an interval of about two weeks,
his abdomen again began to swell.   I again resorted to the diuretic, but this time with by no means such marked effects, the
quantity of urine not being materially increased, and, after using

it about two weeks, it was abandoned. I then made trial of the digitalis, squill and colchicum internally, which was attended by complete failure.

"On careful examination of the patient, and from a consideration of his antecedent history, I diagnosticated chronic (perhaps scrofulous) inflammation of the peritoneum, with, perhaps, obstruction to the portal circulation. The fluid continued to increase, and tapping was had recourse to, in order to relieve him. About three gallons were drawn off. It re-accumulated rapidly, and the patient died on the — April. At the necropsy, we found extensive and violent inflammation of the visceral peritoneum; slight enlargement of several of the mesenteric glands; and, lastly, an obstruction to the circulation of the blood through the vena portæ, caused by two large tubercular or scrofulous masses.

"From the lesions observed after death, (and which confirmed my diagnosis,) it is obvious that the diuretic could have been of no permanent benefit.

"Case II. Peter Rose was admitted into the Hospital, March 31st, 1851, laboring under intermittent fever. Being at the time sick, Dr. F. P. Porcher, who visited it for me, succeeded, in a day or two, in checking the fever. On resuming my duties, a few days after, I found that his abdomen began to swell, and I soon detected fluctuation—ascites—due, in all probability, to the engorgement of the liver and spleen, resulting from the repeated paroxysms of the fever. Being encouraged by the success that attended their exhibition, the first time, in case No. 1, I immediately resorted to the use of the diuretics externally. The effect was very prompt in this case as in the foregoing. In less than forty-eight hours, the quantity of urine was notably augmented, and, by the fourth or fifth day, he was passing upwards of a gallon per diem. The hydropic accumulation had entirely disappeared by the ninth day. This patient I exhibited to several of the Counsellors of the South .Carolina Medical Association.

"Case III. George Bond was admitted, January 22d, 1851, to be treated for congestion of one or both kidneys, with the ordinary symptoms, such as discharge of blood, etc., the result, apparently, of cold. Cupping, blistering, soda, sweet spirits nitre, watermelon seed tea, digitalis, colchicum, etc., variously combined, were used, as counter-irritants, and as depletives of the kidneys, but with partial effect. I then substituted the vegetable astringent, tannin, without any decided benefit. I gave him turpentine, and, in a few days, the hemorrhage ceased. From time to time, however, it returned, from imprudence on the part of the patient, such as a fatiguing walk, getting the

fect wet, etc., showing that the congestion had not been completely resolved. In this state of the case, I thought that the
diuretics, externally applied, might be of some service. They
were used, consisting of the substances above named, with the
addition of colchicum, which suggested itself to my mind as
likely to assist the action of the other ingredients. Its effect was
soon shown by an abundant discharge of urine ; but, so great
was the action set up in the kidneys that it recalled the hemorrhage, which ceased on the discontinuance of the diuretic."

I have also used it in two other cases, with decided advantage : the one an old lady, who had an almost complete suppression of urine, from indigestion ; the other, a lady of middle
age, who had anasarca from the impoverishment of the blood
in chronic diarrhœa.

A medical friend informs me that, at my suggestion, he has
employed it in a case of scarlatinal dropsy, and in three other
cases of effusion, from various causes, with happy effect.

The external application of diuretics possesses, it seems to
me, a manifest superiority over the internal use in this, that it
may be employed in all states of the system, without causing
any general or local disturbance, even if it does no good.
Every one is aware that the stomach is sometimes so irritable
or weak, or the bowels so relaxed, etc., no medicines can be
retained by it, or, if retained by the stomach, they may increase
the action of the bowels. Beyond this, no advantage is claimed
for the external over the internal use. It appears, however,
from one of Prof. Christison's cases, that the diuretics succeeded externally, when the same combination failed internally.

I have watched closely the action of the diuretics, when applied externally, and have observed but the single effect upon
the kidneys.

The combination recommended by Prof. Christison is a good
one ; but other substances may be added, or they may be combined in different proportions. To the tinctures of soap, digitalis
and squills, may be added vin colchic., tinct. cantharides, etc.

I have deviated somewhat from the quantities and the intervals spoken of by him. He used but ʒii. or ʒiii. of the compound, rubbed upon the abdomen three times daily. In two of
the cases above reported, I ordered from ℥ss. to ℥i., four, five,
and even six times in the twenty-four hours. In one case, Prof.
Christison simply applied a linen rag, saturated with tincture
digitalis, upon the abdomen, and with equally marked benefit.

I have observed, while experimenting with diuretics in this
way, the fact that, when they fail *externally*, (as they have, in
two or three instances, since the above cases were treated,)
the same, or other combinations, invariably fail *internally*.

In mentioning this circumstance to two medical gentlemen of this city, they remembered that the same thing had occurred in their trials with them. Thus, it would seem that the kidneys are sometimes wholly insusceptible of the influence of this class of agents.—[*Charleston Med. Jour. and Review.*

On a Novel Method of Treating Diseased Joints. By Mr. GAY.

[The following synopsis of a paper read before the Medical Society of London, November 15th, 1851, bears so close an analogy on a mode of treatment set forth in previous numbers of this Journal, that we are constrained to copy it entire, as we find it in a late number of the London Medical Gazette.— *Ed. N. Y. Jour. Med.*]

Mr. Gay commenced his paper by observing, that to the present time there was no department of surgery in which the powers of art have been comparatively so feeble as when applied to the relief of those diseases of the joints, which, from their results, might be termed destructive. Hence, let the articular surfaces of the joint be bereft of their cartilages, a sinus or two be formed around it, and the health of the patient show symptoms of exhaustion, and the joint, and probably the whole limb, is doomed to amputation. He adverted to the causes of the removal of the cartilage from joints, and gave it as his opinion, that in addition to primary synovial and osseous disease, the cartilages were sometimes removed by absorption, in consequence of degeneration of their own tissue, without any traceable affection of the contiguous textures. In all cases of removal of cartilage the tissue degenerates into a kind of fibrous texture, antecedent to the final process ; and as portions of cartilage were sometimes observed to be removed without any apparent disorder of either the synovial or osseous surfaces, and, moreover, as cartilage was known to be inadequate to its own repair, Mr. Gay thinks it most probable that the portions of cartilage so removed had first spontaneously degenerated, and then become absorbed. Mr. Gay went on to remark, that if a series of joints be examined in which the removal of the cartilages is taking place, the appearances will be as follows: If it be presumed to follow disease of the synovial capsule, the cartilage will be found in some to maintain its connection with the bone, whilst it is thinned by absorption at its free surface. In others, however, the bone is found inflamed at various points of its connection with the cartilage ; and at these points the cartilage is loose, and may be peeled off, so that portions of thin attached and unattached cartilages are found in the

same joint.   When entirely denuded, or almost so, the surfaces
of the bones may exhibit simply a state of increased vascularity,
which precedes the effusion of plastic lymph for the purposes
of reparation by anchylosis, or may be observed to be in a condition of ulceration.   This ulceration may exist as a simple
abrasion, or be of considerable depth ; but there is generally a
uniformity in this respect over the whole surface.   With this
state of ulceration there is also a softening of the osseous structure, and frequently disintegration ; the contents of the joint
consisting of broken up cartilage, and osseous and other debris
together, or osseous matter, with ichorous or sanious discharge.
When the disease originates in the bone, as in by far the greater
number of cases, in Mr. Gay's opinion, it does, the separation
of the cartilage is effected by another process, which he terms
" shedding," and the cartilage is then reduced to the condition
of a foreign body within the joint.   Shreds of cartilage thus
situated in a joint may be observed after months and even years
of disease ; and as, on the other hand, its separation from the
articular extremity of the bones may be accomplished in an
almost incredibly short period of time, it is fair to infer that the
time thus passed must have been occupied in the process of its
extrusion from the joint, and that this is accomplished, neither
by ulceration nor absorption, but disintegration by, and solution in, the discharges of the joint.   But the bone itself being
diseased, adds its exfoliated or disintegrated particles to the
cartilaginous debris, which, with its own discharges, constitute
generally the contents of a joint in which the disease commenced in its bony elements.   The result of these discharges is
to set up inflammation in the sound textures contiguous to the
joint, and general systematic irritation.   Sinuses form around
the joint ; the disease extends itself ; the ligaments become ulcerated ; the spongy tissue of the bones infiltrated with pus,
and broken down ; osteophytes form around the heads of the
bones ; abscesses extend themselves into the surrounding soft
parts, separating the different structures, and setting up unhealthy and destructive action amongst them ; and, in short, a
climax is arrived at in which the local mischief reacts upon the
constitution, and life is only to be preserved at the sacrifice of
the joint or of the limb.   Mr. Gay inferred from these remarks,
of which only an imperfect abstract has been given—

1. That there appears to be no reason why disease effecting
the constituents of a joint should be slower in their course of
reparation than diseases of any other part or structure.

2. That the removal of cartilage from its osseous connection
in a joint is occasionally effected by absorption, but most frequently by a process of "shedding," or exfoliation.

3. That cartilages thus shed become, by their being pent up in a joint, sources of local and constitutional irritation, and thus promote disease in the osseous and other structures appertaining to a joint, supposing that such affections do not exist primarily ; and in case they do, these cartilages, by the same influence, maintain and extend these diseases also.

4. That the natural outlets for these discharges, the sinuses, are inadequate for that purpose.

5. That therefore the exfoliated contents of a diseased joint have to be minutely broken up by, or dissolved in, the discharges of the joint, in order to their removal ; processes which are necessarily of a very protracted order, and which account for the tardiness in general characteristic of joint diseases.

6. That the exfoliated contents of a joint, after its cartilages have been removed, and even after extensive diseases has been set up in the bones and other textures, have only to be completely removed, and processes of reparation will, in the majority of instances, immediately commence.

Mr. Gay then alluded to the usual modes of treatment, and remarked, that the operation of resection of a joint is not only a useless but an unphilosophical mode of treatment for diseased joints.   In the first place, primary disease is generally limited to one of the articular extremities of the joint ; it is therefore a useless mutilation to remove more than that disease, supposing the operation were for a moment admissible.   But, moreover, dissections show that disease originating in bone, when arrived at that stage at which the operation of resection is generally employed, has extended itself far beneath the surface, and frequently along the shaft for a third of its whole length, so that resection cannot accomplish its purpose, which must be manifestly the removal of all disease.   The plan Mr. Gay recommends, then, is free and deep incisions made along each side of a joint, so as to lay open its cavity freely, and to allow of no discharges being by any possibility retained within its cavity. They should be made of such a length, and so treated, that they do not heal into the form of sinuses.   They should be made, if possible, one on either side of the joint, and in the direction of the long axis of the limb.   They should extend into the abscesses in the soft parts so as to lay them open.   If sinuses exist, the incisions should be carried through them, if this can be done without departing from a slight curve.   If either of the bones be carious or necrosed, the incisions should be carried deeply into such bones, so as to allow the dead particles of bone to escape.   Ligaments which stand in the way of free discharge from the joint should be cut through.   Of course important vessels should be avoided. The wounds should be kept open by pledgets of lint, and free sup puration encouraged. The constitutional powers have in each case rallied immediately after the operation; and as the discharges from the joint have altered in character and become healthy, which they in general do in the course of two or three weeks, these become invigorated, and improve with the improving joint. Mr. Gay then narrated some cases in corroboration of his views: Peter D——, aged thirty-eight, admitted into the Royal Free Hospital in 1842, for diseased elbow joint of three years' standing, with ulceration of the cartilages and sinuses. The joint was opened on either side, and healed in eleven weeks. The next was a case of disease in the articulation between the first and second phalanges of the thumb of eighteen months' standing. Cured in six weeks. The third case was that of a man with "long standing" disease of the tarsal articulation. One sinus led to the interior of the joint. Incisions were made on each side of the foot, and complete anchylosis followed. The fourth case was that of a little boy with strumous constitution, with disease of the knee joint consequent upon suppuration of the bursa behind that joint. The little fellow was reduced by fever to a very low ebb, so that bed-sores formed on parts of his body. The joint was opened; anchylosis took place at the end of four months, and the knee bent on the thigh. The fifth case was that of a German, with disease of the wrist joint, which had resisted treatment. One sinus led into it. One incision was made at the back of the joint, and anchylosis followed, but was not observed to be perfect for six months. The sixth case was that of a young Irishwoman, with disease of the tarsal articulation, following upon traumatic erysipelas of the leg and foot. She was reduced to an exceedingly low condition, and from cough with bloody sputa, night sweats, (according to Dr. Heale,) the physical symptoms of the chest, and extreme emaciation, she was supposed to be phthisical, and so diseased, that amputation, which was supposed to be the only remedy for the disease, so far as the joint was concerned, was forbidden by the authority of Dr. Heale. Mr. Gay made an incision on either side of the foot in this case, and the change both in the joint and constitution was remarkable. Her health rallied from that moment, and the joint assumed a more healthy aspect. In a fortnight the joint was fixed by the exudation of lymph between the bony surfaces, and in five weeks perfect anchylosis had taken place, and the wounds had healed. She soon after left the hospital, and was, a week or two since, to Mr. Gay's knowledge, in perfect health. The seventh case was that of Highley, a report of which has been published. The eighth case was that of a little boy with disease of the articulation of the first and second phalanges of the thumb. In this case the cure was not accomplished. The incisions re-solved themselves into sinuses, and after several months the necrosed phalanx came away."—[*N. Y. Journal of Medicine.*

Observations on Iodo-Hydrargyrate of Potassium. By Thos. J. Garden, M. D., of Wylliesburg, Va.

The February and August numbers of the American Medi-cal Journal for the years 1834 and 1840 contain papers on a combination of iodine, mercury and potassium, by Doctors Channing of New York, and Hildreth of Ohio. These papers present some discrepancy of opinion with regard to its effects in diseases of the chest and some other acute affections. Both, however, describe it as an agent of no ordinary power, admitting of a wide range of applicability in the treatment of diseases. I was lead by these papers to make trial of the agent; and as its virtues are not generally understood in this country, I have been induced to present you for publication some cases of disease I have been enabled to relieve through its agency within the last fifteen years. The remedy is an *universal alterative*, and seems to be an excitant of particular organs and functions.

The judicious practitioner will bear in mind, (in imitating the practice which was so successful in the cases now reported,) that numerous exceptions are to be found. Disease is an integer, and each individual case must stand for itself.

The invaluable agent which is the subject of this paper has been prescribed by myself almost monthly for the last fifteen years, and is certainly a signal instance of the power and effi-cacy of combination. The formula for its preparation is as follows: ℞ Deuto-iodide mercury grs. iv; distilled water ℥ i; iodide potassium ϵ i. Mix. The solution is of a beautiful straw color. The medium dose 5 gtt., taken three times per day in some bitter infusion to disguise the strong metalic taste. This dose to be gradually increased until its morbid effects are man-ifested. A suspension of its use for a day or two will quiet these morbid effects; but when it is recurred to, begin with the medi-um dose of 5 gtt., and gradually increase. In very many cases, susceptibility to its action is enhanced by the system being once brought under its influence, so that even a reduction of the me-dium dose is required.

Dr. Channing asserts, that under such circumstances the one-four hundredth part of a grain administered during the day evinced the most indubitable action.

The morbid effects demanding a suspension of its use, accor-ding to my observation, are nausea and vomiting, griping and purging, giddiness and a peculiar sensation of heaviness about the frontal region.

The remedy being an *all pervading*, universal alterative, it has been recommended in a variety of pathological conditions, amongst which may be enumerated chronic bronchitis, amenor-rhœa, leuchorrhœa, diabetes, aptha tonsilitis, pharengitis, chron-ic gastro-enteritis, habitual constipation, dyspepsia, ascetis, ana-sarca, herpes, scrofula, chronic eczema, and a variety of others.

CASE I. John, a colored man, carpenter, aged 40, of athle-tic frame, had gonorrhœa some years ago, which was treated by an early resort to astringent injections and followed by her-nia humoralis; complains of weakness and pain in the region of the lower lumbar spine; frequent micturition; skin dry; pulse full and strong—not accelerated; tongue coated with a short white fur; loss of appetite; costive bowels. He was cupped over seat of pain. Ordered rest, abstinence, alterative mercu-rial aperients, followed by infusion of buchu. This treatment followed by no good results. Upon a more rigid investigation, I ascertained that he not only had frequent desire to pass wa-ter, but that the quantity of urine passed daily greatly exceeded the standard of health; and that the case was one of renal disease, with diabetic symptoms. Having but little confidence in the treatment usually recommended for diabetes, and be-lieving that in this intractable affection some active modifier of the system of nutrition was plainly indicated, I determined to try the deuto-iodide of murcury, and at once to test its efficacy fairly and fully. Five drops were accordingly directed three times per diem for one week; the second week the dose was in-creased to 8 gtt. per diem, and so on, increasing one droy every day until the morbid effects of the agent presented themselves.

The use of the agent was now suspended for a few days until these latter subsided, when its use was again resumed without being able afterwards to bear as large doses as he did at first. Under this treatment all the symptoms were improved, and under its steady use for two months they entirely disappear-ed, without any adjuvant whatever. I find that according to Dr. Channing's uniform observation, diabetes is more promptly benefitted by this agent alone than any other known treatment.

This case occurred thirteen years ago.

This man was again sent to my care in September last to be treated for hydrocele of the tunica vaginalis testis, attended with the same renal and diabetic symptoms that had existed before to a more moderate extent. I gave him 2 oz. of sol. deuto-iodide of mercury, with directions for its use.

Under its use the symptoms entirely disappeared. About Christmas these symptoms were reproduced in a modified form by exposure and excesses. A resort to the remedy again gave relief, and he is now in enjoyment of perfect health.

In describing the symptoms of this man's case in his first attack, thirteen years ago, I omitted to mention in its proper connection, that he labored under functional, though complete impotence, and that the remedy displayed its powers in a most happy manner in restoring his virile powers; but I shall offer other evidences of its efficacy, in another case of the same character more in point.

Case II.   This was a case of chronic eczema; patient aged 35; disease had existed for a number of years, and been treated by a number of physicians.   The affection of the dermoid tissue was seated on the outside of the right thigh, from the hip to the knee joint, embracing about half the circumference of the leg.   The pruritus and burning pain at night were almost insupportable.   General health bad; dyspeptic symptoms of ancient date; complexion sallow; bowels costive; tongue loaded; considerable emaciation.   The patient had strong prejudices against the use of mercurials; he was purged efficiently with blue pill, and placed under the use of deuto-iodi. mercury.   Its action was manifested by copious purging of dark, offensive matters.   His general health improved rapidly, with manifest improvement of the local disease.   An ointment of the salt was now applied.   (Deut. iodide mercury, grs. xv, lard 2 oz.)

This treatment was continued two months; an astonishing improvement followed; he fattened 25 pounds in a short time, and the skin affection has given him but little trouble since.

Case III.   This is a case of complete impotence, occurring in a young man in his 19th year, of perfectly sound constitution, perfect genital organs and chaste habits.   I was unable to trace his defect to any satisfactory cause.   Without entering into a detailed mode of the treatment in this case, (it being similar to the plan pursued in the cases already reported,) suffice it to say, his virile powers were restored to complete and full vigor in the space of four weeks, under the exciting agency of the sol. deut. iodi. merc.   This case occurred during the summer of 1851.

Case IV.   This is a case of vicarious menstruation of four years' standing, and is a signal triumph over disease. Miss ——, aged 19, had never had but one natural menstrual period, the stomach performing the double function of digestion and menstrual secretion.   The regular periodicity of the menses was often lost, and this distressing deviation from health attended by the most frightful train of nervous symptoms.   The patient had been under the care of different practitioners, and after a long course of medication, abandoned as hopeless.

I found her with most distressing symptoms of indigestion; feeble and sallow; bowels constipated; altogether a pitiable example of human suffering.   An examination per vaginam re-

vealed no deviation from nature in structural formation, and
no pathological degeneration. The lactiferous apparatus, and
other external concomitants of the puberic age, were present.
I suspected the existence of ovarian disease. The dyspeptic
symptoms being most urgent, I made trial of argent. nitras,
acet. morphine, and subnitrate of bismuth successively without
any manifest amendment. The deuto-iodide of mercury now
presented itself to my mind as an article worthy of trial, and
more likely to meet the varying indications of the case than
any other with which I was acquainted. Six weeks' use of
the deuto-iodide of mercury restored the catamenia, quieted a
most refractory and rebellious stomach, imparted tone and vigor
to the nervous system, removed the œdema, improved the appetite, and there is every encouragement to hope for a permanent cure of the case. She is still under treatment, but has been
rid of all her distressing symptoms for the last three months,
and is now anxious to discontinue farther treatment.

I would add at the conclusion of this paper, that for the last
12 years I have been constantly in the habit of prescribing this
agent in chronic gastric derangements unaccompanied with
serious structural lesion, and have been seldom disappointed in
the results. If sufficiently persevered in, together with proper
dietetic measures, it will seldom fail of relief. Dr. Hildreth
reports a case of dyspepsia of 20 years' standing, in which the
remedy was in use for three or four months with unequivocal
benefit. In these cases it should be taken after meals and in
medium doses, as its salutary effects depend upon administering
it *so as to avoid* its morbid action.—[*Stethoscope.*

---

*On the treatment of fractures in the vicinity of the ankle-joint ;
with observations on the practice of tenotomy, as facilitating
reduction of the broken bones.* By RICHARD G. H. BUTCHER,
F. R. C. S. I., Examiner on Anatomy and Physiology in the
Royal College of Surgeons of Ireland, Surgeon to Mercer's
Hospital, &c., &c., &c.

In the Dublin Quarterly Journal of last month, there is a
practical paper by Mr. Butcher, illustrative of the treatment of
fractures in the vicinity of the ankle-joint. A number of instances are recorded, some of them of the most complex nature,
yet, by the treatment laid down, and the apparatus recommended, the "integrity of the limb and its normal functions were in
every instance preserved to the sufferer." Space will not
permit a lengthened detail of the several cases and their management, but the concluding observations on the practice of

tenotomy in similar cases, we shall transcribe in the author's own words :—

"One of my chief reasons for wishing to place these cases on record is the practice lately brought into requisition in London, in the management of the special fractures under consideration. I allude to *tenotomy*, the division of the exten-sor tendons, to facilitate reduction, as practised by Meynier, Berard, Laugier, and other French and German surgeons. A lengthened discussion not long since took place before the Medico-Chirurgical Society of London, on the practice of tenotomy, in some cases of fracture, when Mr. C. De Morgan related some cases in illustration." In the first cited, the ten-don was not divided until the day after the accident. 'The second case occurred in the author's own practice. The patient was a female, aged 66, of drunken habits, and was admitted into the Middlesex Hospital in March, 1849. She had been knocked down by a cab, and both bones of one leg were frac-tured a little above the ankle.' The report goes on to say :—'The author divided the tendo-Achillis on the ninth day, with instant relief to the suffering of the patient, and immediate re-moval of all untoward symptoms.' A very important feature in the management of these cases has been omitted altogether : the manipulation adopted for the reduction of the fracture, and the position in which the limb was placed afterwards. In the second case, it is stated that 'the tendon was divided on the ninth day.' I can easily understand that this might be requisite, if the fracture, with its attendant deformity, was left unreduced for that length of time ; failure of the therapeutic means em-ployed ; and the spasmodic actions of the extensor muscles thus prolonged ; for if fractured bones be left unreduced for such a lengthened period as this, *permanent* spasm seizes on the muscles and becomes established ; a fact clearly pointed out and insisted on by Sir A. Cooper. Mr. De Morgan goes on to say :—'In the case related, the chasm between the divided portions at first did *not* exceed a quarter of an inch, that being sufficient to get the bone into position ; and in a short time after there was no appreciable space at all.' This admission goes still further to proclaim that there is no necessity for di-vision of the tendon to effect reduction, if the case is seen early ; for, by flexing the thigh as I have recommended, we can relax the extensor muscles more than 'the quarter of an inch, that being sufficient to get the bone into position.' I am of opinion that, in ninety-nine cases out of a hundred, there will be no necessity for division of the tendon to effect reduction, if the limb be treated as I have advised ; nay, on the contrary, I think, in some instances, the division of the tendon would be

very injurious, as removing the support posteriorly from the
ends of the broken bones, and thus permitting displacement in
that direction.   The mode in which the fracture box, which I
have described, supports the leg in a horizontal line, with the
thigh slightly flexed, padded, and cushioned, as illustrated by
the foregoing cases, meets every requirement of the surgeon.
Dupuytren's splint, in conjunction with these means, as used in
some of my cases, is a most admirable adjunct ; but, taken by
itself, it will not answer as well for the management of the
form of fracture under consideration ; for if the limb be done
up as directed by Dupuytren, and placed flexed upon its side,
some lateral displacement will take place ; or if, with the splint
so applied, the leg be allowed to rest upon the heel, it is unsteady, and rolls about, and the entire limb is in the extended
position—a posture very objectionable, as making tense the
tendo-Achillis.

From a review of these cases, and the observations upon
them, the following facts are, I think, deducible :

1st. That by proper position of the limb, and early reduction,
co-aption of the broken fragments can be effected, and spasm
averted.

2nd. As the result of the broken bones being kept in accurate position, irritation is subdued, excess of callus prevented,
and the motions of the joint left unimpaired ; a fact of great
practical importance here, for the experiments of M. Cruveilhier
prove that various forms of irritation will make the periosteum
and ligaments ossify, and it has been ascertained that in some
cases of fracture near the joints the ligaments have sometimes
been converted into bone, and M. Rayer has observed, from
numerous interesting experiments, that a similar change may
be exerted not only in the fibrous but also in the cartiliaginous
structures.

3rd. That tenotomy is not called for in the vast majority of
cases, being perhaps only admissible when permanent spasm
has located in the extensor muscles, owing to neglect of early
reduction."—[*Canada Medical Journal.*

Note on Sulphate of Bebeerine. By HENRY S. PATTERSON,
M. D., Professor of Materia Medica in Pennsylvania Medical College.

At a time when the discovery of a substitute for Sulphate of
Quinia is a topic of general discussion, it may not be inappropriate to call the attention of the profession to a substance,
heretofore noticed, but too generally neglected.   The Sulphate
of Bebeerine has been shown, by Dr. Maclagan, of Edinburgh,

to be a medicine of very considerable anti-periodic power, closely resembling the corresponding salt of Quinia, and in many respects equal to it, possibly superior. It is obtained from the Bebeeru or Green-heart (*Nectandra Rodiei*) of British Guiana, a tree of considerable size and extremely abundant. The bark yields the alkaloid largely, but it is particularly abundant in the nut. A decoction of the latter is the ordinary popular remedy for intermittent fever in Demarara, and, as I am informed by an intelligent gentleman of that place, seldom, if ever, fails to arrest the disease. The nut may be collected in almost indefinite quantities, and could be obtained here, if a demand were created, for little more than the expense of collection and transportation. The process for separating the alkaloid is almost identical with that for quinia, and not more expensive. If, therefore, it proves on trial equal in efficacy to that alkaloid, we will have a cheap and effective substitute within the reach of all. The subject certainly deserves a more extended investigation than it has hitherto received. The object of the present communication is to invite attention to it, and induce the profession, in miasmatic districts, to give the remedy a fair trial.

Sulphate of Bebeerine occurs in shining brown plates, (sometimes with a greenish tinge,) is inodorous, and has a bitter, harsh, somewhat astringent taste. Like the Sulphate of Quinia, it requires an excess of acid for its perfect solution. It may be given in pill, solution, or powder. That it is a good general tonic, in small doses, is very evident. In the full anti-periodic dose it is more apt to disturb the stomach than the same quantity of Sulphate of Quinia, and occasionally vomits; but it possesses the advantage of being much less stimulating, and does not affect the head as that salt does. Dr. Maclagan asserts that it is "not so liable to excite the circulation or affect the nervous system," and Dr. Meligan adds, that "this conclusion is fully borne out by his experience." The patients who have used it under my care expressly state that it did not occasion in them the same headache and vertigo as the quinia had previously done. Its dose is stated at gr. i.—v., three or four times in the day. Neligan directs it made into pill with conserve of roses, or in solution, with the addition of a few drops of Acid. Sulph. Arom. The anti-periodic dose may be stated at gr. xv.—xx.

A letter from my friend and former pupil, Dr. H. J. Richards, of Grey Town, Nicaragua, of the date of March 25th, 1852, contains the following: "I have used the Bebeerine, as you suggested, with uniform success in quotidian intermittents. I have since had no opportunity to prescribe it in remittents.

All the intermittents of this coast, however, are comparatively easily treated at this season, and yield readily to both quinine and arsenic. The remittents and even intermittents of the fall months, are more virulent and often speedily fatal." Those months will certainly furnish a fairer test of Bebeerine ; but it is something to know that, under existing circumstances, it produces the same effect as the Quinia.

Dr. Watt, of Demarara, thinks that it is tardier in its effects than the Quinia, not interrupting the paroxysms so immediately, but he also thinks that its effects are more permanent. The cases in which I have had an opportunity of using it, seem to confirm the latter opinion.

1st. A gentleman residing in Blockley township consulted me in September last concerning an obstinate and constantly recurring tertian intermittent, under which he had labored for a length of time. He stated that the Quinia always interrupted the disease, but that it inevitably recurred in two or four weeks. I gave him Sulph. Beheer. ℥ss. dissolved in ℥viij. water, a table-spoonful to be taken every four hours during the apyrexia. The next paroxysm was prevented, and he has had no return of the disease up to the present time (April).

2d. A. J. applied to me in October last, with a very similar statement. While residing in New Jersey, about six years since, he had a violent and protracted "bilious fever," since which time he has had, every month or two, an attack of "intermittent fever," which has been generally speedily arrested by quinine. Such was his account of the case. I found his tongue furred, his eyes icterode, his breath offensive, his urine scanty and high colored. The anorexia was complete and thirst considerable. He had a daily slight chilliness, followed by considerable fever and a slight sweat. I gave him a mercurial purge, and on the next day fifteen grains of the Sulphate of Bebeerine. He complained of some nausea, but no disturbance of the head. The same quantity of Bebeerine was given on the two succeeding days, when, the paroxysms no longer recurring, it was discontinued. He remains free up to this period (April), and says that he enjoys better health than he has done for years.

If the permanent character of effect, which these cases seem to indicate, should be established by a more extended experience, we will have in the Bebeerine an agent of very great value, adapted to cases which have hitherto seemed uncontrollable, except by arsenic, to which there are so many objections. It is also much more speedy in its effects than the arsenic. Bouchardat (Ann. de Therap.) expresses his surprise that the Bebeerine has been so entirely neglected in France, where trial is daily made in agues with substances of inferior efficacy. I trust that the same remark may not long be made with regard to the American profession, but that the precise value of the medicine may soon be established by an adequate extent of observation.—[*Medical Examiner.*

On Bandaging the Abdomen after Delivery. By W. B KESTEVEN, Surgeon.

[Mr. Kesteven, although sensible that the weight of opinion is against him, records his conviction that too much stress has been laid upon the importance of the bandage after delivery, and that the rationale of its usefulness has been misunderstood. In order to arrive at a correct conclusion on the subject. he examines it under the following points of view :—1st. The alleged object to be gained by the bandage. 2d. Its real effects. 3rd. Its proper object, and the right period for its application. With this intent, he thus proceeds :]

1st. The objects alleged to be gained by the application of the roller directly after the completion of labour, are :—*a*, to promote the contraction of the uterus ; *b*, to lesson the severity of the after-pains ; *c*, to prevent hemorrhage ; *d*, to prevent syncope ; *e*, to protect the patient against the consequences of sudden alteration of the balance of the circulation, by which syncope, inactivity of the uterus, hemorrhage, and subsequent diseases, have been produced.

On examining, at the bedside, the validity of these several objects, it may be observed, in the first place, that all or any, of these supposed ends may be gained without the use of the bandage.

a. In the vast majority of cases the uterus contracts rapidly, firmly, and permanently, directly upon delivery, without the aid of bandaging. That such is the case a very short experience among the *labouring poor* will soon convince the clinical student. The poor women who are delivered by midwives, and the hundreds, ay thousands, who are yearly delivered without any aid, would, were it not so, have all the dangers of uncontracted uterus to contend with. That such is rarely the case admits of no doubt.

b. That measure which shall promote the contraction of the uterus can hardly be seriously recommended as a means of lessening the severity of the after-pains ; the contradiction is too manifest to require further comment.

c. For the prevention of hemorrhage the application of a roller certainly possesses no claim. Every practitioner who has diligently applied the bandage has had to remove it, in order to apply that efficient pressure to the uterus which is most important in promoting its contractions, hemorrhage having taken place in spite of the compression that had been made by the bandage. In fact the tightly bandaging the hypogastric region with the addition of pads, compresses, basins, &c., &c., has probably frequently given rise to hemorrhage by interfering with the gradual tonic contraction of the uterus. The early application of a binder and compress is a complete obstacle to that vigilant attention to the state of the uterus after labour, which it is the wisdom as well as the duty of the medical attendant to pay for some little time after delivery. Where pressure is properly made, hemorrhage is not frequently met with. The very officious accoucheur, who loads his patient's abdomen with divers pads, and other similar contrivances, must frequently have had occasion to remove them. Without these, the earliest signs of hemorrhage may be recognised ; with them, they are often concealed ; without these hindrances, therefore, the occurrence may be arrested at its outset. It is not the purpose of the present communication to dwell upon the treatment of uterine hemorrhage, but the above hints may serve to show that the bandage has few claims for adoption on that score.

d. The prevention of syncope is undoubtedly an object of paramount importance ; it calls, therefore, for very full examination, as obtainable by the use of the bandage after labour. The indication for its use in reference to the prevention of syncope is theoretically deducted by analogy from the necessity that exists for the application of abdominal compression during the operation of paracentesis. Here, although an analogy does undoubtedly exist, the cases are far from parallel—the conditions not identical—at least not in labour unattended with flooding. When hemorrhage from the uterus occurs, the heart is then physiologically affected in the same manner as where a large quantity of dropsical effusion has suddenly been removed from the abdomen. The removal of the pressure from surrounding vessels in the one case being performed in the upright or sitting posture, suddenly empties the heart of its blood, in the same way that it is emptied by a sudden gush from the uterus. In natural labour there are these points of physiological difference : the heart is not suddenly deprived of a quantity of blood, because the mass of blood previously circulating in the enlarged vessels and hypertrophied structure of the uterus is thrown back upon the aorta *pari passu* with the diminution of the tumour by the contractions of the uterus. The consequent removal of pressure from the surrounding vessels is therefore compensated by the non-abstraction of blood from the arterial system, which so far may be regarded as the equivalent of the compression which is had recourse to for the purpose of obviating the sudden change in the state of the circulation that takes place in tapping. Cases of excessive quantity of liquor amnii, triplet and quartet cases, form instances in which the analogy with the effect of tapping becomes closer. The difference in position must also be borne in mind, when an analogy is attempted to be drawn between these two conditions. In tapping, the position is erect—in labour, it is horizontal. To this rule of difference, however, exceptions occur, parturition sometimes occurs so rapidly, and so unexpectedly, that delivery takes place before the parturient woman can assume the recumbent posture. That such exceptional cases do not invalidate the rule is sufficiently shown by their rarity, and also by the evil consequences that often follow thereon. It may be remarked then for these reasons, that it is obvious that women after delivery have not to thank the bandage for their exemption from syncope. The writer has never seen a case of mere syncope occurring after labour, where the horizontal posture has been carefully observed for some hours, although he has systematically neglected to apply the bandage. He has occasionally seen it, and has heard of even fatal syncope where this precaution of the horizontal position has been violated.

e. Having above disposed of the futility of the argument for the use of the bandage to prevent hemorrhage or syncope, other evils supposed to be consequent upon a disturbance of the circulation are obviously as likely to be benefited by that contrivance.

The second division of this subject is next examined.

2d. The real effect of bandaging the abdomen after delivery.

a. It affords support to the abdominal walls, if applied moderately firm.

b. It gives comfort to the patient, and meets her wishes or prejudices with reference to the preservation of the figure. Among its effects, which are not so harmless as these, are its aggravation of after pains, and the inducement of irregular contraction of the uterus; its obstruction to manipulations; its interference with the action of the diaphragm; its displacing the uterus, and causing obliquity, prolapsus, &c., of that organ; its interference with a most valuable means of controlling uterine hemorrhage, viz: the compression of the aorta. All these are highly important matters, and are to be found among the consequences of the tight bandaging which is adopted by some practitioners.

3d. The consideration of the two preceding topics leads to that of the third,—the proper object of, and right period for

the application of the bandage.   The first point may be very
briefly expressed in the words of Dr. Blundell.   It is to be applied "with that degree of tension which may yield a sense of
grateful support."   This is the whole truth of the question—
the sole object of the bandage is to afford a comfortable degree
of support; it is not to effect forcible compression of the abdomen.

The proper period for its employment is therefore not until
the uterus has firmly contracted, the patient having been left
to undisturbed rest for at least two hours, has had her linen
changed, and is being "put to bed."   Before this period it, as
has been shown, is but an incumbrance.   At this time the bandage will afford "a sense of grateful support," and will meet
the patient's prejudice with reference to the preservation of
her figure—a prejudice which may in this way be harmlessly
humoured; it being emphatically impressed upon the minds of
the patient and her attendants, that the application of the bandage is of infinitely less importance than quiet rest; that the
contraction of the uterus is more effectually and naturally induced by the child's mouth at the nipple, than by all the screw-
ing and squeezing machines that ever were contrived.

If the necessity of any proceeding may be measured by the
end it is intended to serve, most assuredly the importance of the
abdominal bandage has been much over-rated.   The preceding
remarks have shown that its alleged objects are not obtainable,
even if they are desirable; that its real effects are either trifling,
or evil; that its proper object is of a very subordinate character, and pertaining rather to the functions of the nurse than to
those of the medical attendant.—[*Medical Gazette.*

On the Varieties of Alvine Discharges in Children.   By Dr.
Merei.

[The intestinal discharges mentioned by the author are:]

1. The *yellow* discharge.   This is the regular kind of stool
in infants.   It is a mixture of intestinal secretions with bile.
As children advance in age, and begin to take substantial food,
the colour of their regular discharge becomes more and more
of a light brow colour.

2. The *mucous* discharge.   With mucous matter, more or
less thick or liquid, and mixed with serum, sometimes with a
proportion of bile.   This discharge is preceded by but moderate
pains, and frequently by no pains at all.   It denotes a catarrhous, sub-inflammatory, or irritable state of the intestines,
and is almost always of local, and not of sympathetic, origin;

in general it is not dangerous, and at its commencement is easily manageable by opiates, warm poultices, and convenient hygiène. If neglected, it becomes pertinacious and severe, and not seldom connected with swelling, softening, or granules of the mucous membrane, or ulceration of the follicles. If stripes of blood are mixed with the mucus, and pain be present, it denotes a higher degree of inflammation, in particular of the follicles. The highest development in this direction constitutes enteritis or colitis (dysentery.)

Sometimes we find among the mucus, consistent *plastic concretions* of a more or less tubular shape, similar to those of laryngeal croup, but larger in proportion to the volume of the intestines. This is the strongest degree of the catarrhous process which I might term the *croup of intestines.* Among the whole number of my little patients, which may be about 30,000, I met with this discharge perhaps only twenty or thirty times. The discharge is effected with very painful efforts at a stool.

3. The *serous.* In general, after more or less severe pains, the discharge takes place with a certain rigidity and noise, after which the pains lessen or subside. It consists of an abundant quantity of serous liquid, dirty whitish, yellowish, or greenish, as besides mucus, bile is the most common mixture with the serum. The serous diarrhœa is commonly the effect of rheumatism in the peritoneum, in the serous and fibrous membranes, or in the nerves of the intestines. I found in these cases the abdomen very hot. If a great deal of mucus and some blood are mixed with the serum, we may suspect parenchymatous enteritis; if the serous membrane alone enters into the state of acute inflammation, frequently transudation takes place on its free surface.

. I have seen cases of profuse serous discharge, in a very short time, even in less than twenty-four hours, produce collapse and death, and in some of these instances necroscopy could not discover an adequate alteration either in the mucous or in the serous membrane.

. . The serous species of discharge is frequently merely a product of sympathetic secretion. I observed it sometimes connected with large transudations in the chest, and with chronic hydrocephalus.

. Speaking in general, serous diarrhœa, if even arising from rheumatism, is more difficult to manage than the mucous. Very minute doses of calomel, with Dover's powder and mustard poultices, are frequently beneficial.

Pure serum, like ricewater, is a less favorable quality than the dirty-white or yellowish. Dark-brown serum frequently denotes a disorder in the portal system, present in some severe gastric or typhoid fevers, but I have seen a similar quality also in chronic affections of the brain, and very frequently in scrof-ulo-impetiginous children. This is worthy our attention, in particular if eczema or impetigo has disappeared from the head and face. This brown and fetid discharge accompanies some-times the commencement of chronic hydrocephalus. I treated it successfully, in this last case, with high but very diluted doses of iodide of potash.

4. *The green bilious discharge.* If pure bile, then the voided matter is in general not abundant. In young children it is of a more yellowish than green colour. The essential character of bile is, to be *of a greenish colour* (in infants it is voided green) *at the very moment of its evacuation.* This kind of discharge is very frequently present in acute inflammatory and febrile affections ; if dependent upon an affection of the brain, then we may find the colour to be rather brown, and the abdomen re-tracted. If a similar source produces abundant serous-bilious discharges, then we find the abdomen much collapsed. But I must observe, acute affections of the brain are almost always connected with constipation, only in some cases of chronic hydrocephalus I met with the mentioned diarrhœa. Bilious discharge, as arising from bilious fever, or from derangement of the liver, is rare in young children. In this case the right hypochondrium will be more or less bloated up. We must be careful not to confound the green bilious discharge with the following :

The *discharge, like chopped eggs,* mixed with mucus, some clots of bile, and caseous coagula of indigested milk, or other kind of food, accompanied almost always by gripes and flatu-lence ; its smell is disagreeably acid, and the whole matter, some minutes after being discharged and *exposed to the atmos-phere, becomes green.* We know not exactly the chemical change which produces this coloration, it seems to be an oxy-dation of some of the elements. Then the essential character of this discharge is, that it is yellow at first, and becomes green by exposure to the atmosphere, whilst bile is green at the mo-ment it comes out. I shall call this *the acid saburral discharge,* which is the most obvious before the sixth month of age, in particular if the sucking child takes, besides the milk, some farinaceous food. Practitioners commonly prescribe in this case rhubarb, with magnesia. For my part I prefer, in tender infants, to rely more upon a convenient change in the diet, and as a remedy, aromatic frictions of the epigastrium, and internally bicarbonate of soda, dissolved in mint water.

6. The *bloody discharge.* Pure red blood is seldom dis-

charged by children ; in some rare cases I have seen half or one table-spoonful come out, as the product of active congestion and hemorrhage.   Very frequently, on the contrary, blood, is combined with the mucous discharge, and in this case, if it is preceded by pain, without tenderness, it denotes an inflammation in the upper parts of the intestinal tube, at least not near the rectum.   Tenesmus signifies that the seat of the inflammation is in the lower parts of the colon, or in the rectum.   This form is commonly called *dysentery*, not dangerous, if it is without bilious complication and fever, and if treated in its early stage with Dover's powder, some doses of castor oil, and warm poultices ; in a stronger degree leeches at the anus ; but if neglected in the commencement, it becomes dangerous to the life of the child.   Professor Rokitansky, of Vienna, describes most exactly what he calls the " dysenteric process," in three gradual degrees of anatomical change.   The highest degree, presenting a dirty red and gray marbled surface, with considerable thickening, granulation, and ulceration, I never saw in the tender age.   Young children die before this stage is developed.

Passive hemorrhage of the intestines very seldom occurs in children.   I have seen, however, some cases where, without adequate pain, a considerable quantity of dark thin blood was discharged.   Lastly, we have seen in this town, with Mr. Wilson, a case in a child six years old, where, during the course of a gastro-typhoid fever, more than one pint of carbonized blood was discharged in two days.   The case recovered.   The boy is affected with an enlarged spleen.

Moderate quantities of red blood, discharged without pain, frequently occur, mixed with mucus, and are, without signification, sometimes even connected with the advance of recovery from gastric affections.   This is the same case as with epistaxis.

Golding Bird and Simon state, as the result of chemical analysis, that some dark green stools of children owe this colour to blood which has suffered a certain chemical change ; but those chemical inquiries are not yet arrived at a satisfactory exactness ; we do not even know exactly what kind of green discharges were the subject of these inquiries.

7. *Calomel stools.*   Green, more or less thick, or mixed with serum, and in this case more abundant, produced by full doses of calomel.   Calomel stools resemble bile, and contain much bile, but they contain also some particular chemical elements which we do not exectly know.   In many instances it happens that the calomel diarrhœa commences some days or weeks after the use of mercury, and we must be aware of this, and not confound it with the primary bilious discharge.   In the

former case the region of the liver is in general softer than in
the latter.   A clever practitioner will never try to stop directly,
and with astringents, a green discharge, whatever be its origin
and nature.

Calomel stools sometimes contain blood.   After what I have
seen in dissection, I incline to attribute this circumstance to a
sub-inflammatory state, with superficial erosions of the mucous
membrane, which sometimes take place in children after the
continued use of calomel.

[The author states that he considers all these qualitative and
physical distinctions of the discharges of children as very imperfect outlines of a sketch, which, by farther physical and
chemical inquiry can become corrected and perfected.]

[*Provincial Med. and Sur. Journal.*

*Peculiar Effects of the root of the Podophyllum Peltatum or
May Apple; and its Alcoholic Extract.* By CHARLES W.
WRIGHT, M. D., of Cincinnati.

Having been called upon to make an analysis of some cocoa,
which it was supposed had been poisoned by having been pulverized in a mortar in which cantharides had been reduced to
powder a short time previously, and which it was believed had
not been properly cleansed ; but, being unable to detect the
presence of cantharides by any of the proposed tests or the
scales by means of a microscope, I was induced to attribute the
symptoms of poisoning to the presence of some other agent ;
and upon investigation the following appears to have been the
cause of the symptoms observed :

Upon inquiring of the person who pulverized the cocoa
beans, it was found that the mortar, a short time before, had
been used to pulverize the alcoholic extract of the podophyllum
peltatum, called by the self-styled eclectic practitioners *podo-
phylline,* and by whom it is almost exclusively used, being their
substitute for calomel.

Now it is found that if a person take the powdered root, or
the alcoholic extract of the May apple for a considerable period
of time, a peculiar papular eruption makes its appearance on
the scrotum, accompanied by an irritation of the neck of the
bladder, especially when the dose is not sufficient to produce
free catharsis.   This eruption not unfrequently makes its appearance on those employed to pulverize the root, and occurs
so frequently in the practice of the eclectics that they have
given it the name of *Scroteritis.*

All of those persons who used the cocoa containing the extract of May apple, were affected with irritation of the neck of the bladder and tenesmus; and in some of the cases the pain was so severe that they would lay hold of the nearest object for support until it subsided.

The powder of the root and extract is excessively irritating to the eyes, producing, in considerable quantity, an inflammation which is extremely difficult to treat.—[*Western Lancet.*

On Amputations in Children. By M. Guersant.

The amputations at the *Hôpital des Enfants* are of frequent occurrence, not less than from eighteen to twenty taking place annually; being usually performed for white-swelling or other chronic disease. M. Guersant is, however, no advocate for hasty operations in such cases, as the lymphatic habit upon which the disease of the joint depends may often be ameliorated, and a valuable though an imperfect limb be preserved. Much depends upon the social position of the parents. The working-man has not at his command those resources which may be required for years during an endeavour to preserve the limb of the child; and after the operation the latter may be apprenticed to many trades, even though he has a wooden leg. The child placed in easy circumstances can command prolonged medical attendance, sea-air, change of climate, or whatever may be deemed beneficial, and amputation need not be performed until all other means have been exhausted. After a long period, however, all the chronic disease in a scrofulous child suffering from arthritis seems to concentrate itself in the diseased joint; and upon the removal of this, his health may become re-established. Amputation frequently succeeds better in debilitated than in very strong and vigorous children.

Whenever possible, M. Guersant prefers the months of May, June, and July, for the operation, as unfavorable complications are of more common occurrence in the cold and changeable seasons of winter and spring. The child requires but little preparation; the means which have already been employed for the improvement of its general health, is iodine, bitters, cod-liver oil, &c., all placing it in the best condition for undergoing the operation. If a large eater, the food should be somewhat diminished two or three days before; and any existing diarrhœa must be arrested by anodyne injections and bismuth.

M. Guersant sometimes employs the oval operation, but hardly ever the circular. In most cases he prefers the flap, which renders the co-operation of the assistants easier, occasions little inflammation or suppuration in children, frequently allowing of union by the first intention, and affords a better covering for the bone. Chloroform is employed, and the principal artery of the limb carefully compressed, so as to avoid hæmorrhage. In very hot weather, the edges of the wound are united by some points of suture, and the stump left exposed to the air. When bandages are employed, the stump is dressed daily. On the evening of the operation a little broth is allowed, next day a stronger soup, and the day after that sometimes a little roast-fowl.

By observing these rules, M. Guersant finds, as a general rule, that eight or nine cases in ten recover. If erysipelas occur, leeches are applied to the nearest lymphatics; and if these do not suffice, a circular blister is placed around the stump; emetics and purgatives, but especially the former, being given. In cases of purulent resorption, he has obtained some benefit from aconite. If the surface of the wound takes on a greyish colour, and becomes covered with false membranes, chlorined water or lemon-juice is the best application. When union by the first intention does not take place, the inner lip of the wound should be stimulated, and then strapping applied ; and when fistulæ occur, they will usually be found dependent upon small portions of bone tending to necrosis.—*Gaz. des Hop.*

[A writer in the *Bull. de Thérap.* (tom. xl. p. 81) observes, that M. Guersant did not lose a single case of amputation during 1850, though the thigh, arm, foot, and shoulder, were among the parts removed. The great success of operations on the young has long been known, and is usually attributed to the greater vitality of childhood and the absence of mental disquietude. However this may be, M. Guersant's especial success is probably, in a great measure, due to his habit of ordering good, nutritious diet as soon after the operation as possible. Under the influence of this, the children rapidly recover strength and flesh, the wound assumes a healthy aspect, and the colliquative diarrhœa, so common prior to the operation, ceases. Abstinence is ill-borne at this tender age, and most of these children have become exhausted by suppuration prior to the operation.]—*Medico-Chir. Review.*

Treatment of Varicose Veins.

An entirely new method is coming extensively into vogue, in England, in the management of enlarged veins of the lower limbs, that merits the attention of American surgeons. An India-rubber stocking is manufactured in Liverpool, expressly to meet this particular condition of the veins. It is a loose net-work, reaching to the knees, but which uniformly compresses the vessels, supports their outer wall, and yet gives no sensation of tightness, or otherwise any unpleasant feeling. We examined a gentlemen, a few days since, who is habitually wearing one of these stockings, which he represented as a great comfort. Some years ago, Dr. Mott, of New York, operated on one of the largest veins, but with no particular benefit. Till the India-rubber stocking was drawn on, he was haunted with an apprehension of the possibility that some of the over-distended vessels might burst. This has been completely prevented by wearing this article, and fears of a contingency of that kind are now entirely gone. This pain and sense of weight, after being on foot through the business fatigues of the day, and not felt, and the patient urges upon sufferers from the same affliction, to procure the simple palliative of an India-rubber stocking.—[*Boston Med. and Sur. Journal.*

Wine and Honey in Infantile Marasmus.

Dr. Baun states, that in the marasmus of infants he has derived truly remarkable benefit from the employment of a mixture consisting of one part wine and two or three of honey, giving several tea-spoonfuls daily. Not only Madeira but good Burgundy may be so employed, or when diarrhœa is not present, the Rhenish wines. Refreshing sleep, and an increase of animal temperature, are the first effects, and an improved digestion a latter one.—[*Journ. für Kinderkrank. Medico-Chir. Rev.*

Treatment of Asphyxia Infantum.

Dr. Tott states, that he has often succeeded in restoring life in the *asphyxia asthenica infantum* after the failure of the usual means, by causing a person to stand on a table, and pour cold water from a tea-kettle on to the pit of the stomach. In this way Professor Hasselberg saved many lives.—[*Ibid.*

Purgative Syrup of Jalap. By M. Viel.

Take of powdered jalap, an ounce ; alcohol, $3\frac{1}{2}$ fluid ounces ; water, $26\frac{1}{2}$ fluid ounces ; sugar, 30 ounces. Digest the jalap in the water and alcohol, previously mixed in a flask, during five or six hours, at the temperature of 90° to 100° F., filter, add the sugar and dissolve it, aromatise and preserve for use.

This syrup, which is an agreeable purge for young children, may be given in tea-spoonful doses.—[*Jour. de Chimie Méd. Amer. Jour. of Phar.*

Solution of Aloes and Soda. By Professor Mettauer.

In this preparation the aloes is held in solution and its action
modified by the presence of bicarbonate of soda.   It is a useful
aperient for persons of costive habit, and may be employed
without the unpleasant effects that sometimes result from the
employment of aloes alone.

Take Socotrine Aloes,	two ounces and a half, *troy;*
Bicarbonate of Soda,	six ounces ;
Compound Spirit of Lavender,	two fluid ounces ;
Water,	four pints.

Macerate the mixture for two weeks with occasional agitation,
and filter.

The dose is from a fluid drachm to a fluid ounce half an hour
after meals.—[*American Journal of Pharmacy.*

Disulphate of Quinia rendered soluble by Tartaric Acid.

M. Righini has proposed to substitute tartaric acid for sulphuric acid to render the commercial sulphate of quinia soluble
in water when directed in solution by prescriptions, as being
less austere and disagreeable to the taste.   M. Casorati, of Tu-
rin, gives the following formula: Sulphate of Quinia, *six
grains;* Tartaric Acid, *three grains;* Syrup of Oranges, *a
fluid ounce.*—[*L'Abeille Médicale.,* and *Ibid.*

Gentianin recommended as a substitute for Cinchona.

Dr. Kuchenmeister affirms that impure and uncrystallized
gentianin can be substituted for sulphate of quinia, and he has
noticed : 1st, that this substance acts on the spleen at least as
efficaciously as sulphate of quinia.   2d. Its action is not less
rapid.   3d. That it is sufficient to administer 15 to 30 grains
twice a day ; and 4th, that gentianin constitutes probably the
most valuable substitute for Peruvian bark.—[*Jour. de Chimie
Méd.,* and *Ibid.*

Antidote for Poisoning by Corrosive Sublimate.

The Boston Medical and Surgical Journal contains the details of a case in which a large quantity of the Bi-chloride of
Mercury had been taken, and which was successfully treated
by Dr. Cummings, with repeated draughts of a solution of
salæratus.   The alkali deprived the mercury of its acid, and
thus rendered it inert.   The whites of eggs were also given.

ﬞ iscellany.

American Medical Association.—We are indebted to the politeness of the Editor of the "Stethoscope" for the Proceedings of the fifth meeting of the American Medical Association, recently held in Richmond, Va., from which we condense the subjoined details. The meeting having been called to order by Dr. Moultrie, President, and twenty-three States being represented by two hundred and seventy-five Delegates, the following officers were elected for the present year: President—Beverly R. Welford, M. D., of Virginia; Vice-Presidents—Jonathan Knight, M. D., of Connecticut; James W. Thompson, M. D., of Delaware; Thomas Y. Simons, M. D., of South Carolina, and Charles A. Pope, M. D., of Missouri; Treasurer—D. F. Condie, M. D., of Pennsylvania; Secretaries—P. C. Gooch, M. D., of Virginia, and Edward L. Beadle, M. D., of New York.

The Committee on Prize Essays awarded the prize of $500 to Dr. Austin Flint, of Buffalo, for his essay "On Variations of Pitch in Percussion and Respiratory Sounds, and their application to Physical Diagnosis."

The Report of the Committee on the Medical Botany of the United States for 1850–1, was presented by Dr. A. Clapp, and referred to the Committee on Publication. The reports of the regular standing committees were then called for in order, and were severally laid over or continued.

Dr. Pinkney, of the Navy, read a memorial he had prepared to present to Congress, on the subject of assimilated Rank—which was referred to a committee. It was then resolved, that no member should speak more than ten minutes at a time, nor more than twice on the same subject. Dr. T. Y. Simons offered a preamble and resolutions in reference to the evils of crowding emigrants on ship-board. Dr. Storer vindicated himself against certain attacks as chairman of the committee on Obstetrics. Dr. J. B. Flint proposed the establishment, by the Association, of a Quarterly Journal, instead of issuing a volume of Transactions—which was laid over to the next meeting.

Dr. Hays, chairman of the Committee on the Constitution, made a Report, and Dr. Yardly a counter Report, both of which were referred to a committee of three, for the purpose of reconciling the differences between them, if possible. The City of New York was then selected for the next meeting of the Association. A communication from the New York Academy of Medicine, in reference to the "College Cliniques," was read and referred to the committee on Publication.

The Report of Dr. H. Adams, of Massachusetts, on the " Action of Water on Lead Pipes, and the Diseases resulting from it," was also referred to the same committee. Dr. Williman, of South Carolina, read the Report of the Committee on " The blending and conversion of the Types of Fever," and Dr. Hayward, of Massachusetts, read that of the Committee " on the permanent cure of Irreducible Hernia—both of which reports were ordered to be printed. The application of the representative of the late Dr. Horace Wells for the appointment of a committee to inquire into and report on the claims of the contestants for the priority of the discovery of Anæsthesia, was laid upon the table.

It was determined that, in future, all Reports, &c., exceeding ten pages, must be accompanied with a synopsis of the contents, which may be read before the Association.

The following amendments to the Constitution were read and laid on the table for farther action :

ARTICLE I.—*Title of the Association.*—This institution shall be known and distinguished by the name and title of " The American Medical Association." It shall be composed of all the members of the medical profession of the United States of good standing, who acknowledge fealty to and adopt the code of ethics adopted by the association ; and its business shall be conducted by their delegates or representatives, who shall be appointed annually in the manner prescribed in this constitution.

Strike out the whole of Article II, referring to " Members," and insert the following :

ARTICLE II.—*Of Delegates.*—§ 1. The delegates to the meetings of the association shall collectively represent and have cognizance of the common interests of the medical profession in every part of the United States, and shall hold their appointment from county, state and regularly chartered medical societies ; from chartered medical colleges, hospitals and permanent voluntary medical associations in good standing with the profession. Delegates may also be received from the medical staffs of the United States army and navy.

§ 2. Each delegate shall hold his appointment for one year and until another is appointed to succeed him, and he shall be entitled to participate in all the business affairs of the association.

§ 3. The county, district, chartered and voluntary medical societies shall have the privilege of sending to the association one delegate for every ten of its resident members, and one more for every additional fraction of more than one half of this number.

§ 4. Every state society shall have the privilege of sending four delegates; and in those states in which county and district societies are not generally organized, in lieu of the privilege of sending four delegates, it shall be entitled to send one delegate for every ten of its regular members, and one more for every additional fraction of more than one half of this number.

§ 5. No medical society shall have the privilege of representation which does not require of its members an observance of the code of ethics of this association.

§ 6. The faculty of every chartered medical college acknowledging its fealty to the code of ethics of this association, shall have the privilege of sending one delegate · to represent it in the association : *Provided*, That the said faculty shall comprise six professors, and give one course of instruction annually of not less than sixteen weeks on Anatomy, Materia Medica, Theory and Practice of Medicine, Theory and Practice of Surgery, Midwifery and Chemistry : *And provided also*, That the said faculty requires of its candidates for graduation—1st. That they shall be twenty-one years of age ; 2d. That they shall have studied three entire years, two of which must have been with some respectable practitioner ; 3d. That they shall have attended two full courses of lectures, (not however to be embraced in the same year,) and one of which must have been in the institution granting the diploma, and also where students are required to continue their attendance on the lectures to the close of the session ; and 4th. That they shall show by examination that they are qualified to practice medicine.

§ 7. The medical faculty of the University of Virginia shall be entitled to representation in the association, notwithstanding that it has not six professors, and that it does not require three years of study from its pupils, but only so long as the present peculiar system of instruction and examination practised by that institution shall continue in force.

§ 8. All hospitals, the medical officers of which are in good standing with the profession, and which have accommodation for one hundred patients, shall be entitled to send one delegate to the association.

§ 9. Delegates representing the medical staffs of the United States army and navy shall be appointed by the chiefs of the army and navy medical bureaux. The number of delegates so appointed shall be four from the army medical officers and an equal number from the navy medical officers.

§ 10. No delegate shall be registered on the books of the association as representing more than one constituency.

§ 11. Every delegate elect, prior to the permanent organization of the annual meeting, and before voting on any question after the meeting has been organized, shall sign the constitution and inscribe his name and address in full, with the title of the institution which he represents.

The Association adopted the following Resolutions presented by the Committee on rank and grade of Navy Surgeon :

1. *Resolved*, That the American Medical Association, representing the medical profession of the United States, reaffirm the resolutions passed at the meetings held in Baltimore in 1848, in Cincinnati in 1850, and in Charleston, South Carolina, in 1851, by pressing their approbation and support of the establishment of the assimilated rank

conferred on the navy medical officers by the regulation of the navy department in 1847.

2. That this association is not aware of any disadvantage attending on the regulation of 1847 ; that they can perceive no just cause for its alteration, and disapprove of the change proposed.

3. That it is the opinion of this association that it would be for the interest of the naval service that this question should be settled definitively during the present session of Congress, and if conformable with the usages of the military service, by legislative enactment, to which request they respectfully invite the attention of the honorable senate and house of representatives.

It was also resolved to memorialize Congress on the subject of publishing the medical statistics of the census of the United States, separately, for distribution to the medical profession.

Resolved, That the Committee on Epidemics be constituted in relation to the division into districts as they were the last year, and that they be continued in service during a period of five years.

Resolved, That the chairman appointed for each district shall have power to select associates, not exceeding four in number, to assist him in his labors.

Resolved, That the several State Medical Associations be requested to use their influence to procure the appointment, by the Legislatures, of Sanitary Commissions.

Dr. Drake read a paper on the " Influence of Climatic Changes on Consumption," which was referred to the committee on printing.

A committee of five was appointed to solicit subscriptions from the members of the association, for the purpose of procuring a suitable stone, with an appropriate inscription, for the Washington monument, now in progress of erection in Washington City.

It was resolved to accredit one member from each State represented in the Association to travel in Europe, and to report upon foreign medical affairs. Also, that the Association hereafter grant two prizes, of $100 each, for the two best essays.

The following reports were then presented, read by their titles, and referred to the committee of publication :

" On the Toxicological and Medicinal properties of our Cryptogamic Plants," by F. PEYRE PORCHER, of S. C.

" On the Epidemics of New Jersey, Pennsylvania, Delaware and Maryland," by J. L. ATLEE, of Pa.

" On the Epidemics of South Carolina, Georgia, Florida and Alabama," by Dr. W. M. BOLING, of Ala.

Together with this report, which was handed in by Dr. DRAKE, of Ky., there was also presented a paper by Dr. D. J. Cain, of S. C.; which was ordered to be appended to the report when published.

"On the Epidemics of Mississippi, Louisiana, Texas and Arkansas," by Dr. Ed. H. Barton, of La.

"On the Epidemics of Ohio, Indiana and Michigan," by Dr. Geo. Mendenhall, of Ohio.

Dr. Stewart, of N. Y., then presented the report of the committee on the amendments to the constitution, and read the following additions which the committee had made since its recommitment:

To section 1, article 2, add "Delegates may also be received from the United States army and navy."

In section 6, article 2, add the words "Comprise six professors and" after "provided said faculty shall."

In section 6, add to 3d requisition on faculties, the words "and also where students are required to continue their attendance on the lectures until the close of the session."

Add section 7. "The medical faculty of the University of Virginia shall be entitled to representation in the association, notwithstanding that it is not composed of six professors, and that it does not require three years of study for its pupils, but only so long as the present peculiar system of instruction and examination practised by that institution shall continue in force."

Add section 9. "Delegates representing the medical staff of the United States army or navy shall be appointed by the chiefs of the army and navy medical bureaux. The number of delegates so appointed shall be four from the army medical officers and an equal number from the navy medical officers."

Special Committees were appointed—"On the Causes of Tubercular Disease; on the Mutual Relations of Yellow and Bilious Remittent Fever; on Epidemic Erysipelas; on Acute and Chronic Diseases of the Neck of the Uterus; on Dengue; on Milk Sickness, so called; on the prevalence of Idiopathic Tetanus; on Diseases of the Parasitic Organs; on the Physiological Peculiarities and Diseases of Negroes; on the Alkaloids which may be substituted for Quinia; on results of Surgical Operations for the Relief of Malignant Diseases; on Statistics of the Operation for the removal of Stone in the Bladder; on Sanitary Principles applicable to the Construction of Dwellings; on Toxicological and Medicinal Properties of our Cryptogamic Plants; on Agency of the Refrigeration produced through Upward Radiation of Heat as an exciting cause of Disease; on the best means of making Pressure in Reducible Hernia; on Cholera and its relation to Congestive Fever—their analogy or identity; on Displacements of the Uterus; on Typhoid Fever; on Epidemics of New England and New York; on Epidemics of New Jersey, Pennsylvania, Delaware and Maryland; on Epidemics of Virginia and North Carolina; on Epidemics of South Carolina, Georgia, Florida and Alabama; on Epidemics of Mississippi, Louisiana, Texas and Arkansas; on Epidemics of Tennessee and Kentucky; on Epidemics of Missouri, Illinois, Iowa and Wisconsin; on Epidemics of Ohio, Indiana and Michigan.

Committee on Volunteer Communications.—Drs. Joseph M. Smith,

Jno. A. Swett, Willard Parker, Gurdon Buck, and Alfred C. Post, of
New York.

Rarity of Repetition of Attempt at Suicide by Fire-arms. By M. H.
LARREY. M. H. Larrey, in a recent discussion, observed, that according to his experience suicidal maniacs may make repeated attempts at
terminating their existence by poison, drowning, or other means of inducing asphyxia, and even by the sword or dagger ; but that individuals who have once attempted to kill themselves by *fire-arms* scarcely
ever renew their suicidal endeavour, but resort eagerly to all surgical
means capable of correcting or effacing the effects of their mutilations.
Among numerous others he might allude to, he referred to two young
soldiers, now at the Val de Grace, who having in vain endeavored
to blow their brains out, have never since shown the slighest attempt
to repeat the act. A case occurred to Dupuytren in the person of a
soldier, who after having in vain attempted his life several times, at
last endeavored to blow out his brains, but only succeeded in mutilating his face. Cured, however, of the effects of this serious accident,
he became also for ever cured of his suicidal mania. M. Larrey inquires, whether the cerebral commotion produced in these cases effects
a salutary perturbation in the mental condition ?

M. Brierre confirmed M. Larrey's statements ; and observed, that
it may be advanced, if not as an absolute, at least as a very general
rule, that individuals who have once endeavored to shoot themselves
never repeat the attempt. Frequently, at the end of several years,
they make new attempts at suicide by other means. Persons, on the
other hand, who have failed in accomplishing their death by the various other means, frequently recur to those among them which they have
already uselessly employed.—[*L'Union Medicale. Medico-Chir. Rev.*

*On the Employment of Sulphate of Zinc for the Preservation of
Animal Matter.* By M. FALCONET.—According to the author, the
substances the most difficult to preserve, as the brain, the intestines,
and other pathological preparations, may be most effectually preserved in a solution of the sulphate of zinc, retaining all their characters
without the least alteration, and, what is very important, not experiencing the contraction observed when alcohol is used. The steel
instruments employed for operating on the substances which have
been injected with the preserving liquid, are not injured even when
immersed directly in the liquid, and left there for twenty-four hours.—
[*Comptes Rendus. Amer. Jour. of Phar.*

Filter Accelerator.—M. Dublanc describes an arrangement to ac-
celerate the filtering process, which consists of a funnel-shaped tissue
of plated or tinned wire on which the filter is supported in the funnel.
It is shaped like a plaited filter, and is made from a flat circular piece
of wire gauze, crimped in plaits running from centre to circumference
so as to give it the shape of a funnel with fluted sides.—[*Journ. de
Pharm., and Ibid.*

SOUTHERN
MEDICAL AND SURGICAL JOURNAL.

Vol. 8.] NEW SERIES.—JULY, 1852. [No. 7.

PART FIRST.

Original Communications.

ARTICLE XXI.

A brief Sketch of twenty cases of Typhoid Fever, successfully treated. By N. H. Moragne, M. D., of Abbeville, S. C.

On the 28th of August last, I was requested to see Lyra, a negro woman, about 30 years old, whom I found in a very low state of fever; skin hot and dry; pulse ranging from 130 to 140; tongue redish on the tip and edges, parched and dry—a brownish fur upon the centre, with distinct papillæ appearing through the coating; the abdomen distended, slight pain from pressure, gurgling sound emitted. On enquiry into the previous history of this case, I learned that "diarrhœa had only supervened a short time back, but that the patient had been sick for three weeks, having a paroxysm of fever every day, slight intermission in the forenoon," her owner having treated her for inter-mittent fever with calomel and quinine; seeing, however, that she grew worse daily, he called in "medical aid," without insti-tuting further examination. I pronounced this fever to be the "slow nervous" of the ancients—the *"febris lens et nervosa"* of Fluxham, or, as it is now familiarly termed, typhoid fever.

My attention was principally directed to the exhausted state of the system, the extreme debility, the high nervous excite-ment, &c. I therefore, without delay put her upon stimulants;

though first prescribing alterative doses cal. and Dover's powder, in order to establish the secretions; having particular
reference to the bowels, not suffering "watery dejections" to
come from them.   Gave the "camphor stimulus" composed
of camph. par. and pepper tea—a very happy formula, I think,
in this disease, owing to its cheapness, and the facility with
which it is obtained; applied mustard poultices to the abdomen,
Dover's powder at night.   Administered sulph. quin., not
however with a view to its anti-periodic effects, but merely as
a tonic.   This case assumed a slow but steady convalescence;
duration 30 to 40 days.

Case II.   On September 1st, was called to see Kinchy, a
girl aged 13, who was attacked with fever two or three days
before.   Pain in head; pulse soft but full, ranging from 90
to 100; tongue red on the edges, brownish fur upon the centre;
papillæ visible; bowels not much distended; no gurgling sound
occasioned by pressure; extreme prostration; inattention; in-
tollerance of light.

This case was a very obstinate one, pneumonia supervening
about the 8th day, came near proving fatal.   I prescribed, in the
first instance, calomel, Dover's powder and ipecac, in alterative
doses, every five or six hours for twenty-four hours; bearing
in mind that none of those evacuations should be produced,
which were calculated to debilitate.   Kept this up every two
or three days until my patient exhibited a better looking
tongue.   For the severe pain in the chest, applied blisters and
mustard poultices; warm pediluvia and Dover's powders at
night.   As I write from memory alone, I cannot give the full
particulars, but only a synopsis of the treatment of these cases.
Notwithstanding my efforts to combat the complication in this
case, the patient grew worse, and had subsultus tendinum, coma,
delirium, &c. &c.

Gave the "camphor stimulus" more frequently, alternating it
with brandy toddy; Dover's powder and warm foot bath still
kept up at night.   In this, and all my cases, when giving Dover's
powder, I did not suffer the patient to be disturbed in order
to give other medicine; finding sleep to be more "refreshing"
than any thing I could administer.   She had a slow but steady
convalescence, duration from six to seven weeks.

CASES III and IV. While attending to the above, I also saw Chloe, a woman aged 30, and James, a man aged 22. I was now satisfied that this fever was prevailing as an endemic on the plantation. These cases presented symptoms similar to the foregoing: pulse compressible; tongue red on the edges, furred; papillæ distinct, &c. &c. They were treated with calomel, Dover's powder and ipecac in alterative doses, camphor stimulus, quinine, &c. They had a paroxysm of fever for twenty days, slight intermission in the forenoon, without any complication.

CASE V. Philip, aged 13, was attacked with fever a week or ten days before I saw him. Severe pain in the head; skin hot and dry; great prostration and aversion to light; tongue red on the edges, thickly coated upon the surface.

This was an extremely obstinate case, not running its course under forty days. His symptoms were not threatening until the third or fourth week, when his abdomen become enormously distended; great meteorism, tympanitis, diarrhœa, and his face and inferior extremities "œdematous."

This is the only case in which I remember observing the "superficial eruption." The tympanitis was relieved by injections of tinct. assafœtida, emolient poultices over the abdomen, &c. The camphor stimulus losing its effect, he was literally fed upon French Brandy. He had a speedy convalescence.

CASE VI. Flora, aged 4. Case VII. Charlotte, aged 11. Case VIII. Prince, aged 8—were all attacked in the same house; but the fever was of a mild type, running its course in twelve days.

CASE IX. Pinder, aged 11. Case X. Primus, aged 8. Case XI. Isaac, aged 6. The fever ran its course with little interruption in two weeks.

CASE XII. Phylis, the mother of the two latter, aged 30, was attacked with fever. For the sake of brevity, we will say that her symptoms were "typhoidal," also her tongue presented the same condition. She had a paroxysm of fever every day for a month, slight intermission in the forenoon. Treated as before indicated. This was the only case in which I was compelled to use injections of nitrate of silver, so much extolled by Dr. Dickson, to check the obstinate diarrhœa which had supervened.

CASE XIII.   Nelly, aged 15; severe cerebral excitement; tongue "typhoidal," parched and dry.   So great was the determination to the brain that she became stupid for several days, extreme deafness, inattention, &c., &c.   Besides the treatment before observed, I applied a blister to the spine, warm foot and hip bath.   Gave the spt. nit. dulc. freely, &c.   Dr. T——, of this District, saw this case, also case 5th.   His prognosis was unfavorable.   She, however, after an illness of thirty days, convalesced.

CASE XIV.   Sam, aged 13.   Case XV. Hannah, aged 11. Case XVI. Chloe, aged 6—were all attacked in the same house with the latter.   The former ran its course with little interruption in twenty days.   Extreme deafness attended these cases: you could scarcely make them hear by raising your voice to the very highest pitch.   Treatment as before indicated with few alterations.

CASE XVII.   Leah, aged 19, living in a house a hundred yards distant from the quarter.   This was a case of typhoid-pneumonia; the complication presented itself doubtless from the severe and sudden change of the weather, which occurred at this time.   Treated as before indicated : blisters and warm mustard poultices to the chest; pulv. Dov. and hot foot bath at night ; leaving orders for the patient not to be disturbed.   She had a slow but steady convalescence.

CASE XVIII.   Grace, aged 13, of a delicate fibre ; nervo-melancholic temperature.   The fever ran its course in twenty days ; she was gradually recovering ; had dismissed her from my care.   Owing to great neglect on the part of her *nurse,* she relapsed ; two or three days afterwards, I was sent for in haste to see her, but too late.   Found her delirious, raving in a low muttering tone; extremities cold ; dry hacking cough, &c. &c. ; learned from some of the attendants that she had been exposed to the inclemency of the weather ; suffered by her nurse to lie out in the rain, for some time, a few nights previous—applied blister to the chest, bowels ; sinapisms to the extremities ; brandy toddy internally.   All in vain, she died.

CASES XIX and XX.   Mr. C——, the overseer, aged 30. Mrs. C——, aged 28, about this time attacked—the former had a severe and obstinate attack ; duration, from six to seven weeks. Owing to imprudence in diet, he relapsed the second time, but recovered by assiduous care and attention. Treated upon the same principle as the foregoing: Dr. F——, saw this case two or three times, concurred with me in the treatment. Mrs. C——, suffered with a mild and benignant attack, which ran its course in eight or ten days. Other cases occurred, but of a mild type, and I shall omit to notice them.

REMARKS.—The above is a very hasty and imperfect summary of twenty cases of typhoid fever, occurring on the plantation of Captain Petigru, upon Little River, in the lower part of this district. In offering them to the Journal, I will only make a suggestion or two. Typhoid fever, for the last few years, has made fearful ravages in this locality : it not only pays us annual, but I may say monthly visits—it has usurped the place of the simple intermittent and bilious remittent of former days—it spreads from hammock to hammock, as the "Simoom sweeps the blasted plains," leaving the mournful truth behind, that some one has fallen a victim to its fury.

I do not presume to give any thing new, or offer any specific in the treatment of this disease. All informed medical men have their minds made up in regard to this matter, that they can palliate, not cure this fever. My only object in reporting these cases, is to state facts as they occurred. It will be perceived that the convalescence in most of them was extremely slow and tedious—this I conceive to be partly attributable to the malignancy of the type, and also to the *inferior nourishment* we were compelled to administer.

Much has been said against the "mercurial treatment" in this fever; but I pursued it here as elsewhere, with success, which the result of my cases will abundantly testify. "The statistics of France show a mortality of one-third." It is with a careful hand though, I should advise calomel to be measured out to the prostrated invalid ; also, a close investigation as to its effects. And last, though not least, a prying search in the *nursing department*, which in many cases, is the only "plank of safety in the wreck."

Extracts from the Records of the Physicians' Society for Medical Observation, of Greene and adjoining Counties. Georgia. By D. C. O'KEEFFE, M. D., of Penfield, Ga., Secretary.

MARCH 8th. *Lobelia Inflata*, by Dr. J. E. Walker, of Greenesboro'.—Dr. Walker, in directing the attention of the Society to this article of the materia medica, said: I am aware that I am running some risk, if not of censure, at least of ridicule ; but my motto is *"je prends le bien où je le trouve."* I stand upon the broad platform of medical science, and care not from what source, or by whom discovered or recommended, my remedies are, if after a faithful trial they fail me not, then, independent of all sectarian feeling, I shall use them, and will feel bound as a member of our liberal profession, to recommend them to my brother practitioners. Laying aside, then, all prejudice, let us examine briefly the therapeutic properties of the plant which heads this article.

From a youth I have had much opportunity of observing the effects of lobelia upon the human as well as the brute system, and although I have seen it used in almost every form and variety of disease, and without the least discretion, still I have never seen the first accident or ill-result from its use, but in a majority of cases, decided benefit.

As an antispasmodic, lobelia stands unrivalled, when its power and safety are considered. There is scarcely a practitioner of any experience who has not witnessed its beneficial effects in that distressing affection, spasmodic asthma. I have often tried it myself, not only in asthma, but in spasm of the stomach and bowels, and have found nothing equal to it. And here I may also state that I have administered it to horses and seen it frequently used by others, for colic in that noble animal, and I have not known it fail, in a single instance, to give speedy and entire relief. In spasmodic croup and hooping cough, I know of no substitute for it ; in truth, for spasm, of whatever character, I know of nothing which I could use with equal confidence. I have not seen it used in tetanus, but have reason to believe it might be of service in the treatment of that fearful disease.

There are many nervous affections in which its beneficial effects are manifest : in hysterical convulsions, even when deglutition was impracticable, I have seen the convulsions cease upon pouring the tincture between the teeth, so as to bring it in contact with the tongue and fauces. In one individual who has periodical attacks, simulating epilepsy, the tincture of lobelia will not only cut short an attack, but (if taken when the first symptoms appear) will entirely prevent one. So true is this statement, that for several years past, this patient has not suffered, except when without the medicine—in which event she seldom escapes. From this circumstance, it is reasonable to infer that lobelia exerts no curative agency, but averts the attacks by its anti-spasmodic power. I have no doubt, however, that if this patient had used the lobelia, when she first became subject to the disease, and continued its use in her youth, the habit might have been broken in upon, and entire exemption have been the result. In further illustration of its antispasmodic properties, I will adduce another case.

On Saturday morning, 23d August ult., I was called to see Martha, a negro woman about 24 years old, and found her affected with some very strange hysteroidal disease. There was complete spasm of the œsophagus extending partially to the tongue and jaws. She had not swallowed a particle of any substance since the Sunday evening before. Previously to my seeing her, another practitioner was called in who treated her for five successive days and yet was unsuccessful in restoring deglutition. Cups were used and blisters to the spinal column and epigastrium and temples—the blistered surfaces dressed with morphine—all to no purpose. She remained in *statu quo.* The indications were obvious—to relax the spasm was the paramount object. I felt confident that if I could effect emesis, that result would follow; but how to get an emetic into the stomach was the question for my decision. I concluded to give lobelia a trial, by pouring the tincture into the mouth, and holding the head in such a position as to bring it in contact with the tongue and fauces. I took the precaution to combine with it 5 grs. sulph. zinci, to insure speedy vomiting, if she should swallow the mixture. After it had remained a short time in the mouth, the spasm gave way, she swallowed the mixture, free emesis ensued, and there was no return of the spasm. Under the use of tonics and a nourishing diet she had a speedy recovery, except that there remained complete aphonia, which persisted some days after all other symptoms had subsided. I removed the tonsils which were enlarged, gave her quinine, used local stimulants and galvanism. Under this course she entirely recovered and has had no return, although she had been obnoxious to them for several years.

As an emetic, I seldom use lobelia, unless its relaxant effects are desired. I much prefer ipecac, over which lobelia possesses no advantage as an evacuant of the stomach, or for revulsion to that organ. In strangulated hernia, I have no doubt it is a valuable medium, preferable to many articles in common use. Dr. Eberle used it successfully in a case where tobacco seemed to be indicated. The relaxation resulting from the free use of lobelia, is, in my opinion, sufficient almost for any emergency. I am sure I would never use a tobacco enema, if I could obtain lobelia.

I now proceed to notice one of the properties of lobelia, which has escaped the notice of experimenters generally, viz., its power as an antidote for poisons. And since lobelia has been denounced as a narcotic poison itself (its narcotic properties, if it have any, being very feeble) I fear this announcement will startle some of my brethren. I have seen great prostration, but never narcotism, follow repeated doses of it, when it was not vomited ; and before I conclude, you will see what opportunities have been afforded me for gaining some knowledge of the effects of this article. So far from being a poison of such virulence as many have supposed, lobelia certainly possesses antidotal qualities. The following experiment will serve to corroborate the above statement. Some years ago, I had two favorite dogs which were both bitten by the same moccasin, one in the mouth, the other upon the foot. (I mention the locality of the wounds, to show that one must 'have been more unfavorable than the other.) They both were very sick, and seemed as if ready to die. Having heard of the success of lobelia in snake bites, I determined to try it on my dogs, and accordingly mixed half an ounce of the pulv. seeds with a sufficient quantity of milk, and offered it to the one least affected, (the one wounded on the foot)—he however refused it, and I could devise no means by which to introduce it into his stomach.   I then gave it to the other, whose head by this time was swollen to nearly twice the normal size; he drank it all, as if by instinct, and by next day was entirely relieved, while the other was no better, nor did he recover for many days.

The success of this experiment has induced me to make further trials.   I have used it with the best results for the sting of the common bee, and other poisonous insects, and confidently recommend it to be kept in every family—in these cases I apply the tincture to the affected parts.   In the eruption following the Rhus Toxicodendron, the tincture is equally successful. For diseases of the skin generally, and especially those of the scalp, it makes an excellent wash,* and to foul and indolent ulcers it imparts a peculiar stimulus, and favors the process of healing.

Lobelia also possesses *febrifuge* powers.   I have known many cases of intermittents relieved by it alone, when administered in small and oft-repeated doses, so as to keep up a continual nausea for several hours before the expected paroxysm. It is not so good as quinine, but is much cheaper and deserves a trial.   It also possesses, in an eminent degree, expectorant properties, and is especially useful in pleurisy and pneumonia— not however from its expectorant properties alone, but from a peculiar influence which it exerts over the circulation.   I may truly say of lobelia, in this respect, what Dr. Norwood has said of the American hellebore.   I have used nothing which so completely controls the circulation, equalizing it by relaxing the whole system; with a pleasant, soothing sensation that extends over the entire system it produces gentle diaphoresis— hence its value in inflammatory diseases.   It has been stated by some that lobelia acts as a cathartic, but this statement

---

* Since the reading of this essay before the society, we have used the tincture of lobelia in a case of lepra; after a few applications, the inflammation of the derma was arrested, the hypertrophy diminished, and the scales of morbid derma thrown off and never replaced.—(*Secretary.*)

needs confirmation. I have had much opportunity of testing that point, but I have had no reason to believe it ever acted in that way. Having stated that my opportunities for observing the effects of lobelia on the system were numerous and good, I would remark that, for more than half my life, it has been extensively used in my neighborhood, and in the family in which I have lived ; for twelve years, scarcely a week passed but some member was taken through *a course*, and while suffering from continued fever, I have myself taken twenty-seven emetic doses in as many consecutive days. Now I do not consider that was judicious practice, and yet I cannot say it was in the least detrimental.   It is a matter of much regret, that this valuable article should have been brought into disrepute by a set of empirics, to such an extent that Allopathists are almost afraid to pronounce its name. " This ought not to be." The indiscriminate use of the article, by those who are self-constituted "Doctors," should not deter us from its prudent employment : their boldness should teach us that it is far less dangerous than has been apprehended. We have no better reason to discard lobelia, than we have to dispense with quinine, opium, and a host of others. If we must leave off the former because "Botanics" use it, and arrogate to themselves and their founder the credit of introducing it into practice, the latter should share the same fate. I would warn these Thomsonian gentlemen, however, to examine some of *our books*, and they may then be able to " render unto Cæsar the things that are Cæsar's."

Allow me, in conclusion, to urge a trial of lobelia upon the members of this Society : in inflammatory diseases, I employ an infusion of the dried plant ; in spasmodic affections I use the tincture.

Drs. Park, Rea and King spoke very favorably of the lobelia.

The Spontaneous Origin of Scarlet Fever, by Dr. B. F. Rea, of Greensboro'.—It cannot be denied that we *country physicians*—as we may correctly term ourselves—occupy a more advantageous position for the investigation of *some* subjects, connected with the ills to which flesh is heir, than those dwelling in cities. It has occurred to me, that the origin of that large and important class of diseases denominated contagious, is one of these; for, moving in a community where all are individually known to each other, where the modes of living, habits, and intercourse of all are understood and freely commented upon, it will consequently be in his power, often, to trace a contagious disease to the cause producing it—to ascertain when and where it has been imbibed, and decide in regard to its spontaneousness.

My observation leads me to believe that, in *many* instances, those diseases supposed to be wholly the result of contagion, have a spontaneous origin.   I am aware that, upon this subject, I differ with many, who are disposed in every instance, to suppose that exposure to, or even contact with a diseased subject must have taken place, before the disease made its appearance—although when and where the exposure occurred, they are unable to affirm.   Such seem to forget that all diseases *must* at *some* previous time have been spontaneous—at some point in the history of the human race, I care not how remote the period, they had an origin.   A combination of circumstances, internal or external, or both combined, produced them ; and the question arises, did this combination occur but once ?—and have the diseases then produced, been transmitted ever since by the subtle influences of contagion ?   Is it not more reasonable to suppose, that the *causes* then producing a disease, *may* have occurred *again* and *again*, and that the physician will many times meet with similar cases?

I am inclined to think so, for we have instances recorded, and in our own experience, where individuals living in isolated situations, remote from all exposure, have become the victims of small-pox, scarlet fever, &c.

The principle of contagion is, I know, very subtle.   It is transmitted many times, doubtless, by ways and means of which we have no cognizance; but, as I before said, I cannot see why the causes which were *once adequate* to produce a disease, may not be found *always so ;* nor can I believe that these causes have only once existed.   The most violent poisons are sometimes generated within the systems of animals, without apparent extraneous aid.

No one will deny that, Rabies—incorrectly termed hydrophobia in the canine species—and Equinia, in the quadrumana, may originate spontaneously, as well now, as at any former period. Nor can their contagiousness be denied; and "may it not be reasonably inferred, by analogy, that all the poisons to which the human system is liable, may occasionally be generated in the same way?" I see not why the inference may not be drawn: nor can I see that scarlet fever, measles and small-pox, (and some others might be mentioned,) should always be ascribed to contagion.

I will proceed to mention a case of *Scarlet fever*, the origin of which I believe to have been *spontaneous*. I presume others among you may have met with similar cases, in which no apparent opportunity for contagion existed.

This case occurred last May in the family of Mr. J., residing eight miles from town. His family of children consisted of four boys. On the night of the 27th inst., his third son, "four years old, was taken with fever, nausea and vomiting, &c., and on the following morning his tongue was coated with a thick white fur. Some purgative medicine was given to him, and he seemed to be a little better through the day." I will remark that, he was noticed to be unusually dull during the day preceding his attack. On the following night, the youngest son, æt. 15 months, "was attacked in precisely the same way," and the next day, 29th, I was called for the first time to see them, when I received from the father the above statement. The first case grew rapidly worse, becoming in a few days so deaf, that the loudest calling, with the mouth placed close to his ear, could not make him hear—the deafness taking place before any coma had appeared. At the same time, there was a copious and steady acrid discharge from the Schneiderian membrane. He died on the seventh night of his attack. The other case, the youngest, had a very protracted recovery—a general *anasarca* following, and desquamation continuing irregularly for some weeks.

In seven days, (counting from the time the disease appeared in the first case,) two negro children, who had not been in the room occupied by the first cases, though they had been in the house, were attacked about the same time, and in a day or so thereafter the eldest son of Mr. J. was attacked; and in two or three days, the second son took the disease; then, at intervals of a few days, others of the negro children were attacked till some twenty had it—some having it very lightly, with scarcely any efflorescence; but in *every case* there was more or less *soreness* of the *throat* complained of. A number of the children, although exposed, escaped entirely.

Very little treatment was required in the greater number of the cases, and the disease, in each case, progressed regularly to a favorable termination. I should not neglect, however, to mention, that the plan first proposed by Taylor, viz., that of *inunction*, was pretty freely used, especially in the cases occurring among the negro children; but as these cases were generally mild, I cannot say whether it did much good or not.

Now two questions arise here: Did the first case originate spontaneously? or, was it the result of specific contagion? The latter question, I think, can be fully settled in the *negative*, when I affirm that there was not a case of scarlet fever, at the time, within fifteen miles of the family, nor had there been, in twelve months, that I could ascertain by careful inquiry; nor had any of the family been exposed at any time to the contagion, either by visiting from home, or by being visited by any one, having this, or an analogous disease. Indeed, so far as I could ascertain, there was no scarlet fever prevailing in any of the adjoining counties.

As to the question of the spontaneousness of it, which I am compelled to believe, I leave the society to form their own opinion.

Cazenave says, "Scarlet fever is the result of an unknown contagious principle." Churchill says, "It is very difficult to say whether the disease may originate spontaneously by any combination of predisposing causes. The best writers think not, and seems to me unlikely."

Now the two authors above cited, reside respectively in the large cities of Paris and Dublin, where the disease in question is, perhaps, at all times prevailing to a greater or less extent; for "its appearance is confined to no particular season"— hence their opinion that it is the result of contagion, which is certainly true to a very great extent; but the disease may have a spontaneous origin, as well in a city as in the country. Professor Dunglison, of whom I am an unworthy pupil, whose opportunities for observation have been second to but few, says: "It is probable that the disease (scarlatina) arises, at times, from other causes than contagion. It can scarcely be maintained, that its universal mode of propagation is by some specific miasm disengaged from an individual labouring under the disease, and that no combination of influences can now arise, capable of generating it *de novo.*" So we see a difference in the opinion of these authors.

The opinion ef Cazenave, as of most authorities, that "scarlatina is most contagious during the period of desquamation," seems not to hold good in the above cases.

The first case, you will observe, was attacked on a certain night, and the second case on the night immediately following, *before any desquamation, according to the nature of the disease,* could have taken place, which, in the mildest forms, does not usually begin till the *seventh* or *eighth* day.

A different question arises here, which is, to me, very interesting—viz: Did the second child, which was attacked twenty-four hours after the first, contract the disease from the first, or was it also of spontaneous origin? I know the period of *incubation* in scarlatina is stated in books to be *one week*, but this is by no means strictly true. Dr. C. A. Clark has shown that this may be, in some instances, only *three days*, (New York Med. Times, for Feb.,) and in the case I refer to, it could have been only *twenty-four hours*, at farthest, admitting that the second case was contracted from the first, and that the *poison* was taken into the system of the second at the very time the disease manifested itself in the first.

That the "contagion" of eruptive fevers is given off, in the majority of cases, during the desquamative period, may be true, but I do not believe it is essentially necessary that there should be any *desquamation*, nor even *eruption*, to render these diseases communicable, especially *scarlatina* and *rubeola*, for we may have either of these, without apparent *eruption;* yet, under favorable circumstances, such cases, I am inclined to think, are as transmissible as the more completely developed forms.

I believe the *morbid poison* or the "*contagious something*"—call it what you wish—which exists in the blood, is given off by the lungs, in the expired air, &c. We may reason so, at any rate, from analogy; that is, if I am correct, when I say that, in mumps, hooping-cough, and perhaps some other diseases which are contagious, I believe their *contagious poison* is given off in this way.

We may more reasonably believe this, than that the contagious principle emanates from the surface of the body; for, in the latter diseases, there never is any eruption. We must infer that the blood is fully charged with the poison; for, in the exanthemata, we have several well authenticated instances of their having been propagated by inoculation with the blood.

In numerous instances, also, children have been born with scarlatina. "Dr. Gregory mentions that a child of his own was born with it;" and it is through the blood of the mother alone, that the disease is communicated to the fœtus *in utero*, unless we say it originated spontaneously.

Upon the conclusion of Dr. Rea's essay, a lengthy discussion ensued concerning the nature of scarlatina, in which several of the members participated. Dr. Walker considered it of spontaneous origin. Dr. Randle was firmly of the opinion that it was not a contagious disease, for he had frequently inoculated healthy persons with the secretions from scarlatina patients, and no propagation followed: he considered it an epidemic, and he had met with numerous mild epidemics. In reply to Dr. Randle, Dr. Rea said it was epidemic, and also contagious, and thought that many of the epidemics which Dr. Randle had seen were not genuine scarlatina, but what some of the German authors describe under the head of *Falschen Masern*, or spurious measles, which has some resemblance to both measles and scarlatina—a sort of intermediate disease which he (Dr. Rea) has seen, and which is not a protection against either.

Various opinions were expressed on the treatment of scarlatina. Dr. Rea spoke favorably of anointing the surface with bacon rhind. Dr. Foster stated that he had never found any benefit from blisters or emetics. Dr. Randle's experience led him to follow the expectant plan—do as little as possible. Dr. Callaway spoke with confidence of sponging the surface with whiskey and water.

Dr. R. S. Callaway, of Public Square, mentioned a case of congestion or oppression of the brain, to which he was called on the night of the 31st of January. The subject was a negro man, aged about 35, and was found in the following condition: Appearance, that of a person in a deep sleep—could not be aroused by shaking or calling; pulse about 75, rather feeble; surface cool; respiration sonorous, deep and rather slow: his sensorial system in a state of perfect stupor.

Prescribed: Sinapisms to spine and epigastric region extensively. These means restored sensibility sufficiently to enable the Doctor to administer an emetic of ipecac, which operated well in the course of an hour, causing the ejection from the stomach of at least *one pound* of new bacon, with almost entire relief to the brain. A dose of ol. ricini completed the cure.

Dr. R. H. Randle, of Penfield, detailed the symptoms of a case of what he considered "misplaced rheumatism." On his first visit, the symptoms (rational) were those of pneumonia; but at the second and future visits, he had to treat an attack of acute rheumatism in the joints of the inferior extremities.

ARTICLE XXIII.

Cases occurring in the Practice of Professor Dugas. Reported by H. Rossignol, M. D., of Augusta, Geo.

Case I. *An Eye destroyed by a bird-shot.*—Mr. ——, was hunting birds on the 11th March, 1843, when, in order to secure their game, he took one side of the field and his brother the other, the distance between them being supposed sufficiently great not to incur any risk in firing towards each other. His brother fired, and a single shot seems to have reached Mr. ——. This passed through the cornea and lodged within the globe of the eye. There being but little pain, and several days passing without much inflammation, the patient flattered himself that the accident would not prove very serious. The pain, however, began to be acute, inflammation rapidly increased, the eye swelled out enormously, and the patient was finally relieved by excision of the cornea, which allowed the disorganized humors to escape with the shot in their midst. Recovery took place in the usual time, and a glass eye was substituted, which very effectually obviates the deformity.

The reporter finds in the Southern Medical and Surgical Journal, for 1838, (vol. 2, p. 647,) several cases recorded, in which Prof. Dugas resorted to excision of the cornea for the purpose of relieving great local pain and constitutional disturbance consequent upon a disorganization of the contents of the eye. Whenever the eye is irretrievably lost and proves a source of serious annoyance, Prof. D. thinks that it should be at once emptied, both as a measure of relief, and as a security against sympathetic disease in the sound organ. He has never found any bad effects from such a course.

CASE II. *Ex-ophthalmia caused by a tumor in the orbit.*— Peter, a negro boy about 5 years of age, had been suffering for a number of months with pain in the left eye, and with a gradual impairment of its vision. Placed in charge of Prof. Dugas on the 6th January, 1848, the eye was found to protrude so much that the eye-lids could not cover any portion of the cornea; this was opaque and the conjunctiva highly injected; vision was and had been for some time entirely lost. The opacity of the cornea prevented the condition of the humors of the eye from being seen. The boy suffered incessantly most excruciating pain in the eye and in the front of the head, which, added to febrile excitement, loss of sleep and impaired appetite, had very much reduced him.

After watching the case for a few days, Prof. D. determined to excise the cornea and to empty the eye. This was followed by only temporary relief. In a few weeks the sunken eye began to protrude again; the pain in the forehead returned, and increased in severity, if possible. The boy became delirious, and gradually comatose, and died in March, after being apparently at the point of death for a month.

The existence of a tumor of some kind behind the eye became evident, upon the reprotrusion of this organ, but its nature was uncertain, and the brain had become too much implicated to warrant an attempt to relieve the patient by extirpation of the contents of the orbit.

Post-mortem examination revealed the presence of a fibrous tumor in the orbit, which, in pressing the eye forward, had put the optic nerve very much upon the stretch. Within the cra-

nium the optic chiasm was found drawn towards the affected
side, and surrounded with a stratum of pus which extended
beneath the whole of the anterior lobes of the cerebrum.   The
brain itself did not appear to be softened, nor otherwise affected.

CASE III.   *Gunshot wound of the face.*—Mr. Beal, being on
a hunting excursion on the 17th November, 1850, was passing
through an old field with his gun in the trailing position, when
a vine catching the trigger, fired off the gun, and wounded the
carrier in the face.   He was brought to town (a mile distant)
and seen by Dr. Dugas and myself immediately upon his arrival.
The gun was charged with bird shot, nearly the whole of which
appeared to have been received by the right side of the face.
The upper lip was torn from the angle of the mouth to the
nostril; the entire nose, from its attachment to the frontal bone
down to its lower extremity, including the septum, was thrown
over upon the left side of the face and hung by the skin of that
side alone, leaving a frightful chasm in its stead.   Some of the
shots had passed through it, but it was not as much lacerated
as might have been expected.   One shot penetrated the right
lachrymal caruncle, and other minor wounds were to be seen
about the face.

The face and wound being well cleansed, the nose was replaced and secured with stitches and adhesive plaster; bits of
lint were rolled up and placed in the nostrils; and lastly the
lip was secured by sutures and plasters.   A linen handkerchief
was now dipped in cold water and placed over the face, with
orders to keep it cool.

Under this treatment the case progressed without any unpleasant accident whatever.   Nearly the whole wound healed
by the first intention, and the remainder was well in ten days.
The patient was so little disfigured that no one, on seeing him
after recovery, could form any adequate idea of the hideous-
ness presented by the wound prior to its having been dressed.
This case is reported merely as an illustration of the extraordinary restorative energy of the system in some persons.   It may
not be amiss to add that the patient was intoxicated at the time
of the accident.

ARTICLE XXIV.

Wounds of the Small Intestines: Recovery. By L. A. Dugas,
M. D., Professor of Surgery in the Med. Col. of Georgia.

Mr. W. T., the subject of this case, is about 25 years of age, of
spare habit and not robust health. Being in a state of inebria-
tion on the 12th of April last, (1852,) he got into an alterca-
tion with another man, and at 4, P. M., was stabbed in the
abdomen with a bowie knife an inch and a half in diameter.
The abdominal walls presented but one wound, which was of
the diameter of the knife just described, and situated about
midway between the umbilicus and left anterior-superior spinous process of the ilium. After receiving the wound, he walked
three or four hundred yards to the office of Dr. E. Girardey,
where I found him a few minutes after, lying upon a bed, with
a mass about the size of a common fist protruding from the
wound. His face was extremely pallid, his surface covered
with cold sweat, his pulse small and frequent, and his stomach
very irritable. He had eaten a hearty dinner, which he threw
up, strongly impregnated with alcoholic liquor.

Dr. Girardey and myself examined the protruding mass,
which proved to be a portion of the small intestines with a little of the omentum, in a state of partial strangulation. At one
point, the intestine was almost completely severed in two; at
another, about half its circumference was cut open, and at a
third, there existed another and still smaller cut, about an inch
long. These three intestinal wounds were transverse, and
there were other scratches which did not transfix the coats.

After cleansing the parts, the intestinal wounds were neatly
closed by Dr. G., with the glover's stitch. Feeling the importance, in such cases, of animal sutures, which would be readily
dissolved and absorbed, we used a violin string of the smallest
size, previously softened with water. The protruding mass
was then returned into the abdomen, the external wound
stitched with good silk, and covered with an adhesive plaster,
over which a compesss was placed and secured with a roller
bandage.

The patient was now carried home upon a litter and put to
bed, with strict injunctions to keep the abdomen continually

covered with a napkin dipped in cold well water as often as necessary to keep it cool. These directions were effectually carried out by having two napkins in use, which were alternately applied to the body, and thrown into a bucket of cool water every five minutes during the first six days, and gradually at longer intervals until the twelfth day, when the process was discontinued.

A full dose of opium was given in the evening, and ordered to be repeated, if he did not rest well. Cold water allowed, in small quantities at a time.

13th April. Passed a very uncomfortable night—took the opiate freely, but was continually annoyed with nausea and painful efforts to vomit, and could not sleep; no febrile excitement; pulse less frequent. At 10 o'clock this morning the matters vomited began to assume a stercoraceous character, and continued so during the day. A little mint tea, essence of peppermint, or cold water alone, were occasionally taken, and the mouth rinsed with vinegar and water to correct the unpleasantness after vomiting.

14th. Resorted again to opiates during last night, with better effect—stomach still irritable, and ejected matters stercoraceous and very offensive. No febrile excitement; pulse better. Same treatment continued.

15th. Vomiting ceased this forenoon; slight febrile reaction; pulse better; skin warmer and of a better color. Drinks still used sparingly.

16th. Feels very comfortable; pulse and temperature natural; passes flatus from the rectum.

17th. Still improving; would like a little nourishment, but is not allowed to take it.

29th. On the 18th he was allowed chichen broth in small quantities at a time, and afterwards his diet was gradually though cautiously improved. Opiates were occasionally given until the end of the first week. To-day an inclination being felt to evacuate the bowels, this was facilitated by an enema of tepid water, which was followed by a good, natural and fecal discharge, without pain; the first since the reception of the wound.

It is particularly worthy of remark that the abdomen did not

at any time become tumefied ; that it was at no time tender
upon pressure, except in the immediate vicinity of the wound,
where it was a little so for a few days.   After the third day the
pulse remained at 80 beats per minute.

On the 1st of May, he dressed himself and walked about the
room.   On the 3rd, diarrhœa supervened in consequence of
exposure or of the atmospheric constitution, bowel affections
being then very prevalent in the city.   The diarrhœa changed
to dysentery on the 5th, but was checked by an anodyne enema.
Since then he has had no other difficulty, and is now (1st June,)
attending to his business, apparently as well as ever.   He is
made to wear a truss bandage over the seat of the wound in
order to prevent the tendency to hernia, which usually follows
such cases.

In conclusion, I may be permitted to add that the singular
exemption from general peritonitis, and the ultimate success of
this case may very reasonably be attributed to the use of animal sutures instead of silk, and the free application of cold water to the abdomen.

I cannot let the opportunity pass without complimenting my
young associate in this case for his skill and attention.

· PART II.
Eclectic Department.

On Healthy and Morbid Menstruation.   By J. Henry Ben-
nett, M. D., late Physician-Accoucheur to the Western
General Dispensary, etc.
[Continued from Page 355.]

Menorrhagia.—By menorrhagia is meant profuse, prolonged,
and too frequent menstruation, and uterine hæmorrhage generally in non-pregnant females, when not occasioned by the
existence of uterine tumors, or by malignant disease.

From this definition it will be perceived that the forms under
which menorrhagia may manifest itself are varied.   Thus, it
includes menstruation normal as to duration and periodicity,
but hæmorrhagic in quantity ; menstruation normal as to periodicity and the amount of blood lost during a given time,
but hæmorrhagic from its being prolonged beyond the physiological duration ; and menstruation normal as to quantity and

duration, but too frequent in its return.   Again, all these modes
of hæmorrhagic manifestation may be combined, and menstruation may be too profuse, too prolonged, and too frequent ; or
the hæmorrhage may be continuous, with irregular or periodical
exacerbations denoting the menstrual nisus.   In a word, a
marked increase in the quantity of blood usually lost during
the menstrual flux by the individual in question constitutes
menorrhagia.   It must, however, be borne in mind, that, as we
have already seen, there is no *general standard* by which the
menstrual flux can be measured, and by which the normal
state can be separated from the abnormal.   What is normal in
one woman would be hæmorrhagic in another, and *vice versa.*
The only standard for each individual female is her own condition, when indisputably in health.

Menorrhagia is generally considered to be the result of an
active or passive state of congestion of the uterus, existing independently of local disease, and connected with or occasioned
by general conditions of the economy.   This, the opinion of
both ancient and modern pathologists, is founded on ignorance
of the facts elucidated in my work on Uterine Inflammation.   In
reality, the quantity of blood lost during menstruation is seldom
increased so as to constitute hæmorrhage, and the menstrual
periods are seldom morbidly approximated, *for a continuance,*
(apart from tumours, polypi, and cancer,) unless there exists
some chronic inflammatory disease of the cervix or of the body
of the uterus, or unless menstruation be finally disappearing.
Idiopathic menorrhagia, except at the change of life, is as rare
as hæmorrhage from the lung under the influence of mere congestion, apart from any organic disease, tubercular or other.
In the uterus, as in the lung, there is nearly always some organic
lesion which produces the congestion that precedes hæmorrhage.
This assertion is not the result of theory, but of scrupulous
observation, and must become equally evident to all practitioners who will accurately investigate the state of the uterine
organs of patients so affected.   Congestion of the uterus exists,
it is true, in confirmed menorrhagia, but it is all but invariably,
with the exceptions above made, the result of uterine inflammation, and assumes an active or passive character, according to
the natural constitution of the patient, and to the amount of
reaction produced by the disease and by the loss of blood on
the system at large.   If the uterine inflammation is of an active
nature, and has not had time sympathetically to debilitate the
patient, hæmorrhage is considered active or sthenic.   If, on the
contrary, the local disease has long existed, and has produced
great anæmia, and been attended with great hæmorrrhage, the
hæmorrhage is said to be asthenic.

Accidental Menorrhagia.—The above remarks, however, apply only to *confirmed* menorrhagia, and not to those cases in which menorrhagia appears in a casual and evanescent form, under the influence of some accidental and temporary cause, such as mental emotions or violent exertion. Under such influences the mentrual flux is not unfrequently increased in quantity, prolonged in duration, or morbidly approximated, in the absence of local disease. This is more especially observed in those females who are habitually menstruated profusely, and with whom menstruation presents the extreme physiological duration. These casual hæmorrhagic manifestations, however, very rarely become permanent, ceasing without treatment; the function, as it were, soon righting itself.

Inflammatory Menorrhagia.—Menorrhagia originating in chronic inflammation of the cervix or body of the uterus, occasionally persists after the removal of the morbid condition which at first occasioned it. When this is the case, its persistence is generally the result of a torpid, languid state of uterine circulation, giving rise to obstinate congestion; a not unfrequent sequela, as I have elsewhere stated, of long-neglected uterine disease. This congested condition of the uterine circulation may or may not be connected with chronic enlargement or hypertrophy of the body of the uterus. I have, however, met with such enlargement in most of the cases of menorrhagia which have obstinately persisted after the subdual of local inflammatory disease. In these cases, the uterine hypertrophy did not appear to be connected with actually existing inflammation of the body of the uterus, but to be traceable to a previously diseased state of the cervix or uterus, which had prevented the latter organ returning to its normal size after parturition. Indeed, I think I may state, as the result of observation, that the *actual existence* of chronic inflammation in the tissue of the body of the uterus, generally diminishes the menstrual flux, and retards its appearance, whilst inflammation of the cervix renders it more profuse and more frequent than usual. Inflammation of the mucous membrane lining the uterine cavity, on the contrary, is often a cause of hæmorrhage.

A congested state of the portal circulation, connected with hypertrophy and passive congestion of the liver, or with other abdominal lesions, has occasionally, in my experience, given rise to obstinate uterine hæmorrhage, especially in cases in which the tone and contractile powers of that organ had been simultaneously weakened by chronic inflammation.

Menorrhagia from Ovaritis.—Sub-acute inflammation of the ovaries may no doubt sympathetically re-act on the uterus, and produce menorrhagia. Notwithstanding, however, the intimate physiological connexion between the ovaries and the function of menstruation, I have not often been able to trace, clinically speaking, menorrhagia to such disease, unaccompanied by uterine lesions. At the same time, it is quite possible that the irritable state of the ovaries, which inflammatory disease of the uterus so very frequently induces, may re-act on the menstrual function, and contribute to exaggerate and pervert it. In these cases, however, the uterine lesion is generally according to my experience, the primary and principal cause of the menorrhagia ; on its removal the ovarian irritation disappearing along with the menorrhagia.

Menorrhagia at the Dawn and Close of Menstruation.—Menorrhagia is occasionally met with at the dawn and close of menstruation, from mere uterine congestion, apart from any local inflammatory disease.

Thus, the first manifestation of the menses may be characterized by a severe attack of hæmorrhage, the subsequent periods being physiological ; or the menses may continue to appear hæmorrhagically at irregular intervals for several months. This latter type of menorrhagia, however, is much less frequently met with than the first. When, also, the menses are about to cease definitively, and become physiologically irregular, profuse menstruation, amounting to flooding, is not unusual, as a result of mere congestion. Thus the menses will disappear for two or more months, and then return with excessive abundance. It is very seldom, however, even at this period of life, that hæmorrhagic menstrual fluxes occur frequently, and assume a continued character, in the absence of tumours or malignant disease, unless there be inflammatory ulceration of the cervix. In nearly all the instances of very obstinate hæmorrhage at the change of life which I meet with, I find, on examination, that the congestion and hæmorrhage are kept up by inflammatory and ulcerative disease. Indeed some of the very worst instances of protracted and severe hæmorrhage that I have ever seen, have been cases of this description ; and what satisfactorily proves that the inflammatory affection is the cause of the continued hæmorrhage is, that when it is cured the hæmorrhage generally ceases. This is not, however, invariably the case. I have occasionally met with females at the critical period of life, in whom hæmorrhage obstinately persisted after the removal of the inflammatory and ulcerative disease of the cervix, which had probably in the first instance given rise to it. In several of these cases, however, time or dilatation of the cervix has subsequently proved that the hæmorrhage did not proceed from a sound uterus, but was connected with the presence of a polypus, or of a fibrous tumour, so small and obscurely situated as not to have been recognized at first.

Menorrhagia during Pregnancy.—The periodical hæmorrhages which occasionally occur during pregnancy, are considered by some writers to be of a menstrual character.   Without
denying the possibility of a true menstrual flux taking place
from the cervical canal during pregnancy, I would mention,
that in nearly all the cases of this form of hæmorrhage—not
merely temporary, and not proceeding from separation of the
ovum—that have come under my observation, I have discovered inflammatory ulceration of the cervix.   This fact certainly
offers the most natural explanation of the presumed menstruation of pregnant women, at least in the majority of instances.
On examining these patients, I have generally found blood escaping from the ulcerated uterine neck, the ulcerations presenting the peculiarly turgid and luxuriant appearance which I
have elsewhere described as characteristic of such leisons during pregnancy.   When a pregnant female suffering from
ulceration of the cervix is instrumentally examined, the ulcerated surface bleeds freely on the slightest touch, and women in
whom abortion or premature confinement is brought on by such
disease are very frequently found, on inquiry, to have experienced repeated hæmorrhagic fluxes during the pregnancy, which
are often mistaken for menstrual periods.

Menorrhagia after Parturition.—The continued and obstinate hæmorrhage which is often observed after parturition, both
before and after the return of menstruation, is nearly always
complicated with and occasioned by inflammatory ulceration
of the neck of the uterus, with or without disease of the body
of the uterus.   This form of menorrhagia may be protracted
for months after the labour, until the patient be reduced to the
last stage of anæmia, if the real cause is not discovered and efficiently treated.

In the various forms of menorrhagia occurring in the non-
pregnant females, and accompanied by ulcerative lesions, does
the blood escape from the lining membrane of the uterine cavity,
as in ordinary menstruction, or from the ulcerated surface ?   I
believe that both these surfaces are often simultaneously the
sources of the hæmorrhage, although sometimes it may proceed
from one only.   I have frequently seen the blood oozing from
the diseased surface under all the circumstances mentioned,
and have often checked it instantaneously by freely cauterizing
with the solid nitrate of silver the *entire* ulcerated surface, both
internally and externally to the os uteri.

Treatment.—The views and facts which I have above developed are of extreme practical importance.   Not only do
they render unnecessary, in the immense majority of cases, the
hair-drawn distinctions of pathologists with reference to the

constitutional state of the patients suffering from menorrhagia, but they also greatly simplify treatment. The hæmorrhage being in reality nearly always the result of local disease, the latter is in most cases, the real element to be attacked and subdued. Instead, therefore, of an intricate and complex system of therapeutics, founded on a host of indications, the practitioner has, generally speaking, merely to *bring to light and treat* the disease which causes the mischief. By so doing, he removes the morbid condition which keeps up the hæmorrhagic state, and menstruation spontaneously returns to a natural state.

In those forms of menorrhagia in which the absence of any local disease is evident, or at least to be presumed,—at the beginning and termination of the menstrual function, for instance, or when the hæmorrhage occurs in an accidental manner from some easily assignable cause, mental or bodily,—very little medicinal treatment is, generally speaking, required. If the patient is kept at rest in a horizontal posture, and the cause be removed, the hæmorrhage will generally subside of itself, without leaving any trace in the general health beyond temporary debility, which quiet and a moderately nourishing dietary soon remove.

This is not, however, always the case; the hæmorrhage may, even under these circumstances be so severe and so prolonged that it would be imprudent to trust to the unassisted efforts of nature. When such is the case, the indications are, to moderate the activity of the circulation by the means of sedatives, such as opium, hyoscyamus, digitalis, hydrocyanic acid, Indian hemp, and other medicinal agents similar in their action ; to modify the plasticity of the blood by the administration of vegetable and mineral acids; and to exercise a revulsive action on the intestinal canal by the means of saline purgatives. The application of cold to the lower abdominal region, and the injection of cold astringent injections into the vagina, may also be resorted to, should these means fail. It is as well, however, to wait, unless the hæmorrhage be excessive, until the normal duration of the menstrual flux in the patient have passed, lest the impression of cold should suddenly arrest the excretion of blood whilst the physiological flux towards the uterus is still in force, as extreme congestion, and even inflammation, might ensue. This appears to me a desirable precaution, and one which I usually adopt, although the direct impression of cold to the uterine organs during menstruation, does not appear to be in reality as dangerous as it is usually considered.

In this the most simple form of menorrhagia, it is seldom necessary to resort to those medicinal agents which have a direct influence upon the uterus, such as ergot of rye and savine. It must not, however, be forgotten that they are very valuable anti-menorrhagic remedies, and often succeed when all other medicinal means fail to arrest the hæmorrhage. As a last resource, we can resort to plugging the vagina; but this is a means of treatment which may be said to be scarcely ever necessary in mere accidental menorrhagia, and which may be kept in reserve for the more formidable forms of hæmorrhage, of the treatment of which we have yet to speak.

Should the antecedents of the patient, carefully scrutinized, reveal the existence of any decided uterine symptoms, or lead to the impression that uterine disease may exist, as soon as the hæmorrhage has stopped or has been temporarily arrested by the means above-mentioned, the state of the uterus and of its cervix ought to be investigated—firstly, by the touch, and secondly, by the speculum, should the finger detect disease, or a suspicious condition of the uterine neck and of its cavity. In those cases in which the hæmorrhage is continuous, or all but continuous, it is not necessary to wait for its entire subsidence to examine the patient. When the exacerbation which corresponds to the menstrual epoch in the patient has passed, and the hæmorrhage has abated, the state of the uterine organs should be ascertained without delay.

When inflammation, and more especially inflammatory ulceration of the neck of the uterus, is discovered, and the absence of cancerous lesions or fibrous growths has been ascertained, the practitioner may consider that, in nineteen cases out of twenty, he has found the key to the menorrhagic state, and that the most efficacious and prompt means of treating it is to treat the disease he has discovered. From that moment he may look upon all medicinal anti-hæmorrhagic agents as mere adjuvants —useful no doubt, but of very secondary importance compared with the treatment of the local disease. Very often the hæmorrhage stops as soon as the irritability of the inflamed surface is modified, and long before the disease is cured.

The menorrhagia, however, may persist with more or less intensity, notwithstanding the gradual improvement of the local disease. It is with such patients more especially that great advantage may be derived from the administration of ergot of rye in substance or infusion, of savine in powder, of gallic acid and of the other medicinal agents mentioned. I generally begin with scruple doses of the ergot or savine two or three times a day, gradually increasing the dose if required.

In those cases in which, as we have seen, the hæmorrhage persists after the entire removal of local disease, owing to enlargement of the uterus, to the presence of a small unrecognised polypus or uterine tumour in the cavity of the uterus and its neck, or from the mere hæmorrhagic habit, I have of late resorted with encouraging success, to plugging *the os uteri it-self*, instead of the vagina.   It occurred to me that the usual plan of filling up and distending the vagina by pieces of sponge or a handkerchief, was a very clumsy, painful, and inefficient mode of opposing mechanical resistence to the exit of blood from the undeveloped uterus, when its orifice could be so easily brought into sight.   Acting on this idea, I have, in several in-stances, brought the cervix uteri into view, and passed inside the os two or three small pieces of cotton, tied to a piece of thread, which I wedged in firmly, covering the whole cervix with two or three larger pieces left in close contact with it on the withdrawal of the instrument.   In most of the cases in which I have resorted to this plan, I have easily arrested the hæmorrhage.   Indeed this modification of the ordinary practice appears to me so simple and so consonant with common sense, that I cannot but think it will be adopted in severe cases.   In the ordinary operation of plugging the vagina, that canal has to be distended by a large mass of sponge or linen, soaked with clotted blood, which often interferes with the functions of the bladder and rectum, is always a source of great discom-fort to the patient, and is not always efficient ; whereas, by the plan I describe, the end proposed is much more effectually en-compassed, with scarcely any annoyance to the patient beyond that which the use of the speculum occasions.

Owing to the natural contractility of the cervical canal, and the pressure of fluids from behind, if the cotton is not well pushed in, it is soon forced out.   The plug may be left without renew-al twenty-four or even thirty-six hours ; but in the latter case it is generally expelled spontaneously.   A small piece of sponge may be used and is more likely to remain *in situ*, owing to its expansion ; but as it must necessarily be very small, it is more likely to be permeated by the blood. If sponge is used, great care should be taken to extract the piece passed into tho os, to which a small piece of thread should always be tied, as the os uteri might not be able to expel it alone, owing to its great expansion.

In the class of cases of which we are now treating, I have occasionally found that a few leeches applied after menstrua-tion to the cervix uteri, have arrested the hæmorrhage.

I need scarcely add that any disease of the abdominal viscera that appears to favour the hæmorrhage, should he treated, and that the debility occasioned by menorrhagia must be met, du-ring the intervals of the attacks by as nourishing a diet as the patient will bear, and by those tonics which are suited to her state.   It must, however, be borne in mind that when the hæ-morrhage is accompanied or occasioned by inflammatory uterine lesions, the stomach is generally sympathetically affected, and unable to digest much food, so that a free dietary may be positively injurious and increase the mischief.

I have not spoken of the hæmorrhage that is observed in fibrous tumours and polypi of the uterus, and in cancer, because it is so much a symptom of these diseases, that it can only be properly treated of in connexion with them.

[To be Continued.]

Bright's Disease.

" Bright's Disease and its Treatment" are still among the *vexatæ questiones* of pathology and therapeutics, and as Dr. Frerichs is so well known and highly esteemed in this country on account of his physiological inquiries, we feel assured that an analysis of his pathological researches will be more welcome than any lengthened critique upon their results.

It is not easy to condense into smaller compass a work so crowded with facts as that before us ; but, limiting ourselves to the observations and opinions of its author, and placing in the most prominent position those which have the greatest share of novelty, the probability of his receiving justice at our hands will be greater than if the attempt were made to weigh the merits of his treatise with those of others who have preceded him.

The first chapter contains an " historical retrospect," into which it is not necessary to enter, as the facts are more or less familiar to every student of pathology. It is interesting to observe the early date at which groups of symptoms were recognized as bearing more than an accidental relationship to each other, and it is still more so to perceive that the links connecting them were discovered only when inquiry proceeded upon the truly inductive method,—for we are conscious that there is in it the germ of a power which will eventually be great enough to grasp facts apparently more widely separated, and penetrating enough to perceive their bonds of union.

The anatomical changes in the kidney are divided into three forms, which may also be considered as stages of the process of disease.   They are the following :—

I. The stage of hyperhæmia, and of commencing exudation.

II. The stage of exudation, and of its commencing transformation.

III. The stage of degeneration—atrophy.

In the first of these, which is frequently attended by hæmorrhagic effusion from the glomeruli, from the capillary plexus surrounding the urinary tubuli, or from the veins upon the surface of the cortex, the epithelium of the tubuli is not essentially changed, although the canals themselves, especially those of the cortical substance, are commonly filled with coagulated fibrin. These coagula are sometimes perfectly simple, and present themselves in this condition as casts of the tubes in which they were formed, while at other times parts of the epithelial lining, or more or less changed blood-corpuscles, may be found imbedded in them. This condition is not often met with anatomically (20 times in 292 *post-mortem* examinations,) and is then the accompaniment of an acute, violent illness. The disease when chronic is rarely fatal at so early a period.

In the second stage the progress of exudation increases, while the hyperrhæmic condition becomes less marked. Metamorphosis of the exuded matter follows; the epithelium and the fibrinous-casts of the tubuli break up into fatty molecules. In the Malpighian corpuscles similar exudation and fatty matter are seen lying between the capsule and its contained glomerulus, and then these bodies are raised above their natural size; but as long as the stream of secretion, poured from the glomeruli, is sufficiently powerful to remove the coagula of fibrin, this increase of dimension is not observed. In the urinary canals, especially those of the cortical substance, important changes are in progress; the epithelium undergoes complete transformation, losing gradually the form of its cells, presenting fatty infiltration to a variable extent, and ultimately losing its characteristic appearance and function, and becoming replaced by granular detritus and fat. This second stage was found in 139 in 292 examinations. It embraces the 1st and 2d forms of Bright; the 2d, 3d, and 4th of Rayer and Rokitansky; the 2d, 3d, 4th, and 7th of Christison; and the 2d and 3d of Martin Solon.

In consequence of the degeneration of fibrin in the urinary tubuli and the Malpighian corpuscles, and the removal of this with the more or less transformed epithelium, the walls of these structures collapse, and part of the kidney is atrophied. It is this which constitutes the third stage of Bright's disease. This atrophy is brought about in some cases by the contraction of plastic matter, when the latter has been exuded into the interstitial textures. This is rare, however, and when present is only a co-operative cause of atrophy. This 3d stage of Frerichs corresponds with the 3d of Bright, the 5th and 6th of Rayer, the 5th and 7th of Rokitansky, and the 4th of M. Solon.

Among the not constant anatomical changes of the kidney, Frerichs enumerates and describes—1. Apoplexy; 2. Suppuration; 3. Cystic formations; 4. Calculous deposits; 5. Tubercle, etc. In the paragraphs upon the chemical changes in the kidney, the amount of solid constituents is given, and the proportion of fat in a hundred parts of dried kidney substance. In health the latter varies from 4·4 to 4 05 per cent. In morbus Brightii, it was found varying from 4·40 to 13·9. Generally speaking, the quantity of fat was greater when the disease had advanced to the third stage, but this is not invariable ; and the fact, that by chemical examination the quantity is often found so much less than microscopic observation would lead us to expect, must, according to Frerichs, be considered as a proof that we are not justified in naming as fat all those globules which resemble it in form. In the kidney of a cat, and in that of a dog, the fat was found by Frerichs to vary from 27·20 to 32·50 percent. Both animals were perfectly healthy ; their urine contained not a trace of albumen, a sufficient proof that morbus Brightii cannot be considered dependent solely upon fatty degeneration.

A statistical report, and tabular representation of the changes found (*post mortem*)in other organs, concludes the second chapter of the book. The cases are gathered from Bright, Christison, Gregory, Martin Solon, Becquerel, Rayer, Bright and Barlow, Malmesten, and the author's own observation.

The third chapter presents a short account of the general course of the disease in its two forms, acute and chronic ; and we pass from it to the fourth, entitled " Special Symptomatology." In this the appearances (merely sketched before) are described in detail,—their frequency given numerically,—their causation examined,—and their clinical value in respect of diagnosis, prognosis, and treatment, pointed out.

The symptoms are treated under the following heads :—1. Those of disordered uro-poësis,—embracing, (a) pain in the region of the kidney ; (b) percussion and palpation ; (c) frequency of micturition ; (d) changes of the urine. 2. Those of changed blood. 3. The habitus of the patient. 4. Dropsy. 5. Changes in the action of the skin. 6. Uræmic intoxication, (chronic and acute.) 7. Disturbances in the functions of the primæ viæ. 8. Pseudo-rheumatic pains.

It would be impossible to present anything but the most unsatisfactory analysis of this chapter, if we attempted to embrace all its contents. We shall limit ourselves to those included under the 6th and 7th heads ; and we shall do so simply because the statements there made have more of novelty than the others.

1. *The Chronic Form of Uræmia.*—This steals slowly and unobservedly upon its victim, and is in almost every instance fatal. In the early stages of Bright's disease, there is a peculiar dulness, or sleepiness, in the expression of the face, and in the demeanor of the patient. He complains of dull headache,—a " light" feeling,—the eyes are expressionless,—the whole physi-

ognomy is depressed in its features,—he is forgetful, and listless.
These symptoms diminish if the secretion of urine becomes
more abundant, and sometimes they disappear entirely for a
time.   In other cases they gradually increase in intensity ; the
sleepiness passes into stupefaction ; the patients, who at first
can be roused by speaking to them loudly, or by other means,
and will then give rational replies, now sink into everdeep-
ening lethargy ; it is impossible any longer to arouse them ;
respiration becomes stertorous, and is replaced only by the
gurgling of death.   They generally lie perfectly still, without
speaking.   Delirium is rare ; when it does occur, it is of the
low muttering description ; the patients repeat, times without
number, a few words or sentences.   Death is often preceded
by convulsions; trembling of the hands: distortion of the features, becoming quickly followed by clonic spasm, extending
over the whole system of voluntary muscles.   This is the
more common form of nervous disturbance in Bright's disease.
It may last for a longer or shorter time, and is often capricious
in its course.   Nevertheless, it is more to be dreaded than any
other complication, for it is the most certain herald of a fatal
termination.   Differing from it in its manner of appearance,
and very essentially different in respect of prognosis, is the
    2. *Acute form of Uræmia*, which commences suddenly, and
in a short time reaches its full intensity.   It appears to attack
the patient in one of three ways, the first symptoms being either
those of depressed cerebral function, of irritation of the spinal
cord, or of a combination of the two.   Frerichs confirms, from his
own experience, the statement of Dr. Addison, that when (under depressed cerebral function) the respiration becomes stertorous, there is not the deep guttural tone heard in hæmorrhagic
apoplexy, from the movements of the velum palati, but that the
sound is of higher pitch, and is caused by the passage of air
against the hard palate and the lips.   He also adds his testimony to that of Dr. Bright with regard to the persistence of
consciousness in some cases where uræmia has evidenced itself
first by convulsion.   Although the prognosis is more favorable
when the attack has this acute character, inasmuch as it generally follows a sudden suppression of the urinary secretion, yet
it may prove fatal in a few days, or even hours; and the result
must be anticipated as very unfavorable when acute uræmic
intoxication occurs, as it does not unfrequently, during the
course of chronic Bright's disease.   A sudden change in the
quantity or quality of the urine, disturbances of the organs of
sense, etc., are insisted on as of importance in the light of
warning symptoms.   There are cases, however, where these
are entirely wanting, and the diagnosis may be attended with

great difficulty. A very constant, and in the earlier periods of
uræmia, a prominent symptom, is vomiting. Altered ingesta
are thrown up at first, but subsequently a thin, watery substance only. Its re-action, seldom acid, is generally neutral or
alkaline; it emits frequently a sharply ammoniacal odour; and,
if a glass rod dipped in hydrochloric acid is brought near it,
copious white fumes are developed. If the inodorous, neutral,
or even slightly acid fluid is heated with liquor potassæ, the
presence of an ammoniacal compound is demonstrated. Frerichs has frequently sought for undecomposed urea in the vomited matters, but always without success. Artificial uræmia,
induced in animals by extirpating the kidneys and injecting
urea, is attended by the vomiting of similar matters containing
a large quantity of carbonate of ammonia, but no undecomposed
urea. The decomposition of urea into carbonate of ammonia
does not (according to Frerichs) take place in the stomach
through the action of the gastric fluid, (as Bernard and Barreswil maintain,) but it is brought about in the blood within
the vessels.

This form of vomiting must not be confounded with others,
which are very common in the course of morbus Brightii, and
which have their origin in chronic catarrh of the stomach,
simple perforating ulcer, the misuse of spirits, etc., etc. The
characters described serve to distinguish them from that of
true uræmic character.

Serious disturbances of the nervous system appear to be in
many cases delayed or altogether avoided by this vicarious
excretive process. This has, however, been too confidently
asserted to be a general rule by Bernard and Barreswil. In
the stomachs of animals whose kidneys have been removed,
ammoniacal compounds are constantly found; but the uræmic
condition is not thus delayed in the majority of instances. It
gives evidences of its presence at the time that the described
change takes place in the secretion of the stomach. Ammoniacal salts are then found in nearly all the secretions, and
compounds of that base may be discovered in the expired air.
The relation of diarrhœa to uræmia requires further elucidation,
and Frerichs does not give his opinion upon the subject.

The conditions of the perspiration and of the expired air are
then closely examined. The former has been tested principally by the noses of pathologists, and is left doubtful; in the
latter, the presence of ammonia is established; and in artificial
uræmia, it was not until this base could be detected that any
signs of disturbance in the nervous system were observed.
Pathological anatomy is then shown to throw no certain and no
constant light upon the nature of uræmic intoxication; and it

is believed, that in the condition of the blood the key to the
mystery is to be found. Its physical properties, in respect of
consistence, colour, odour, etc., present no unvarying change
of character. Its chemical relations are altered, and the alterations are essential. In all cases where the symptoms of uræmia
presented themselves, carbonate of ammonia, and, in addition,
undecomposed urea, were found in the blood. The quantity
of the former is variable to a high degree ; but in no one
instance did it remain undetected. Frerichs gives another
historical sketch of the theories of this branch of his subject.
For a long time the opinion has been almost universally held,
that the cause of these symptoms was to be found in the retention of some urinary elements in the blood. Osborne and G.
Owen Rees form the exceptions ; the former being of opinion
that arachnitis was the cause, to which pathological anatomy
returns the most satisfactory answer ; and the latter, question-
ing the influence of urea in the production of coma, etc., from
the perfectly correct observation, that the appearance and
intensity of such symptoms in morbus Brightii, hold no constant
relation to the quantity of the urinary secretion ; and further,
that the blood may be surcharged with urea, and yet cause no
symptom of uræmic poisoning. Rees considered hydræmia
as the essential condition ; but this cannot be so important as
he would make it appear, since coma, convulsions, etc., occur in
acute morbus Brightii, during either the earlier or later stages
of scarlet fever, typhus, etc., without there being any evidences
of such thinning of the blood. The question remains to be
answered, in what way suppression of urine exerts the influence
assigned to it, and which of its elements is the active agent ?
By the experiments of Vauquelin, Ségalas, Bichat, Courtin, and
Gaspard, repeated with additions of his own, Frerichs proves,
that the presence in the blood of a large quantity of urea,
of uric acid, or of urine itself, with extractives and salts,
cannot cause the symptoms commonly observed when suppression of the secretion takes place. The result of a course of
inquiry undertaken by Frerichs in 1849 and 1850, is that for
the production of uræmic intoxication, the presence of any or
all of these substances is insufficient, but that the urea must be
decomposed through the agency of a peculiar ferment substance,
and carbonate of ammonia set free within the blood-vessels.
The production of this decomposing agent in febrile affections
is not difficult to suppose, and the rapidity with which symptoms of uræmia are developed when morbus Brightii supervenes
upon scarlet-fever, typhus, etc., together with the suddenness
of their appearance in a person whose blood has been for a
long time overladen with urea (without them) lend support to

the view. The injection of carbonate of ammonia into the blood induces all the symptoms of uræmia, and without defining the precise nature of the ferment body, but asserting that a very slight modification of one of the normal elements of the blood would be sufficient for the purpose, Frerichs, by a course of experiments, considers that he has established his theory with regard to uræmia.

It would be impossible, within the limits of this review, to follow our author closely through the minutiæ of the concluding chapters. We can but indicate the topics which form their basis, so that our readers may form some estimate of the book.

In the chapter upon the *complications* of morbus Brightii, the several diseases of the heart, arteries, veins, liver, and spleen, &c., &., are examined and described. The *frequency* of Bright's disease, its *duration, course,* and *terminations,* are then considered; and separate chapters are devoted to the questions of etiology and pathogenesis, essence of the disease, diagnosis, prognosis, varieties (forms,) and therapeia. An Appendix, containing clinical reports of sixteen cases, and the results of a series of experimental researches, concludes the volume.

Frerichs describes the following forms :—1. Simple. 2. Cachectic. 3. That of the drunkard. 4. That occurring in acute blood-disease, (cholera, scarlet fever, measles, typhus, &c.) 5. That accompanying pregnancy.

In the chapter upon treatment, the disease locally and generally, its more constant and its occasional complications, are severally dwelt upon. The author does not commit himself to the system of depletion, of strengthening, of continually produced diuresis, purgation, or diaphoresis, but gives the moderate and judicious employment of all the various agents mentioned a position in his list, the peculiarities of the case under consider-ation leading to the choice of that which is most suitable.

In respect of the treatment when uræmic intoxication is present, Frerichs recommends acids, which should form innocuous compounds with ammonia in the blood, such as the vegetable acids.—[*Medical Times.*

On the Catarrhal Pneumonia and Lobar Pneumonia of Children. By MM. Trousseau and Lasegue.

Catarrhal (or lobular) pneumonia is a disease as distinct from simple (lobar,) as variola is from erythema. This is seen in their respective mortality. Of twenty children who have been admitted to the hospital clinique, suffering from *simple pneumonia,* in six months all have recovered ; of nearly thirty who were attacked with *catarrhal pneumonia*, not one survived. Most of the first class of cases exhibited an excessive degree of acuteness which burnt out like a fire of straw ; while several of the second, notwithstanding their fatal termination, commenced with very mild symptoms.

Simple · pneumonia hardly ever affects a child below two years of age, and rarely those of two or three, but becomes of more and more frequent occurrences as the child approaches adolescence. Its cause and symptoms resemble those of the adult, with some modifications. After twenty-four or thirty-six hours, the souffle and bronchophony can alone be heard ; the crepitant râle, which is often observed in the adult when the patient coughs, even when much souffle is present, is hardly ever heard in the child. So afterwards, from day to day, without the crepitation of resolution, the souffle disappears, leaving only a feeble respiration. The progress of the disease is also more rapid than in the adult. In the mild form of the disease, recovery takes place rapidly, and in large proportion ; but in its grave form, many cases are lost by any mode of treatment. M. Trousseau generally bleeds the child, gives it an emetic of sulphate of copper, and then a mixture, containing Kermes mineral and extract of digitalis.

Catarrhal pneumonia commences with a catarrh, which rapidly extends to the small bronchi, and then we hear numerous and small sub-crepitant *râles* disseminated over both lungs, and especially posteriorly. These *râles* may persist for four, six, eight, or fifteen days, without any *souffle* becoming manifest ; but sooner or later we hear a *souffle*, the resonance of the cries or the voice, or at least a prolonged respiratory murmur. While these latter sounds, common to simple and catarrhal pneumonia are thus manifesting themselves, we find, by the subcrepitant *râles*, that the capillary catarrh is still persisting in the rest of the lung. The disease has extended from the mucous membrane to the parenchyma of the organ. Febrile action is less than in ordinary pneumonia, being predominant at some portions of the day, and entirely ceasing at others ; and these alternations of better and worse may continue for fifteen, twenty, or thirty days ; the disease being originally a pulmonary catarrh, and partaking of the obstinacy and uncertainty of catarrhal complaints. As more and more of the parenchyma becomes implicated, the fever becomes more continuous and intense, and the respiration more difficult, until the children die exhausted. In other cases, in which the bronchial phlegmasia was very intense from the first, and the lung became rapidly invaded over a great extent, death takes place with rapidity. The progress of the disease has usually been more rapidly fatal, when it has succeeded to measles, chronic disease of the skin, or laryngitis. All means of treatment that have been tried have proved impotent.

These two affections may be compared, *exceptis excipiendis*, with erysipelas and phlegmon. Erysipelas traverses the surface like the catarrh ; and when it persists too long, it induces ulcerations of the skin, furuncles, and circumscribed subcutaneous abscess, just as the capillary catarrh induces suppuration of the lobules, little abscesses of the lungs, and circumscribed pneumonias. Simple pneumonia, on the other hand, progresses like simple phlegmon, violent in its febrile reaction, but terminating abruptly and rapidly.

· It must not be supposed, from what has been said, that catarrhal pneumonia is almost invariably fatal. Although this is the case amidst the miamata of an hospital, which exert effects at once so terrible and so difficult to avert, it is not so in private practice. In this, one-half the patients may be cured by repeated vomiting, flying blisters, antimonials, and digitalis ; but how terrible are the ravages of a disease, which, under the most favorable circumstances, kills one-half its subjects !

[*L'Union Médicale. Med. Chir. Rev.*

On the Simultaneous Occurrence of Hyperæsthesia and Anæsthesia of the Skin in Neuralgia. By Dr. TURK.

During or after an attack of severe neuralgia, there is sometimes a more or less considerable amount of hyperæsthesia of the superficial layers of skin seated over the affected parts, so that not the least contact can be borne. Much oftener, however, the contrary is the case—viz, anæsthesia of the superficial layers over the points of deep-seated pain. The degree of this superficial anæsthesia is proportionate to the amount of pain in the deeper layers of the skin ; and it is sometimes so considerable that nipping the skin with the nails, or blistering it by the application of heat, is unfelt. These opposite conditions of the same part may be observed for some time after the attack of spontaneous pain has disappeared. The two conditions do not always observe the same limits. Sometimes the most superficial layer of the skin only is anæsthetic, and the formation of a moderately thick fold of skin causes pain ; while at other times the chorion is anæsthetic throughout, and thick folds of the skin may be pinched up, pain being only felt at the subcutaneous layers.

The intensity of the anæsthesia diminishes in proportion to the distance from the site of the spontaneous pain. An entire side of the body has been observed to be anæsthetic ; but the

insensibility has usually become so diminished towards the
boundary, as to be incapable of being tested by irritation by
the finger, though readily so by the application of hot or cold
bodies.   This hemiasthænia· sometimes extends to the wall of
the mouth, and side of the tongue.   Oftentimes it has been only
observed over the greater part of half the body, certain portions
of the trunk or head being exempted.   In some cases the functions of the s,·nses have also been found disturbed.

The hyperæsthesia of the deeper layer of the skin rarely assumes such an extension as the anæsthesia of the superficial
ones; though cases have been observed in which it, too, has
occupied one entire half of the body.   In double-sided neuralgia, the anæsthesia and hyperæsthesia are also double, being
more intense on one side than the other, if that is the case also
with the neuralgia.   In some cases, both sides of the body are
affected symmetrically, having their limits then drawn horizon-
tally.

Besides the occurrence of these conditions in neuralgia, it
not unfrequently happens, according to the author's experience,
that in typhus there is a more or less intense hyperæsthesia of
the deeper layers of the skin in various parts of the body, especially the calves of the legs.   It is sometimes so considerable,
that the half-soporose person utters expressions of pain under
the influence of even but moderate pressure.   Examined after
the fever had run its course, no abnormal conditions of sensibility were observed in some of the patients; but in other spontaneous pains, accompanied by hyperæsthesia and anæsthesia of
different parts (especially the leg and foot,) and in different
degrees, remained for weeks.—*Froɪiep's Tagsberichte. Ibid.*

External Use of Chloroform.

Dr. Channing read the following paper on this subject:—
" I have made some trials of the external application of chloroform.   It has often been entirely successful in the present relief
of pain.   In some, the relief has been permanent.   This use of
the remedy of pain is not new.   It has been said that a free
application of chloroform to a part on which a surgical operation is to be done, will render such part insensible to the
violence done it.   Thus, immersing a finger in chloroform
will prevent the suffering which accompanies the deep cuts
which some of the diseases of this member require, and which
are described as exquisitely acute.   These statements rest on
good authority.   In such use of chloroform consciousness
remains unimpaired, the brain not being at all affected by it.

Having frequently applied chloroform externally for the

relief of pain, in many and various cases, and often with speedy, and generally with continued relief, I propose to present some of them to the Society :—

CASE I. 1848. Mrs. ——, about 30, has children. For some years has had symptoms of uterine disturbance. Among these, have been suffering on intercourse, leucorrhœa, tumoral pains in and about the pelvis, always increased by walking, and which, except pain in the spine, are relieved by lying down. For the uterine conditions the usual means were faithfully employed, and her complaints there were entirely and permanently removed. The dorsal trouble, however, was·as great as ever.

For this I recommended the external application of chloroform over the whole course of the spine which was involved in the disease. The effect was immediate and complete. I saw this patient, a few days since, Nov. 1851, and found her well in regard to the back, and speaking of herself as very well in all respects.

In this case, the pain in the spine was doubtless the result of the reflex function, the womb being the original seat of the malady. But when the uterine affection was relieved, the sympathetic dorsal difficulty remained, and only yielded to the use of chloroform. The quantity used was an ounce.

CASE II. Mr.——, aged 22. A very feeble man in appearance; very thin in flesh; pale; and an almost constant sufferer from headache. This pain occupied but a small part of the head arc, and most frequently the right temporal region. It was accompanied by constant nausea, frequent vomiting, great prostration of strength, and demanding for its present relief firm pressure over the part affected.

The last attack, which happened a few weeks since, I applied chlorform to the seat of pain. A few drops were applied by means of a handkerchief. The immediate effect was redness of the skin and a tingling sensation in the spot. The pain was at once relieved. He raised his head from a friend's shoulder, opened his eyes, looked round, and expressed his utter surprise and deep pleasure at the entire relief which had followed the use of such apparently simple means. He called on me the next morning, and reported himself perfectly well. I have not been called to him since.

The relief in this was *sudden* in its occurrence, as it had been in others. It has not been less permanent on that account, or in such cases. It has acted at once to remove pain, and with a rapidity which distinguishes the relief entirely from that which follows etheaization by inhalation. The brain does not seem to have anything to do with the matter. Local pain is abolish.

ed, and at once ; and the nerves have no story of suffering to
tell to the brain.   The sentinel is at his post, but his function is
not needed.   The part does not lose its natural sensibility at all.
On the contrary, it feels the tingling, the irritation of the chloroform, just as distinctly as at first.   Nothing has been lost of
natural power and healthful function.   All that has happened is
this : the pain has ceased, and the patient is well.

CASE III. 1851. Mrs. ——, aged 36. Has long suffered
from uterine disturbance.   The most exhausting and annoying
symptom was leucorrhœa.   This was a perpetual drain, and
made her exceedingly uncomfortable.   I was occasionally consulted in this case ; but as her general health continued tolerably
firm, no systematic attempt at recovery was thought necessary
by the patient.   She became pregnant, and supposed herself
between two and three months advanced in that state, when
hemorrhage and severe uterine pain occurred, on account of
which I was desired to see her.   She had lost a great deal of
blood before I saw her.   I found her perfectly blanched—lips
and whole face ; skin cold ; hands bloodless ; faint ; almost
pulseless.   Various means were used, and the hemorrhage was
stopped.   I considered her case, however, so pressing, that I
passed the whole day in the house.   She now began to complain of pain in the back.   This had exacerbations in the night,
becoming too severe to allow of sleep, and continuing three or
four hours without mitigation.   For this I recommended chloroform, which was applied by means of a handkerchief, and with
excellent results.   After three applications, on as many days
or nights, the pain ceased, and has not now, at the end of some
weeks, returned.

CASE IV. Mrs. ——, aged about 40. Last child, thirteen
years old.   I was called in consultation in this case, because
of vomiting, attending pregnancy, of about three months standing.   The vomiting ceased under treatment, and food was
taken in sufficient quantities, and was well borne by the stomach.
A comatose state supervened, which increased, with entire
abolition of mind, and death was its consequence.   The termination of cases of fatal vomiting by coma has occurred in
many instances which have come under my notice or knowledge.   I do not, however, recollect a case in which apparent
recovery has been followed by coma ending in death.

This case is reported here, because of the use of chloroform
for one of its symptoms.   This was pain in the back, in the
course of the spine.   It was very severe, taking the lead, in
distress, of all the rest.   For this pain I prescribed an ointment,
if so liquid a substance as was produced by the union of lard
and chloroform deserves the name.   It was applied twice or

thrice a day, and with most excellent effects, the pain entirely disappearing. It was used in the same way in the first of these cases.

CASE V. Mrs. ——. Has had four premature labours; the first at about five months, the fourth at about the eighth. They were all still-born, or neither of them lived over an hour or two. The fifth pregnancy was terminated at the full time by the birth of a living, healthful male child, on the 17th October, 1851. I visited her for the usual time after delivery, and left her in rapid progress towards perfect recovery. I was called to see her on the 27th October, and found her apparently very ill. Pulse rapid; skin hot; face flushed; much pain in head and in both breasts, making all attempts at nursing absolutely agonizing. A thick eruption had appeared over the whole chest. Upon examination, the breasts were found exquisitely sensitive, not bearing pressure at all. Sufficient pressure, however, was made to enable me to ascertain that there was no unusual hardness, or, in short, any other sign of disease in either organ. The pain was confined to the skin, and seemed to involve its whole tissue. The eruption proved to be a very full crop of sudamina of unusual size, resembling exactly an exaggerated form of the same kind of eruption in typhoid fever. Various means had been used before my visit, but without any good effect.

I recommended chloroform, and with the best effects. I regret I had not used it in combination with lard or rose ointment, both of which I have used, and for the reason that it may in this way be more extensively applied, with more continuous benefit, and with less of the unpleasant tingling which so generally accompanies the uncombined substance.

On what did this aching pain depend? It resembled that which at times makes *shingles* so very distressing. Was it owing to the eruption? I have never known the skin in sudamina to be complained of as the seat of pain, and I have examined it when covered by this eruption after a manner to have produced pain had morbid sensibility existed. In Mrs. ——'s case, the pain was persistent, being much aggravated by handling, though never so gently. The pain in this case subsided, under the use of chloroform, long before the eruption disappeared.

CASE VI. Mrs. ——, aged 25, married very young, and had a premature labour within a year or two afterwards. I was desired to see her, October, 1851, on account of an enlargement of the abdomen, on the left side, and for various signs of ill health. The tumour was found to be an excessively enlarged spleen. It filled the left hypochondrium, extending forward to the epigastrium, and downward to Poupart's ligament. Its anterior boundary was the linea alba. From this point or line it extended laterally and backward, filling accurately one whole side of the abdomen. She has been always regular in regard to the catamenial function. with the exception of the last two periods. Nausea, vomiting, and other unusual and disagreeable feelings have led to a suspicion that pregnancy may exist. She has recently taken a fatiguing journey of three days, and has suffered much since. The pain has been most troublesome in the head, and in the seat of the tumour. Diarrhœa and flatulence, with general anasarca, involving the face and head, are also present. Chloroform to the forehead and to the seat of the tumour has given her much comfort, more than has been derived from any other means used.

Case VII. Mrs. —— was delivered of her second child, a daughter, December 25th, 1850. Since that event she has been liable to diarrhœa, which, however, has not impaired her general health. She has long been annoyed by a spasmodic catching of her breath, almost resembling hiccup, but producing more general agitation of the body than does that. After her last confinement, this affection was for some time unusually troublesome.

I was called to see Mrs. ——, October 6th, 1851, and found her apparently very ill. She was hot ; feverish ; pulse rapid ; severe pain in head, which it was attempted to relieve by bandage, and different washes ; vomiting large quantities of watery fluid, colourless, having floating in it masses of a dense, white substance, resembling coagulated milk. No milk has been taken for some time. Copious diarrhœa, with very severe, intermitting pain around the umbilicus. No sleep at night, and for a week or more has suffered many of present symptoms. Means were used to check vomiting and diarrhœa, but without any useful result, and I determined to try chloroform externally. Its effects were most grateful. The head, stomach, and bowels became easy. They were, in short, relieved of all their trouble. This was in the evening. At my morning visit, I found Mrs. —— up and dressed, nursing her child ; and, except weakness from so much suffering, and forced total abstinence, in her usual health. I forgot to mention above, that, during this very severe attack, the catching respiration revived, as it does, I was informed, whenever she is at all indisposed, and continued till she recovered.

Case VIII. Mr. ——, of strongly-marked nervous temperament ; very *impressible ;* an excellent mesmeric subject. I was called to this gentleman on account of violent pain in the head, and to which he was very liable. I found him in bed.

He could not sit up at all, and any noise in the room, or house, or jarring of the furniture, increased the pain to agony. Pressure to the head gave some relief. While I was examining his case, he said he could bear his sufferings no longer ; that he must get up, and walk round the room ; do anything which might afford some relief. He was hot ; skin dry ; pulse rapid. I sent for leeches ; but before they could be got, and because of the increased suffering, I made a free application of sulphuric ether to the forehead. The relief from its use was soon apparent. It was strongly expressed, until, worn out by his long agony and sleeplessness—and now relieved—he fell asleep ; and, after long and perfectly quiet rest, awoke without pain, and next day went to his business.

The relief here was quite as striking as from chloroform. A good deal of ether was used, indeed, and the patient may have found some of the relief he experienced in the unavoidable inhalation of the ether vapour. This was not at all the case in the instances in which chloroform was applied. The quantity was very small, hardly damping the handkerchief beyond the limits of a twenty-five cent piece, and with the wet surface close to the skin, and often under the bed and other clothes. This case is reported, not on its own account only, but also to allude to another mode of employing local etherization. A professional friend of the highest reputation amongst us, and very cautious in forming opinions concerning the direct effects of remedies, once told the writer that he had been much gratified with the agency of sulphuric ether in procuring sleep in cases in which he was desirous to avoid the employment of opiates. His method was gently to have the forehead and face wiped with a cloth damped with sulphuric ether, and very often most grateful sleep followed this use of it.

CASE IX. Mrs. ——, aged 19, in seventh month of pregnancy. Of excellent health before marriage, she has suffered, in an unusually severe form, the signs and diseases of pregnancy. Vomiting occurred very early, and such was its excess that it seemed impossible that she could live through its ordinary continuance. To this succeeded ptyalism, which has been quite as uninterrupted and severe as was the vomiting. She is constantly in bed, having no power to sit up. Violent headache ; pain in abdomen ; in back ; in short, pain occurring in all possible localities, has made her life, for months, wretched. Having tried the ordinary means of diminishing these troubles, I have at length applied chloroform. The pain in the head has entirely ceased since she began this course. All other means are omitted. Pains elsewhere are sensibly diminished. She has no nausea, no vomiting, and the ptyalism is less. She bears milk, in small quantities, quite well on her stomach. As the pain in the back and abdomen continues to recur when the effects of the chloroform have passed away, I have to-day, November 10, 1851, directed an ointment of chloroform, two drachms to an ounce of lard, to be applied to the spine and to the epigastric region.

CASE X. This case occurred in the person of the writer. The disease was toothache. It was in one of its severest forms; had continued many hours; extended to the temple and lower jaw, and made the least application to it, a touch merely, exquisitely painful. Chloroform on a handkerchief was applied to the third branch of the fifth pair, where it passes out upon the face, and to its ramifications, and especially to that part of the cheek which was over the diseased tooth. The usual sense of tingling and burning was experienced, and the skin became slightly red. After a few minutes, a most grateful sense of relief was experienced. The pain disappeared as entirely as it does after an aching tooth has been drawn. No tenderness remained. The tongue or finger could be freely pressed against the tooth, and without producing any uneasiness. Chewing was possible and grateful. Cold water gave no agony. It may be inferred that I have exaggerated the suffering. Said a patient to me once, to whom I had suggested the idea that she might be in error as to her suffering, " *Sir, I know by my feelings how I feel.*" I can say that what I have said of the pain, and of the relief from chloroform, need not to be questioned. I felt and understood both.

Relief continued for some time. Pain recurred, but it was at once treated as above, and was at once relieved.

REMARKS.—I have written off these cases that I might report them to the Society, because I think this method of using anæsthetics may often be useful. It is not on account of the novelty of this mode of application of chloroform that the cases are presented, for the suggestion of such use will be found elsewhere. They are read because they present a number of cases, of facts, in which it has been a purpose to afford relief by the remedy, and especially by a faithful trial of it.

Another reason: These cases are sufficiently numerous to furnish some basis for generalization. By adding to them, they may at length authorize the establishment of rules of practice, which may not only contribute to the comfort of the sick, but exert important influences over disease.

Again. This use of chloroform is perfectly safe. Not the least disturbance of system or organ has been produced by the external employment of this substance. Consciousness remains undisturbed. The pulse, breathing, temperature, are natural. The expression of relief is very striking. In other uses of chloroform, or ether, consciousness is more or less abolished, and we know nothing of the relief but what comes of absence of complaint. From its external use we learn at once the whole story of the comfort, the extreme pleasure which is experienced.

Again. I present these cases in the hope that others will be induced by them to seek for their patients' relief from other sources than those ordinarily employed, and which so often do little more than occupy a certain amount of time in a self-limited disease. These cases show that we have the means of shortening this time, nay, of giving relief at once, and thus of anticipating recovery. I have used chloroform externally but once in acute inflammatory disease—puerperal peritonitis. In this case, after-pains continued until the fourth day from delivery, with retention of urine, and pain in the lower part of the abdomen, which broke sleep and produced extreme discomfort. This case was some miles from town, and I was attending in consultation. I advised a trial of chloroform to the part, and used it as above described. Its effect was not agreeable. The skin had been sodden with hot rum, brandy, hop-bags, &c., and had been made so tender that unusual smarting, tingling, and heat were at once produced, so as to make it necessary to remove the chloroform. There were recent leech-bites near the seat of pain, and these may have been irritated by the application. Should I again use chloroform externally in similar cases, I would combine it with some ointment, say rose ointment, in proportion of one or two drachms to the ounce of the ointment, and apply it on cloth, or, which would answer better, sheet or woven lint.

Has not our subject important physiological and therapeutic relations? The nerves, under ordinary circumstances and in their healthful state, convey at once to the brain morbid occurrences whenever or wherever such happen, and thus most important information is given of the state of the system, or of a part of it. So, when the body in every part of it is in health, the nerves communicate the knowledge of this fact to the brain and mind. The result of such agency is that consciousness of universal physical soundness—health—which constitutes the highest enjoyment of life. But chloroform, as we have seen and said, abolishes pain—we do not say cures disease—and, in this freedom from suffering, leaves it to the nerves to aid in such living processes as are themselves tending to the recovery of the diseased organ to health, and to aid the therapeutic powers of medicine. The mind remains ignorant of the state of the diseased part, so far as pain has given it knowledge of such state; but recovery is not thus delayed. We believe, on the contrary, it is hastened.

Of the mode of applying chloroform endermically, a word. A handkerchief fresh from the drawer, and a phial of chloroform, are all that is needed. Apply the handkerchief to the open mouth of the phial, and invert the latter so that the chloroform may wet a spot in the centre of the cloth. Do this two or three times, and then apply it to the seat of pain by moderate pressure and without friction. Let it remain till it is dry, and then wet and apply it again if need be. Ordinarily, the pain soon becomes less, and will even be found often to disappear entirely, with no further application of chloroform. Some redness is commonly produced, and some tingling or smarting. These, however, disappear when the handkerchief is removed. To prevent evaporation, and especially to prevent inspiration of the chloroform, always cover the cloth which contains it with another dry one.—[*Amer. Jour. of Med. Science.*

On the Treatment of Cancer by the Lactate of Iron taken by the Mouth and injected into the Veins. By DANIEL BRAINARD, M. D., Professor of Surgery in Rush Medical College, &c.

About two years since I communicated to Prof. Mussey, Chairman of the Committee on Surgery of the American Medical Association, some reasons which I had for supposing that the lactate of iron was possessed of more influence over cancer than any medicine yet known.

I have, since that time, had occasion to prescribe it often with results which, while they confirm the views expressed in regard to its efficiency in checking it, have not shown that it was capable of entirely curing it. This result was to me neither surprising nor discouraging, as I have already formed and expressed the opinion that to effect a cure "the whole of the solids and fluids of the body must be brought under its influence." That this is not effected by the simple introduction of medicines into the stomach is sufficiently obvious, and indeed to be expected, since the medicine, used in that way, is subjected to the action of the same nutrition and absorption under the influence of which the disease has originated. It is necessary to go behind this; and one of the means of doing so is by injecting it into the veins. It is only recently that I have had an opportunity of putting this method to the test of practice.

CASE. December 13th, 1851. Wm. H. Plumb, æt. 56 years, Englishman, applied to me on account of a tumour of the left orbit.

He gave the following history of his disease : About 25 years ago he had a disease of that eye, called by his physician cataract, which entirely destroyed the vision, but for which no operation was performed. About five years ago he received an injury of that eye from a stick striking against it, which was slight and gave but little pain. About seven months after this blow, he noticed a tumour, no larger than a pea, at the inner canthus "sending off roots into the eyeball." At this time, the tumour and eyeball were removed together by Prof. Smith, of Baltimore. The wound cicatrized well.

He remained in pretty good health about four years, when a tumour made its appearance at the lower and inner part of the orbit ; which, in eight months, attained the size of a large hickory nut. It was then operated upon again, but at the end of six weeks recommenced to grow, and, at the time of this examination, was of the size of an orange, filling up the whole of the orbit and projecting in front of it. Its surface was nodulated, elastic, pulsating, ulcerated to a great extent, and from this point there oozed a bloody serous fluid. He was thin but not sallow, and his health was not very much impaired. He complained, however, of acute lancinating pains through the orbit and head.

16th. Extirpation was performed in presence of the hospital class. It was found so firmly attached to the lower part of the orbit that it was necessary to remove the periosteum with it, and at the back part it could not all be removed. There remained a muscular mass which bled profusely, and which was so soft as to break under the forceps or tenaculum. After several ineffectual attempts to apply a ligature the actual cautery was resorted to and succeeded. The wound was dressed with lint. No inflammation followed. There was a copious discharge of red serum for a day or two, which gradually became yellow, and afterwards changed to pus. He was put, from the day of the operation, on the use of lactate of iron gr. v, three times a day in solution.

31st. Injected into his viens f$\mathfrak{Z}$j of the following solution : Ferri lactis gr. viij ; Aq. dist. $\mathfrak{Z}$j. Carefully filter through paper.

Jan. 3, 1852. Injected $\mathfrak{Z}$ij of same solution ; 6th, f$\mathfrak{Z}$iij thrown in ; 14th, $\mathfrak{Z}$ijss injected ; 22d, $\mathfrak{Z}$ij ; 26th, $\mathfrak{Z}$ij ; 28th, $\mathfrak{Z}$ij.

Feb. 3d. $\mathfrak{Z}$ij injected ; 9th, $\mathfrak{Z}$ijss.

During the whole of this time the wound cicatrized rapidly. At first luxuriant granulations sprang from the surface, which were repressed by the application of nit. silver. Lancinating pains continued for some time, but gradually diminished and at length subsided.

In six weeks from the operation the cicatrization was nearly complete. In eight weeks he returned home perfectly well. ·

The question whether the diseased mass was cancer I do not hesitate to decide in the affirmative. Its history and appearance sufficiently indicate this; its interior perfectly resembled the brain of an infant in a vascular state, and under the microscope it exhibited the most perfectly formed cancer cells. Dr. Johnson, resident physician, fully coincided in this point.

Whether it would have cicatrized without the use of the lactate of iron cannot be determined with the same degree of certainty. Taking into consideration the return, when last extirpated, with the fact that it was afterwards impossible to remove the whole of it, I think the probability of obtaining cicatrization by ordinary means was slight. I should not, however, have thought of performing, or attempting extirpation, but that the patient (who is intelligent and trusting) expressed his desire to be submitted to the treatment when it was explained to him.

I am aware that many surgeons, under the influence of preconceived opinions, may regard such treatment as hazardous. I had fully convinced myself that such was not the case. I have repeatedly thrown gr. x lactate of iron, imperfectly dissolved in an ounce of water, into the veins of a small dog without, in any case, peculiarly bad results.

It will be seen that gr. iij was the largest quantity thrown in at a single time. It was passed in gradually and cold, and, as soon as sensible effects were produced. it was stopped. The effect noticed was a flush of the face, a fullness of the veins of the head, and a tendency to sneeze, which all passed over in a few seconds. The circulation otherwise was unaffected. If the case had not progressed favourably, and it had seemed advisable to change the nutrition more profoundly, I would have had the solution warmed and put it in slowly until its effects were perceptible, then, allowing it to pass over, have repeated it as far as appeared safe.

Up to the time of his departure the injection had been performed nine times, and grs. xix in the aggregate injected. When the activity of the salt is considered, it will be conceded that such a quantity is capable of having an effect on the system by being thrown into the blood.

In addition to that he has during this period, eight weeks, taken ℥ xix of the lactate by the mouth, to what extent this may have been absorbed and carried into the circulation, or what changes it may have undergone, it is impossible to determine.

In case of a cancerous disease seated upon an extremity I should in addition to the two methods of administration resorted to in this instance, infiltrate the whole of the diseased and the healthy tissue about it with a weak solution of the medicine. This can readily be effected by putting a ligature moderately tight about the member until it becomes œdematous, when by the aid of frictions the infiltration and maceration may be effected. I had omitted to mention that all the injections were made into the veins at the elbow.

In submitting this case to the profession, I am far from claiming for it any merit which it does not possess, or drawing inferences which no single case could warrant. It is offered as an evidence of the practicability and safety of maceration through the medium of the blood systematically pursued with active substances, and to invite attention to other means of treating this inveterate disease than those which hitherto have been admitted by consent to be unsuccessful.—[*Amer. Jour. of Med. Science.*

Amputation of the entire Lower Jaw, with disarticulation of both Condyles. By J. M. Carnochan, M. D., Professor of the Principles and Operations of Surgery in the New-York Medical College, Chief Surgeon to the New-York Emigrants' Hospital, &c.

Notwithstanding the repeated instances on record of large portions of the lower jaw having been lost by accident or dis. ease, surgeons appear to have been slow in admitting the possi. bility of practising amputation, either partial or total, of this bone. To Dupuytren was reserved the glory of having, in 1812, first removed, by a methodical operation, a portion of the body of the inferior maxilla ; but since the innovation of the celebrated French surgeon, the operation for the partial exsec. tion of this bone has been repeatedly performed. In the annals of surgery, there is an *allusion* made to the amputation of the *entire* lower jaw, by Walther, of Bonn ; but I have not been able to trace the truth of it to an official source.

The following case will prove that this operation can be per. formed with success ; and that the patient, although deprived of the chief instrument of mastication, may survive, and enjoy the usual condition of health.

Nicholas Donegan, aged 43, a farmer by occupation, was admitted into the New-York Emigrants' Hospital, March 7th, 1851. He was treated for some weeks, in the Medical Divi. sion, for typhus fever, and was afterwards transferred to the Surgical Department, under my charge. Upon examination of the patient, his face presented much tumefaction, and he complained of great pain, seated chiefly in the region occupied by the inferior maxilla. Upon carrying the examination further, the lower jaw was found to be extensively affected with necrosis. All the external appearances denoting a cachectic condition of the constitution, with extreme debility and general prostration of the vital functions were present. The patient stated that, during his recent voyage to this country, he had received a severe blow upon the lower jaw and side of the face. This circumstance, coupled with the cachectic condition following the attack of fever, appears as far as can be learned, to have been the origin of the disease of the bone.

A tonic course of treatment was prescribed for him, and various local applications and lotions were resorted to, in order to allay the irritation in the mouth, and abate the fetor emanating from the disease. In a short time the teeth became loose, and had to be extracted ; the alveolar ridge became partially denuded; the swelling increased towards and over the rami and condyles; and the patient complained of excruciating suffering and depression. Nutritious diet and the various therapeutic agents, proper to improve and renovate his system, were persevered in ; and soothing and astringent lotions and applications were unremittingly used. This plan of treatment was pursued for about three months ; at the expiration of which time, it became evident that the disease of the osseous tissue was too deeply rooted to be affected by mere remedial agents. In fact, they were found to be entirely unavailing. The disease had now apparently seized upon the entire jaw ; pus was abundantly secreted into the cavity of the mouth; the saliva was also thrown out in great quantity; and the fetor became almost intolerable to the patient himself, and to those around him in the ward. Constitutional irritation and hectic of a grave character had also set in ; diarrhœa made its attack ; and the patient was gradually sinking under the complications of his disease, and the terrific pain by which he was unceasingly tortured. It was apparent to me that the speedy death of the patient could only be avoided by removing the source of such intense suffering and constitutional derangement. The integuments over the disease, although much tumified, œdematous, tense and red remained free from ulceration; the vitiated secretions taking their exit by the cavity of the mouth.

On the 13th of July, a consultation was held, and an operation for the removal of the bone decided upon. The formidable nature of the operation proposed, together with the debilitated and cachectic condition of the patient, induced me to enter into full explanations, and to inform him of the great risk that would attend it. The matter was then left to himself, and at his urgent request, I proceeded to use my efforts for his relief. It was not thought expedient to administer either chloroform or ether, on account of the liability to asphyxia from the passage of blood into the wind-pipe.

The patient being seated on a chair, and the assistants properly arranged, an incision was first made, commencing opposite the left condyle, passing downwards towards the angle of the jaw, ranging at about two lines in front of the posterior border of the ramus, and extending thence along the base of the jaw, to terminate by a slight curve on the mesial line, half an inch below the free margin of the lower lip. The bone was now partially laid bare, by dissecting upwards the tissues of the cheek, and by reflecting downwards, for a short distance, the lower edge of the incision. The tissues forming the floor of the mouth, and situated upon the inner surface of the body of the bone, were separated from their attachments from a point near the mesial line, as far back as the angle of the jaw. The attachments of the buccinator were next divided. The facial artery, the sub-mental and the sub-lingual, already cut, were then secured by ligature. It was now seen that the bone was partially separated at the symphysis, and that the necrosis was complete from that point to the inferior portion of the ramus. The ramus itself was found diseased; the periosteum externally was inflamed, and in some parts easily detached. The tongue was now grasped and held forwards, while the attachments of the genio hyo-glossi muscles were divided. A double ligature was passed through the anterior part of the root of the tongue, and entrusted to an assistant, in order to prevent its retraction upon the superior orifice of the larynx. A fatal case from the falling backwards of the tongue, occurred a few years ago, in the practice of an eminent surgeon of this city; and a similar misfortune should always be guarded against, when the muscular attachments of the tongue to the posterior part of the bone behind the symphysis are divided. A slight force exercised upon the left half of the body of the jaw, broke the connection at the symphysis and at the angle, and this part was easily removed. The next step consisted in the removal of the left ramus. The external surface of the branch of the jaw, and of the temporo-maxillary articulation were exposed, by dissecting the masseter upwards, as far as the zygomatic arch. Seizing the ramus in order to pull the coronoid process downwards below the zygoma, it was found that the temporal muscle was rigidly and permanently retracted. This circumstance presented an unexpected difficulty, which was increased by the unusual development of this apophysis, and by the retraction also of the pterygoid muscles. Passing the forefinger along the

inner aspect of the ramus, the situation of the internal and external carotids was sought for and recognised.　The insertion of
the pterygoideus internus was then felt and cut, grazing the
bone in doing so; the lingual nerve, here in close proximity,
being carefully avoided.　Passing still higher up, the orifice of
the dental canal, indicated by an osseous projection, could be
felt; and the instrument, still guided by the finger, divided the
dental artery and nerve.　The knife was thus made to separate the tissues attached to the inner face of the bone, as high up
as a point situated above a line below the sigmoid notch, between the condyle and the coronoid process.　On a level with
this point. at the posterior margin of the ramus, the transverse
facial, internal maxillary and temporal arteries form a kind of
tripod, the two last named branches of which should not be
divided, if possible.　It now became necessary to detach the
tendon of the temporal muscle.　As the coronoid process could
not be depressed, I proceeded cautiously. by dividing the lower
attachments of the tendon, by means of blunt curved scissors;
and by using them and a probepointed bistoury, alternately—
keeping close to the bone—a considerable portion of the tendon
was divided.　Deeming it not prudent to use freely a sharp
cutting instrument, deep in the temporal fossa, where the coronoid process was situated, I made use of a pair of bone scissors,
curved flatwise; and by passing the blades of this instrument
over the process, as far as its position would permit, the temporal muscle was detached; a small portion of the apex of the coronoid process being cut through.　The ramus, now movable,
could be made use of as a lever to aid in the disarticulation of
the bone.

In order to effect safely the disarticulation of the condyle, I
began by penetrating into the joint, by cutting the ligaments
from *before backwards*, and from *without inwards*.　The articulation was thus opened sufficiently to allow the condyle to be
completely luxated.　Blunt scissors were now used to cut carefully the internal part of the capsule and the maxillary insertion
of the external pterygoid muscle; and by a slow movement of
rotation of the ramus upon its axis, the condyle was detached,
and the operation was completed on this side.　By proceeding
to disarticulate by the method here described, injury to the temporal artery, as well as to the internal maxillary, was avoided.

To effect the removal of the other half of the lower jaw, the
same incision was made on the opposite side, so as to meet the
first on the mesial line.　The dissection was also similar; and
by disarticulating the second condyle in the same manner as
had been observed for the first, I was successful again in avoiding lesion of the temporal and internal maxillary arteries.

The object I had in view, in shaping the external incisions, in such a way that an inverted V should be formed in front of the insertion of the genio-hyo-glossi muscles, was to leave a portion of integument so fashioned, that the suture-pins could be passed through the integument, and, at the same time, through the root of the tongue, at the point where its muscles had been detached from the inner surface of the lower jaw. The several tissues becoming thus incorporated in the resulting cicatrix, served to form a new bridle, somewhat analogous to the natural muscular attachments of the tongue to the genial processes.

The amount of blood lost was inconsiderable; the arteries divided, besides those mentioned, where the transverse facial, the anterior masseteric, the anterior parotidean, &c., and these were secured as soon as divided. The bone being disarticulated, the flaps were adjusted, and the lips of the incision united, by eighteen points of twisted suture. The tongue was retained forwards after the dressing, by attaching the ends of the ligature already passed through its base, on each side, to a bandage passed vertically around the head. Forty-eight hours after the operation, the first dressing was removed. Union by first intention had taken place, and eight of the suture-pins were taken out. In ninety-six hours, the wound was again examined. Union was found to be entirely competent and the remaining pins were removed. On the seventh day, it was thought safe to remove the ligature from the tongue. On the tenth day, the arterial ligatures came away; and on the fourteenth day, the patient was pronounced cured; not having had an untoward symptom since the performance of the operation.

The operation occupied fifty-five minutes, the patient having been allowed intervals of repose to recruit. It was performed in the presence of a number of professional gentlemen; and I was ably assisted by my colleague, Dr A. V. Williams, by Drs. Dewees and Dixon, of New-York, and by Drs. Thompson, Whitehead, Smith and Bailey, resident assistants attached to the surgical staff of the Hospital.

The present appearance of the patient, presents much less deformity than might be expected from the severe mutilation which he has undergone. His general condition and health are good; and he is now able to perform any ordinary vocation. The ducts of Steno, on both sides were necessarily divided in the superficial incisions; but there is no salivary fistula, the saliva taking its course into the mouth. The division of the branches of the facial nerve has not been followed by paralysis of the face; although for a time after the reunion of the incision the orbicularis palpebrarum of the right side appeared to have

lost its action to some extent. In grasping the chin, a thin cartilaginous deposit can now be felt, extending, crescent-shaped,
for about three inches, and occupying the position at which the
bone was most diseased. Higher up. toward the glenoid cavity
no deposition of bone or cartilage has taken place. Injury to
the bag of the pharynx, during the detachment of the soft tissues
from the angle of the jaw, was carefully avoided, and fluids
could be swallowed, in small quantities. immediately after the
·operation. Deglutition is now effected without difficulty. Articulation is sufficiently distinct to render his words intelligible,
and although unable to masticate, he does not complain of difficulty in eating, breaking up, as he says he does. his food between
the tongue and the palatal vault of the superior maxillæ.

[*New-York Jour. of Med.*

Successful removal of the Knee-Joint. By A. J. WEDDERBURN,
M. D., Professor of Anatomy in the University of Louisiana.

George Chandler, born in England, aged 18 years, was admitted into the Charity Hospital, January 9, 1852, with a painful enlargement of the knee-joint—had only been attacked
about a month previous to his admission. His health had
previously been very good ; attributes his attack to exposure
alone, having received no injury. The tumor being fluctuating,
the usual remedies for hydrarthrus having been resorted to,
without effect, and the enlargement progressing, I determined
to settle an opinion, by the introduction of an exploring trocar
regarding its being an abscess of the joint ; about two ounces
of its contents were removed by this method, containing a
large proportion of pus. Being satisfied that the disease had
progressed so far as to have produced at least a partial destruction of the cartilages. and not being willing to defer an operation
longer until the character denoting the true nature of the disease should be more distinct, rendering the success of an
articular exsection much more doubtful, and having taken fully
into consideration the advantages of a stiff leg over the loss of
the same from amputation, I determined upon the former, and
made the operation on the 18th day of February.

Operation by the H. incision, the transverse part of which was
made immediately at the lower portion of the patella. The flaps
were turned back, the joint bent at right angles, and the lateral
ligaments divided with a probe-pointed bistoury. directed by
the forefinger of the left hand, which was passed respectively
beneath both, and under the surface, next the cavity of the

joints. The divison of the ligaments having been effected, rendered it easy to project the articulating surface of the femur so far forward as to facilitate the passage of an amputing saw from a line above the incrusted part of the joint—from its anterior to its central portion, and in an oblique direction down-wards, removing by this section something more than one half of the articulating surfaces belonging to the two condyles of the femur. The next stage in the operation was to divide the crucial ligaments from their two points of attachment, and then to dissect them away together with the greater part of the synovial membrane of the joint which was very much thicken-ed, and elevated by the sub-synovial cellular tissue; the patella was removed also in the progress of this dissection. The pos-terior half of the articular surfaces of the condyles were then removed by the chain saw, in such an oblique direction fiom behind, forwards and downwards, as to occasion a loss in the length of the bone not exceeding three-fourths of an inch. A very slight dissection was then made around the head of the tibia upon its anterior and lateral surfaces, and the entire articulating surface removed by the passage of an amputating saw from before and backwards.

The constitutional symptoms following this operation were violent for a few days, but since there have been no bad symp-toms. Without entering into a description of the different methods by which this operation has been done, I will only state that there will be, from the manner of this, only a' short-ening of something less than an inch, and a much larger surface exposed for the formation of callus. The different methods by which the knee-joint has been removed will be found in Vel-peau's *Operative Surgery*, by Mott.—[*N. O. Medical Register.*

Morbid habit of swallowing Hair; Prolonged sojourn of the foreign bodies in the gastro-intestinal canal. Evacuation of Packets of Hair by vomiting and alvine dejections. (Under the care of Dr. CRAWFORD, Middlesex Hospital.)

Dr. Thompson has alluded. in this journal, to the case of a girl who used to swallow her hair, and had lately vomited pack-ets of it. The patient has, since then, passed, per anum, a large mass of the same organic product; this circumstance induced us to inquire more minutely into the case, and we learned from the girl the following facts.

She is a servant, twenty-three years of age, now pale and thin, but formerly ruddy and stout, and was admitted Nov. 16, 1851, under the care of Dr. Crawford, with very obstinate

constipation.   The patient began to menstruate at the age of
twelve years, and at thirteen, while in a comfortable situation,
contracted the habit of picking off her hair, biting, chewing,
and at last swallowing it.   She went on satisfying this depraved
taste for four or five months, when, being reprimanded, she
gave it up. and has never resumed the custom since.

Soon after this, the patient began to feel a pain under the
false ribs, on the left side, just over the spleen and the large extremity of the stomach.   She was treated in various ways, and
at different hospitals and dispensaries, during several years, for
this pain, no one, nor herself, suspecting that the above-mentioned habit was the source of her malady.   The general belief
was, that she suffered from a tumour in the vicinity of the
spleen ; pain in that region, constipation of bowels, and wasting,
being the principal symptoms.

At last, about a fortnight before admission, she was seized
with fits of vomiting, and, among the rejected matters, a solid
concretion, about the size of a walnut, was noticed ; but this
attracted no attention, until a second and much larger one was
likewise brought up in the hospital.   The nature of the affection became now apparent, but the constipation was very obstinate, and went so far as to produce stercoraceous vomiting.
No more hair was noticed after these symptoms abated. until
Jan. 26, about nine weeks after admission, when a very large
hairy concretion was discovered in the fæces.   It was of the
size of the dilated rectum, measured five inches in length, and
was of a deep black colour.   (The girl's hair is of a light tint.)
The patient states that she felt this in the right iliac fossa, and
she is now under the impression that more hair will be evacuated.   The health has of late been rather weak. but the appetite
is pretty good, and the intellect clear ; but the patient complains of flatus, and of the bowels rolling in knots.   This is
another and very striking example of the difficulty of treating
disease, when we do not know *every particular* of the history.
[*London Lancet.*

---

*On the Treatment of Ununited Fracture by the sub-cutaneous
perforation of the bone, with a Case.*   By DANIEL BRAINARD,
M. D., Professor of Surgery in Rush Medical College.

No one acquainted with either the literature or the practice
of surgery, will doubt that our knowledge of the treatment of
false joint is extremely imperfect.   The published cases and
statistical tables prove this ; but it is rendered still more evident
by the far greater number of uncured and unrecorded cases to

be met with in practice, in the more remote sections of our country. ·These, but a small proportion of which fall under the notice of a single person, would form, if they could be collected together, an array calculated to weaken our confidence in the means usually resorted to for their cure. I have been led to the conclusion from having, during the last fourteen years, met almost yearly with one or more cases of the kind, and from having found that they present themselves to such of my professional friends as I have had opportunity of consulting on the subject.

These cases are in this country almost invariably treated by the seton, and when this is unsuccessful they are given up as hopeless. Of four cases which have presented themselves to my observation during the current year, two were of that kind. One of these, of the arm, was of eleven years standing, the seton had been used a year without benefit ; the other will be given in detail.

It is greatly to be regretted that Dr. Physick, whose experience with the seton must have been extensive, did not have a record of its results. It is asserted on the one hand he lost confidence in it. This is denied on the other hand by Norris, who had every means of information, who says : "We have authority for stating that up to the period of his death Dr. Physick *always* advocated the treatment of these cases by the seton." * Nevertheless we find in the same article, that "The caustic potash has been successfully used in three or four cases by Dr. J. R. Barton, of this city, in one of which" the leg, "Dr. Physick discouraged the use of the seton for fear of its failure." Gibson also states, that Dr. Physick discouraged its use in cases of fracture of the femur.

I make these remarks not from a disposition to undervalue the seton, which is probably the most useful means yet known, but to show that it is not universally successful or applicable to all cases. Dr. Norris, in the article referred to, which is the best source of information to which I could refer, says that, "in the femur it has often failed." I was myself in the habit, until about four years ago, of abandoning most cases in which the seton had failed, not choosing to resort to resection or amputation. In 1848 I treated a case successfully by passing a silver wire around the ends of the fragments. Further reflections suggested different modes of treatment which I have applied.

A little reflection will, with the aid of our present knowledge of pathology, convince us that the seton is not calculated to be generally successful.

* Amer. Jour. Med. Science, Vol. III, New Series, pp. 55.

The first condition most favorable for the production of callus, is the effusion of a *blastema,* which should not be converted into pus and discharged.

The second is, that this blastema should be in contact with a freshly wounded sufrace of bone—the law of "analogous formation" holding good here.

" The blastema between areolar tissue becomes areolar tissue, at the extremity of divided nerves it forms nervous substance, &c. (Vogel)

Now the seton necessarily causes the conversion of the effused blastema into pus, while its introduction produces no freshly wounded surface of bone ; the case is converted into a compound fracture where it was desirable to only reproduce a simple one.

Can subcutaneous wounds of bones be made without danger of suppuration? To determine this point I at different times perforated all the principal bones of the members of a dog, and did not find that suppuration in any case resulted.

Case treated by perforation of the ends of the bones:

Allcett Barnes, aged twenty-six years, received, June 10th, 1850, a simple fracture from being carried by a belt around a shaft. It was dressed by Dr. Hawley, of Yorkville, Mich., two splints being properly applied. The dressing was changed, perhaps, once a week for eight weeks, when the ulna was found to be united, but the radius was not. A simple bandage was placed about it for four weeks, when he consulted Dr. White, of Kalamazoo, who put on carved splints for a month, when, finding no sign of union, he put through a skein of silk for a seton, which was allowed to remain three weeks. It caused much pain and suppuration. When the seton was taken out, a bandage was put about it for a week, when splints were applied and continued five weeks. They were then taken off and no union found to have taken place. Such was the account given by the patient himself.

Feb. 4th, 1851. Ununited fracture of the radius found above one-third of the distance from the wrist to the elbow, partially overlapped, oblique, moveable, and the hand of little use.

OPERATION.—Having provided several *brad awls,* such as are used by shoemakers, and had them well tempered and tried on dry bones, I carried one of them through the skin opposite the fracture, and by movements of partial rotation perforated both fragments where they overlapped. The awl being then withdrawn from the bone, (but not from the skin,) was directed obliquely upward, then obliquely downward, so as to make three perforations. It was then entirely withdrawn, and collodion put upon the puncture of the skin. The member was dressed with the immovable apparatus. Some tenderness was the effect.

Feb. 17th. The tenderness having subsided, I removed the bandage, repeated the operation in the same manner, choosing a different point of puncture, and re-applied the dressing.

March 11th. Repeated the operation again, and dressed as before; mobility scarcely perceptible.

March 21st. Dressings removed, union perfect.

The dressings were in this case continued on near seven weeks, but it is probable the last perforation and dressing might well have been omitted.

The occurrence of union in so short a time where the seton had failed, and with no operation which interfered with the comfort or amusement of the patient, was a most favorable result, but not different from what was anticipated. I do not know that this sub-cutaneous perforation had been used by any one. Perforations by incision and inserting pieces of metal have been tried. I, myself, treated a case in this manner. It was on a man thirty-six years of age, who had long deposited phosphatic gravel in the urine, and in his youth been affected with necrosis of the femur. It was near the middle of the femur, and the fragments extremely moveable.

Sept. 20, 1850. I made an incision an inch in length over the false joint and down to the bone. I then perforated the extremity of each fragment with a *bitt*, and putting in a director from a pocket case dressed the limb in the angular apparatus for the lower extremity. The director was taken out in about ten days.

In this case the dressing was removed in eleven weeks, and the patient was able to walk at the end of four months. At the present time, (Jan. 1852,) he is pursuing an active occupation with a good limb.

Notwithstanding the favorable result of this case. it must be admitted that the symptoms were severe, like those resulting from resection. Such were they also in the case treated by the wire, so that although it seems probable that in both these cases the result was at least as favourable as could be expected from resection, it is also true that the danger incurred is not materially less.

In all these cases the operation is severe, while the sub-cutaneous perforation is free from danger, and reasoning from the analogy of simple fractures, or judging from the result of a single case, promises to be much more efficient.—[*North-Western Med. and Surg. Journal.*

Chloroform applied locally in Fractures and Dislocations.
By H. N. HURLBUT, M. D., of Chicago, Ill.

Messrs. Editors—Permit me to call the attention of the profession to the local application of chloroform to remove pain and induce insensibility of parts to be operated upon.   I have made use of it for two years past as a local remedy. with the most happy results.   In cases of comminuted fractures, producing as it does insensibility and relaxation of parts, it enables the surgeon to overcome the resistance of muscles, and to reduce the fractures without pain or suffering to the patient.   In dislocations, I have no doubt its local application would be attended with the same happy results.   I have used it in a similar manner in felons, neuralgia, &c.   The best mode of application I think is to saturate a cloth with it, apply immediately, and over that a piece of oil silk (to prevent evaporation), allowing it to remain some four or five minutes, which will be sufficient. A second application may be necessary in fractures of the superior third of the femor, or in dislocation of the same bone.

The frequent deaths reported from the inhalation of chloroform has induced me to call attention to its local use.   If in the hands of others it shall prove as safe and efficient a remedy as it has in mine, I shall be amply rewarded.—[*Ibid.*

Cold Water in the Treatment of Croup.

(Translated for this Journal)

Dr. Hauner, of the Children's Hospital at Munich, having pretty generally seen leeches, emetics, calomel, &c. fail in the treatment of genuine croup, has had recourse for several months to the employment of cold water.   The cases below will show this method of treatment.

CASE I.   A girl, 4 years of age.   In this case cold affusions were used every three hours, to the neck, back and chest, then the patient was wrapped up for a half or three quarters of an hour in wet sheets and put in a large blanket.   Every half hour cloths wet with ice-water, were applied to the neck, and these covered with dry ones.   At the end of 12 hours there was a very marked improvement: the cough was looser; portions of membrane were thrown off by expectoration and by the bowels. She took alternately warm and cool water.   Two injections were administered per day. The child recovered, but remained hoarse for a length of time.

Case II. A boy, $2\frac{1}{2}$ years of age and of strong constitution, was suddenly taken with croup. Four leeches were immediately applied, and as soon as they fell off the cold applications were applied to the neck as above, and renewed every half hour. In 12 hours the patient was out of danger, but the applications were continued for two days.

The method employed by M. Hauner may act powerfully as a perturbating cause and thus prevent the formation of membranes, but we think that the other known remedies in croup, particularly emetics and calomel, might well be combined with it.

[*Jour. des Con. Medico-Chir.*

Miscellany.

New Treatment of Deafness.—" One of the latest efforts to restore to a deaf ear its original functions, consists in applying a cup that fits closely to the side of the head, round the outer ear, and exhausting it with an air-pump. A common cupping apparatus answers every purpose, provided the glass will fit so well as to prevent the ingress of atmospheric air under the edge. In a variety of cases, the simple process of carrying on this exhaustion till a new sensation is felt, something like extreme tension in the lining membrane of the meatus externus, is represented to restore the organ to its normal state Under such circumstances the theory of the remedy is, that deafness results from an impoverished flow of cerumen, in consequence of the inertia of the excretory ducts; and by taking off the atmospheric pressure, their proper fluid oozes out upon the tube and instantly modifies the condition of the mechanism, exterior to the drum. Having thus been roused from a state of torpor and suspended activity, they continue afterwards to act with energy. If they subsequently fall partially back to their abnormal condition, the pump must be re-applied, as occasion may suggest. As there is no witchcraft about it, and almost every practitioner has a breast-pump or similar contrivance, by which an experiment could be made, and there being no hazard attending it, it may be worth a trial, and it is very possible that one out of a dozen cases might be essentially benefited by this simple operation."

The above notice taken from the editorial department of the Boston Medical and Surgical Journal, will serve the purpose of directing attention to a new remedy for deafness; but we cannot transfer it to

our pages without comment. In the first p'ace, deafness being a common symptom or result of various and very dissimilar pathological
conditions of the auditory apparatus, it is evident that the remedy
cannot be applicable to all cases. Nor are we prepared to admit with
our respected brother editor that there is "no hazard attending it."
It is highly probable, nay certain, that by undue exhaustion of the
cups, the membrane of the tympanum may be ruptured. We have
not tried the "experiment" upon the dead body so as to determine
what force may be necessary to produce this rupture, nor do we know
how much may be borne by the living without giving pain. Deafness
is sometimes the consequence of an inflammatory condition, more or
less acute, of the organ, in which state of things it is difficult to conceive how the process can be otherwise than injurious.

When there is a defect of circulation or an atony of the parts,
cupping, judiciously resorted to, may be useful. It may possibly
be advantageous in cases in which the membrane of the tympanum is
already ruptured, for then it might tend to dislodge matters contained in the cavity of the tympanum, by drawing a column of air
through the Eustachian tube, and even to re-open this tube if it were
obstructed.

A similar procedure has been somewhere suggested for the treatment of impaired vision. It may be remembered that a few years
ago the newspapers were filled with the discovery, attributed to the
venerable ex-president John Quincy Adams, of a simple method by
which the use of spectacles might be dispensed with by the aged. This
consisted in the frequent, though gentle, compression of the sides of the
eye-ball, by placing the thumb upon the external angle of one eye
and the middle finger upon that of the other eye, and slowly approximating them towards the root of the nose, so as to elongate the axis of
vision. We know persons of intelligence who affirm that they have
been thus very much benefitted. Whether the relief be attributable
to the effect assigned or to the tonic influence of the combined pressure and friction, is not the question before us. For the purpose of
elongating the visual axis, however, an india rubber cup has been
invented and is to be found in the shops. It is simply a half globe
which when flattened and applied to the orbit, reacts by its elasticity,
and in resuming its original form tends to draw out the eye by the
vacuum thus occasioned. Now this little instrument must have the
effect of producing a congestion of the eye which is not without risk,
especially if often repeated.—[EDITOR.

BIBLIOGRAPHICAL.

We are indebted to publishers, societies, colleges, and other institutions, for a large number of works and documents, for which we
return our grateful acknowledgements, and hope that we may be able
to notice them more particularly. The following books received
through our booksellers, Messrs. J. A. Carrie & Co. and T. Richards & Son, are kept for sale by them:

The Principles of Surgery. By JAMES MILLER, F.R.S E , &c., &c.
3d American from the 2d and enlarged Edinburgh edition. Illustrated with 240 engravings on wood Revised, with additions by
F. W. SARGENT, M. D., &c. Philadelphia: Blanchard & Lea.
1852. Pp. 751.

The very high estimation in which the surgical works of the distinguished Edinburgh Professor are generally held, will insure for
the present improved edition of his "Principles of Surgery" a cordial
reception by the profession in America. The numerous *illustrations*
add very much to its value, especially for students, and will make it a
popular text-book for college classes.

*The History, Diagnosis, and Treatment of the Fevers of the United
States.* By ELISHA BARTLETT, M. D., Prof. of Materia Medica
and Medical Jurisprudence in the College of Physicians and Surgeons of New York, &c , &c. 3d edition, revised. Philadelphia:
Blanchard and Lea. 1852. Pp. 595.

We are happy to find that this truly American work has been so
well appreciated as to require a third edition. It is decidedly the best
treatise on fevers in our language, and the only one adapted to the
necessities of this country. It ought to be in the possession of every
practitioner.

*An Analysis of Physiology: being a condensed view of its most
important facts and doctrines—designed especially for the use of
Students.* By JOHN J. REESE, M. D., Lecturer on Materia Medica
and Therapeutics in the Medical Institute of Philadelphia, &c , &c.
2d edition, revised and enlarged. Philadelphia: Lindsay & Blakiston. 1852. Pp. 368.

A very good manual of Physiology—remarkably well adapted to
the wants of first course students.

*Elements of Chemistry; including the applications of the Science in
the Arts.* By THOMAS GRAHAM, F. R S., Professor of Chemistry
in University College, London, &c., &c. 2d American edition,

from an entirely revised and greatly enlarged English edition—with numerous wood engravings. Edited, with notes, by ROBERT BRIDGES, M. D , Professor of Chemistry in the Philadelphia College of Pharmacy, &c., &c. Philad.: Blanchard & Lea. 1852.

We feel assured that all cultivators of chemistry will be gratified to learn that Graham's Classical work is being re-published, "greatly enlarged," by such a house as that of Blanchard & Lea. It is to be issued in two parts—the first of which we have received. The elegant style in which it is presented is a just tribute to the intrinsic merits of the work.

Astringent or Anti-diarrhœal Mixture.

Tinct. Catechu, two parts.
Tinct. Opii,
Tinct. Camphoræ,
Tinct. Myrrhæ,
Tinct. Capsici, of each one part.
Mix—dose, fiom one to two teaspoonfuls.

This is a prescription we have been using constantly for the last ten years in the treatment of ordinary cases of diarrhœa and cholera morbus, with such marked success that we have been very frequently applied to for it. It should not be given until the discharges have been sufficient to empty the bowels completely. In most cases of diarrhœa a teaspoonful given in a wine-glass full of water morning and night, or three times a day, will speedily arrest the disease. In cholera morbus the dose should be doubled. If it be borne in mind that it contains one part of laudanum in six, the dose may be easily graduated for children. To a child one year of age we usually give from 12 to 24 drops, and by its timely use may generally arrest the attacks to which they are so subject in spring and summer. The remedy is rarely useful in dysentery.—[EDITOR.

Georgia is, we believe, the only State in the Union, that has drawn upon its Treasury for the encouragement of quackery. The last session of her Legislature appropriated five thousand dollars to the Thompsonian or Botanic School, located at Macon.

We have quite a number of communications on our table, which will be attended to in due time.

SOUTHERN
MEDICAL AND SURGICAL JOURNAL.

| Vol. 8.] | NEW SERIES.—AUGUST, 1852. | [No. 8. |

PART FIRST.

𝔒riginal 𝔔ommunications.

ARTICLE XXV.

A Synopsis of Reports made in 1848 *to the Parisian Academy of Medicine, by eminent Surgeons, upon Gun-shot wounds.* By JURIAH HARRISS, M. D., of Augusta, Ga.

Accidents attending gun-shot wounds are so varied in their form and position, and so serious in their nature, as frequently to demand a large amount of anatomical and surgical knowledge to meet them with discriminating promptitude. Many of them require immediate and decisive action on the part of the surgeon, without allowing time to consult authorities or to call in additional counsel. A limb may be heedlessly and rashly removed, or an individual's life be sacrificed, by injudicious delay or indecision. In this day of advancement, when the facilities for medical education and improvement are so multiplied, ignorance is considered a crime by the public, and declared such by law.

It is in consideration of the interest, importance, and many difficulties that accompany the treatment of gun-shot wounds, that I ask the indulgence of the readers of this Journal, while I lay before them the experience and results of the practice of many of the first surgeons of France upon this subject, as reported by them to the Academy of Medicine. If their experience and observations are worth any thing, they must be valuable; and as their individual reports cannot reach the profession generally in this country, I have presumed to give a synopsis of them. Their observations, owing to recent struggles in France, have been vast, and will probably induce improvements in military surgery, from which civil surgeons may draw useful instruction.

It is to be regretted, that surgeons are so divided as to the mode of treating gun-shot wounds and their consequences. Military surgeons disagree upon nearly every point connected with gun-shot wounds; but the greatest discrepancy exists, between military and civil surgeons, upon the question of immediate amputation and the attempts to preserve the limb.

The questions which elicited most discussion among the reporters to the Academy of Medicine, were—

1st. Should gun-shot wounds be enlarged by incisions so as to reduce them as nearly as possible to simple incised wounds?

2d. Should free incisions be made to extract foreign bodies and fragments of bone, or should these be left to be expelled by suppuration?

3d. Are refrigerants, as ice, suitable applications to gun-shot wounds?

4th. The comparative advantages of immediate and secondary amputations.

1st. *Should Gun-shot Wounds be enlarged by Incisions.*— M. Larry and the early French military surgeons recommended this practice almost universally and without discrimination. In latter days, says M. Roux, surgeons not only doubt their utility, but presume to reserve them for exceptional cases. M. Roux raised the question of incisions only in relation to simple wounds, where the object is solely to enlarge them for the escape of pus and the debris of sloughing. Incisions for extracting foreign bodies, arresting hemorrhage, &c., he discusses in their proper places. The question, he thinks, does not extend itself to consecutive incisions that are made for the exit of pus, after it is known that it has been formed and burrowed in the soft parts. As to their propriety there can be no doubt; they are warranted and sanctioned by all surgical authority. M. Roux is of the opinion that there are but few cases in which incision of simple gun-shot wounds is advisable : they seem to him to be but useless complications.

M. Baudens, the chief surgeon to the Military Hospital of Val-de-grace, in Paris, rejects incisions entirely, and believes that no circumstances will warrant them.

Blandin, I think, more philosophically, takes the medium ground between the contending parties. He neither agrees with those who contend that all gun-shot wounds should be incised, nor coincides with those who universally blame this practice. He reserves incisions for those cases in which the thickness and strength of the aponeurosis will probably constrict the part, and by its resistance will not give room for the distension of the tissues, which is so common in inflammation, and which so frequently leads to gangrene. He contends that in such cases they lend no complication to the wound, as the superficial aponeurosis alone act as constrictors, and the incisions are therefore always superficial and not at all serious.

M. Velpeau, with Blandin, reserves incisions for exceptional cases. He says, afterwards that they have generally, perhaps, no other inconvenience than being useless. M. Jobert is most decidedly opposed to them. It will be perhaps remembered that J. Hunter strenuously objected to them.

· 2d. *Should free incisions be made to extract foreign bodies and fragments of bone, or should these be left to be expelled by suppuration ?*—The acts of the economy, when a foreign body, such as a ball, has penetrated the tissues, are among the most beautiful processes of nature. The presence of the body causes inflammation in the part, the latter condenses, and an effusion of plastic lymph forms a sac and becomes more or less organised, and thus the tissues accommodate themselves to its volume, weight and presence. This is the case even with some of the most vital organs, such as the lungs. I recollect a case in which a ball entered and buried itself in the brain so deeply that it could not be extracted. There was a large opening in the cranial bones, through which could be seen the distension of cerebral masss at each contraction of the heart and the rise and fall of the brain during the acts of respiration. This patient lived six weeks, and such was his condition at this

time, that the Surgeon, M. Michon, expressed very decided
hopes of his recovery. He died suddenly, in attempting to
raise himself in bed. There is yet another process of nature
in such cases, which has been very graphically described by J.
Hunter, and styled by him the "ulcerative process." When
a foreign body is deeply imbeded in the soft parts, says this
author, it gradually and without constitutional disturbance
makes its way near the cutaneous surface and there forms an
abscess, at which time it can be easily extracted. They but
seldom cause an abscess when deeply imbeded in the soft tissues. The abscess in such cases usually forms in the subcutaneous cellular tissues. The sufferer is not, however, always so
fortunate. The foreign body frequently induces intense pain
and constitutional derangement, and finally carries the patient
to his grave.

M. Roux, with other surgeons, adopts the rule, that if the
ball or other body is easily extracted, if the position of the body
is well detected and can be reached by a direct passage, without interesting too much the soft parts, its extraction should be
attempted, but not otherwise. M. Roux recommends large
and free incisions. All surgeons agree that splints of bone
should be removed immediately. This is a well established
precept.

M. Jobert agrees with Hunter, in considering foreign bodies
as almost inoffensive to the tissues, with which they are in contact. Out of 17 foreign bodies in different persons, he extracted only 3, and these were immediately beneath the integuments.

3rd. *Are refrigerants, as ice, suitable applications to Gun-
shot Wounds?*—The object of these applications is to prevent
too great inflammatory action and suppuration, which always
have a tendency to exhaust the patient and cause constitutional
disturbance. M. Roux objects to them, but there can be no
doubt, that they are in many cases far preferable to the warm
poultices which he usually applies. They not only subdue or
prevent excess of inflammation, but are generally more agreeable to the sufferer. Where cold applications are desirable, the
roller bandage is objectionable; the more simple the dressing
the better. A compress lossely applied so that it can be re-

moved, and moistened at pleasure, and that allows the wound to be inspected without inconvenience to the patient is much preferable. M. Velpeau does not use cold applications in general. His remarks upon this point in his report are excellent and we will give them in full. "The object and effect of the refrigerant treatment in gun-shot wounds are to prevent or cut short the inflammation, but it must be remembered that a certain degree of inflammation is necessary to heal a wound of this nature. The contused layer of tissues cannot be expelled save at this price. Besides the temperature is not modified by ice to the same degree, through the entire thickness of the wounded limb ; hence the external part of the wound is cool, while the internal preserves its great heat. This produces an inequality in the inflammation, which is evidently less favorable than a frank and regular phlegmasia. There is thus produced a bastard inflammation, a sanious and badly elaborated discharge, and the wound consequently marches slowly to cicatrization. If there is a flap, if the circulation of the member is already embarrassed, ice will manifestly favor mortification. I have even seen refrigerants produce eschars upon the healthy skin. The only cases in which refrigerants are advisable, are those in which there are violent pains, or a sensation of great heat, without much swelling or inflammation. They may perhaps be advisable in very warm weather." M. Velpeau reasons well, as he always does, even when upon the wrong side. He urges that a certain amount of inflammation is necessary to heal a gun-shot wound. This is very manifest and is quite true in every variety of wounds. I presume, that the same course of reasoning induces him never to attempt to heal a wound of any description by the first intention. He never calculates upon this result, and is always surprised when the wound heals without suppuration.

4th. *The comparative advantages of immediate and secondary amputation.*—The question of amputation is the most complex and difficult in the whole range of gun-shot wounds. Rules in regard to the character of the wounds requiring amputation, and the time at which operations should be resorted to, are far from being determined. Indeed it would seem, in reading different authors, that each surgeon lays down his own rules. There can be little doubt, but where an operation is or will probably be necessary that it should be primary or immediate. Secondary amputations have this very decided inconvenience, that the suppuration and sloughing debilitates the patient to an incalculable degree, produces an immense amount of constitutional disturbance and thus lessens the chances of final success. It is unquestionably in accordance with well established rules of surgery, to operate early, when an operation is necessary, before suppuration debilitates the system and the efforts of nature are exhausted in attempts at reparation.

M. Malgaigne enters more largely upon amputation than the other reporters, but confines himself more particularly to amputations of the thigh. We will translate some of his remarks, as they are very concise. He says that, " it is a very generally accepted doctrine, especially among military surgeons, that fractures of the femur by projectiles from a gun require amputation."

Larrey contended that if the femur be fractured in the lower fourth or even third, the limb may be saved, but if in the centre or superior third, amputation is indispensable.

Ribes expresses himself thus upon this subject : " However serious a gun-shot wound of the superior extremity, the limb may be attempted to be saved, and that without endangering the life of the patient,* but in the inferior extremities, when the bones are broken, the least hesitation may cost the life of the individual." He confirms the doctrine of Larrey in regard to the middle and superior part of the femur, but also extends the rule to the inferior part of the bone. He adds, "the fracture of the inferior part of the bone is about as serious as that of the centre." Upon 4,000 patients, Ribes did not see a single consolidation of the femur, when fractured by projectiles from a gun. At Toulouse there were 47 amputations and 9 died.

Dupuytren, in 1830, (at Hotel Dieu,) had 12 fractures of the femur not operated upon, 5 cured, 7 died.

There is another very important question to be determined, that of immediate or secondary amputation. Guthrie, at the

* This is a practice taught by Guthrie. London Lancet. April, 1852.

battle of New Orleans, performed 45 immediate amputations, 7 died or 1 in 7. Upon 5 secondary amputations 3 died.

M. Malgaigne ends his report by repudiating the doctrine of military surgeons, and says that he never amputates but for urgent necessities, and nearly always attempts to save the limb, believing that there is not so much risk in this attempt as in amputating it.

The following is the result of his practice in 1848.

5 Fractures of thigh,		2 cured,	2 died. 1 sec. amp.
6	do.	of leg,	2 cured,	4 died.
2	do.	of tibia,	2 cured,	0 died.
3	do.	of fibula,	1 cured,	2 died.
3	do.	of arm,	1 cured,	2 died.
5	do.	fore-arm,	5 cured,	0 died.
2	do.	metcarps,	1 cured,	1 died.
			14 cured,	11 died.

Hemorrhage.—This subject is discussed by some of the reporters. Hemorrhages are divided into primary and secondary. The primary are rare in gun-shot wounds; 1st. because the yielding and elastic properties of the large vessels allow them to give away to the force when applied to them; and secondly, when they are wounded, the contusion is so great as to cause a coagulation of the blood, which closes the wounded orifice of the artery.

M. Roux states that in all the gun-shot wounds he has had to treat, he has never seen a primary hemorrhage of any importance. When they do occur, he is of the opinion that the bleeding vessel should be immediately secured and ligated at the point of injury. This is a disputed point among surgeons, many believe that the main trunk should be ligated above the point of hemorrhage.*

According to M. Roux, consecutive hemorrhages are more frequent than primary ones. If the soft parts are alone interested, the hemorrhage occurs from the 7th to the 10th day, rarely later. When the bones are fractured they occur later still; from the 12th to the 20th day after the receipt of the

* Guthrie says, that both extremities of the wounded artery should be secured. See London Lancet. February 1851.

injury.   The reason of this, he remarks, probably is that the
spiculæ of bones irritate and keep up the inflammation much
longer, and when in the vicinity of blood vessels, increase the
chances of the ulceration of their coats, to say nothing of their
sharp points penetrating directly the vessels.

Anel and Hunter have proposed to ligate the vessel above
the point of hemorrhage.   Roux coincides with them, urging
that in secondary hemorrhage the difficulties of finding and
securing the artery are immensely increased at the seat of injury.   He makes a distinction in the treament of primary and
secondary hemorrhage.   In the first he prefers applying the
ligature at the point of injury and in the latter above.

The generally accepted opinion is that gun-shot, like lacerated wounds, do not bleed, save in exceptional cases.   M. Blandin, however, more exact in his observations and minute in
his descriptions, affirm that primitive hemorrhage is the rule,
for in all of his cases the patients clothes were bloody.   Such
is also his experience in lacerated wounds.   Hemorrhage, according to this surgeon, takes place before nature can provide
against it, as she soon does by retraction of the wounded vessels, formation of clots, &c.   He admits that large primitive
hemorrhages are rare, he having seen but one case that required
the immediate ligation of the vessel.   May not these small
hemorrhages, occurring immediately after the receipt of the
injury, be from the veins, and particularly the small veins?   I
think I have observed in lacerated wounds, that while there
was no hemorrhage from the larger vessels, there would be
slight bleeding from the venous radicles occurring drop by
drop.

M. Blandin prefers, in secondary hemorrhages, to ligate the
artery above, and at a distance from the wound, thus adopting
the precept of Hunter.

Some of the reporters referred to the question of the relative
size of the openings of entrance and exit of a ball.   This is an
interesting question, and if it could be determined with precision, would be a considerable step gained in a medico-legal point
of view.   The belief that the opening of exit is larger than
that of entrance was universally sustained until 1830, when
Dupuytren advanced the contrary opinion.

M. Blandin says, that experience and extensive observation have led him to side with Dupuytren, and advocate his position. He gives the reason why the results should be as he has been induced to believe they are :—"When a ball strikes the body, it encounters the skin supported by the subjacent soft parts, and traverses it immediately without distending or allowing it a play of its elasticity ; hence the opening will be about the size of the ball. But, on the contrary, after the ball has traversed the soft parts and comes in contact with the skin upon the opposite side, it pushes it out, distends and finally passes through it, only after having put in play its entire elasticity ; and, consequently, the opening ought to retract proportionately to the distension and the elasticity of the integuments."

M. Velpeau thinks that no rule can be established upon this point, inasmuch as the ball is not always round, but sometimes flat, pointed, or irregular, before it comes in contact with the skin. Again : if circular, when it strikes the integuments, it may become flattened or irregular by striking a bone before its exit. It will be easily seen, then, that if a ball enters by its point, and passes out by its base, that the opening of exit will be the larger, and vice versa. The mobility, elasticity, &c., of the parts should be taken into consideration upon this point. He concludes with the statement, that the opening of entrance is generally larger than that of exit, but frequently smaller.

ARTICLE XXVI.

Application of Cold Water to the Head in Narcotism from Opium. By E. J. HARRIS, M. D., of Fayetteville, Ala.

Interchange of medical opinion is one of the principal sources from which the physician derives his knowledge of the treatment of disease; deprive him of this, and all his knowledge must be confined to the narrow sphere of his own observations. There is no physician, of much experience, who has not met with some case or cases, the history of which would be interesting to the profession. Were he to give them publicity, which is certainly his duty, our medical journals would then be filled with practical matter, and our physicians thereby made acquainted, not only with the various diseases afflicting different sections and localities of our country, but also with their treatment. In a word, in doubtful and difficult cases, we could call to our aid all the skill and experience of the land; thereby inspiring us with confidence and, no doubt, lessening the mortality. It is certainly the duty of every physician who is a friend to suffering humanity, and loves his profession, to contribute his *mite*—even if he should not be *learned in the law*, and happen to be in error, it will present an opportunity of having that error corrected and he enlightened—and if right, he will have the satisfaction of knowing, that probably he has done some good.

I do not present to the profession the treatment of Narcotism from opium by cold water to the head, as anything new or original, but for the purpose of calling attention to it as a remedy always at hand and of easy application. In the American Journal of Medical Science, for April, 1852, Dr. J. Young, of Chester, Pennsylvania, reports two cases, the lives of whom were no doubt saved by this simple remedy. The first was that of a child two years old; the mother had given it a portion of "Baker's Specific." The poison had been in its stomach six hours when the doctor saw it—it was as limber as a rag—all muscular contraction had ceased, and it had lost the power to swallow—it could not by any means be aroused. The doctor called for a pitcher of water and poured in one continuous stream on the crown of its head, until a gallon had been used, by the time the child showed signs of muscular contraction; the water was continued a little longer and the child roused up, cried lustily and soon got well.

The second was that of a negro girl aged 18 years, who had been in the habit of taking laudanum for some time past, in increasing doses, for the purpose of producing exhilerating feelings. On this occasion she had bought a two ounce vial full and drank it all at three draughts; in two or three hours she was unconscious, and the muscular system completely released. Cold water poured on the back of her head for five minutes completely restored her, and nothing further was done but a dose of oil to open the bowels. Immediate relief was obtained, and probably life saved in both these cases by cold water alone.

These two cases of doctor Young's brought forcibly to my recollection three cases which came under my own observation, and which I treated in the same manner, long before I had heard it recommended by any one else. In the winter of 1844, while I was practicing my profession on the Yazoo River, in Carrol county, Mississippi, I was summoned early one morning to see an aged lady. A profuse diarrhœa, with which she had been attacked the night previous, was fast wasting her little remaining spark of vitality; extremities cold; pulse weak; quick and steady; tongue and mouth dry and parched; thirst great; skin hot and dry over the abdomen. Prescribed, mustard sinapisms to the extremities, with hot brick to the feet; $\frac{1}{4}$ gr. morphine in a little warm brandy toddy, to be repeated every four hours if the bowels required it; a teaspoonful of laudanum in six oz. decoc. kino by enema, if the morphine should fail; mustard sinapisms to the spine to arouse the dormant energies of the spinal nerves. I then left my patient, with a promise to see her again that night. Shortly after my departure, two or three pretty profuse discharges from my patient alarmed her friends: in consequence, they gave the morphine about every hour and a half, at the same time using the enema, so that in four hours after I left she had taken $\frac{3}{4}$ grs. morphine and two teaspoonfuls of laudanum. This arrested the diarrhœa, but it was well nigh at the sacrifice of her life; she became so drowsy that it was with difficulty she could be aroused: the relatives, thinking "death was on her," sent after me in great haste, as though I could stay the hand of Omnipotence, and ward off at will the "king of terrors." On my arrival, I found her completely narcotised, lying on her back, eyes half open and turned back; muscular system completely relaxed, so that the under jaw hung down, bathed in a profuse perspiration; breathing deep, and very slow, not more than four or five times in the minute; lips and face somewhat livid and could not arouse her by any means in our power. Noticing the temporal arteries were completely on the strut, and thinking that cold water might produce contraction of these vessels and drive off the superabundant quantity of blood thrown to the head by the opiate, I called for a pitcher of ice water, had her head held off the bed and poured it on in one continuous

slow stream. By the time the contents of the pitcher were exhausted, she spoke and called for water. I gave her coffee as an
anti-somnolent. We thus continued the cold water for half an
hour, when she seemed completely restored. In half an hour
after we stopped the water, she seemed to be sinking again
into her narcotic slumber. The water again relieved her, and by
keeping it up occasionally as the symptoms indicated, she was
permanently relieved in three or four hours after I commenced
its use. I, also, during all this time, gave her frequently hot
coffee to drink, without cream or sugar, at the same time keeping the spine and extremities well burnt with mustard. Some
good probably resulted from the coffee and mustard, but the
principal relief is attributable to the cold water. She had no
more diarrhœa; nothing ailed her but debility, from which she
gradually recovered and got quite well.

In 1845, I was called to see Mrs. S——, aged 30, married
10 years; no children; suffered much with dysmenorrhœa; tall
and spare made; scrofulous diathesis, subject at times to cramp
colic. On the morning of my visit, she had had a more violent
attack than usual of this painful affection, for which she had
taken something over a teaspoonful of very strong laudanum;
she was talking wild and incoherent; had a vacant expression;
tossing her head from one side to the other; throwing her
hands about—in a word, she was perfectly deranged. I applied
the cold water to her head and in fifteen minutes she was per-
perfectly restored to consciousness—the water was re-applied
whenever she began to " feel strange," as she expressed it, and
always with the same happy result, until the opiate influence
wore off, when she was as well as ever.

In 1849, in this place, Fayetteville, Fayette county, Alabama,
Miss M. W——, in her 18th year, was attacked with dysentery.
I prescribed for her pills composed each of 1 gr. opium, 2 gr.
camphor, ½ gr. calomel, 1 gr. ipecac: one to be taken every
four hours. This was early in the morning. In two hours after
taking the first pill she had a mucous discharge from her bowels,
and being much pained she took another. In one hour after
this, she took a third, and feeling no better in two hours more,
she took *two* others, and continued to take them every hour or
two until by four o'clock in the evening she had taken *eight.*

At six I was summoned to her bed-side, when I found her perfectly distracted. The pills had seemed to exert no influence until five o'clock, when they took effect and seemed to exert as powerful an influence as though all had been taken at once. She remained in this frenzy state about an hour, when she sunk into a deep stupor, from which nothing could arouse her but cold water, and whenever this was discontinued 15 or 20 minutes, she would again become comatose. It was kept up through the night, and by next morning she was as well as ever, except weakness.

In all these cases the great beverage of nature evidently relieved much suffering and probably saved life. I have noticed in all the cases of narcotism from opium that the patients got well of their dysentery or diarrhœa immediately after their recovery from the narcotism. Does the opium produce a change in the determination of the fluids?

ARTICLE XXVII.

On the Cutaneous Eruption induced by the internal use of Tartar Emetic. By P. M. KOLLOCK, M. D., of Savannah.

In the June No. of the Southern Medical and Surgical Journal, I read the description of two cases, by John S. Wilson, M. D., of Airmount, Ala., of a "Specific Cutaneous Eruption produced by the internal use of Tartar Emetic." Being thus reminded of a similar case, which occurred in my practice some years since, and, like the author of the communication, never having seen any notice of such effects of the drug in question in books, I send you a copy of the note which I made of the case at the time of its occurrence.

September 1, 1848. Saw Mrs. C.'s little girl, about three years old. Incipient laryngitis—to which disease there is a strong epidemic tendency at this time in the city. Her mother had given her castor oil previous to my being consulted. The disease proved extremely obstinate, but yielded to treatment, consisting of vomiting with "Turpeth Mineral," 2 grs., repeated at intervals of 15 minutes (two doses producing vomiting); purging with calomel; small doses of calomel and ipecac; and, lastly, a solution of tart. antim. gr. i. to water ʒi., gtt. 10 every two hours. Of this last, she took in all ʒss. of the solution, which broke up the remains of the disease. Two blisters had been applied, one on sternum, the other on dorsal spine. I intended this last to be confined to nucha; but owing to her restlessness, its effects had extended over a much larger space. She seemed, however, to be entirely relieved of the catarrhal disease, and to have nothing more to contend with than the irritation produced by the remedies. A little febrile excitement continued. At this time an eruption, resembling prickly heat, broke out all over the body; the blistered surfaces became very much inflamed, and seemed very much disposed to ulcerate, although I was assured by the mother that the blisters had not been applied more than two hours. About the 6th or 7th, as the fever seemed to exhibit a paroxysmal tendency, I commenced giving sulph. quinine. She took one grain, when the stomach became exceedingly irritable and incapable of retaining any thing whatever. The eruption on the skin became pustular, and extended all over the body, and the blistered surfaces continued to look badly in spite of the free use of chlor. sod. She died on the morning of the 9th, and the eruption on the trunk assumed a purple color. Previous to death she bled from the nose.

ARTICLE XXVIII.

Catalepsy Relieved by Ether Inhalation. By JOHN S. WILSON, M. D., of Air Mount, Alabama., (formerly of Georgia.)

Since the introduction of Ether and Chlorform, the various medical journals have contained numerous reports of their successful use in almost every variety of nervous and spasmodic disease; but never having seen a case of that rare disease, Catalepsy, included in any of those reports, I have concluded that the following case might not be uninteresting to the profession, and that it might suggest a valuable resource in a form of nervous disorders that is so unusual and so little noticed by writers as to produce some embarrassment in its treatment.

CASE. On the 6th of March last, I visited a negro woman,

the property of Mr.•W., for the purpose of deciding as to her "soundness"—Mr. W. having recently purchased her. I found on examination per vaginam, that her uterus was prolapsed, and that it was fixed in the pelvis, possessing but slight mobility—it seemed moreover to be somewhat indurated. On the 9th I was called again, about 9 o'clock, A. M., when I learned from her owner that he had called her early that morning, but receiving no answer, he went to her, and found her speechless and motionless. He could not tell how long she had been in that condition.

When I saw her, she presented the following symptoms : Pulse slow and full—respiration the same, and without stertor—muscles rigid, but no convulsive movements—except a slight twitching of the muscles of the eyes and lips. Sensation was almost wholly abolished ; none being manifested on pinching and pulling the skin, and very little on the application of a live *fire-coal*—the arms retained any position in which they were placed, as in the mesmeric state.

Treatment. I first abstracted a small quantity of blood, for the purpose of removing or preventing cerebral congestion ; I then used the Sulph. Ether freely, by inhalation, with the view of resolving the tonic rigidity of the muscles.

After continuing the remedy about 20 or 30 minutes, and when she had inhaled near 2 ozs, the muscles became gradually relaxed : the Ether was then discontinued, and soon afterwards consciousness returned : she then sat up and looked about with a bewildered expression ; and on being questioned as to the manner of her attack and her previous condition, she could not give any satisfactory answers, expressing entire ignorance in reference to the experiments made to test her sensibility, while in the cataleptic state, and also, with respect to the bleeding. Up to this date she has had no other attack. My object in reporting this case having been already mentioned, it is needless to say more :—I would merely observe that every one who has seen a subject in the "mesmeric state," will, on seeing a case of catalepsy, be strongly impressed by the remarkable analogy existing between those two singular phenomena of the nervous system.

PART II.

𝔈𝔠𝔩𝔢𝔠𝔱𝔦𝔠 𝔇𝔢𝔭𝔞𝔯𝔱𝔪𝔢𝔫𝔱.

On Healthy and Morbid Menstruation. By J. Henry Bennett, M. D., late Physician-Accoucheur to the Western
General Dispensary, etc.

[Continued from Page 417.]

Amenorrhœa.—By amenorrhœa is meant the absence, when
physiologically due, or the sanguineous discharge by which
menstruation is *externally* manifested.   The menstrual function
consisting, as we have seen, not merely in the periodical secretion of blood from the interior of the uterine cavity, but
also in the maturation and elimination of ova from the ovary,
it is necessary to make the above distinction.   Ova may, by
exception, be matured and evolved from the ovary in the
human female, as well as in the lower animals, without any
sanguinous discharge taking place, as is evidenced by the repeatedly recorded facts of the conception of young females who
have never menstruated, and by the pregnancies which occur
in women who are nursing, without menstruation having returned.   Thus, the external excretion of blood can no longer,
in our present state of knowledge, be considered as comprising
the entire function, although, as the rule, its manifestation is the
evidence of the existence of those all-important ovarian phenomena with which it is generally connected.

Amenorrhœa may be studied under two principal forms : in
the first which we will call " constitutional amenorrhœa," menstruation has never taken place ; in the second, which may be
termed "accidental amenorrhœa," it has manifested itself, but
has been suddenly or gradually suppressed.

Constitutional Amenorrhœa.—In order to appreciate this, the
first form of amenorrhœa, we must recall to mind some of the
principal facts connected with the physiology of menstruation
noticed in a former paper.   Thus we must recollect, that the
first appearance of this function follows no strict rule, oscillating
in health, between the ages of eleven and nineteen or twenty,
an interval of nine or ten years; and that the average age of
fourteen or fifteen is obtained by the inclusion of the exceptionally extreme cases.   We must also bear in mind that, apart
from constitutional and family peculiarities, the acceleration or
delay of menstruation appears to be more the result of favourable or unfavourable hygienic conditions than of climate, as
was formely taught and believed.

Such being the physiological conditions of memstruation, it
is evident that its non-appearance after the average age of four-

teen or fifteen is not to be considered a morbid state, as long as the delay is unaccompanied by any symptom of disease or ill-health. Thus we occasionally meet with young females, non-menstruated, of the age of seventeen or eighteen, or even older, whose frame is well developed and healthy, and who complain of no ailment beyond an occasional headache or backache, and sometimes not even of that. With them, menstruation is mere-ly late in its manifestation : they are not suffering from amenor-rhœa.

In a considerable proportion, however, of the young females who reach the age of eighteen or more without being menstrua-ted, the delay is either attended with great discomfort and dis-tress, apart from any physical deficiency ; or is connected with defective general and sexual development ; or is occasioned by some local or general morbid condition ; or is prevented by some physical impediment. Each of these states may be said to constitute a distinct form of amenorrhœa.

In those who belong to the first category, we find a well-formed frame, properly developed breasts, as also the other exter-nal signs of puberty ; but the patient suffers from constant head-ache and flushing of the face, severe pains in the back and loins, extending to the lower part of the abdomen and down the thighs, and often form a leucorrhœal discharge. It is evident that the changes that precede and accompany menstruation, both in the internal and external organs of generation, have taken place, but that the function has a local difficulty in establishing itself : thence an irregular state of circulation, determination of blood to the head and face, congestion of the uterus, vagina, and ovaries, with consequent pain in the uterine regions, and the leucorrhœal discharge. This state is not unfrequently connec-ted with a plethoric condition of the system, and may last from a few months to several years. The advent of the menstrual hæmorrhage generally relieves the patient at once, although she may still continue to suffer at times as above described, if menstruation fails to establish itself regularly.

. The second division comprises non-menstruated females, who, although they have attained, or even passed, the ordinary age of puberty, do not present that development of the mam-mæ and other external organs of generation, by which this period of life is usually characterized. They remain thin, angular, and flat-chested, and retain all the characteristics of girlhood, mental as well as bodily. It would appear as if in these cases the ovaries remained dormant, and as if the general stimulation which their progressive maturation imparts to the economy were not supplied.

We have seen that, physiologically, menstruation is retarded by bad living and unfavourable hygienic conditions; whereas, its advent is accelerated by good living and favourable hygienic conditions. From this fact alone, we might conclude that all diseases that debilitate the economy would have a tendency to retard the menstrual flux; and such is really the case. Phthisis, scrofula, chlorosis, fevers, indeed all diseases that weaken, produce this effect. None, however, more frequently occasion amenorrhœa than chlorosis, a disease of the blood, in which the solid constituents of the vital fluid are diminished, and the fluid or serous increased. The delay or suppression of the menses, under the influence of this malady, is so prominent a feature in its history, that many writers have very erroneously connected it with the uterus, and have described it as a uterine disease. In reality, the state of the menses is a mere symptom of the anæmia and debility occasioned by the morbid state of the blood. It is only in a few exceptional cases that I have found chlorosis connected with actual uterine disease.

Lastly, the menstrual secretion may have taken place, but the excretion may never have occurred, owing to congenital or accidental closure of the genital passages. The os uteri, the vagina, and the hymen, may be all closed together, or they may be each closed separately. If the closure exists at the os uteri, the menstrual fluid accumulates in the cavity of the uterus, and gradually develops it, so that the enlarged organ rises out of the pelvis, and appears above the pubis, simulating pregnancy. If it is the lower part of the vagina or the hymen that is imperforate, the menstrual fluid first accumulates in the vagina, which it distends to an extreme degree before it enlarges the uterine cavity. If the fluid collection reaches the hymen, it generally pushes it forward, and forms a tumour, which appears between the labia. This distention of the internal uterine organs is generally attended with great suffering, both local and general, and is marked by periodical exacerbations, corresponding to the monthly periods.

Accidental Amenorrhœa.—The second class of cases comprises those in which menstruation has existed, but has been suddenly or gradually suppressed.

The sudden suppression of menstruation is generally the result of exposure of the body, and especially of the feet, to cold or to the wet; of a mental shock, from fear, grief, pain, or anxiety, &c.; or of a sudden attack of disease. It not unfrequently occurs, for a time, as a result of a sea voyage or of change of climate, without giving rise to much distress, and without requiring medical treatment, the return taking place spontaneously. The sudden suppression of the menses, under the influence of the other causes mentioned, is often followed by the development of inflammation in the uterus, ovaries, or lateral ligaments. Even when suddenly suppressed, however, the suppression may be unattended with any unfavorable symptom beyond slight pain in the back and hypogastrium, flushing, and headache. Amenorrhœa, thus suddenly induced, seldom extends over more than one, two or three periods, under proper management, although the suspension may be much more lengthened, and is sometimes indefinite.

A gradual suspension of menstruation is sometimes observed in those females in whom the function has set in late and with difficulty, without there being any evident cause, general or local. It would appear as if the ovarian and sexual vitality were anomalously low; and after making one or more efforts, at irregular periods to establish itself, menstruation ceases, not to return, except under the influence of treatment. When this occurs, the health is scarcely ever good, the constitution generally remaining delicate and weak.

In such cases, however, we are warranted in suspecting ovarian or uterine disease. Generally speaking, in the absence of the chlorotic or tubercular cachexia, the gradual suppression of the menses is connected with such disease. The development of the various tumours to which the ovaries are liable, frequently entails amenorrhœa; and the chronic inflammatory affections which are so often observed in the neck and body of the uterus, may have the same result. Menstruation first becomes irregular, being delayed days, weeks or months, and then ceases completely. I have often been consulted for amenorrhœa by females who were labouring under these forms of disease and in whom it had evidently come on subsequently to the uterine affection.

When menstruation does not return, the uterus, and especially its cervix, even in the absence of positive disease, appear sometimes to be the seat of a kind of permanent congestive irritation, which ultimately may bring on hypertrophy and induration of the latter region. I have seen the cervix become thus enlarged, under my eyes, as it were, in the course of four or five years, although there was never any really tangible disease during that time. In one instance, that of a married woman, now twenty-eight, the menses, which from the first had been irregular, stopped immediately after marriage at twenty-three. Soon afterwards she began to suffer from uterine symptoms, and when she consulted me, I found the cervix inflamed and ulcerated, but not hypertrophied. The disease was soon subdued, but the menses have only returned once or twice. The uterus has appeared to remain in a state of semi-congestion, and the cervix has gradually enlarged. This female remains delicate

although in very tolerable health, free from pain, and not suffering under any other morbid state.

Suppressed menstruation, either sudden or gradual, is not
unfrequently followed, even when uterine inflammation is not
developed by serious general symptoms, obstinate vomiting,
severe hysteria, and sometimes by the establishment in the
economy of a supplementary hæmorrhage, to which the name
of "vicarious menstruation" has been given. The mucous membrane of the nasal fossæ, of the lungs, stomach, and bowels, are
the most ordinary seat of this hæmorrhage, which takes place
in some instances with the regularity of normal menstruation,
and in others at irregular periods. All the other mucous membranes, as also the skin itself in various regions, have been the
seat of vicarious menstruation. It has not unfrequently been
observed from the surface of wounds or sores. Such being the
case, it is evident that hæmorrhage occurring from any of these
sources in a young female in whom the menses are suppressed
has not that importance which it would have under other circumstances. The hæmorrhage may be, and probably is, merely an effort of nature to establish a supplementary issue for the
menstrual secretion, which has not taken place.

Treatment.—The rules which should guide the practitioner
in the treatment of amenorrhœa must be drawn from an attentive consideration of the causes by which it is occasioned, and
must vary as they vary. In a general point of view, however,
the indications are, 1st, to give tone to the economy if tone be
deficient, and to remove general or local disease if such disease
be present; 2ndly, to favour and promote, within reasonable
and judicious limits, the menstrual function. We will now
briefly see these indications are best carried out in the various
forms of amenorrhœa above described.

When the advent of the menstrual flux is retarded in well-
developed young females, who evidently suffer, both generally
and locally, from the delay, a little judicious management will
often determine its appearance. The state of the health should
first be carefully scrutinized, and any general or functional
derangement remedied by proper treatment. If the patient is
weak and delicate, the various preparations of iron, with a generous dietary, are often of great use. If on the contrary, she
is plethoric, and subject to headache and flushing of the face, a
light diet, gentle exercise, and alterative or saline medicines
are indicated. A young female suffering in this way is better
at home, under the eye of a devoted and attentive mother,
should she be fortunate enough to possess such a parent, than
in a public school, where the rigid discipline usually enforced
renders it difficult to pay that attention to her state which it

requires.   Under the influence of these general means, the mem-strual function usually manifests itself, and becomes regularized in the course of a few months.   Should they prove inefficient, slight periodical stimulation of the uterine system should be resorted to.   The plan I most frequently adopt is, the applica-tion of large mustard poultices to the breasts and inner and upper parts of the thighs, alternately, night and morning, during five or six days, every four weeks.   The mustard poultices should be allowed to remain on until the skin reddens and begins to feel painful, but not long enough to blister it, as that would prevent their being replaced the following day.   The feet may also be put in hot water night and morning, for a few minutes, and if there is any pain in the hypogastric or ovarian regions, large warm linseed poultices, sprinkled over with laudanum, may not only afford relief, but also promote the menstrual excretion.   When the symptoms of local congestion are very marked, the application to the vulva of a few leeches every month, or about the fifth day of the local treatment, may be of great assistance.   The commencement of this local treatment should be made to coincide with the menstrual nisus, when it manifests itself periodically.   When it does not, a certain date should be taken, and adhered to at the interval stated—that is, every twenty-eight days.   In such cases the medicines known as emmenagogues, which exercise a special influence over the uterus, are scarcely in my opinion, admissible, the object being to *gently* promote the natural function, and not to violently stimulate, and probably irritate, the uterine organs.

In amenorrhœa connected with deficient uterine and bodily development, the local treatment should be conducted on the same principles only it generally requires to be carried out more perseveringly and for a greater length of time.   In addition to the means mentioned, I have also derived great benefit from electricity, the electric current being carried through the pelvis from the hypogastric to the sacro-lumbar region, for an hour night and morning, during the week that local means are resort-ed to.   In these cases it is evident that the non-development of the body is often in a great measure the *result* of the dormant condition of the uterine organs, inasmuch as I have repeatedly succeeded in rousing them to action by the local treatment above detailed, when the most judicious and perseveringly general treatment had failed.   In these cases I have invariably seen the bodily structures subsequently develope themselves with great rapidity.   At the same time, the knowledge of this fact must not for a moment prevent our employing every possi-ble means of invigorating the general health, of vitalizing econo-my, and of promoting the regular play of the various functions.

After removing any morbid functional condition which a careful scrutiny may detect, recourse should be had to the mineral and vegetable tonics, and especially to ferruginous preparations, to which should be added a generous diet, moderate food, or horseback exercise, cold bathing or sponging, early hours for retiring and rising, and residence in the country, if possible.

When amenorrhœa can be traced to a debilitating disease, such as chlorosis, phthisis, scrofula, &c., the best treatment is the treatment of the disease to which it is referrible. Thus, in chlorosis, the menstrual flux gradually diminishes, and may finally cease altogether under the influence of the progressive deterioration of the blood, without there being any uterine disease or any other uterine symptom than the scantiness and final disappearance of the secretion. As under appropriate general treatment the blood becomes healthy, menstruation returns or again becomes gradually more and more normal, without any local treatment being necessary in the immense majority of cases. The same may be said of scrofulous and other forms-of constitutional debility. In pulmonary phthisis, the falling off and final disappearance of menstruation is a symptom of much more serious import, as it is generally connected with the more advanced stages of the disease, and with an amount of tuberculur deposit, and of consequent marasmus, through defective nutrition, which renders the chance of a recovery very problematical.

Amenorrhœa from physical obstacles can only be remedied by surgical means. If the hymen is imperforate, or the lips of the vulva are adherent, and the menses have collected behind, a crucial incision in the center of the bulging hymen, or vulvar protuberance, in all that is required. Care, however, should be taken, once the menstrual fluid has been evacuated, that the divided surfaces do not unite and cicatrize. This is to be prevented by the use of small sponge or cotton tents for a few days, or by the application of the nitrate of silver to the edges of the incisions—a more painful but equally efficacious process. When the vagina is partially or wholly absent or closed, either congenital or by adhesion from accidental causes, the case is a much more serious one, and more difficult to remedy. If there is merely adhesion of the walls of the vagina, this adhesion can generally be removed by the dilatation of the vagina, coupled with the gradual and careful division of the adherent surfaces. When the vagina is partially or entirely absent, the symptoms produced by the retention and accumulation of the menses in the uterus may be sufficiently serious to render it imperative to attempt to form an artificial passage by surgical means, of the distended uterus. In such cases the difficulty and risk of the operation depends on the distance that separates the vaginal cul-de-sac or the imperforate vulva from the uterus, the operator having to make his way between the rectum and the bladder. Considerable assistance in diagnosis is derived from a careful rectal examination. It is of great importance to find a vent for these uterine accumulations of menstrual fluid, as, in addition to the suffering endured, there is positive danger to life. Cases are on record in which the distention of the uterus extended to the Fallopian tubes, and in which death occurred from the peritonitis occasioned by their rupture.

Occlusion of the os uteri, as a congenital occurrence, is rare; but since I first recommended the use of potassa cum calce as a last resource in obstinate inflammatory disease of the cervical canal, I have seen several cases in which its use had been followed by all but complete occlusion, and by partial retention of the menses, or at least their difficult excretion. This was evidently owing to the want of due caution at the time of application and during the period of healing afterwards. The tendency of the tissues thus treated to contract being very great, it should be counteracted, if necessary, by the occasional use of wax bougies, until the process of repair has been fully accomplished. The possibility of this accident occurring through the want of caution of the operator, does not in the least invalidate the utility of the remedy as an exceptional and ultimate one. I have generally, but not always, found this form of occlusion easy to remove by progressive dilation. Should occlusion of the os uteri exist congenitally, once recognised it is easily remedied by a slight incision in the region of the os, and by subsequent dilatation.

When menstruation is accidently arrested or prevented, by exposure to cold and wet, by illness, or by any other of the causes enumerated, the amenorrhœa is seldom of long duration. The condition in which it originated having ceased to obtain, the function generally rights itself; the only treatment usually required being that which is most calculated to restore the general health of the patient. In some cases it may also be necessary to resort to the local means already detailed, when menstruation appears to have a difficulty in re-establishing itself.

The catamenial function appears to be more especially liable to arrest from accidental temporary influences in those females who present the low degree of sexual vitality to which allusion has been made in the first part of this paper, and with whom menstruation appears late and with difficulty. In such constitutions, indeed, it sometimes stops for many months, or even permanently, if no treatment be resorted to, without any apparent cause. Under the influence of decided general and local treatment, the menses will often return for a time, but flag and cease as soon as the treatment is suspended. If there is no positive disease of the uterus or ovaries, the emmenagogues, such as ergot of rye, savine, &c., may be cautiously tried. I have known also the married state, especially if followed by conception, produce a complete change in the functional activity of the uterine system, and menstruation become regular and natural. It is in these cases that the application of the nitrate of silver to the cavity of the uterus, or the scarification of its mucous surfaces, has been proposed. I must confess, however, that I do not think we are warranted in thus interfering with so delicate and sensitive a region of the uterus for such a purpose. In the unmarried female the application of leeches to the vulva, and in the married to the neck of the uterus, answers every purpose without being open to the same objection.

The development of inflammatory disease in the neck or body of the uterus, or in the ovaries, and of cystic and scrofulous tumours in the ovaries, is one of the most frequent causes of amenorrhœa in those in whom the function has once been fairly established, and especially of partial amenorrhœa. When such lesions exist, they generally give rise to other symptoms which an attentive and well informed observer may easily recognize. This remark, however, applies more to the uterus than to the ovaries, for important morbid changes are not unfrequently found after death in the latter organs, which, during life, have given little other evidence of their existence than the modification or arrest of the catamenial functions.

In all these cases, the amenorrhœa is merely a symptom of the ovarian or uterine disease. The latter is the condition to be treated, the only indication the amenorrhœa itself supplies being the advisability of having resource to such local means as are calculated to promote menstruation, whenever nature appears to be making the least effort to establish the menstrual flux.

In vicarious menstruation, our first effort ought to be directed to the restoration of the integrity of the uterine organs, if it be impaired. We should then, by all the means enumerated, attempt to divert the molimen hæmorrhagicum of menstruation from its abnormal to its normal seat. The most important of these means is the abstraction of blood from the vulva or cervix uteri, which should be resorted to every month, a day or two before the vicarious menstruation is expected, and may be treated after it has begun, should the strength of the patient admit of such a step. By this treatment the menstrual nisus may be diverted into its natural channel ; whereas, any attempt to stop the morbid hæmorrhage, by means, applied directly to the organ from which it takes place, might be productive of mischief to the system at large.

On the Chlorosis of Pregnancy.   By M. Cazeaux.

M. Cazeaux recently read, at the Paris Medical Society, a paper, the object of which was to show "that hydræmia or serous polyæmia is the most frequent cause of the functional disturbances in advanced pregnancy usually attributed to plethora." The analysis of the blood of pregnant women exhibits a diminution of globules and an increase of water, differing indeed only from that of chlorosis by containing an increased quantity of fibrine. The quantity of fibrine is far less than in phlegmon, and the buff it gives rise to has been often observed in the chlorotic. The functional disturbances of pregnancy resemble those of chlorosis, many of these indeed being common to plethora and chlorosis. The effect of treatment confirms this view of their nature; for while here, as in chlorosis, depletion may prove a temporary and fallacious means of relieving serous plethora, it is from the employment of animal food and iron that real benefit is obtained; and this even in cases wherein local bleeding may be deemed advisable. M. Cazeaux does not, however, deny that true sanguineous plethora may be met with occasionally, and especially in the early months.

During the animated discussion which followed, M. Duparcque admitted that pregnancy may occasionally induce a condition analogous to chlorosis; but he referred to the marked power of venesection in arresting threatened abortion from active uterine congestion; and believes that the practice followed by our predecessors of bleeding at the middle of pregnancy, on account of the then active disposition to abortion, may often be advantageously imitated. A similar plethoric determination takes place at the seventh and ninth months; and when the mother does not suffer ill effects from this, it may produce cerebral apoplexy, or that state of general congestion termed asphyxia, in the infant—the plethora killing the child, though it spared the mother, when precautionary venesection had been neglected. Puerperal convulsions might often be prevented, if bleeding were instituted for the plethoric condition in which they so frequently originate. In judging of the presence of plethora, too much weight has been attached to the highly-coloured condition of the skin, especially that of the face and its adjoining mucous membranes, and to the projection of the veins. But it is very common to see persons who are constantly plethoric, and who are liable to phlegmasiæ, congestions, and hæmorrhages, exhibiting so colourless a condition of the tissues, that from their mere aspect, we might believe them subjects of chlorosis. Such persons bear losses of blood, which those of a higher colour and apparently eminently sanguineous temperament, could not endure.

M. Jacquemier stated that he had examined the blood of about 200 women, in the eighth and ninth months of pregnancy, most of them being persons from the country. The so-called inflammatory crust was not met with so often as is usually supposed; but occurred much oftener in winter (when many of the women suffered from bronchitis and influenza) than in the summer; it being met with at this latter period only once in six or even in nine cases. Most frequently when the buff did exist, the clot was pretty large and softish, and the serum was not in excess; the hard, retracted clot, covered with a thick buff, and bathed in a large quantity of serum, as seen in inflammation and chlorosis, being rarely met with. According to his observations, the excess of fibrine, whether absolute or relative to the diminution of globules, is not considerable enough to habitually give rise to the production of the inflammatory crust. The diminution of globules is infinitely greater in a chlorotic person than in a pregnant woman; and all the analogy that can be traced between the two conditions may be stated in the fact, that a considerable number of women, after the middle period of pregnancy, exhibit the commencement of anæmia. Clinical observation does not favour the view of the identity of the two conditions. Among many hundreds of women auscultated at the Maternite, during the last two months of pregnancy, M. Jacquemier only met with the carotid *souffle* in two or three.—[*Rev. Médical. Medico-Chir. Review.*

On the Management of Women after the Cessation of Menstruation. By Dr. E. J. Tilt.

[The superabundance of blood and nervous energy after the cessation of the menstrual flow may be safely and effectually kept down by the habitual use of small doses of purgatives; and, as they may have to be continued for some length of time, it is best to consult the patient as to what medicine would be best tolerated. The purgative to be used depends upon the constitution of the patient. Perhaps the best is some mild purgative which has been found to agree with the patient. Dr. Tilt continues:]

I frequently prescribe the soap-and-aloes pill of the Edinburgh Pharmacopœia, ordering five or ten grains to be taken with the first mouthful of food at dinner. Hemorrhoidal affections I have never seen *caused* by this frequent use of aloes, but I have seen them *relieved* by it; and as I read in Giacomini's 'Treatise of Materia Medica' my experience on this point is confirmed by that of Avicenna, Stahl, Cullen, and his own, so I think there must be some exaggeration as to the extraordinary property generally ascribed to this valuable drug, which can be associated with hyoscyamus, and is thus said to be less liable to induce piles. Kemp and Hufeland recommend the following powder to be given to those who are advanced in years, and who complain of a tendency to vertigo :—Guaiacum resin, cream of tartar, of each half a drachm, to be taken at night. This, no doubt will sometimes be found a useful laxative ; so will the popular remedy called the Chelsea Pensioner, of which Dr. Paris has given the following formula in his excellent Pharmacologia : —Of guaiacum resin, one drachm ; of powdered rhubarb, two drachms ; of cream of tartar and of flour of sulphur, an ounce of each ; one nutmeg finely powdered, and the whole made into an electuary with one pound of clarified honey : a large spoonful to be taken at night. I generally administer the flour of sulphur alone, or else to each ounce of it I add a drachm of sesquicarbonate or biborate of soda, and sometimes from five to ten grains of ipecacuanha powder. One to two scruples of these powders taken at night in a little milk, is generally sufficient to act mildly on the bowels, and I consider such combinations as very valuable when a continued action is required.

I feel obliged to class sulphur amongst purgative remedies because such is its visible action, but I believe that it owes its chief value, in diseases of cessation, to another action, much more difficult to understand, and which has long rendered it so valuable both in hemorrhoidal affections, where there is an undue activity of the intestinal capillaries, and in skin diseases marked by a morbid activity of the cutaneous capillaries. Whether sulphur cures by acting on the nerves or on the blood-vessels, or by modifying the composition of the blood itself, is difficult to tell, but it does certainly cure the diseases I have enumerated. It forms part of many popular remedies for the infirmities of old age, was recommended by Hufeland, and is lauded by Dr. Day in his work ' On the Diseases of old Age ;' but its utility is not generally known in all derangements of the menstrual function, at whatever period of life they may occur, and particularly at the change of life, where, if required, its action may be continued with impunity for months and years.

[*Provincial Med. and Surg. Journal.*

On Leucocythemia. By Professor BENNETT, Edinburgh.

[In the first article of our last volume (vol. 23) the reader will find a very interesting paper on the subject of white cell blood (Leucocythemia,) which is a proper introduction to the present

one.   Prof. Bennett has established the existence in the blood
of an excess of the colourless corpuscles; a condition highly
important to the pathologist and physiologist.   He says:]

The blood may be loaded with a multitude of cells, exactly
resembling those of pus ; that such blood may circulate in the
human subject for months, or even years, without destruction to
life, and that this condition is always associated with disease in
those organs, the functions of which have hitherto been involved
in the greatest obscurity, constitute facts which seem calculated
to exercise an important influence on many views that have
been long agitated in science.   The constitution of the blood
itself; the origin of its morphological elements and chemical
proximate principles; the importance of the lymphatic system ;
the functions of the spleen and other blood glands ; the nature
of purulent infection, and other diseases of the blood, may be
expected to be more or less elucidated by a study of the accompanying phenomena, causes, and results, of leucocythemia.
With a view, then, of stating as succinctly as possible the conclusions which may be legitimately derived from the thirty-five
cases previously recorded, I shall divide this part of the inquiry
into several sections, in which all these important topics will
be shortly considered.

I. *Symptoms observed in individuals affected with Leucocythemia.*—The symptoms have been very carefully observed in
several of the cases recorded in the first part of this memoir,
but we have great difficulty in referring any of them to the
mere alteration in the blood.   Several of those which were
most constant and best marked in advanced cases, were apparently caused by the increased size of the spleen or liver, as
they have been seen to occur in other cases where these organs
have been enlarged, without the occurrence of leucocythemia.
No doubt the peculiar change in the blood of which we are
treating has been discovered in individuals affected with enlarged spleen ; but this may arise from the circumstance, that
the circulating fluid has been more frequently examined in persons laboring under that complication.   When leucocythemia,
however, is more generally studied, it will very probably be
found associated with enlargement in other organs, especially
of the thyroid, thymus, supra-renal capsules, and lymphatic
glands.   Hence, I am persuaded, no systematic history of the
symptoms connected with this morbid state can be given in the
present state of our knowledge ; and I shall therefore merely
content myself with an analysis of those observed in the cases
recorded.

Of the thirty-five cases which are given in the preceding
pages, leucocythemia was demonstrated to exist, by careful

microscopic examination, in twenty-five.   The facts presented by these may be afterwards compared with those offered by such cases as were doubtful, or by those in which, associated with large spleen, it was proved that the blood was quite healthy.

Sex.—Of the twenty-five cases, sixteen occurred in males and nine in females.

Age.—The youngest case in which leucocythemia was observed was in a girl aged 9, and the oldest in a woman aged 69 years.   In two cases the ages are not stated, but in the remaining twenty-three they may be arranged as follows : Under 10 years, one case; between 10 and 20, two cases; between 20 and 30, three cases; between 30 and 40, seven cases; between 40 and 50, four cases; between 50 and 60, three cases; and between 60 and 70, three cases.   So far as this analysis goes, the diseases would appear to be most common in adult life, and more frequent in advanced age than in youth.

Abdominal swelling.—Greater or less swelling of the abdomen was present in twenty out of the twenty-five cases,— evidently dependent, in the majority of these, on enlargement of the spleen and liver, singly or united.   In five cases ascites was also present.   In several of the cases there was more or less abdominal pain or tenderness, while in a few the enlargement only produced inconvenience, from its size or weight.

Respiration.—The respiration was more or less affected in twelve out of the twenty-five cases.   Of these dyspnœa existed in eight.   The respiration is said to have been hurried in one ; short in a second ; laborious in a third ; and slow in a fourth. The disordered respiration appeared to be dependent in some cases on enlargement of the abdomen, and corresponding compression of the pulmonary organs, in others (five cases) it may have resulted from disease of the lungs themselves.

Vomiting was present in seven cases.   In two at the commencement, in three it was occasional, in one there was hematemesis, and in one it was connected with ulcer of the stomach.

Diarrhœa was present in twelve cases, and in some was the leading symptom throughout the progress of the disease.   In Tinlay, for instance (Case 2,) during the six months he was in the Infirmary, the bowels were opened from eight to twelve times a-day for weeks together.   In other cases this symptom only came on latterly, and in a few was not urgent.

Constipation is said to have existed in five cases.

Hemorrhages.—Extravasation of blood occurred in fourteen out of the twenty-five cases.   Of these there was epistaxis in

six cases ; hematemesis in one case ; hemorrhage by stool, including hemorrhoids, in four cases; hemoptysis in one case ;
flooding after delivery in one case, and bleeding from spongy
gums in one case. In some of these cases bleeding from the
gums or bowels was associated with epistaxis, and this last
symptom was observed in some of the best marked cases of
the disease, with enlarged spleen.

Dropsy was present, more or less, in thirteen cases, generally
dependent on the abdominal tumour. There was anasarca in
two cases, ascites in four cases, and œdema of the lower extremities in seven cases.

Fever.—More or less fever was observed in eleven cases,
indicated by increase of pulse, loss of appetite, thirst, and heat
of skin. It was occasionally present at the commencement, at
other times at the termination of the disease. In no case did it
exist to any extent, or was long continued. From the frequency
of splenic enlargement, it might be supposed by some that the
disease was connected with intermittent fever, but that this ever
occurred is very doubtful. It is said to have preceded the disease in three cases. In Case 8 the report says, that four months
previous to admission there had been intermittent fever, but
Dr. Walshe adds, " this point was not sufficiently inquired into."
In Case 10 there had been repeated attacks of ague, the last of
which occured nine years before he came under observation,
and seven years before the abdominal tumour was perceived.
In Case 19 the patient also had laboured under intermittent
fever, but seventeen years previous to the commencement of
the abdominal swelling. So far as the recorded cases are concerned, therefore, there is every reason to believe that intermittent fever is in no way concerned with the production of
leucocythemia.

Pallor of the surface.—An unusual pallor of the surface was
observed in many cases, resembling that of anemia. The conjunctivæ, also, were of a peculiar light blue tint.

Jaundice.—In one case only of all those in which the liver
was affected, was jaundice observed.

Emaciation.—In most of the fatal cases emaciation was extreme.

Complications.—Disease of the lung was present in five
cases, including one case of bronchitis, one of phthisis, and three
of pneumonia. Bright's disease existed in two cases,—cerebral
hemorrhage in one case ; cancer was present in three cases,—
in one, in the form of an undescribed abdominal tumour (Case
10,) in a second, there was a cancer of the thyroid body and
neighbouring lymphatics, and in a third, cancer of the liver,
with ulcer of the stomach, stricture of the urethra, and hydro-

cele. All these diseases were characterised by their peculiar
symptoms, or physical signs during life.

It must not be supposed that the above numerical account of
the symptoms exhibits even an approximation to the proportion which any particular one holds to the number of cases on
record. Owing to the imperfection with which many of these
are described, important symptoms in some not being even
alluded to, this is obviously impossible. Statistics are no more
applicable to this subject than to any other in medicine, where
the cases have not been expressly drawn up in reference to
such an injury.

II. *Condition of the Blood in Cases of Leucocythemia.*—Of
the twenty-five cases of undoubted leucocythemia, it was detected after death only, in ten; during life only, in six; and
both during life and after death, in nine cases. Thus it has
been detected in the living body in fifteen cases, and in the dead
body in nineteen cases.

On examining the blood of living persons (which is most
readily accomplished by extracting a drop from the finger by
pricking it with a needle, and then examining it between glass-
es under the microscope in the usual way), the yellow and
colorless corpuscles are at first seen rolling confusedly together,
and the excess in number of the latter over the former is at
once perceived. This, however, becomes more evident after a
short time, when the coloured bodies are aggregated together
in rolls, and leave clear spaces between them, which are more
or less crowded with the colourless ones. Means are altogether
wanting to enable us to determine with exactitude the relative proportion of the two kinds of corpuscles in different cases.
In some the colourless corpuscles are only slightly increased
beyond their usual number. In one case they are described
as five times as numerous as those in health. .They are also
said in particular instances to be "greatly increased," "one
third as numerous," and "as numerous" as the coloured corpuscles. In all these statements there is nothing exact. Perhaps the best method of judging is to regard the spaces or
meshes left between the rolls or aggregations of yellow blood
corpuscles. When these are completely filled up, the colourless bodies do not, in fact, amount to one-third of the coloured
ones, on account of the large number of the latter which may
exist in a small space, in the form of rouleaux.

The size of the colourless corpuscles in the various cases giv-
en differs considerably. Even when at first sight they appear
to be of tolerably uniform size in any one case, it may be observed, when they are magnified, highly and carefully measured,
that some are twice the size of others, with all the intervening

sizes between them. In some cases, though comparatively few in number, they are described as being three or four times larger than the coloured corpuscles, and in two cases recorded, they were in one about the same size, or somewhat smaller, and in the other of two sizes, one larger and the other decidedly smaller.

In the nineteen cases in which the blood was carefully examined after death, the same variations with regard to number and size of the colourless corpuscles were found to exist, as have just been referred to in blood drawn fresh from the finger. It was always observable, however, that they were most numerous in the clot ; and when they existed in any number, as in Cases 1 and 2, they communicated to the colourless coagulum a peculiar dull, whitish look, and rendered it more friable under pressure. When less numerous, portions of the colourless coagulum from the heart and large vessels might be seen to present a dull cream colour, easily distinguishable from the gelatinous and fibrous appearance of a healthy clot, and such altered portions always contained a large number of the colourless bodies. This was especially observable in Case 34.

There is one remarkable fact which has been strongly impressed upon me by careful observation of the preceding cases. In no one instance has the condition of the blood been observed to undergo any marked change after the excess of white cells in it was discovered. In no case has this condition of the blood been seen to appear and progress gradually, as is observed in so many other lesions. In the case of Tinlay (Case 2,) the patient was under medical observation for a period of eighteen months, and the same excess of colourless corpuscles existed at the end of that time, as at its commencement. In the case of Kerr (Case 19,) the corpuscles were only slightly augmented in number, and yet at the end of eleven months they were not more numerous than when first examined. Cases are still to be met with, therefore, in which the commencement and progress of leucocythemia are to be observed. Such can only be expected to be found when the microscopical investigation of the blood is more generally practised in clinical investigation, as it is commencing to be in the Royal Infirmary.

III. *Chemical Composition of the Blood in cases of Lecocythemia.*—The chemical analysis of white cell-blood has been undertaken in only five cases, a number far too few to arrive at any important results. One cause of this is, that the majority of the twenty-five undoubted cases were only discovered after death, when any analysis of the blood in reference to the relative proportions of all its constituents cannot be determined. Another cause is owing to the circumstance, that several of the cases observed during life were so weak and exhausted, that the abstraction of even two oz. of blood, for the purpose of analysis, could not be safely ventured upon. Of the five analyses, three were performed by Dr. William Robertson, of Edinburgh, one by Dr. Parkes, of London, and one by Dr. Strecker, of Giessen. Dr. Robertson also analysed the blood of a sixth case (Case 28,) in which there was enlargement of the spleen without leucocythemia. The following is a tabular view of these analyses, the inferences from which will be given on a future occasion :—

ANALYSES OF THE BLOOD.

Case.	Sp. Grav.	Sp. Gr. of Serum.	Fibrin.	Serous Solids.	Globules.	Total Solids.	Water.	
No. 2.	1041·5	1026·5	6·0	72·0	67·5	145·5	854·5	Leucocythemia.
3.	1036·0	1023·0	2·3	67·0	49·7	119·0	881·0	
8.			7·08	75·22	101·63	183·93	816·07	
Later analysis.			4·75	77·52	97·93	180·2	819·8	
19.	1049·5	1029·0	5·0	95·0	80·0	180·0	820·0	
29.			4·46	82·35	97·39	184·2	815·8	
28.	1042·0	1025·5	3·9	75·7	76·3	155·9	844·1	

IV. *Morbid Anatomy of individuals affected with Leucocythemia.*—Of the twenty-five undoubted cases of leucocythemia which have been recorded, the body has been examined after death in nineteen. The information obtained from this source may be still further extended by a consideration of four cases in which the existence of this condition of the blood is highly probable; of seven cases recorded by Dr. Hodgkin of enlargement of the spleen and lymphatic glands, and of two cases examined after death where the spleen was hypertrophied without leucocythemia. In all, thirty-two dissections.

The organs which have been found to be most uniformly diseased are the spleen, the liver, and lymphatic glands, and of these I shall speak separately. The other lesions found in the brain, lungs, heart, kidneys, &c., alluded to in Section I., under the head of complications, were evidently accidental or consecutive, and need not be alluded to especially, in this place.

Condition of the spleen.—Of the nineteen cases of leucocythemia in which the body was examined after death, the spleen was found to be more or less enlarged in sixteen. In the other three, although it was healthy, the pulp in one, is said to be " a little more compact than usual ;" in a second its condition after death is not alluded to, although an encephaloid tumour occu-

pied the left side of the abdomen ; and in a third the spleen
was " healthy."

Of the sixteen cases in which the spleen was increased in
volume, it weighed above 7 lbs. in three ; above 5 lbs. in two ;
above 3 lbs. in two ; above 2 lbs. in four ; and nearly 1 lb. in
one case. In four cases it was not weighed. The greatest
weight of a spleen was 7 lbs. 13 oz., and the largest measurement 16½ inches long, and 9½ inches broad. The texture of
the organ varied in different cases, in some being of unusual
density, in others natural, and in a third case more or less soft
and pulpy. In a few cases it contained yellowish masses, apparently a form of deposit, but in reality degenerated tissue. The
structure was examined microscopically in seven cases, in all
of which it was demonstrated that the cell and nuclear elements
were increased, while the fibrous portion of the organ was apparently normal.

In four cases in which the existence of leucocythemia is probable, changes similar to those just stated occured in the spleen,
and in Dr. Hodgkin's cases similar lesions were found associated with enlarged lymphatic glands.

It is clear, however, that mere enlargement of the spleen is
not necessarily connected with white cell-blood, for in case 27
it was simply hypertrophied and weighed three pounds and a
half ; and in numerous other cases where this organ has been
undoubtedly enlarged, it has been proved by careful examination that the blood was normal—(Cases 26, 28, 35.) It remains
to be ascertained what are the structural differences in the spleen
existing between cases like these last, and those in which
leucocythemia exists.

Condition of the Liver.—Of the nineteen cases examined
after death, the liver was diseased in thirteen. In the other
six it is distinctly stated to have been healthy in five, while in
one it is not noticed in the report.

Of the thirteen cases, the liver was cirrhosed in two,—one
in its incipient and one in the advanced stage of that disease. In
a third case there was cancer of the organ, and in the ten others
the liver was more or less hypertrophied. Of these it weighed
above 13 lbs. in one ; above 12 lbs. in one ; above 10 lbs. in
one ; above 6 lbs. in three ; and above 5 lbs. in two cases. In
two cases, though much enlarged, the weight is not stated. In
these cases the organ was more or less congested, and its consistence varied from great firmness to a degree of softening
amounting to diffluence. The minute structure of the liver
was carefully examined in four cases, and found to be unaffected in three, while in the fourth it was infiltrated with cancerous
exudation.

In the six probable cases of leucocythemia, it is said that the liver was greatly hypertrophied in four. In the other two its condition is not stated.

Condition of the lymphatic glands.—Of the nineteen cases examined after death, the lymphatic glands were more or less diseased in eleven. Indeed, it is very probable that they were affected in a larger number, as in most of the other cases they were in no way alluded to, and may possibly have escaped observation from an unacquaintance with the importance which, as we shall see, ought to be attached to them.

Of the eleven cases, the lymphatic glands throughout the body were greatly enlarged in four, and more or less cancerous in three others. The mesenteric glands were especially affected in two; the thyroid and epigastric glands in one; and the solitary and aggregate intestinal glands in one. In some cases they were soft, presenting on section a granular whitish appearance, and yielding a copious turbid juice on pressure. In other cases they were more indurated; and in one there were slight calcareous deposits. The glandular structure was carefully examined microscopically in eight cases, and in all exhibited increase of the normal tissue, the juice abounding in cell or nuclear elements. In two cases, cancer cells were mingled with the healthy textures of the glands.

In the 17th volume of the Medico-Chirurgical Transactions, Dr. Hodgkin has recorded seven cases in which the lymphatic glands were more or less enlarged, and at the same time associated with increased size of the spleen. He considers the enlargement of both structures to be allied, and to depend upon a primary lesion unconnected with inflammation or adventitious structures. The appearance of a bloody serum in the thoracic duct and absorbents struck him in two of these cases, but the blood itself was not apparently noticed. At the time Dr. Hodgkin wrote (1832), the microscope was not much employed in pathological investigation, but had the blood been examined in these cases, I cannot resist the conviction that the discovery of leucocythemia would not have been reserved for the year 1845.

In the concluding portion of this memoir, it will be my endeavour to establish from the foregoing facts, and from numerous other observations and experiments:—

1. That the coloured blood-corpuscle is derived from the colorless one.

2. That the colourless blood-corpuscles are derived from the glands of the lymphatic system.

3. That the lymphatic glandular system is composed of the spleen, supra-renal capsules, thyroid body, thymus (pituitary pineal ?) and lymphatic glands, and that these constitute an ex-

tensive apparatus for the formation and elaboration of blood-corpuscles.

4. That the fibrin of the blood is derived from the solution of the blood-corpuscles, and the effete matter resulting from the disintegration of the tissues.

5. That these propositions concerning the origin, development, and disintegration of the blood-corpuscles are now as a consistent theory advanced for the first time, receive proof of their correctness from the cases of leucocythemia previously detailed, and are in harmony with the facts elicited by the labours of Hewson, Nasse, Wagner, Richert, Gulliver, Zimmerman, Wharton Jones, Simon, Kölliker, Milne Edwards, Goodsir, and others.—[*Monthly Jour. of Med. Science.*

On Chronic Rheumatism. By JOHN CARGHILL.

[The following paper, read before the Newcastle and Gateshead Pathological Society, comprises an analysis of one hundred and forty-three cases, one hundred of which were treated by the nitrate of potash in large doses, and the remaining forty-three by colchicum.]

These cases have been treated during a period of nearly six years, *i. e.* between 1842 and 1848, and they have been nearly all in-patients of this Hospital, so that I have had them constantly under my own eye, the few not so situated having been out-patients.

I have compared the cases together under as equal circumstances as possible, and have endeavored to attain as much accuracy as I could by carefully registering them at the time; this register comprises the following features:—Age, sex, duration of malady previous to admission, seat of pains, dose and combination of remedy, time of its employment, result, disturbing or other effects on the system, temperament of the patient, and concomitant treatment.

I shall first consider these points in reference to what was observed in the colchicum patients, and then in those treated by nitrate of potash, and shall conclude by recording certain deductions, which I think have unfolded themselves from the various facts, and likewise mention the views I entertain of the pathology and intimate nature of rheumatism.

Of the forty-three cases treated by colchicum, fourteen only were cured, or about one-third, and the average duration of the treatment was fifteen and a half days; the average duration of the malady before admission being seventy-three days. In addition to the fourteen who recovered entirely, there were twelve relieved, whilst twelve remained no better. In one the complaint appeared to be worse, and in the other four, circumstances arose which prevented any positive conclusions from being arrived at.

Dose and combination of the Colchicum.—In rather more than half of those cured, that result was effected by the vinum seminum colchici in the dose of from fifteen to thirty drops thrice a day, with a little magnesia and sp. etheris nitrici. In a very few intances ten grains of Dover's powder were given a few times at bed-time. In six out of the forty-three, the colchicum was given in powder in four grain doses thrice a day; in one case it was given in six grain doses thrice a day, and in one case in two grain doses thrice a day, all combined with pulvis cretæ. In all but the last named it produced vomiting, griping, and diarrhœa in two or three days' time, and had to be left off for the vinum with magnesia. Of this latter combination, the dose before mentioned, viz: ℥xv. to xxx. with fifteen grains of magnesia, and ℨss. of sp. eth. nit. was the most effectual, and the best borne. When the vinum was given by itself it seemed slower in its curative effect, and when given in ℨjss. doses of ℨj. doses thrice a day, either alone or combined (a measure in a few instances adopted,) it invariably had to be left off, from its producing very speedily its usual severe physiological effects, with great depression, and often cramps, the disease remaining at the same time unaffected. I should add, that these results followed even when the above doses were attained to very gradually.

Concomitant treatment.—In seventeen out of the forty-three cases the warm bath thrice a week was used, and in fourteen out of this number manifest relief was obtained. In ten cases out of the forty-three, Dover's powder was given in from ten to fifteen grains each night, and in six of these cases it was followed by beneficial effects. Cupping was occasionally used, and generally with benefit. Bleeding from the arm was scarcely ever practised, and calomel, Epsom salts, blue pill, or colocynth, were used as preliminaries, if constipation existed. As to the seat of the disease, it was in the several joints and muscles. In four cases wherein the rheumatism existed along with sciatica as its chief feature, the treatment by colchicum was fruitless.

II. *Chronic Rheumatism treated by Nitrate of Potash in large doses.*—Of the one hundred cases treated by this method, there were sixty-one cured, being more than six-tenths of the whole, and the average duration of the treatment was thirteen and three-quarter days. In addition to the sixty-one cured, there were twenty who experienced great relief, but were not entirely cured at the time of dismissal; there were five who experienced very slight benefit only, three received no benefit, and three got worse. In the remaining eight cases no positive conclusions could be arrived at.

Dose and combination of the remedy.—The usual dose to begin with was Ðij. thrice a day in barley water; this was adhered to in many cases throughout, but in a large number it was increased to ʒj., ʒiss., ʒij., thrice a day, and in one case ʒiij. every four hours was begun with and continued without intermission for twelve days, without the smallest inconvenience to the patient, who was cured in that period. This was a bad case of two and a half years' previous duration. The dose was often begun with and continued at ʒj., and with no disagreeable effect; sometimes ʒj. thrice daily, and sometimes ʒj every four hours consecutively.

Being desirous of ascertaining whether the duration of the malady might be shortened, or good in other ways obtained by combining the nitre with sp. nit., antim., tart. and tinct. opii, I adopted this in a considerable number of cases, and the result has shown me that no advantage is derivable from this practice. The dose of sp. of nitre was generally from ♏xv. to ʒss. or more; that of the vin. antim. ♏xv., and that of the tinct. opii. ♏v. to each dose of the pot. nit. Sweating and diuresis were equally produced by the nitre alone as when given in the above combination. Of the three, the tr. opii alone appeared useful by frequently assuaging the severe pain.

Disturbing effects.—It is of great importance to remark that this remedy was invariably administered in a large quantity of warm barley water—not less than ʒviij. to each dose. When given in the above large dose, without a diluent and demulcent like barley-water, it produces intense griping, with pallor of the countenance and cold perspiration, the pulse and heart's action flagging and coming down, and the greatest anxiety being experienced. This is followed by a dry red tongue, with enlarged papillæ and much thirst. This I had an opportunity of seeing to an intense degree in one case wherein the nitrate of potash in those doses had been administered several times without any diluent by the oversight of a nurse; she gave it in ʒiss. of plain water. I was on the point of applying numerous leeches to the epigastrium, fearing that gastritis was coming on, when the symptoms at last yielded to diluents and warm external applications, leaving no appreciable effects behind.

I shall now mention what were the *disturbing effects on the system* observed to be produced by large doses of nitrate of potash in cases *where it had been duly taken* with barley-water, but had not been well borne by the system. Those effects were seldom manifested, the medicine, when properly diluted, seeming to act mildly and efficiently.   When it is not tolerated, however, its effects are primarily on the nervous system.   They are these : general debility of the limbs, especially the lower extremities, and the knees, too, particularly complained of.   I have seen this carried to an extent which made the patients believe that they were seized with general paralysis; the whole body seemed to be made of wood, and for some hours it was impossible for them to rise from their seat or to move hand or foot.   To this were conjoined general tremblings, and the speech was affected ; occasionally the names of things were forgotten or mistaken ; there was also giddiness, and a painful rushing sound in the ears.   I never in these rare instances saw any distortion of the features, and the symptoms subsided in a few hours by diuretics or copious perspiration.   In the event of such results occurring, the chief remedies I should recommend would be hot diluents and hot blankets.   The subjects of them will be found generally of the purely *nervous temperament*, especially if associated with feeble power of the constitution.   When the sanguine or bilious temperament is combined with the nervous, the remedy is better borne and may be pushed farther ; and it agrees with my observation that the bilious lymphatic temperament, with its firm, harsh, muscular development, is the one in which this plan of treatment the oftenest succeeds, and may be used the most fearlessly, as it is the one on which chronic rheumatism, when once established, displays itself with perhaps the greatest relentlessness.

The *concomitant treatment* was simple, and most generally dispensed with altogether (with a view to ascertain more accurately the value of the nitrate of potash itself), except in cases of severe complication, in which the need for additional means, chiefly local, was urgent.   It consisted in occasional warm baths and vapour baths.   Cupping and leeching were had recourse to in such cases as showed a concentration of the disease in particular joints, as evidenced by swelling, redness, and acute pain not shifting its seat.   In dull chronic pains localized, occasional blisters were applied, and often with benefit ; and, towards the termination of the cases, a liniment of ammonia and turpentine was frequently useful in restoring tne natural suppleness of the parts.   When the pains were so great as to prevent sleep, and to harass the patient in an unusual manner, a draught of muriate of morphia, with solution of acetate of ammonia and water, was given at bed-time   The bowels were kept free by means of occasional light cathartics; and the treatment was generally commenced by giving a dose of calomel and colocynth, followed by a draught of infusion of senna with sulphate of magnesia.

The *diet* enjoined was nutritious, being the ordinary diet of the house—viz., meat once a day, milk, rice, broth. In such cases as presented symptoms verging on the acute, low diet was prescribed—such as milk, tea, sago, &c. In all old standing chronic cases generous diet was found the best, accompanied even by ale, porter, wine, or gin.

In the above 100 cases, the *duration of the malady previous to admission* was widely different—so much so, that no analytic average could be struck with a view to results that would not have a tendency rather to conduce to error than to elucidate truth. I may state in general terms that the length of time in these cases, previous to coming under the above treatment, was from seven days to ten years, whilst there were a few who could remember no period of their lives in which they had not been victims, more or less, to the complaint. Two months, five years, six years, six months, one year, were the most common periods cited; and it should be remarked that nearly all the cases were of an unusually severe character, and had been under all manner of practitioners; for many, despairing of a cure otherwise, had committed themselves to the tender mercies of unprincipled quacks, from whose fiery ordeal they had emerged with the conviction that now nothing but a residence in an infirmary with the reputation of our own could avail to benefit them!

Sex.—It is remarkable that, of the whole 143 patients, 17 only were women, the remaining 126 being men. The average age of the women was $35\frac{3}{4}$, that of the men $37\frac{1}{3}$. From this it appears that, in this part of the country, men are about $8\frac{1}{2}$ times more liable to be affected with chronic rheumatism than women, or for one woman attacked with chronic rheumatism there will be between eight and nine men. This is in all probability owing to the greater exposure of men to cold and wet; for I have found that in all of these cases the exciting cause, when any could be given, was invariably cold and wet, or sudden transitions from a high temperature to the opposite. On referring to MS. notes of M. Louis' clinical lectures on this subject, taken down by me at the time of their delivery at the hospital of La Pitié, in 1835, I find his experiments the same as to the exciting cause—invariably exposure to cold air or draughts (un vent frais).

The difference as to the *frequency of rheumatism* in France and England seems to be very great. Louis says that, out of 100 cases of all sorts treated by him, he only found one of rheumatism; and in the Paris hospitals, during two years, it was rare that rheumatism, whether acute or chronic, ever fell under my observation. That the difference is great among us will appear from the following fact:—On analysing, a good while ago, a number of cases of all sorts, nearly all of them chronic, treated by me in this hospital, embracing a period of five years, and amounting to 959, I found that 86 were cases of chronic rheumatism, being, on an average, one in eleven and a sixth of the whole number. From this I think we may infer that climate exercises an immense differenc in this disease; and doubtless the same cause is, in regard to all other diseases, more powerful than we are generally aware of. How else can we explain the entire exemption of some countries from certain maladies? In India and Egypt phthisis is unknown.

I will take the opportunity of stating here, that I believe heart affections to be very uncommon associates with chronic rheumatism; nor do I think that this malady is apt to be *followed* by cardiac disease. In the cases above analysed it was constantly found that such of them as showed heart disease, had been preceded by rheumatic fever, and the heart affection could be traced to that period of acute disease. This is in conformity with the opinion, now, I believe, generally entertained—viz: that acute rheumatism is frequently accompanied by endocarditis, and without very vigorous measures, is apt to be succeeded by permanent disorganisation of the heart. I have seen this hold to the full extent admitted by Dr. Hope, though not perhaps to the degree maintained by Boullaud. In chronic rheumatism properly so called, heart disease is, in my opinion, a rare occurrence.

In speaking of acute rheumatism I would record here my experience that in patients *under the age of puberty* acute rheumatism seldom or never happens without most seriously involving the heart; and the younger the patient (I have known it occur at five years) the more certainly fatal is this heart affection. I have never seen a single subject in the above category who eventually shook off the heart affection and recovered. And, in addition to the ventricular hypertrophy and dilatation constantly present in these cases, as well as the valvular disease, I must mention a morbid appearance perhaps equally constant, and which I think has been overlooked by pathologists, or only casually if at all mentioned—viz: a tough, dense, false membrane lining the general interior of one or other of the dilated auricles, generally the left, obliterating the musculi pectinati almost entirely, and so converting the auricle into an uncontractile sac: thus furthering mitral regurgitation, and, by its undoubted effect of congesting the lungs and brain according to the auricle affected, mainly producing the frightful dyspnœa and brain symptoms which constitute the worst features of the malady.

Of what value is the nitrate of potash in large doses in *acute rheumatism?* I have had no experience of it myself in *acute* rheumatism, trusting as I have done to calomel, opium, Dover's powder, antimony, and, in the worst cases, bleeding; but my friend, Dr. Fenwick, of North Shields, who afforded me valuable assistance in preparing the first series of the above cases, when clinical clerk in this house some years ago, as did also Mr. Gibb, informs me that he has adopted it to a large extent in private practice in Shields, and has found it to answer in a remarkable manner. I would also refer you to Dr. Basham's cases of the acute form, and his treatment by the nitrate of potash in large doses—a paper read to the Royal Medical and Chirurgical Society of London, and published in the 'Medical Gazette,' Nov. 24, 1848. His success was great, the urine acquiring a high specific gravity, and the salt being detected in it. The specific gravity was raised to 1030 and 1040, which he thinks was owing to the nitrate, though Dr. C. B. Williams attributes it to the urea and the lithates which are by its agency made to be present in the urine. Dr. Basham states his belief that, owing to its agency in acute rheumatism, there is a certain degree of *exemption* from disease of the heart.

I will conclude this paper (already too long) by recording certain facts and deductions which have manifested themselves to me from the careful investigation I made of the above cases.

In nine cases out of those wherein no relief or only slight relief was obtained, there were either *purulent collections* somewhere, or the usual *common inflammations* which precede suppuration—such as testitis, obstinate conjunctivitis, erysipelas. Are we entitled to deduce from this the general therapeutic principle, that in chronic rheumatism, when it is in that aggravated form in which we have pus circulating in the blood, the treatment by nitrate of potash is not to be depended on, and must be relinquished for another?

Again, in 81 out of the 100, the cure was almost or altogether effected in 14 days by the nitrate of potash in large doses, and these were cases wherein, though severe, there was no suppuration, nor ordinary inflammation of particular organs. It has been before laid down that nitrate of potash acts primarily on the nervous system. May we not infer, then, that those 81 cases were cases in which the nervous system was alone at fault? And, from the two considerations taken together, may we not look at rheumatism as a disease composed of two varieties—viz., that in which its assaults are expended on the nervous system alone, and that other more severe one in which pus circulates in the blood? Various observations and reflections have led me to take this view of the subject. Rheumatism is

first a nervous and then a blood disease, and it maintains a distinct individuality in both these phases in a manner more singular than other complaints.   In what I call its nervous form
it is a kind of Harlequin inflammation, and less mischievous
than it seems.   A little energy will knock it out of the system:
if uncontrolled, it undergoes ·a transmutation, becomes grave,
enters the blood, and changes it, and walks into the heart itself,
the citadel of life.   At present we want a set of careful microscopic experiments on the blood in all the varied conditions of
rheumatism.   Last year, at my request, Mr. Gibb took for microscopic examination small portions of the blood of several
patients affected with different diseases.   In the blood of one
who had no trace of inflammatory disease of any kind we
found, to our surprise, numbers of pus globules.   In a few days
there was developed in this patient a severe erysipelas, which
finished by becoming phlegmonous.   Here, then, inflammatory
disease existed in the blood for a certain time without betray·
ing its presence, until at length its increase became such (*vires
acquirit eundo*) that nothing but an acute attack upon the skin
sufficed for its elimination.

3. In cases wherein *mercury* has been previously extensively
taken, and cases where there is syphilitic malady present in the
system, whether mercury has been taken or not, the nitrate of
potash is without power.   The remedy is the *hydriodate* of
potash.

4. In cases of general chronic rheumatism, in which *sciatica*
is the most painful feature, the nitrate of potash will banish the
complaint from the other parts, but will not avail against the
sciatica.   In this event, *arsenic*, where it is borne,·is the most
powerful remedy.

5. In cases wherein the symptoms are doubtful, being circumscribed though severe, and simulating such other common
inflammations as pleuritis, peritonitis, ordinary cerebral or·spinal
meningitis, and even spinal irritation and hysteria, the *state of
the tongue*, if it appear as if overlaid with a coat of deep or light
white paint, so constant in the rheumatic condition, will most
essentially guide the diagnosis.—[*Med. Gazette.*

On Hæmaturia.   By Dr. G. Owen Rees, F.R.S., &c.

[Blood may exist in the urine in different degrees; either in
such quantities as that the red globules colour the urine by
their quantity, or they may be so minute in quantity as to require the microscope for their detection, or the paler parts of
the blood may be present, requiring chemical means for their

detection. If it be effused in any quantity, the conditions of the various parts of the urinary apparatus must be considered. The treatment of the diseased conditions of these parts is so much within the province of the surgeon that Dr. Rees counsels physicians to remember this whenever hæmaturia cannot be satisfactorily explained on other grounds. There are one or two points to be noticed connected with the examination of urine containing blood. And first, with respect to the recognition of the blood corpuscles under the microscope.]

These bodies, as they float in urine, are seldom seen precisely as they appear in serum. They are thicker at their edges, and the colouring matter within them is paler. This condition is caused by the entrance of urine into the corpuscle—an effect which occurs in virtue of the law of endosmosis. The blood-corpuscle naturally contains within its membrane a fluid of the same specific gravity as the liquor sanguinis; and when therefore, it comes in contact with the urine, which is far below the specific gravity of the liquor sanguinis, endosmodic currents are immediately set up, an interchange takes place between the contents of the corpuscle and the urine without, and as the urine is of less specific gravity than the contents of the corpuscle, the interchange takes place in such manner that it enters the corpuscle in greater proportion than the contents pass out; and thus the body becomes distended.

I shall hereafter have occasion to allude to the presence of pus and mucus in the urine, together with blood, and to the importance of detecting them, inasmuch as we are thereby greatly assisted in all our diagnosis in certain obscure cases of hemorrhage; and I will therefore now describe the appearances presented by pus and mucus when so observed. Pus and mucous corpuscles are both larger than those of the blood: they are colourless, and variegated on their surface: whereas the blood corpuscle is smooth and of a light yellow colour. The pus corpuscle very closely resembles the mucous; but if carefully examined, we observe that it is dotted and granular rather than variegated on the surface, and of looser texture than the mucous corpuscle. The reactions of urine containing blood are easily appreciated; and there is but one source of fallacy to which it is necessary to direct your attention. This consists in a condition of urine which will seldom be present to confuse you, and I have not seen it more than twice. I allude to the brilliant red colour sometimes produced in urine by certain articles of diet. Many vegetable matters colour the urine of a fine amber colour; the pyrola and sumach possess this property in a marked degree. Sometimes this colour will nearly approach to red; and occasioaally, when beet-root has

been eaten, the colour observed in the urine is so completely that of blood, that it is impossible to discriminate without
having recourse to the use of reageants.   The distinction is
easily made, however.   If the urine be tested by the liquor potassæ, a dirty brownish precipitate is produced if the colour be
owing to blood ; but in the case of vegetable colouring matter,
the urine will become of a fine green tint.

When blood is present as a deposit in urine, in any quantity,
we may be-sure that albumen exists in solution ; and it is important that we should know, within certain limits, the corres-
-ponding degree to which we may expect the urine to be albuminous for any given quantity of red corpuscles which may
appear in it.   An approach to tolerable exactness may be
attained by practice and attention to this point ; and it is one
of great value in the diagnosis of urinary diseases.   When we
boil urine containing albumen, if it be acid, as is generally the
case, a precipitate is produced.   Now when blood is present,
you will be surprised how much of it is required to produce an
amount of albuminous precipitate such as characterises cases
of ordinary albuminuria.   Unless, indeed, the urine present the
appearance of being made up in very large proportions of blood,
the amount of albumen will generally be trivial.   This will
not appear extraordinary to those who are in the habit of observing how much show a little blood can make ; and the quantity of albumen in the urine of morbus Brightii may well appear
comparatively great, when it often amounts to as much as indicates the disintegration of several ounces of blood per diem ;
and one ounce of blood will make a great show in the quantity
of urine passed in twenty-four hours.   The importance of paying attention, then, to this point, principally consists in our being
able occasionally to detect the morbus Brightii by showing an
amount of albumen in the urine far above that indicated by the
red corpuscles present.

Returning to the pathology of the subject, let us now assume
that careful examination of the bladder and prostate gland has
satisfactorily shown that the kidneys or ureters are the source
whence the blood contained in the urine must be derived, and
consider to what condition of those parts the hemorrhage should
be attributed.   First, as regards idiopathic hæmaturia.   This
bleeding from the surfaces of the kidney, without any special
cause beyond exposure to cold or to the vicissitudes of climate
in warm and damp localities, has been considered as rare by
most writers.   For my own part, it has so frequently occurred
to me to detect the cause of such hemorrhage in lesion of some
organ, that I am much inclined to deny hæmaturia ever occurs,
except as an indication of decided disease of the kidney or

other part of the urinary apparatus. It is true, idiopathic hæmaturia sometimes occurs, together with hemorrhage from other mucous surfaces, in those who ascend to great heights, and who consequently suffer the loss of that amount of atmospheric pressure which preserves the conditions of equilibrium necessary to the safe circulation of the blood; but we may at once exclude such cases as these from the consideration.

With respect to the appearance of the urine, Dr. Prout considered that, when blood tinctured the whole fluid, appearing equally dissolved throughout it, that the kidneys were generally involved. This is an observation which experience certainly verifies. When such an appearance is observed, however, it co-exists or alternates generally with blood as a deposit, and we may conclude that there is calculus in the kidney, or that the organ is the subject of other diseased condition, attended either with great congestion, granular deposit, or malignant disease. The detection of the real state of matters becomes very important in such cases. The symptom is a prominent one, and the patient's friends are sure to press the practitioner urgently for his prognosis. Now, though in most cases, if calculus be present, the history or severity of symptoms will assist us at once to the truth, yet it sometimes happens that such evidence is not afforded; and this is more especially the case when oxalate of lime calculi are contained in the kidneys. Under these conditions the urine may be bloody, and no other symptoms observed beyond dull lumbar pains. If oxalate of lime crystals exist in the urine, there is also pain in the penis, which does not affect the glans penis, as in stone in the bladder; but, on the contrary, is most plainly felt at the root of the organ.

Now, though in these cases the hemorrhage will generally follow upon some unwonted exertion, still it is not always so, and the case is thus greatly obscured; for we lose a most important adjuvant to our diagnosis. If the hemorrhage is the result of any of those chronic states of disease to which the name "morbus Brightii" has been given, we may easily detect that it is so, for then the hemorrhage which may occur will soon be found to give place to other conditions, in which the colourless matters of the blood alone become effused. We have here only to wait; and, whenever the urine may be excreted of its natural colour, to test it for the presence of albumen; and if this principle then be present in any quantity, without the colouring matter of the blood, we may be nearly certain that the further progress of the case will be marked by the continued exertion of natural coloured urine containing albumen, and not by hemorrhage, and that the patient is suffering from some form of the morbus Brightii.

If, however, the urine, on becoming of its natural colour after an attack of hæmaturia, does not prove to contain albumen, then we may feel nearly sure that the hemorrhage proceeded either from a calculus in the kidney, or some malignant disease of the organ.

The diagnosis between these two conditions must depend on the observation of the following points :—

1st. In malignant disease the blood is generally passed in larger quantity than in calculus of the kidney.

2ndly. There is more frequent tendency to nausea *on slight occasion* than in calculous disease.

3rdly. Microscopic examination of the urine will frequently show pus or mucus in excess, if there be calculus ; whereas, in malignant disease, this sign does not so frequently exist.

4th. The appearance of those suffering from malignant disease of the kidney, is nearly always indicative of a state of anæmia more or less advanced.

5thly. In calculus, hæmaturia generally follows upon some unwonted exertion.

6thly. Careful examination of the abdomen will frequently lead to the detection of tumour if there be malignant disease of the kidney.

To sum up, I should say, in the first place exclude from the consideration, cases of what has been called idiopathic hæmaturia, which can scarcely exist under ordinary barometrical conditions ; secondly, determine that the case does not belong to the morbus Brightii, by ascertaining that when the red particles cease to appear the albumen also leaves the urine ; and, thirdly, when the hemorrhage observed is placed within these limits, determine whether it be owing to calculus in the kidney, or to malignant disease, by especial attention to the following points :—The appearance and complexion of the patient; the presence or absence of nausea on slight occasion ; the presence or absence of pus and mucus in the urine mixed with blood corpuscles ; and, lastly, by careful exploration of the abdomen for the detection of tumour.

Now as regards the treatment of the two forms of hæmaturia I have been speaking of,—viz : that produced by calculus in the kidney, and that which is the consequence of malignant disease.

From what I have already brought before you with respect to the treatment of alkaline urine, as produced by irritation of the urinary mucous surface, you will at once perceive that the condition brought about by the existence of a calculus can never be benefitted by the exhibition of other than demulcent and alkaline remedies. It matters not how the calculus may

be composed,—be it uric acid, oxalate of lime, or phosphatic,—
be it soluble in acids or alkalies,—we cannot treat it chemically
while in the kidney. Our object must be to render the urine
as unirritating to the mucous membrane as possible, and enable
that membrane thus to bear the presence of the calculus with
as little inconvenience as possible. There is another indication,
however, which we answer by this alkaline and demulcent plan,
and a most important one. It consist in the relaxation of the
spasm of the canal. By effecting this, a small calculus may be
often brought away, which otherwise might remain to increase,
and perhaps destroy the patient. It is with this view that we
should combine our demulcent and alkaline remedies with such
sedatives as the patient can bear without disturbance of stomach. Our most favourable result, of course, will be the expulsion of the calculus. Next to this we must hope that it will
become encysted, and, by being so fixed in the kidney, cease
to cause irritation ; while we have to fear, as the worst result,
the setting up of inflammatory action in the body of the kidney.
This may terminate in the effusion of lymph in the tissue of
the organ, and in a subsequent contraction of the inflamed
part ; and sometimes the patient may be so fortunate under
these circumstances as to have the calculus which has caused
the acute nephritis should it be a small one, impacted in .the
kidney, so as to create no further irritation. In a great many
of these cases, however, the acute nephritis terminates in suppurative disease ; and if there be any constitutional imperfection dependent on strumous or syphilitic taint, this is the way
in which we may generally expect the case to end. All we
can do under these circumstances is to support our patient,
exhibit opiates, and render the renal secretion as unirritating
as possible. It is absolutely necessary that such persons should
avoid exercise in any way beyond that necessary to walking
gently, or exercise in any easy carriage. Neglect of this dou-
bles the danger to the patient, while the difficulty of enforcing
the injunction is often very great.

With respect to the treatment of cases in which the hæmaturia depends on malignant disease of the kidney, of course we
cannot proceed with any hope of cure ; but much may be done
by attention to the general health, and by relieving those symptoms which arise as the result of the hemorrhage and the impaired state of the chylopoietic viscera. The anæmia so often
noticed in these cases, which causes dyspnœa on slight exertion,
and restless nights (from the facility with which any error in
diet produces palpitation and throbbing of the carotids,) may
be to a great extent combated by the exhibition of iron in some
palatable form. Perhaps the best preparation for the purpose

is the tinctura ferri sesquichloridi, taken in doses of from ♏x. to ♏xx. three times a day, the bowels being watched the while, and kept regular by the exhibition of mild and aromatic laxative medicines.

It may be objected to the use of iron that it frequently tends to produce hemorrhage, and that we ought scarcely, therefore, to exhibit it; and it is quite true that care is necessary on this point. Watch the effects of the remedy, however, and you will constantly find you can exhibit it with advantage; that it will not induce hæmaturia, and especially if it be exhibited in the form of the sesquichloride of iron tincture. With regard to the use of styptics, they frequently appear useful in cases where the disease is not much advanced. One of the best I know, and which I have used several times of late, is the tannic acid, exhibited, if necessary, at intervals between the doses of iron in the form of pill. The dose should be from four to eight grains three times in the day. I may here remark, with respect to the use of this remedy, that, if you wish it should reach the stomach as tannic acid, you must not exhibit it in solution. You may, if you do so, have the good luck to give the first dose before it becomes changed; but tannic acid is rapidly converted into gallic acid when dissolved, and the best means of exhibiting it unchanged is in the form of pill.—[*Med. Gazette.*

On Nitric Acid in Hooping Cough and Asthma. By F. C. T. Arnoldi, M. D., Lecturer on Midwifery and Diseases of Women and Children, St. Lawrence School of Medicine, Montreal, &c., &c.

The few following remarks I take the liberty of communicating to the profession, through the pages of this excellent Journal, feeling perfectly confident they will be read with pleasure, inasmuch as they are somewhat novel as regards the alleviation of hitherto supposed intractable diseases, viz: hooping cough and asthma. The modus operandi of the remedy I will not at present attempt to explain, but from the results of my own practice and that of my medical confrères who have watched it and adopted it, I confidently recommend its application to all such as meet with similar cases. In hooping cough, at whatever age, whether it be a child at the breast, or a full grown adult, I administer nitric acid in solution, as strong as lemon juice, sweetened ad libitum. I had given to a child of two years of age, as much as one drachm and a half of concentrated nitric acid, in the above manner per diem, and I have never known the disease to resist its use beyond three weeks. In one instance, that of a child at the breast, only seven months

old, the disease disappeared within eight days. In another instance of a young lady fifteen years of age the paroxysms were
subdued within the first twenty-four hours, and the disease disappeared within ten days. Again, in the cases of two boys
about ten years of age living at a great distance from one
another, who had had the cough for several weeks, and to such
a violent degree, that both of them had the circumference of
their eyes ecchymosed as though they had been pummelled in
pugilistic combats, the acid acted positively like a miracle. A
medical confrère of mine had four of his children severely affected with the same disease in the middle of winter, and although
they had to be kept in-doors owing to the inclemency of the
weather, they were nevertheless all perfectly cured within three
weeks. I might go on to cite a hundred similar instances, but
these, I am satisfied, will prove sufficient to induce the profession to adopt this treatment. As regards asthma, the use of
nitric acid has proved not only in my own practice, but in that
of others who have adopted it, truly marvellous, and I trust
that the profession will remain satisfied by my quoting two
special cases. One is that of an elderly person, who had been
for five years a frequent inmate of the Montreal General Hospital, a thorough victim to this disease. He generally remained
under treatment the winter, and used to be discharged when
the disease seemed to have exhausted itself. This patient,
about eighteen months ago, was again admitted into the Hospital, under the care of my friend Dr. David, who, observing the
obstinacy of the paroxysms, resolved on trying the use of nitric
acid, the result was that the first night was passed tolerably ;
the second night he slept well ; the day after the third night he
reported himself perfectly convalescent, and on the fifth day he
was discharged at his own request, since which he has never
been heard of. The other case is that of a stout plethoric servant girl, about thirty-five years of age, who applied to me in
the early part of December last. She was then labouring under
very severe asthmatic distress, and told me that she had been
a martyr to repeated attacks, equally severe for four or five
years past; that she had consulted many medical men, but
could never obtain any relief, until, as she said, the disease had
spent itself. I gave her a prescription containing half an ounce
of concentrated nitric acid, and I have never seen her since,
but during the New Year holidays, happening to call at the
house where she served, I made enquiry about her, when I was
told, much to my merriment, that the reason why she never
came back to see me was that she thought that I had bewitched
her. She had often taken medicines which gave her no relief,
but that the very first night after taking the acid, she slept per-

fectly sound, and had not, up to that time, had any return of the symptoms. Now, these are obstinate facts, and I trust that this familiar method of communicating them will not diminish their value, nor need any of the profession to be too sceptical to follow the treatment.—[*Canada Med. Jour.*

Turpentine in Dysentery. By John Long, M. D., of Pleasant-ville, Kentucky.

For more than twelve months past, I have been in the habit of using Turpentine in the treatment of Dysentery, as it has occurred in this section of country, and find it to be a most valuable remedy in this often formidable disease. I have employed it in cases where the irritation or inflammation seem-ed to be confined to the lower portion of the bowels, as well as such as were complicated with typhoid fever. Dose, ten drops of the turpentine combined with twenty drops of lauda-num, for an adult every eight hours—with mucilagenous drinks and farinaceous diet. In obstinate cases it is necessary, in con-junction with the above, to resort to the ordinary enemata of laudanum and starch. Other remedies, as mercury, quinine or astringents, may also be used as circumstances require.

I was first induced to resort to turpentine in the treatment of dysentery, at the suggestion of Dr. Wood of Philadelphia, who recommends it in typhoid fever.

During the past summer, I treated thirty cases according to the above method, twenty-nine of which recovered and one died; the latter resided fifteen miles off, and I did not see him but once.—[*St. Louis Med. and Sur. Journal.*

On the remedial virtues of Nitrate of Silver in Chronic Diar-rhœa. By Professor A. H. Cenas, M. D.

. On taking charge of the Obstetrical department of Charity Hospital in November last, I found in the wards several chil-dren, between the ages of two and four years, laboring under Chronic Diarrhœa.

As they had been treated in the usual manner, viz: with astringents, absorbents, opiates, etc., etc., without success, I resolved to try the efficacy of Nitrate of Silver in solution and by the mouth. The good effects of the remedy are shown in the following cases.

Case I. This child, a girl, aged about two years, came un-der notice 6th November, she had been laboring under diarrhœa for nearly two months, and was very much emaciated, anemic and ulcerations in the lower extremity. Bowels were moved about twenty times in the course of twenty-four hours and the discharges were thin, glairy and greenish, and voided with considerable tormina.

> ℞. Nt. Argent Chrys. gr i.
> Mucilag Acac, oz. iss.

Ordered a tea-spoonful of this solution to be given after each stool. Diet, chicken broth; drink, toast water.

Nov. 7. Decidedly better, discharges from bowels reduced to twelve in twenty-four hours; less tormina, but stool of the same character. ℞. cont. treat. and diet.

Nov. 8. Improving rapidly, only eight stools in last twenty-four hours, no tormina, stools of better color and constitution, child more sprightly, complexion improving. R. cont. treat. and diet.

Nov. 9. From this date until the 15th improvement progressive, medicine gradually withdrawn and child discharged well on the 16th.

CASE II. The child, also a girl, and aged about two years, had been ill about two weeks; condition and symptoms pretty much as above; not, however, so many discharges from bowels, being, as well as nurse could ascertain, about fourteen or fifteen in twenty-four hours. R. Nit. Argent., as in the preceeding case, with entire relief in four or five days.

CASE III. This case, a boy, nearly four years old, had been laboring under diarrhœa for more than two months, was very much reduced in flesh, and so debilitated as not to be able to rise from bed; about fifteen stools in twenty-four hours, which were serous and almost inodorous, but acid, excoriating the anus and neighboring parts.

R. Nit. Argent, as above, chicken tea, drink, toast water.

Nov. 21. A shade better; passages not quite so frequent; nurse thought only two or three less than before medicine; child expresses himself as much easier. R. cont. treat. and diet.

Nov. 22. Decidedly better, only eight stools since last visit, which were of better color, and constitution otherwise improved, disposed to set up. R. cont. treat.

Nov. 23. Still improving; only four evacuations in last twenty-four hours, and these were fecal in constitution and odorous; appetite improving, strength returning. From this date he continued to improve, getting out of bed for a few hours daily and was finally discharged on the 28th.

CASE IV. Nov. 24. Also a boy aged about three years; this child had been laboring under lienteric diarrhœa for several months, with tumid abdomen and enlarged mesenteric and cervical glands. Highly unfavorable symptoms, indicating an advanced degree of marasmus and scrofula.

Thus this case was decidedly unfavorable, and I had no expectation of affording relief; still, as the diarrhœa was incessant, everything the child drank running through him, I ventured on the solution, giving him the usual dose and in the usual manner. Without detailing the case from day to day, I will state that for the first few days it acted like a charm, reducing the number of evacuations from more than twenty daily to only two or three, and otherwise so greatly improving the little patient that I began to hope for something permanent ; when, however, on the fifth day of the treatment, the efficacy of the remedy failed and the little patient fell rapidly back to his first condition, in which he lingered for a few days longer.

Case V. Occurred in female practice : the patient a little girl aged about fourteen months, had been labouring under choleriform diarrhœa for nearly three days before I saw her. I found her, April 3d, pale, cold, and with a frequent pulse, and having about twenty thin serous and fetid evacuations in the twenty-four hours. I commenced the treatment of the child by a few of the ordinary remedies, and continued them for nearly twenty-four hours, when perceiving no amendment, I resorted to sol. of Nit. Silver as in the above cases, with the satisfaction of restoring my little patient in the course of forty-eight hours.

I could enumerate other cases, but I think the above sufficient to show the advantages of Nit. Silver exhibited in the manner indicated, viz : in solution and by the mouth. I have used the agent before under similar circumstances per anum, but with indifferent success. This was principally owing to the inability on the part of the infant of retaining the enemata, or it may be to the want of precaution of the nurse in administering it. By the mouth these objections vanish, the medicine being tasteless, and any mother or nurse can properly administer it.—[*New Orleans Med. Register.*

Suppositories. By A. B. Taylor.

As our National Dispensatory gives no account of this valuable class of medicinal applications, (*suppositoria*) a brief notice of their preparation, in the "American Journal of Pharmacy," will perhaps be serviceable to some of its readers. Though hitherto but little employed in this country, suppositories have long been extensively used in France. They have recently, however, attracted the attention of some of our physicians, and bid fair to grow into much more general demand.

They may be described as medicated compounds of a stiff consistence, designed to be introduced into the rectum, and serving the purposes of the ordinary clysters or injections:

(*Enemata.*) They are applicable in all cases of constipation, or of irritability, or inflammation of the lower intestines; and have the advantage over liquid injections of more easy intro- duction, as well as of greater comfort and cleanliness; and they may sometimes be retained, when liquors would not. There is, perhaps, no substance so well adapted to serve as the vehicle of these applications as the butter of cocoa, (*oleum cacao*,) as no combinations of suet, spermaceti, or wax, &c., combine in so great a degree the proper hardness or firmness of substance, with the requisite fusibility.

The following formula, is a prescription of Dr. S. W. Mitch- ell and has been considerably used.

Take of Cocoa Butter, ℥ iss.
        Powdered Opium, gr. xii.
Mix and make into twelve suppositories.

The butter of cocoa is to be melted by a gentle heat. The opium is then to be well rubbed up with a small quantity of the fluid, until thoroughly incorporated, and the remainder of the melted butter gradually added. When cool and slightly thick- ened, the mass, being well stirred, should then be poured into paper cones. * If the cocoa butter is too fluid when transferred to the moulds, the opium will settle to the apex of the cone, and not be properly diffused through the substance. When perfect- ly hard these cones should then be pared or scraped at the base, until they weigh just one drachm,—giving one grain of opium to each suppository. Practically, therefore, it will be necessa- ry to make one less than the required number,—reserving the parings for another operation.

The following formula has been prescribed by Dr. Pancoast:

Take of Cocoa Butter, ℥ i.
        Extract of Krameria, ℈ ii.
        Powdered Opium, gr. v.
Mix and make into ten suppositories, as above.

It is stated that cocoa butter is much esteemed in France, for its supposed healing qualities, and is a favorite application in cases of piles. With powdered galls, or tannic acid, this sub- stance would therefore probably form a useful substitute for the ordinary pile ointment. The proportions to be employed, would of course be regulated entirely by the physician's order.

In DORVAULT'S French work on "Practical Pharmacy," sup- positories are described as varying from the size of the little finger, to that of the thumb; and weighing, from ℥ i¼ to ℥ ii½; (five to ten *grammes*.) The author gives as a formula for the

---

* These moulds should be made of sized or writing paper, and may be con- veniently placed in shallow boxes of sand, to preserve their position.

vehicle, butter of cocoa melted with an eighth part, by weight, of white wax : or as an inferior substitute, and one less used, common tallow mixed with the same proportion of wax.   Soap suppositories are formed by simply cutting soap into convenient shapes.   Suppositories are also prepared from honey, by boiling down this substance till it becomes sufficiently hard to retain its shape.   There are also formulæ given for anthelmintic, anti-hemorrhoidal, astringent, emmenagogue, laxative, and vaginal suppositories ; as well as belladonna, calomel, cicuta, mercurial, and quinine suppositories.

In Gray's "Supplement to the Pharmacopœia," there is given the following formula for a suppository ; taken from the *Codex Medic. Hamberg*, 1845.

℞. Aloes,	ʒ vi.
Common Salt,	℥ iss.
Spanish Soap,	℥ iss.
Starch,	℥ viii.

Mix and make into a mass with honey, and then form into cones of the required size.—[*American Jour. of Pharmacy.*

Charcoal Cushions for Deodorization.

A. S———, a patient under my care in the Hackney Union Infirmary, has for some time "passed every thing under her," and thereby become a nuisance and cause of complaint to the other patients in the ward.   Eleven days ago, I adopted the plan of placing beneath her a calico bag two feet square, partly filled with Irish peat-charcoal, so as to form a sort of a cushion and absorbing medium.   It has had the happy effect—which continues even now, without any necessity for changing the charcoal—of completely neutralizing all unpleasant odor ; and if the bed becomes partly wet all the offensive ingredients are absorbed and neutralized by the charcoal, which thus is a most simple means of remedying a great nuisance, and one that requires the most strict attention at best to prevent ; and that attention is often difficult and always expensive to procure.   In cases of incontinence of urine particularly, and indeed all attended with fœtid discharges, cancer, compound fractures, &c., this plan or some modification of it might be adopted with advantage.   I have been informed that some of the same material has been placed in the urinals of the South-Western Railway, with equally good results, in the prevention of unpleasant odor ; and that even after it had been unchanged for some weeks, the fluid that percolates has been found, by chemical analysis, to contain little or no trace of the organic or saline products of urine.   The fact induced me to try it as above.   An argument in favor of its adoption in hospitals and lunatic asylums is, that the peat, after its deodorizing properties are exhausted, becomes more valuable for the purpose of manure, so that its use is without expense —[*Boston Med. and Surg. Journal, from Mr. Howell in London Lancet and Dublin Medical Press.*

Nævus of the Scalp treated by Tartar Emetic.

Anne Shellard, aged nine months, was admitted into the Queen's Hospital, under the care of Mr. Sands Cox, February, 1851, on account of a nævus situated over the right parietal bone, about the size of a half-crown piece. The mother stated that a slight discoloration of the scalp was observed at birth; that it remained stationary for some time, but eventually began to increase, and had during the last two months attained its present size. There was no pulsation evident in the tumor, which was of a bluish cast, and slightly raised above the adjoining integument. The child's general health was good, and all the functions regular; but a branch of the temporal artery was enlarged, and could be traced almost into the diseased parts. On the third day after admission, Mr. Sands Cox ordered the potassio-tartrate of antimony to be applied, which was accordingly done. In two days, the application having been several times repeated, the whole of the discolored portion was converted into a pustular mass, and this with but little or no inflammation or irritation of the scalp. Poultices were now applied, and in the course of a week there was a healthy granulating surface, which cicatrized entirely three weeks afterwards. The patient left the hospital without any appearance of returning disease, and some time after continued quite well.—[*Prov. Med. and Surg. Journal.*

Case of a Large Subcutaneous Nævus cured by Vaccination. By John Woolcott, Esq., M. R. C. S., Surgeon to the Kent Ophthalmic Hospital,

A lady brought to me her infant, a healthy-looking child, nine weeks old, in January, 1848, with an extensive subcutaneous nævus which had existed from birth. The tumor, which was of a blue, livid colour, occupied the whole of the upper eyelid and a small portion of the root of the nose on the right side, and extended upwards upon the brow and forehead as high as the upper border of the orbicularis palpebrarum muscle; outwards and downwards it reached nearly to the tragus of the right ear, and then extended upwards and inwards along the lower margin of the zygomatic process of the temporal bone to the external angle of the orbit, where it joined the morbid product at the upper eyelid ; there was no pulsation in the tumor ; it was soft and compressible, and increased greatly when the child cried, and it then assumed a dark purple color ; pressure on the temporal arteries did not diminish its bulk. The application of ligatures in this case was of course inadmissible on account of the deformity which would arise from cicatrization of the wound causing ectropium. The treatment for the first month consisted in the application of tincture of iodine ; the abnormal growth being freely punctured all over with a fine cataract needle, and the iodine applied over the punctures. The bleeding was considerable, and of arterial character, but it soon subsided on the application of the iodine. These punctures were made twice a week, but the iodine applied daily, except when it caused too great irritation and soreness of the skin, when it was discontinued for a day or two, and then resumed. At the end of the month, the disease remaining unidminished, I altered the treatment and applied vaccine lymph: with a lancet armed with the matter, punctures were made at short intervals all around the circumference of the tumor, and several points in the centre of it ; to insure its taking, I inserted into each puncture a bone-point, also well armed with vaccine lymph ; most of these punctures took, and the irritation they caused was considerable, the child's face and head being swollen enormously. This was attended with fever and much constitutional disturbance, but at the end of a fortnight it had somewhat abated, and at the end of a month the disease was evidently decreasing ; and at the expiration of six months from the vaccine lymph having been used, not the least swelling existed, and the skin was assuming its natural color. I saw the child the beginning of January, 1852, and not a vestige of the morbid structure remains ; and it was only by looking closely for the vaccination scars, that I could tell on which side the nævus had been. I have treated several cases in the same way at the Kent Ophthalmic Hospital, and have succeeded in arresting their growth, but I have never seen so large an erectile tumor cured by this treatment, nor can I remember to have read of any such case. The color of this vascular tumor was venous, the bleeding was arterial.—[*London Lancet.*

Novel Treatment of Aneurism.

We have been much interested during the last few weeks in watching the progress of a case of aneurism of the subclavian artery, under the care of Mr. Fergusson, in which a novel and ingenious method of treatment has been adopted. In imitation

of an occurrence which occasionally happeus by accident in
cases of aneurism, viz., displacement of the mass of fibrine, or a
portion of it, which is usually present in such tumours, whereby,
in consequence of alteration in the current of the blood, a spontaneous cure results, Mr. Fergusson has, by manipulation of the
tumour, thrown loose a portion of the fibrine in the case alluded
to, with the effect of instantaneously arresting all pulsation in
the upper limb. In four days a feeble pulsation at the wrist
could be detected, but the axillary has been pulseless since.
The tumour itself, which was at first about the size of a small
hen's egg, has diminished considerably, and the throbbing within is now little greater than in the subclavian artery of the opposite side, while it has become more solid to the touch.   To
those familiar with the pathology and treatment of aneurism,
and especially the fatal results which have hitherto followed all
attempts at cure by operation on the subclavian on the tracheal
side of the scaleni muscles, we need hardly point out the interesting character of the case now under Mr. Fergusson's care.
[*Medical Times and Gazette.*

*Treatment of Ununited Fracture by the Application of Tinc-
ture of Iodine.* By Professor BLASIUS.

Professor Blasius communicated, in 1847, an account of the
success he had obtained in the external application of iodine in
pseudarthrosis; and in the present paper he furnishes three
other cases.   The first was a healthy soldier, aged 28, who had
suffered a simple fracture of the tibia and fibula.   The ends of
the bones had continued moveable for six months, when the
following tincture was ordered to be applied externally, night
and morning:— ℞ Iodin. Əj, Iod. Pot. 3½, S. V. R. ℥j. In three
weeks the callus was completely consolidated.   In the second
case, the fragments of a fractured femur (occurring in a soldier,
aged 25) remained movable after thirteen weeks; but became
quite firm after three weeks' pencilling with the iodine.   The
third case, occurring in a boy 12 years of age, was equally remarkable.—[*Med. Zeitung.   Med. Chir. Rev.*

On Foreign Bodies in the Air-Passages. By M. JOBERT.

The following is a summary of the principal conclusions with
which M. Jobert terminates a series of papers founded on clinical and experimental observation.
1.   Foreign bodies tend especially to lodge in the right lung,
owing to the direction and dimension of the bronchus of that
side. 2.   They penetrate when the *cordæ vocales* are most

widely separated, and a strong column of air rushes into the trachea, as occurs during the rapid inspirations and expirations in the action of laughing.   3. They traverse the superior aperture of the larynx without raising the epiglottis, which is never closed down upon this, as has been stated.   4. The epiglottis is always raised by virtue of its own elasticity ; and its chief office seems to be to direct the passage of certain articles of food, as along a gutter, during deglutition. 5. The bodies traverse the air-passages rapidly, by reason of the laws of gravity, the impulse of the column of air, and their own nature.   6. They are only temporarily arrested at any particular point, and may change their place, until they have excited the inflammatory process which enables them to hollow out a receptacle, in which they become lodged.   7. A peculiar sound is engendered by their presence ; and the bronchial secretion is always increased, and may become sanguinolent.   8. A louder respiratory sound, and a more extended vesicular murmur, is heard on the *opposite* side, than on the side in which the body is placed.   9. Foreign bodies whose size exceeds four lines in all directions, cannot be expelled by the sole efforts of nature, which are only efficacious in the case of very small ones.   10. In dogs, on the other hand, in whom the glottis is on a level with the upper aperture of the larynx, the expulsion of foreign bodies easily takes place, by reason of the dilatability and dimensions of the aperture.   11. In the dead body, foreign bodies pass the glottis with difficulty, even when aided by the impulse derived from a considerable column of air.   12. In the living body, they have to overcome, not only this passive resistance, but the very active resistance of the constrictor muscles of the glottis.   13. It is only quite exceptionally that the operation of tracheotomy can be dispensed with ; and it should be resorted to as early as possible, in order to prevent inflammation, local changes, and rapid or slow asphyxia.   14. It is a delicate operation, which should be performed by the successive division of all the tissues, and not by an incision comprising all or the greater part of the soft parts of the region at once.   This is the best means of preventing hæmorrhage, the introduction of air into the veins, lesion of the thyroid body, &c.   15. The trachea should be as widely opened as possible, so as to facilitate the escape of the foreign body.   16. We can only be certain that the trachea has been opened, when the air escapes with its characteristic sound.   17. When the foreign body does not issue on the opening being made, we must wait awhile, and excite the sensibility of the trachea by the introduction of a blunt body, so as to cause cough and expulsive efforts.   18. The trachea must be more largely opened, when a foreign body of a nature to swell from moisture has been long retained. 19. Re-union may be obtained by the primary or secondary intention. 20. The union by primary intention may be obtained by simple compression, or by the interrupted suture, this only implicating the *dartroid lamella* that surrounds the trachea. 21. Agglutination may be produced by another procedure, which consists in traversing the walls of the trachea entirely, or in part, leaving the sutures hanging externally, these coming away from the fourth to the thirteenth day. 22. A plastic production serves as the means of union between the lips of the wound. 23. Cicatrization only takes place by means of an intermediate production, and not by the direct fusion of the lips of the trachea. 24. The suture comprising the thickness of the walls of the trachea, may excite inflammatory action both within and without the canal, and give rise to organized fistulæ and encysted abscesses. 25. The suture which only implicates the covering, or a portion of the thickness of the trachea, only induces a plastic inflammation, and is to be preferred.—[*L'Union Medicale. Ibid.*

On the Employment of Tracheotomy in Croup. By M. TROUSSEAU.

In the present series of papers M. Trousseau relates the cases in which he has most recently performed tracheotomy for croup. Adverting to his entire experience upon the subject, he states that he has performed this operation altogether 169 times (11 for chronic disease of the larynx, and 158 for croup;) and that 43 of these cases, or a little more than a fourth, have recovered. Among his last 18 cases, however, there have been 8 recoveries, or nearly one-half. The results obtained at the *Hopital des Enfans* have not been less satisfactory of late; for of 19 cases operated upon, between January and August, 1851, one-half have recovered, and M. Guersant has been as successful in his private practice. M. Trousseau believes that one reason of the greater success in later years is, that now the principles of treatment in these cases are better understood; the children are brought to the hospital in a less exhausted state, their powers not having been lowered by the application of leeches and blisters, heretofore so common. Still more importance, however, does he attach to the modifications he has made in the treatment after opening the trachea. Thus, he has discontinued the application of a strong solution of nitrate of silver to the trachea and bronchi, which he used formerly to insist upon. He now too employs a double canula, so that the inner one may be taken out and cleaned when necessary, without disturbing the other ; and after the wound is dressed he covers all the parts over with a cravat, and thus avoids the difficult expectoration and desiccation of the mucus which occurred when they used to be left exposed.—[*L'Union Medicale.   Ibid.*

On the Gradual Reduction of Herniæ long irreducible.   By M. MALGAIGNE.

In this article M. Malgaigne brings forward two new examples of the efficacy of his plan of reducing old and voluminous herniæ.   This consists in subjecting the patient to a very low diet and purgation, applying ice or cold poultices to the tumour and employing the taxis daily.   One of these cases was an enormous inguinal enterocele, which had remained unreduced for several years, and now equalled in circumference the size of an ordinary hat.   Complete reduction was obtained after continuing the above means for 17 days.   The other was an inguinal entero-epiplocele, which had remained unreduced for 7 years, and was reduced completely in 6 days.—[*Rev. Med. Chir.   Ibid.*

Miscellany.

Anonymous Writers and Personalities.—We took occasion in our May number to animadvert upon the evil of Scientific Journals "allowing their pages to be prostituted by anonymous writers to the grossest personalities and misrepresentations."   We stated, in reference to certain of the objectionable articles, that "their style and general bearing show them to be all written by the same pen, and to have been indited in Georgia."   We mentioned the name of no person in connection with the matter, nor did we indicate the vehicle of such improprieties, preferring to leave both authors and publishers to appropriate whatever they might deem justly applicable to themselves. Of course none would complain but those who found the "cap to fit them."

Since then, we perceive that a Journal published near the frontiers of Canada, is again filled with scurrilities such as could not be surpassed by anything emanating from Billingsgate—a large portion of which is evidently from the same unworthy source as the articles to which we formerly referred.   We understand that this publication has been extensively circulated in this State by being sent to physicians who have not subscribed to it, and who probably never heard of it before. What relates to ourselves, individually, is too palpably malicious and contemptible to provoke any reply; and the prosper-ous condition of the Southern Medical and Surgical Journal, whose long list of subscribers is continually receiving honorable acces-sions, is not to be jeopardized by the vain invectives of unscrupulous calumniators. We would, however, for the honor of the Medical Literature of our country, again appeal to the Editorial fraternity to discountenance such violations of decency and propriety.

Professorial Changes.—Dr. Thomas D. Mitchell has resigned the Chair of Theory and Practice in the Philadelphia College of Medicine.

Dr. John Bell has resigned the Chair of Theory and Practice in the Cincinnati Medical College, and returned to Philadelphia, in con-sequence of delicate health.

Dr. Van Buren has been appointed to the Chair of Anatomy in the University of New York—vacated by the death of Prof. Pattison.

Dr Worthington Hooker has accepted the Professorship of Theory and Practice of Medicine in Yale College, in place of the venerable Dr. Eli Ives, who takes the Chair of Materia Medica.

Dr. Mussey has resigned the Chair of Surgery in the Medical Col-lege of Ohio, and been replaced by Dr. H. W. Baxley. This school has the good fortune to have secured Dr. Daniel Drake in the Chair of Practice, and Dr. Jedediah Cobb in that of Anatomy,— these two gentlemen having left the University of Louisville.

Prof. Benj. W. Dudley has accepted the Chair of Surgery in the Kentucky School of Medicine (Louisville), in place of Prof. Flint, and Prof. Bullitt that of Practice, lately held by Dr. Annan.

BIBLIOGRAPHICAL.

Outlines of a Course of Lectures on the Materia Medica, designed for the use of Students. Delivered in the Medical College of the State of South Carolina, by HENRY R. FROST, M. D. Fourth Edition. Charleston, S. C. Steam-power Press of Walker & James. 1851. 8vo., pp. 384.

We have been favored by the author with a copy of his "Outlines of a Course of Lectures on the Materia Medica," which we think well adapted to the wants of the medical Student. The number of lectures which are daily crowded into the space of a few hours, ren-ders such abstracts of great value to the student, as it enables him, by an effort comparatively slight, to recall many important facts

which otherwise would probably be forgotten. On all the subjects of
which it treats, Prof. Frost's work furnishes all the most important
points, well arranged, and though briefly, yet clearly set forth. But
though we thus commend both the execution and plan of the work, it
must not be concealed that such works are very liable to be abused by
the idle, who manage to procure from them a smattering of the science barely sufficient to squeeze them through the green room.
Nevertheless, it would be unjust to deprive the industrious and ambitious student of such helps, because they are liable to abuse. To
such we cordially recommend the " Outlines." G.

Obstetrics : the Science and the Art. By Charles D. Meigs, M. D.,
   Prof. of Midwifery, &c. in Jefferson Medical College, at Philadel-
   phia, &c., &c. 2d Edition. Revised, with 131 Illustrations.
   Philadelphia: Blanchard & Lea. 1852.

This improved edition of the great work of the very popular Philadelphia professor will be welcomed by the profession as the matured
production of one whose large experience and love of knowledge
must command respect. Prof. Meigs has added much valuable matter to this edition and entirely re-written some of the most important
parts of the work. It affords us much pleasure to recommend this
American book.

Lectures on the Principles and Practice of Surgery. By Bransby
   B. Cooper, F. R. S., Senior Surgeon to Guy's Hospital, &c.
   Philadelphia : Blanchard & Lea. 1852.

This is an eminently practical work, by an eminently practical
surgeon. Although not the equal of Astley Cooper in some respects,
the author is generally regarded as a man of very sound discrimination and as an excellent practitioner. His Lectures constitute quite
a valuable addition to surgical literature and will be read with advantage by all who devote themselves to this department of practice.

*Outlines of the Nerves: with short descriptions. Designed for the
   use of Medical Students.* By John Neill, A.M., M.D., Surgeon to
   Will's Hospital. 2d Edition. Philadelphia : Ed. Barrington &
   Geo. D. Haswell. 1852.

This little work consists principally of plates intended to facilitate
the study of the nerves. The lithographs are, however, so badly
executed that we doubt that they can be of much use to one not already acquainted with the subject.

PHILADELPHIA, June 24, 1852.

Dear Sir :—The " TRANSACTIONS OF THE AMERICAN MEDICAL ASSOCIATION" at its Session of 1852, will, it is estimated, make a volume of nearly one thousand pages. Notwithstanding the increase in size, the Committe of Publication have not, however, considered it expedient to charge the members of the Association, and the several bodies represented therein, a greater price for the forthcoming volume than was paid by them for either of the four already published. They have resolved, therefore, to furnish to the members, and the institutions represented, one copy for three dollars, and two copies for five dollars; provided, the same amounts are remitted previously to the first day of September next ensuing ; after which period the price of the volume will be raised to five dollars.

The Committee of Publication would respectfully suggest the propriety of an early answer to this circular ; the funds in the hands of the Treasurer are insufficient to defray the expense of printing the volume of TRANSACTIONS, and until an additional sum of eleven hundred dollars is received, the Committee will not be warranted in putting it to press.   Respectfully yours,

D. FRANCIS CONDIE, *Treasurer.*

ERRATUM.—*Purgative Syrup of Jalap.*—In the formula for this syrup in the last number of the Journal at page 169 read "*jalap eight ounces*" instead of " *jalap an ounce.*"—[*Amer. Jour. of Phar.*

The above error was copied in our June number, page 381, and should therefore be corrected by the reader.—[ED. SOUTH. MED. AND SURG. JOURNAL.

Hydrargyri Iodium Rubrum.

NEW YORK, Feb. 10, 1852.

Editor of the American Journal of Pharmacy :—

Sir :—Under the article Hydrargyri Biniodidum, the U. S. Dispensatory gives as the dose 1-16th of a grain, gradually increased to grain 1-4th.

Under the same head, Christison's work, edited by Dr. Griffith, ed. 1848, gives the dose from gr. i. to gr. iv.

Has this great discrepancy been before detected, and the error corrected ?—[STUDENT.

[NOTE.—The profession will be obliged by the above hint. We had not observed the error before. Since communicating the fact to the Publishers, Messrs. Blanchard & Lea, they have informed us that the error has been corrected in the unsold portion of the edition. All who have the American edition of Christison should make the correction with pen at once, and all Medical Journals should notice it.—ED. AM. JOURN. PHARM.]

SOUTHERN
MEDICAL AND SURGICAL JOURNAL.

Vol. 8.]   NEW SERIES.—SEPTEMBER, 1852.   [No. 9.

PART FIRST.

Original Communications.

ARTICLE XXIX.

Veratrum Viride. Cases, by E. L'ROY ANTONY, M. D., of Burke county, Geo.

The novel articles from the pen of Dr. W. C. Norwood, of Cokesbury, So. Ca., upon the therapeutic virtues of this article, early and promptly arrested our attention. More recent ones, published with "cases" from every section of the country, attest the professional ardour in the pursuit for the discovery of an agent whose remedial action upon the living organism will produce effects corresponding to those triumphantly ascribed to the Tincture of the Root of the American Hellebore.

We believe its virtues may be mainly attributed to the veratrine contained in the tincture, which we are at this time administering as suitable cases are presented, the results whereof we will, after careful observation, give to the profession. Regularly digested articles have already furnished the profession with Botanical descriptions of the plant, and theories *ad libitum*, of its mode or *modes* of operation.

Individual professional experience is the property of our profession: upon this basis, we propose to record a few cases, illustrative of its adminstration, prophylactic and curative powers. If the results exhibit apparently paradoxical properties, we are in no wise responsible, but remain confident that

its heroic attributes will early win for Norwood historic im-
mortality, and for itself a partition of empire with the lancet
in the domain of Practical Medicine.

CASE I.   *Pneumonia, (typhoid type.)*—Mr. A. W., aged 30,
strumous habit, had been attacked on the 14th April, 1852, with
an indistinct chill, followed by remitting form of a low grade
of reaction, which lasted until the 18th.   Between 10 and 11
o'clock, on the night of the 19th, taken with rigors, upon which
developed a similar grade of reaction, as in the first attack,
accompanied with mucous cough, and free, glairy, uncoloured
expectoration of exceedingly tenaceous mucus, with large globules of air intimately mixed.   These pneumonic indications,
with corded frontal headache—dry, hot, harsh-feeling skin,
(calor mordax); great thirst, and sense of weakness; dry
tongue, brown in the centre; pulse 70, very small, quick and
corded; restlessness, anxiety, and some apprehension as to the
favorable termination of his case.

Under my usual (and somewhat peculiar) treatment, with
no material alleviation, and the supervention of brick-dust
colored sputa, he continued the same until the 27th, 9 o'clock,
A. M., at which time I found the same small, quick, corded
pulse, beating 100 per minute.

This being the first case of Pneumonia occurring in my
practice, after the reception of the tr. veratrum viride from the
hands of Dr. Norwood, I was sufficiently anxious to try it, but
the pulse being heretofore only 70 and 80, I hesitated, and
would not try the lancet, as it had failed to do good in his recent attack of fever; but this morning, the 28th, beginning to
equivocate, myself, as to the termination of his case, the 100
pulse being *tense* and *corded*, though small, I determined upon
its administration, and accordingly prepared—

  ℞. Tr. Verat. Virid. . .   96 gtt.
   Aq. Com. . . . . 12 coch. mag.
   Sacch. Alb. . . .   q. s. ft. M.

Ordered one-twelfth of the mixture every three hours, until
vomiting or purging supervened; in either event, tr. opii. 25
gtt., to be repeated in one and a half hours, and continue the
v. v. in half the quantity first ordered.

April 29th, 11, A. M.   Had vomited and purged, thrice each, between fourth and sixth portions; skin soft and cool, almost *cold;* tongue moist, with light mucous coat; pulse regular, decidedly *fuller,* soft and pleasant to the touch; coughed very seldom during the night; great improvement in the expectoration—says, "if I had taken that medicine at first I would have been well;" and, from the magical alteration in every feature of his case so speedily presented before me, I readily believed him.   Ordered, half table-spoonful (4 gtt. tr. v. v.) of the mixture every five hours—to double the dose if the pulse exceeded 70.

30th.   Passed the night finely; pulse 65, no cough, perfectly comfortable.   Ordered 4 gtt. doses tr. v. v. every six hours, for three doses; then eight hours for three doses, unless he gets worse.

31st.   Pulse 70, soft and pleasant; says he is doing sufficiently well.   Ordered 4 gtt. doses, every ten or twelve hours, for three days.   Discharged.

Case II.   *Acute Pleuro-Pneumony.*—April 28, 1852.   W. G.'s negro woman, Hannah, aged 30; well made, finely developed thorax; saw her at 1 o'clock, P. M.   *Symptoms:* severe frontal cephalalgia extending over the vertex; conjunctivæ injected; face tumid; breathing 36, incomplete and cautious, attended with audible expirations; pulse 130, full and bounding; bathed in profuse general sweat—in fine, general reaction of high synochal grade; sore pain occupying whole dorsal thorax; decubitus, supine; râle crepitant; harsh but moist cough, accompanied with slight pleuritic pain in dorsal pleura; expectoration tenaceous, viscid, yet tolerably frank and partially striated with arterial blood, but occasionally completely ensanguined; had been bled ℥ xx., and bowels thoroughly evacuated—ill two and a half days.   At this time, a large blister, recently applied, was removed from dorsal spine to give the tr. v. v. a fair field. Ordered: ℞. Tr. Verat. Vir.   .   .   96 gtt.

Aq. Com.   .   .   .   .   12 coch. mag.

Sacch. Alb.   .   .   .   q. s. ft.   M.

Dose, 1 coch. mag. tri-hourly until nausea, vomiting or purging supervened.

29th. Vastly better in every respect; pulse 60.

30th. Got up, saying she was as well as ever. Discharged. May 1st, still well.

CASE III. *Puerperal Convulsions before Labour.*—April 29th, 1852. Mrs. A. J. L., age 18: short, and full habit; leuco-phlegmatic temperament; first pregnancy advanced thirty-five weeks; severe cephalalgia for last six or seven days. This morning, at 6 o'clock, had two convulsions. At 10 or 11 o'clock, some one bled her—I dont know how much. By 4 o'clock, P. M., at which time I saw her, she had had ten or twelve violent convulsions: decubitus, flexed on left side; pulse 144, full and hard; profound coma; pupils dilated, but susceptible; pallor; globe of eyes very prominent; whole face and neck swollen; fingers and toes cool; body and head hot. At 4½ o'clock, ordered sinapisms to spine, cold to head, and enemata. Struggling against the indication for the lancet, in person, I attended the administration of 8 gtt. doses of tr. v. v. every three hours. ☞ At 7 o'clock, pulse 120; at 10, pulse 104, spoke incoherently; at 12, (pulse 98,) answering correctly in monosyllables; at 3 o'clock, pulse 75, perfectly conscious; at 5 o'clock, pulse 60, calm, collected, conscious and comfortable, except "I feel sore all over." At 6 o'clock, I left her for home—at 7 was re-called—arrived at 8; pulse 57; had vomited thrice and purged twice; universal surface cool and pleasant; regularly recurring "bearing down" labour pains—touch exhibited second position, crown of Baudeloque entering superior strait—the pains recurring with *perfect regularity.* Expulsion occurred at 10¾, A. M.; fœtus still-born. During uterine contraction, pulse 60—during intermission, 57, uterus contracting finely and firmly. At 11¾, removed placenta from vagina. Ordered ℥iss. ol. ricini, and pulse *to be kept* at 60, for I now believed that the number might be stated, and the pulse put down to it, and maintained there.

30th. General but not severe soreness; surface cool; intellect clear; no after pains; no abdominal tenderness whatever; lochia about right; pulse 65. Ordered 2 gtt. doses tr. v. v. every four or five hours, to be guarded by laudanum, as usual.

May 1st. Perfectly comfortable, except a sore tongue. Milk formed without general reaction. Discharged.

The subsidence of the pulse, the contemporaneous clearing up of the intellect and return of sensation, the accession of labour with the pulse at 57, its happy termination, the formation of milk with her habit, without general reaction—all, with the pulse *far* below its natural standard, present a relationship of cause and effect as striking as beautiful.

CASE IV. *Pneumonia, (typhoid type.)*—April 28th, 1852. B. C.'s female slave, Eliza, age 20, has been ill four days at 12 M. to-day. At this time, suffering with headache; breathing 36, incomplete and hurried; pulse 124, size of a knitting needle, somewhat tense and quick; skin *hot* and *dry;* decubitus mostly on the back and right side, but great restlessness; conjunctivæ icterode; tongue dry, dark and raspish; sordes on teeth; short, jerking cough; expectoration viscid, tenacious plum-juice mucus, frank with occasional sputal ejections of dark-colored nuclei enveloped in healthy-looking mucus; a profound "sore pain" persistent in the right middle lateral thoracic region, increased by pressure on abdomen, but slightly by pressure over the affected spot; crepitous rhonchus: dull sound on percussion over sore spot—had been freely purged on the first day with a black dose. Yesterday, 27th, took Ði. calomel, followed by four copious dark-colored dejecta. At this, my first visit, ordered—

  ℞. Tr. Verat. Virid. . . 96 gtt.
  Aq. Com. . . . . . 23 coch. min.
  Sacch. Alb. . . . . q. s.

Dose, 2 spoonfuls (each containing 4 gtt.) every three hours, until nausea, vomiting, or purging is produced, then 1 spoonful every three hours: if vomiting be obstinate, or more than two alvine dejections in any given three hours, and they be watery, 20 gtt. laudanum, and repeat *pro re nata.*

29th, 12 M. Vomited and purged, three or four times each, last night: is taking 1 spoonful, 4 gtts., tri-hourly; skin *cool* and soft, rather *oily* than moist; expression of countenance good; tongue soft, moist and natural; pulse 76, crow-quill, soft, uniform and compressible, no quickness; no sordes; breathing 20, complete and deliberate; no headache; no soreness at the seat of inflammation, except on abdominal pressure, and then but

slight; sputa collected on sand in a tin pan, so that a fair inspection is impracticable. Ordered, above continued in 4 gtt.
doses.

30th. Apparently well in every respect, except the pulse at
56. Discharged the patient, ordering 4 gtt. doses or 1 tea-
spoonful of the solution of the tincture every six, eight and
twelve hours, for three or four days.

Case V. *Pneumonia, complicated with Eutocia, Flatulent
Colic and Puerperal Peritonitis.*—May 2d, 1852. B. C.'s
slave, Susan, age 20, full habit—had been safely delivered this
morning, at 5 o'clock, of a still-born of 30 weeks: obstinate
constipation of six days; intense keen pains darting through
transverse and descending colon; sense of fulness in epigastrium and left hypochondrium; uterus mounted high in umbilical
region, and somewhat tender on pressure; lochia in abundance,
breasts sufficiently tumid, but not tender; sore, diffused pain in
the left lung; sensation of great weight under the sternum;
short cough, producing great pain in the belly and left side;
expectoration invariably swallowed, and could not be induced
to throw it out; pulse 136, moderately full and quick.

I saw her at 2 o'clock, and learned that these symptoms had
preceded and ushered in labour. Had been bled; quantity
unknown. Ordered, warm fomentations to abdomen; ½ gr.
sul. morphia and ℨi. tr. fœtida; also, ℥ij. ol. ricini to be repeated; warm water enemata, and mustard to entire spine.

May 3d, 5 o'clock, A. M. .Abdomen enormously distended
and exquisitely tender; uterus very tender to external and
internal touch; lochia completely suspended, breasts collapsed;
rigors, headache, no alvine evacuation, discharging large quantities of straw-colored urine; decubitus supine; legs flexed on
thighs and knees widely separated; arms extended, right and
left, at right angles with the body; original pain in the colon
still recognized by her as being present with greater sense of
fulness; countenance anxious; moist, soft and jerking cough;
sore pain in the thorax persistent; pulse 144, very quick, and
not so full as yesterday. V. S. ℥xl., repeated in one and a half
hours, ℥xx. (At this hour, learned she had eaten large quantities of red clay as a substitute for chalk or magnesia.) Intro-

duced 30 inch O'Beirne tube to the colon—met no obstruction, no escape of gas; then threw an enema of warm water and 1 coch. mag. spts. terebinth. into the colon, and repeated; desiring to stool, the tube was withdrawn, and she elevated at an angle of 45°, at which moment a voluminous gaseous eructation from the stomach occurred, continuing ineffectually to throw off more. I had the tube thoroughly cleansed, oiled and introduced into the stomach—a very slight escape of gas, attended with a syphonic discharge of O ij. of greenish colored water: gave O j. melted lard; stomach rejected it.

Knowing it would arrest the pulmonary, I *believed* it would moderate or arrest the intestinal and peritoneal congestion, and perhaps prevent effusion or gangrene. I ordered 10 gtt. doses of the tr. v. v. tri-hourly, until her pulse went to 60; also, 20 gtt. Labarraque's chlor. sod. in half tea-cup of warm water, every two or three hours; gave Ɗi. pil. hydrarg.; vaginal injections of warm water and tobacco enema pr. rect., with turpentine frictions to abdomen, and warm fomentations. Left her at 8½, pulse still 144, but smaller, with same quickness.

May 3d, 12 M., at night. Belly softer; pulse 120, not so quick; no evacuation: had not given the tincture regularly. Ordered epispast., 6 by 7, to abdomen, with 8 gtt. dose of tr. v. v. tri-hourly, *to be given regularly;* also, Ɗj. pil. hydrarg.

May 4th, 5, A. M. Pulse 74; had five or six copious thin slate-colored dejecta, with flocculi of the same, but more consistent; vesication; belly not half the size it had been; slight appearance of lochia; no headache; very little cough; some pulmonary pain; uterus still tender, but allows it handled with some freedom without complaint. Ordered, continuation of tr. v. v. in 6 gtt. doses tri-hourly; Labarraque's liquid 15 gtt. every four or five hours, and 25 gtt. tr. opii. off. Blister dressed with scalded fol. persica.

May 5th. No headache; tongue moist and pleasant, but great thirst; scarcely any cough, can make full inspiration without coughing, but still some thoracic soreness; occasional hiccough ever since yesterday morning; abdominal intumescence contiuue to subside; lochia same; general surface warmer than yesterday; still horizontal, with inferior extremities separated and flexed; pulse 112. (A new nurse having been in attendance the v. v. had been taken irregularly, and only in 2 gtt. doses.)   Two slate-colored dejecta, mixed with portions of red clay.   Suspended Labarraque's liquid, and ordered—℞. Pil. Hydrarg.; Rhei. P. R. *aa* ℈ss.; and continued tr. v. v. in 8 gtt. doses.

May 6th. With the exception of partial retention of urine and lumbar uneasiness, with slight strangury from absorption of cantharadin, she is better in every respect.   Pulse 90, no quickness, more volume.   Catheterism, with replacement of uterus, afforded instant relief.   Continued peach-leaf poultice to the blister, and tr. v. v. in 4 gtt. doses.

May 7th. Bowels moved twice last night, tolerably thin, but of uniform consistency; neither thoracic pain nor soreness; no cough; no colonic pain nor uneasiness; bladder acting finely; lochia in abundance; pulse 90, and skin soft and warm.   I think she will get well.

May 15th. I hear she is up and doing well.

CASE VI.   *Dystocia.*—May 3d, 1852. Mrs. J. M.'s negro woman Lucy.   Saw her at 1 o'clock, P. M., in a small, *close* ill-ventilated log-house, covered with a thick quilt and a blanket, thermometer 92°, a fire on the hearth, and some smoke pervading the room; face and body covered with a profuse active perspiration; carotids and pulse rapid and bounding at 172.   Had the fire extinguished, door unhinged, slats, with which the inside of the house was ceiled, ripped off the side opposite the door, substituted a sheet for the quilt and blanket, gave a light draught of cool water, and bathed her face and breast with some of the same.   In half hour pulse 160; expulsive throes every fifteen or twenty minutes; touch exhibited left arm and pulseless funis occupying pelvis proper in 2d position left arm presentation of Baudeloque; abdominal tenderness on pressure—had been bled freely, and I would have bled her again, but believing from recent experience that I held in my hand the great desideratum, the controller of capillary arterial and cardiac action, I risked her upon it.   The result, I apprehend, will at least speak well for its prophylactic powers.

At 1½ o'clock, gave ½ gr. morphine and 10 gtt. of tr. v. v., preparatory to turning; at 2¼, gave ¼ gr. morph.; at 3¼, gave

8 gtt. tr. v. v. ; at 4 o'clock, she, feeling the anodyne impression and pulse 140, I proceeded to fillet the presenting arm, and
"turn," which I did readily, bringing the feet down to the first
foot Baudeloque by 5½ o'clock ; at 6, removed placenta ; at
6½, pulse 104, surface quite cool.

Ordered, absolute diet ; mucilaginous drinks ; vaginal injections of warm milk and water *bis terve in diem;* soft oiled compress to vulva ; perfect rest, with shoulders slightly elevated ;
also,   ℞. Tr. Verat. Vir. . . 96 gtt.

             Aq. Com. . . . . 24 coch. mag.

             Sacch. Alb. . . . q. s. ft. M.

Dose, 2 coch. mag. tri-hourly, *regularly,* until vomiting or
purging ; in either event, tr. opii. 20 gtt., repeated *pro re nata.*

Dr. Milton Antony, the attending physician, was requested
to note particularly the effects of the tincture upon her pulse,
which I desired to be reduced to 60, and *kept* there for three
or four days, to *prevent,* if possible, the accession of any of
those fatal symptoms so frequently following the maneuvre in
such cases.

May 5th. Received the following from Dr. M. A.

"MAY 4, 1852. *Dear Sir :* I visited Mrs. Moore's Lucy
this afternoon, and found her pulse reduced to 72 to the minute.
She says she is in no pain at all, but complains of being very
sore when moved : she has had three evacuations to-day, one
while I was there, which was *watery ;* vomited several times also.
I ordered Mrs. M. to give the tr. opii., and lessen the dose of the
solution to half table-spoonful (2 gtt. tr. v. v.), as she had already, under your directions, lessened it to one (4 gtt. tr. v. v.)—
continue the mucilage and vaginal injections. She says she
feels much better. I think she is doing finely—much better
than I ever expected : she has a good appetite—wants to eat.
Mrs. M. will give the last dose to-night at 9 o'clock ; so, if you
wish her to continue it send more by the bearer."

I sent more, with a request to *put her pulse* at 60, and *keep*
it there. This last portion did not reach her until eighteen
hours after the first had given out, at which time there was
restlessness, with pulse at 125 ; the re-application of the tinct.
in 8 gtt. doses readily brought her pulse to 65, at which it was
kept for three days.

May 15th. Doing well, except slight soreness at vulva, with lumbar uneasiness.

I would have been pleased to comment lightly upon each of these cases, but the length of this article has already exceeded the limits anticipated.

ARTICLE XXX.

Farther Remarks on Mrs. Willard's Theory of the Circulation.
By Wm. T. Grant, M. D., of Culloden, Monroe county, Ga.

Since writing my last article in the May number of the Southern Medical and Surgical Journal, on this subject, I have been favored by the kindness of an acquaintance, with a copy of Mrs. Willard's small book, entitled "Willard on the circulation of the blood." After reading it, I was more than ever convinced of the fallacy of the position assumed by its authoress, in regard to the circulation.

Her position we will give in her own words: "Expansion is a motive power—the blood receives caloric at the lungs—the blood must therefore expand—if the blood expands it must move." We admit that expansion is a motive power (not under all circumstances, however),—we admit that the blood receives caloric or heat at the lungs, but, we *deny* that the blood expands in consequence thereof. We well know that there is a chemical process going on in the lungs at all times, and caloric is a production of all chemical processes; but the heat is not on that account the *primum mobile* of the blood. The reason is simply this: as soon as heat is disengaged by this chemical action, *it becomes latent immediately*, and cannot therefore produce an expansion of the particles of the blood. That this heat does become latent can be established on good authority,[*] and we deem it unnecessary to say more about it, but pass on to the consideration of some of Mrs. Willard's experiments.

The first experiment of any consequence (figure no. 1 of the above mentioned work) "may be formed by joining three glass tubes by india-rubber into a triangular form, and filling the apparatus with water." This contrivance was then suspended

---

[*] Comstock, Johnston, &c.

and heat applied to one of the sides, and the contained water began to circulate in the tube. By an inspection of the figure and the manner in which the heat was applied, any one can very quickly detect the fallacy. It will be observed that the heat was applied to a side that hung in an oblique direction, and as the air in the water expanded, as well also as the water itself, they began to move *upwards*, and of course began the circulation. If Mrs. Willard had applied the heat to the most elevated part of the tube, the water would never have moved. Besides, in this case the heat is free or uncombined and not latent as is the case in the circulation. This experiment therefore proves nothing.

In her next experiment, Mrs. Willard's object seems to be, to prove that the circulation cannot go on until the heart begins to beat; that is, the heart must begin to beat before the blood begins to circulate. And she proves that it matters not how much heat is applied to the blood in the lungs, yet, if the heart does not begin to beat, the blood will not circulate. Then we are to understand that the heart begins its motions first. If that be the case (and we do not doubt it,) what makes the *heart* move? Mrs. Willard does not and cannot say, and we have to stop in our researches, on this point, for proofs of the new theory.

(The reader would do well to examine Mrs. Willard's book, in connection with the above for a proper understanding of the case as we are confident we have not rendered it very intelligible.)

Having now merely glanced cursorily over these two experiments, we will proceed to relate some performed by ourself on the living animal. There can be no possible cheat or fallacy in them as they were performed on *animals—living animals*, in which Nature's immutable laws must take their course. We shall relate them from notes which we took down at the performance of each experiment.

Exp. I. Took a *toad* and making an incision into the breast, we extracted the sternum. After which we removed the liver. We cut out the sternum and liver, for the purpose of exposing the heart. Having bared that, by these operations, so that we could see it pulsate distinctly, we next cut out both lungs. Now we had the heart *fully* exposed, and had taken out the liver and both lungs. Notwithstanding which, the heart continued its pulsations and the blood its circulation. We let it stay thus an hour and a half or two hours, at the end of which time it still continued to beat. It would be well to state that it was becoming more and more feeble; this is easily explained,— firstly, being exposed to the air it was getting dry and stiff; secondly, the circulation was somewhat impeded by cutting out the liver and lungs, in which we necessarily cut the hepatic and pulmonary arteries; and thirdly, the toad was dying. We think that the roughness of the operation assisted in enfeebling the heart. It were probably well that we state that we pierced the brain of the toad with a small blade of our knife, before doing anything else.

Exp. II. In this case we did not wound the brain of the toad; but bared the heart as in case first, with as little injury to the contiguous parts as possible. In this case the heart beat more than three hours after the excision of the lungs.

Exp. III. In this case, to prevent deception in any way we cut out the whole of the respiratory apparatus, the trachea bronchial tubes, and lungs, and the heart continued its beating an hour and a half; it then became too feeble to pulsate, from the cause mentioned in case first.

Exp. IV. Wishing to remove *every* trace of a doubt as to the correctness of these experiments, we next took a toad, bared its heart as before, without excising the lungs however, and *put it under the receiver of an air-pump.* On pumping out the air, the heart *continued its pulsations.* It was remarked by an eminent gentleman, who saw the experiment performed, "how very tenacious the animal was of life."

Some may object to these experiments because they were performed on so lowly an animal; but we hold them as good as if they were performed on man himself, inasmuch as the toad has lungs, a heart, a circulatory system, and breathes air.

Having now stated these things, we wish to make a few re- marks upon them in connection with the general subject of the circulation. In all of the above experiments, the blood circu- lated as usual, impeded a little perhaps by local obstacles. Now then, the question arises—what causes it to circulate? It is very evident that heat did not do it, as the generator of heat, the air, was excluded. We will answer the question if we can. The cause is to be found in the system, and is galvanism. We can prove that the cause is in the system, but as yet we have to theorize as to its identity. Air is the medium of communication by which everything external produces effects on everything internal. By this we mean that the external things come in *material* contact with the external parts of the body by the air alone. I do not say that we cannot see without air, but I say that a particle of dust, for instance, cannot come in contact with the parietes of the air passages, without air. So then if we exclude air from the body, we exclude everything that is dependent upon the air for a conveyance. In the above experiments we excluded air from the *blood*. Consequently neither air nor any other external material thing did affect the motion of the blood. But the blood circulated; and we are therefore justified in saying that the *air* and other externals do not produce the circulation. Then we arrive at the statement made above, that the cause must be found *internally*. And as before stated that cause can be found in galvanism. There is an experiment, familiar with most chemists, that has some bearing on this point, and shows that a circulation may be carried on through tubes similar to the capillary vessels, by electricity. " We can cause water to flow in a stream through a tube, by running a stream of electricity through the tube with the water, when previously this only went through in drops." There are other things in support of this point that we would like to cite if space allowed, but we fear that we might intrude on the Journal, therefore we conclude by summing up the whole of this article in a few words, viz: we have proved that air is not the cause of the circulation, and that the cause is to be found in the system. And in the end we see that everything points directly to galvanism as being the primum mobile of the blood.

ARTICLE XXXI.

Remarks on the Treatment of Dysentery. By E. F. STARR, M. D., of Rome, Ga.

This being the season for dysentery, it may be allowable to make a few remarks upon its pathology and treatment.

My only apology for this intrusion is that an astonishing number of deaths from this disease occurs all over the country, seeming to justify a repetition of the opprobious language of Macbeth,

" Throw physic to the dogs—I'll none of it."

I am of opinion that *"physic"* is not so much to blame as *physician.* And as I expect to differ practically, if not theoretically, from many members of the profession, let me suggest that we throw aside preconceived and vague notions and opinions which have been acquired by the process of *taking for granted,* rather than by reflection and observation, and that we come up fairly, without prejudice or favor, to the consideration of this interesting, because common, and fatal disease.

To premise: it will be admitted that dysentery consists in an irritated or inflamed state of the mucous membrane of the lower intestines—usually slight at first, having a tendency to increase to a dangerous extent or to diminish to convalescence, according to circumstances. I need not enumerate its symptoms, as these are sufficiently well known; but the question may be asked, is dysentery a primary disease ?—or does it depend upon a depraved state of the secretions ?

I must advocate the former position as generally correct, because I see no good reason for believing otherwise. That the predisposing cause of the disease is a morbid impression made upon the nervous system and reflected upon the intestines, I think very probable; but I must protest against the idea that it depends upon a defective secretion of the neighboring organs. I say this much, because the treatment of many practitioners indicates that they are influenced by a different opinion or theory. Yet, we find in some cases of dysentery a deficiency of the bilious secretion in the alvine discharges; but this no more proves the disease in question to be produced by the want of bile, than it does that the deficiency of bile is occasioned by the disease.

Again: there may be an apparent want of this product when there is no real deficiency. In health there is only a sufficient quantity of bile discharged to colour properly one evacuation per day. How then is it to be expected that in dysentery a dozen discharges in the same length of time will each be equally coloured? In dysentery, we have evident mucous inflammation, more or less intense, producing pain, griping, tenderness, mucous and bloody discharges, &c., &c. The indication is plain, to cure the disease by acting upon it directly where it exists. Have we the remedies to answer this indication? We certainly have. Are they to be found in the catalogue of cathartics? When the physician is called to such a case, the bowels have generally been discharging themselves until there are no consistent matters left, therefore the peculiar service of this class of remedies is not needed. If any cathartic possesses the property of curing inflammation of the mucous coat, I do not know it. I know of none upon which we may rely for this. Why then is so much confidence placed in calomel and other purgatives to the exclusion or partial exclusion of other more efficient and rational remedies? Who does not know that the preparations of mercury in ordinary doses are highly irritating under some circumstances; and that too when such effect is most to be reprehended and guarded against? And will any body believe that an article liable to produce the very effect which we wish to combat is the safest and surest remedy to be used?

Not long since, I happened to hear a man speaking of the prevalence of dysentery in a certain section and of the fatality which attended it, that scarcely any of a number of cases which he had known recovered, that nearly all died Shortly afterwards, I accidentally learned that the practice of a physician who attended among these cases was, to give at first, fifteen grains of calomel at a dose. I did not marvel any more at the tale of mortality. But to come directly to the question, what is the remedy for this disease? I answer emphatically, opium. This should be considered as the leading remedy in its treatment. The chief properties of opium are to relieve pain, produce somnolency and cure inflammation of the mucous membranes ; and I believe I may add, of most of the other tis-

sues. But the most valuable, is that of curing inflammation
and arresting inflammatory tendencies of the system. But,
what ! give opium before you have *cleansed* the stomach and
bowels ?   I say yes, give it, it will cure them, filthy as they are.
Give it, not in quarter grain doses, not in half grain doses, but
in from two to four grain doses, and repeat as often as necessary.
Cure the primary disease and the bile will flow beautifully
again and all will be right.

Thus, then, we have the remedy to answer the plain and un-
mistakeable indication of the disease, which used in time and
in connection with cold water injections, blisters, the astringents,
tannin, lead and zinc, creasote, &c., with the common effervescing soda powder to allay nausea and vomiting, where that
exists, will rarely fail to secure a happy result. Try it, use it
liberally, try it fairly, perseveringly, early in the attack, and
the confidence of the community in the profession will be
strengthened and increased by its success.

A good combination is made of two grains of opium and
from half to one drop of creosote for a dose, to be repeated at
proper intervals ; and for children an emulsion containing two
drops of creosote to the ounce, with the addition of as much
laudanum as may be desirable, to be given in teaspoonful doses
about three times a day.

ARTICLE XXXII.

A Case of Polypus Uteri. By A. F. ATTAWAY, M. D., of
Madison county, Georgia.

Louisa, a colored woman, aged 36 years, the property of
Mrs. M. M., of this county, was committed to my care in the
summer of 1851. She gave birth to a child in the 20th year
of her age, and her health, as reported by her mistress, began
to decline soon thereafter, and continued to grow worse by
degrees, despite of all the aid that could be afforded. She suffered, however, no very great inconvenience until about three
years ago—since when, she has suffered greatly from profuse
uterine hemorrhage, shortness of breath, anæmia, and other
phenomena characteristic of polypus uteri. Upon examination, I found the womb greatly enlarged, the os tincæ consid-

erably dilated, and the cavity of the organ completely filled with a pyriform tumour of a firm, fibrous texture, insensible to pressure, and which was attached to the fundus by a pedicle. From the anæmic and general derangement of the system, I prescribed a tonic and alterative course of treatment to improve her general health.   On the 21st November, I found that half the bulk of the tumour had prolapsed into the vagina. Believing her now to be in as favorable a condition as I would probably find her for the use of the knife or ligature, I proceeded to apply the latter.   The ligature remained until the 26th, being the fifth day of its application, when the tumour was removed.   During the operation, she had the usual treatment. Gooch's double canula was the instrument used.   She has now fully recovered her former health and spirits.   Five months have elapsed without any unfavorable symptoms.

I cannot close this report, without contributing my modicum of praise to the inventor of the invaluable instrument I used.

ARTICLE XXXIII.

A singular Case of Strangulated Hernia, operated upon and reported, by WM. H. ROBERT, M. D., of Orion, Alabama— in a letter to the Editor.

I was recently requested to go 45 miles to see a case of strangulated hernia.   I started on horse back at 6 o'clock, a. m. and at 4 o'clock, p. m. I operated on the man.   I found it a very singular case.   While a fold of the small intestine and a portion of the omentum were very badly strangulated, another very large portion of omentum presented a healthy and normal appearance.   This latter portion of omentum had been protruding so long as to form extensive adhesions to the tunica viginalis testis, and hence its healthy appearance while the other portion was so seriously affected.   I returned the intestine, but the omentum I thought proper to leave where I found it, hoping that it would relieve itself by suppuration.

Eight days after the operation, there was free suppuration from the opening and no constitutional disturbance.   The bowels acted finely (aided by enemas,) in three or four hours after the operation.

PART II.

Eclectic Department.

*Use of Glycerine in the Treatment of certain Forms of Deaf-
ness.* By Thomas Wakley, Esq., F. R. C. S., Eng., Surgeon to the Royal Free Hospital, London.

The class of cases to which I would draw attention in this
report, are those of *cuticular* or *epithelial thickening* of the
meatus, either *partial*, affecting the membrane of the tympanum, or *complete*, being continued over the entire auditory
cul-de-sac.   There is a greater or less degree of deafness,
corresponding with the amount of thickening; cessation of
the secretion of cerumen; frequently tinnitus, or a "singing
and hissing sensation" in the ears, and tickling irritation of the
meatus.   The causes are, constitutional predisposition, advanced age, chronic inflammation, long-continued discharge
following eruptive fevers and the application of escharotics and
irritants.   Amongst the latter, I would mention oily preparations, the globules of which adhere to the sides of the meatus
or membrana tympani, and become rancid, thus producing a
very frequent cause of inflammation.   Upon examination of
the affected ear, we find the meatus shining and inelastic, of a
pearly whiteness, the membrana tympani either clouded or
streaked, sometimes having small elevations upon it.   The
meatus is quite dry, the cerumenous glands being choked up by
the epithelial growth.

The mode of application of the glycerine, when treating this
state of the ear, is as follows:—The meatus is well cleansed
with tepid water, and then dried by means of the forceps and
cotton.   Glycerine is now poured into the meatus, and a plug
of gutta percha, softened in boiling water, made to fit the external opening; this takes the exact form of the ear, becomes
hard, and effectually prevents either the entrance of atmospheric air or the exit of the glycerine.   The ear should be
examined daily and the same process repeated.   The lining
membrane can be examined with a blunt silver probe, passed
gently through the speculum auris, to ascertain the effect of
the glycerine upon the cuticular thickening.   The meatus will
gradually lose its shining pearly appearance, and softened pieces
will fall off, and can be removed either by the forceps, or gentle syringing.   The practitioner should never attempt to tear
them away, but allow them to come away by the means just
stated.   The treatment occupies ordinarily from two to four
weeks, and is generally without any pain or inconvenience of
any kind to the patient, and the results, in some cases, have

been very gratifying. In the after treatment the patients are directed to moisten the auditory canal at least once a week with glycerine, applied by means of a camel-hair brush; this will generally prevent a recurrence of the cuticular thickening.

The *modus operandi* is simple enough—the glycerine being kept continually in contact with the part, acts mechanically, either absorbing or penetrating the epithelial coating, and separating the individual particles.

With respect to the permanence of the relief—some cases always require the presence of glycerine as the best known substitute for the natural secretion of the aural membrane. The frequent introduction of the glycerine tends to restore the external meatus to a healthy condition, and fit it for the healthy transmission of sound.

The mechanical power which glycerine possesses in separating this epithelial growth in some cases is very remarkable. I was consulted about two months since by a lady of rank, a patient of Sir James Clark, for deafness in both ears. In the right ear there was almost total deafness, from an enormous amount of epithelial thickening, which narrowed the calibre of the auditory canal, so that it would not receive the smallest-sized speculum. The depth of the *cul-de-sac* was also much less than normal, from the same cause. The lady was between seventy and eighty years of age, and told me that she had been deaf from her childhood in that ear; and there is but little reason to doubt that the deposit had been accumulating and hardening during nearly the whole of her life. The glycerine was used in the manner already described, and its action was very beautifully illustrated. A short time since, a large mass of the softened growth was removed without any inconvenience to the patient,—a larger quantity, perhaps, than I had ever before separated from the ear. The calibre and depth of the ear will therefore be increased considerably when the swelling of the lining membrane shall have subsided from its having been saturated with glycerine; this will gradually exude and come away. This case is still under treatment, and I shall mention it again at a future period, when the effects of the treatment upon the hearing can be safely declared.

I may mention another case in the family of a nobleman, patients of Sir B. Brodie, where very considerable thickening existed over the entire aural *cul-de-sac*, but which readily yielded to the softening action of the glycerine, although it had previously resisted the use of caustics and various applications of the essential oils, &c., ordinarily employed.

The following cases are examples of the action of the glycerine on this class of chronic diseases of the ear :—

M. R——, a clergyman of Hants, aged sixty-six, applied, June 16, 1851, suffering from deafness of the right ear, which had existed for more than twenty years ; indeed that organ had become wholly useless.   Upon examination, I found the meatus polished and dry, quite inelastic to the touch, and of a dull white colour.   The central part of the membrana tympani presented even more opacity than the other parts, and no secretion could be detected in the ear.   I applied the glycerine after having well cleansed the meatus, fitting the gutta percha plug after the manner already described.   This treatment was repeated every morning, and at the end of fourteen days I was enabled to re- move a large portion of pulpy epithelium.   Again, four days afterwards, more softened skin was taken away.   The ear was well syringed, and all the smaller particles removed.   Upon examination of the ear with the speculum, the meatus was found much improved in appearance ; the membrane slightly swollen, from saturation by the glycerine ; there was still, however, a portion of the cuticular deposition hanging on the left side. Upon testing the patient's hearing with the sonometer, it was found to have improved two degrees.   The same treatment was then continued, and at the end of a week the last piece came away.   The ears were again gently syringed, but with no fur- ther effect.   A small portion of wool was then placed in the external opening of the meatus, and the patient was directed to return to me in four days.   Upon his visiting me as desired, his hearing was again tested by the sonometer, and it was found that he had improved six degress.   There is little doubt that the deafness in this case was owing to the mechanical ob- struction in the passage of sound produced by the cuticular deposition.   When I last heard from this gentlemen, there had been no return of his deafness.

H. M——, a dissenting minister, thirty-eight years of age, consulted me, Aug. 19, 1851, for long-standing deafness of both ears, which he stated would ere long cause him to retire from his profession, as he could hardly hear his own voice.   The meatus throughout had that " parchment appearance" so char- acteristic where cerumen has ceased to be secreted.   The membrana tympani presented a similar appearance.   The same treatment was resorted to as in the foregoing case, and the re- sult was equally successful.   In sixteen days two soft, pulpy, membranous pieces were removed, and in a month his hearing, on being tested by the sonometer, was found equal to the lowest tone but one of the instrument.

During the treatment it was found necessary to attend to the general health of this patient, and preparations of steel and the mineral acids were employed with great advantage.   I am in correspondence with this patient, and he still retains his improved hearing. From the history he gave of his malady I consider that the thickening was caused by constitutional predisposition, or, as he termed it, a "deaf taint" in his family, as several other members, both older and younger, were similarly affected.

H. T—— consulted me at the Royal Free Hospital, (by direction of Mr. Edwards, of Brompton,) Nov. 1851. He had been deaf for twenty-six years, and presented, in every particular, a case of strongly-marked cuticular thickening. He stated that he had suffered from inflammation of the ear, experiencing at the time excruciating pain. This lasted for three or four months. He was told it was neuralgia. As the pain left him, the deafness gradually supervened, increasing daily. This case occasioned me much trouble, from the want of punctual attendance on the part of the patient; at length, however, a considerable mass of almost cartilaginous consistence came away from both ears, with very great relief to the patient's hearing. Caustics had been previously used for the cure of his deafness, to a very great extent; but, as the man said, always making him worse instead of better, causing pain and inflammation of the ear.

This case, in its result, was one of the most successful that has fallen under my notice.

In this report, I feel it absolutely necessary to caution the profession against the use of the impure glycerine in the market. Several samples have been forwarded to me by both surgeons and patients. Upon careful examination of the liquids, I found only one sample to consist of pure glycerine; the others had a low specific gravity, or contained a considerable quantity of lead or of rancid oil, having been manufactured from putrid fat.

Several letters have been sent to me on this subject; the following extract is taken from one that I received from Dr. Houseman, Newcastle-on-Tyne :—

"The use of glycerine in certain forms of deafness is likely to suffer from the impure samples in the market : it would be well to remind the profession of this fact. Messrs. Gilpin, of this town, have supplied me with the preparation pure, and several patients have been cured by the application. Glycerine should be a clear, scentless syrup, intensely sweet, instead of the rancid stuff usually sold under that name," &c. &c.

Thus it is easy to account for failures in many cases that have been reported ; and I would strongly urge surgeons who are treating certain forms of deafness with glycerine to test it themselves, and thus be certain of the purity of their agent.

Pure glycerine should be a white, syrupy fluid, inodorous, specific gravity not less than 1·32, quite free from oily globules and oxide of lead.   The latter may be detected by passing through it a current of sulphuretted hydrogen, which will easily blacken it.   Any fatty matter may be discovered by mixing it with water: the disagreeable smell will at once prove that it has been manufactured from putrid fat.

In conclusion, it may be said, that impure glycerine being so easy of detection, it is desirable that its utility as an agent in the treatment of deafness will not henceforth suffer from the employment of an article that has no nearer affinity to glycerine than the name.—[*London Lancet.*

On Eruptive Diseases of the Scalp.   By CHARLES A. POOLE, Esq., M. R. C. S. E., &c.

On account of the great discrepancy pursued in the treatment of eruptive diseases of the scalp, and indeed of the small degree of interest seemingly evinced in their management, arising probably from the fact of their continuance not endangering life—although one disease at least produces a degree of fatuity—also of their peculiar obstinacy, I am induced to offer a few observations on the *treatment* of these repulsive affections, which tend to render families unhappy, and the afflicted avoided.

Eruptive diseases of the scalp seem always to have been difficult of treatment, which, instead of leading to indifference should stimulate inquiry, with the view of treating these affections on sound rational principles, the want of which too often sends the patient elsewhere for advice, and thus miserably extends the pernicious domains of quackery.

For the suggestion of the following remarks and plan of treatment, I am indebted to Dr. Neligan of Dublin, whose simple and practically efficient division of these diseases into inflammatory and non-inflammatory I have followed, and this I believe to be the true basis on which to build a rational plan of treatment :

Inflammatory—Herpes capitis ; vesicular ; contagious.   Eczema capitis ; vesicular ; non-contagious.   Impetigo capitis ; pustular ; non-contagious.   Pityriasis capitis ; scaly; non-contagious.

Non-inflammatory.—Porrigo capitis; vegetable growth; contagious.

Of course there are other eruptions found on the scalp, but they are in connexion with those generally situated on the other parts of the body, and therefore in this situation require no particular description.

As regards prognosis, this depends more on the length of time any given eruption has lasted, than on any particular kind. When seen early, and properly treated, they are cured in from a fortnight to three weeks, sometimes much sooner; but some old chronic cases require from one to three months. They seem to be curable generally in the following order ;—1st, Impetigo ; 2nd, Pityriasis ; 3rd, Moist Eczema ; 4th, Lupus ; 5th, Dry Eczema.

The treatment is based on the fact of these affections being both inflammatory and constitutional. That they are inflammatory is sufficiently evident; that they are constitutional is almost proved, from the advantage derived from alterative medicines. The absence of this division has formed, I fancy, the chief stumbling-block. Stimulant applications, usually applied in chronic cases, frequently fail, and in recent ones are obviously injurious. As a general rule, in all cases of these diseases, the hair must be cut close with a pair of scissors, and kept so during treatment; shaving, I believe, from the attendant irritation, to be highly injurious; and the head should be covered with an oil-skin cap. The local plan of treatment consists of ointments and lotions of the carbonates of soda and potash, in greater or less strength. The carbonate of potash, being the stronger preparation, is more adapted for the chronic forms, and when the attendant inflammation is slight. The quantities of the carbonates, used as unguents, vary from twenty grains to one drachm, to one ounce of prepared lard, as used in lotions, from half a drachm to one and a half, in a pint of rose or distilled water. The ointment is to be applied three times a day, smeared over the eruption, and washed off each morning with the corresponding lotion. In cases where crusts or scales are found, a linseed-meal poultice applied for twelve hours, and the ointment for a similar period, render them easily removable by washing gently with the lotion. Sometimes the unguents disagree ; in that case, the lotion must be substituted, but used four or five times daily. In the chronic forms, when stimulants are necessary, they are best treated with an ointment consisting of from half a drachm to one drachm of the citrine ointment to one ounce of prepared lard ; this applied at bed-time only, and the lotion during the day. The alterative medicine Dr. Neligan uses is the yellow iodide of mercury (Protoiodide P. L.,) in combination with mercury with chalk, and aromatic powder. To a child six years old he gives half a grain of the iodide, two grains of mercury with chalk, and two grains of aromatic powder, every second morning ; for an older child the same every morning; to a younger child every third or fourth morning; for infants he omits the iodide; but I have found mercury with chalk, aromatic powder, and sesquicarbonate of soda, given more frequently, answer equally as well. During treatment, the child should be kept strictly on milk diet. This plan of treatment I have seen employed, and have used it myself for more than five years with the most unswerving success. I have not seen a single case resist this plan. In illustration, I shall cite a case or two. I might relate many, but do not wish to infringe on your valuable space :—

Charles S———, a fine boy about a year and a half old, has been affected with impetigo capitis since a few weeks after birth; his health not materially affected; appetite bad, bowels constipated; his whole head covered with greenish-yellow crusts, which extend over the forehead, through which is a slight discharge of yellowish matter; the hair matted together; the scalp itchy and hot. A linseed-meal poultice was placed on the scalp for twelve hours, and the following ointment to be applied three times a day :—One drachm of carbonate of soda to one ounce of prepared lard; and the corresponding lotion every morning. The following powder was ordered :—eighteen grains of mercury with chalk, thirty-six grains of carbonate, twelve grains of aromatic powder; into twelve powders, one night and morning. The hair to be cut close, and the child to wear an oil-skin cap. In three or four days the crust had disappeared, and the tendency to heat and irritation entirely subsided; this treatment was steadily adhered to for six weeks, (with the exception of substituting the carbonate of potash in lotion and ointment for carbonate of soda,) when there was not the least tendency to a return of the eruption, his hair was allowed to grow, and the boy to resume his usual diet, having been kept during treatment on milk diet. Although more than a year has elapsed there has been no return of the affection.

H. B———, a lad twelve years old, was brought for advice; his mother states, about a week since he complained of itching of the head, and upon examination she found what she termed little boils scattered over the head; he was affected with impetigo sparsa, the hair slightly matted together, and a little discharge. June 3rd, 1850 : the hair to be cut close, and an ointment of half a drachm of carbonate of soda to an ounce of lard to be applied three times a-day; and powders containing mercury with chalk, soda, and aromatic powder, twice daily. This boy was well in a week, but as a precaution, used the remedies a few days longer.

I might add many more, but it suffices to say that all the eruptions seem equally amenable to the above treatment. If you think this tends to simplify the matter and it meets your approbation, I shall have gained my point, and shall reserve my observations on the remaining (non-inflammatory affections) for another occasion.—[*Ibid.*

On the Employment of the Chloride of Sodium in the Treatment of Intermittent Fever. By W. P. LATTIMORE, M. D.

The discovery of some agent capable of serving as a substitute for Peruvian bark, or for its active principle, quinia, in the treatment of intermittent fever, has long been desired, in consequence of the high price of the sulphate of quinine, and the great adulteration of the salt to which this has given rise.   The amount paid for quinine alone, is no small item in the annual expenses of the country physician ; and this is likely to be increased, as it is said that a company of English druggists have monopolized the entire crop of Peruvian bark for many years to come.

In view of the interest necessarily felt in this subject, we have thought it might not prove uninteresting to the readers of the American Journal, to give the results of investigations made by the eccentric Piorry, upon the use of common salt in the treatment of intermittent fever.   The investigations were commenced at La Pitié, and continued at La Charité, where they were witnessed by the writer.

The attention of M. Piorry was drawn to the subject by a memoir, presented to the French Academy of Medicine, in July, 1850, by Dr. Scelle Montdezert, entitled, *Practical Considerations upon the Treatment of Intermittent Fevers, and upon the mode of action of the Salts of Quinia, and of the Chloride of Sodium.*

In this momoir, M. Scelle Montdezert supposes that every paroxysmal fever is due to the presence of fibrin in the venous blood ; this fluid, in the normal state, being deprived of fibrin by the process of assimilation.   That the salts of quinia owe their efficacy as anti-periodics to the fact that they dissolve this fibrin abnormally present, thus restoring the venous blood to its normal conditions.   In casting about, then, for a substitute, he saw that nature had largely disseminated both potassa and soda, each possessing, in a remarkable degree, solvent properties.   Seeking, among the various combinations of each, that one which, uniting with the divers elements of the blood, should furnish the fewest insoluble compounds, he naturally selected the cloride of sodium, which forms none.   He administered it, and then goes on to say :—

" On account of these considerations we experimented without fear of injury, and we declare with satisfaction that the results of its employment are such that salt may now be considered as sharing with the salts of quinia the prerogative of arresting the paroxysms of intermittent fever. It is sufficient to administer half an ounce of it in the morning, before eating, during the apyrexia, in half a glass of infusion of coffee. Its use should be continued for three days.

" Fortunate results, observed during several years, have confirmed our foresight. It is a counter-proof of our opinion, long since emitted, upon the action of the sulphate of quinine, and one which gives the most satisfactory solution of this therapeutical problem."

M. Scelle Montdezert gives the history of no cases treated by salt, although he alludes to many in which the agent was successfully employed. Under these circumstances the matter came into the hands of M. Piorry, who was one of the committee appointed by the Academy to report upon the memoir, and his cases are the only ones known to us. From these researches it will be seen that the chloride of sodium cures intermittent fever, like the sulphate of quinine, by acting upon the spleen and diminishing its volume, and this sometimes in less than a minute. And in this connection it may be of interest to say a few words in regard to the views of M. Piorry concerning the spleen in intermittent fever, and his method of diagnosticating the disease.

He holds that in all paroxysmal fevers the spleen is enlarged ; that the anatomical lesion is the cause, the fever only the symptom ; that wherever the spleen has a greater length (measuring in a line extending from the middle of the axilla to the anterior superior spinous process of the ileum,) than from 31 to 33 lines, intermittent fever exists. Believing thus, the symptoms for him are zero, while the state of the spleen stands at the other end of the scale, and is everything—percussion (pleximetric) of course, being the *experimentum crucis.*

We cannot resist the temptation of here paying a tribute to the skill with which M. Piorry employs percussion in making a diagnosis. With him *auscultation* is but an infant when compared with its full grown brother *percussion.* By its aid he interrogates the abdominal viscera as frequently as the thoracic, and with no less success, for he has brought it to an almost incredible degree of perfection. With his plate of ivory and his flattened fingers' ends he diagnosticates almost everything—tumours of the abdomen, abscesses everywhere, aneurisms, &c. All acknowledge the delicacy and accuracy of his test, while the looker on is lost in admiration, and wonders whether all his senses are not really concentrated in the ends of his fingers, which by constant drumming have at length become the very reverse of tapering.

Wishing, then, to experiment with salt, a few cases of intermittent fever (old stagers,) contracted in Algiers were selected as subjects.   Behold, then, Piorry at the bedside.   The patient asserts that he contracted the fever and ague several years since in Africa; that he has frequently been cured; but that the disease has constantly re-appeared at the end of fifteen days or one month at farthest.   The type of the fever is tertian. The spleen is percussed and found to be abnormally dull throughout its whole extent; the entire splenic region is sensitive upon percussion, particularly over the dullest points; and each blow is accompanied by marked contortions of the countenance.   This sensibility extends but little beyond the region of dulness, which last occupies an extent of fifty-three lines, measuring in the direction indicated above.   To this patient a drachm of salicine is administered without producing any change in the dimensions of the spleen.   A few minutes subsequently, half an ounce of salt mixed with a cup of soup is given, and upon carefully percussing the splenic region at the end of four minutes this organ is found diminished one inch, from above downwards.   The next day the spleen is found to be of the same size, but upon the administration of a second dose of salt, it suddenly contracts and measures nearly three-quarters of an inch less than yesterday.   The resonance throughout the entire organ has increased while the sensibility has diminished.   The succeeding day, the attack of fever is very slight, and upon giving a third dose, the disease does not return; and when seen six weeks subsequently, the patient is still free from his African enemy.   Thus we see that a diminution of twenty-four lines in the length of the spleen was the result of the medicament, the fever being cured more effectually than ever before; *i. e.,* the patient had remained free from all relapse for the space of six weeks; one month having previously been the longest period of immunity.

We have the notes of seven cases of well-marked intermittent fever, in all of which the administration of the chloride of sodium was followed by rapid decrease in the volume of the spleen and cure of the febrile symptoms.   We also have the record of three cases in which salt was unsuccessfully used; in one of these, the sulphate of quinine effected a cure; in a second it too failed, while in the third it was not tried.   These were all well-marked cases of intermittent fever, such as would pass muster in any of our own malarious districts.

Let it be remembered that most of the fever and ague met

with in the Parisian hospitals, is of long standing, and imported from the malarious districts of Algiers, which generate a form of the disease even worse than that found amid the marshes on the banks of the famed Maumee; that these cases have been treated again and again, have been cured now by the sulphate of quinine, now by arsenic, but only to reappear upon the slightest exposure or imprudence ; in short, to recur as only *the shakes* can recur.

We witnessed many of the experiments of M. Piorry, and in the great majority of them, the fever yielded to salt quite as readily as to the salts of quinia. And as to the theory of M. Piorry, the spleen diminished under the use of the remedy, *pari passu,* with the febrile symptoms, in every case where the disease was cured, proving that this organ really shows the influence of remedies over this class of fevers—that it is, as it were, a febro-barometer—for the diminution of the spleen is a constant phenomenon accompanying the cure of the disease, whatever be the curative agent employed.

M. Piorry's method of administering the chloride of sodium is, to give half an ounce in a cup of thin soup during the apy-rexia and fasting. It usually agrees with the stomach perfectly well, but in some few cases we have seen it excite vomiting and diarrhœa. Three doses commonly suffice to effect a cure, the first two to be taken on succeeding days, and the third after an interval of one day. Should the spleen be undiminished in volume by the first dose, we may be sure that the remedy will not cure the disease ; and the same is true of all the antiperio-dics. Excepting in rare cases, the diminution of the spleen occurs immediately upon the administration of the remedy (salt or sulph. quinine,) and may frequently be detected within one minute, after which the organ remains stationary until a second dose of the medicament be administered.

Is the chloride of sodium as efficient an antiperiodic as the sul-phate of quinine? Are the cures effected by the one as per-manent as those effected by the other? The first question can only be answered by those possessing a larger field of observa-tion than the writer. May we not hope for a solution from those of our profession who observe the disease too largely either for comfort or pleasure ? In regard to the permanency of the cures, we apprehend there is not much difference, be the medication what it may ; for relapses are only too common after the greatest care and most patient attention.

Should the discovery prove as useful and applicable as it promises, the benefit accruing from it will be immense. If it be capable of taking the place of the sulphate of quinine in the majority, or even in one-half the cases of intermittent fever, therapeutics will be largely the gainer.—[*Amer. Jour. of Med. Science.*

On Chordee. By John L. Milton, Esq.

[There are two facts to be noticed as to the cause of chordee as bearing upon the treatment; viz., that there is spasm, and that this is attended by pain, caused, primarily or secondarily, by the condition of the mucous membrane. The following appear the best known and most commonly employed methods of treatment:]

Mr. Lagneau says, "for the inflamed chordee, bleeding from the arm, hot bathing to the perineum, lavements, eighteen or twenty leeches to the canal of the urethra, two or three times repeated, and when the pain is severe, gr. i. of the watery extract of opium, and gr. ii. of camphor," which he recommends giving in the evening. He winds up this energetic treatment by a solemn warning not to plunge the penis into cold water, as it may be, and has been, followed by a metastasis of the complaint of the bladder.

M. Ricord recommends gr. iiss. of camphor, and gr. ss. of opium in a pill, of which two or three may be taken every night.

· Richter recommends that the patient sleep on a hair mattress, and very cool, or else on a canopy, and do not turn on his back. Eisenmann that the parts should be exposed to the influence of narcotic vapours; or that infusion of camomile or cherry-laurel water be injected or dropped into the urethra. He found sedatives of no avail. He recommends the patient to make water more frequently than necessary, because a distended bladder irritates the vesiculæ seminales and the neighboring parts. He objects, also, to dipping the penis in cold water, and then recommends soothing injections, or poultices; opium being less useful. Peyrihe recommends ammonia and injections of soap ley. Iodine, the empyreumatic oil of tartar, and blue ointment, have also been praised.

Mr. Hunter says, "he has known twenty drops of the tinctura thebaica take it (painful erection) away for a whole night, and that the cicuta has likewise some powers in this way." For the chordee, he recommends opium joined with camphor, praises local bleeding with the free use of hot vapour to the parts; poultices with camphor; while the effused lymph which remains may be removed by mercurial ointment in friction. He has seen the cicuta of service.

Mr. Wallace recommends calomel and hippo,* with opium and camphor.

Such are the general outlines of the practice pursued by surgeons, as we find it recorded in books. These plans bear a pretty strong resemblance to each other, and are nearly all calculated to lead to one point—the allaying of pain by the use of sedatives. The idea of attempting to remove it by the pure antispasmodics, does not seem to have been worked out or even entertained, although everything seems to show that it is more amenable to them than to opium. I will add but one more remedy, as remarkable for its originality as any I know, and which was, I believe, first recommended in writing by Dr. Colles. It is, that when the patient finds the chordee coming on, *he do turn over, and balance himself on his knees and elbows till the chordee goes off.* The reader can easily imagine what effect such a remedy would produce. Let him figure to himself an exasperated patient struggling in the middle of the night to get ease in this way! Verily, this is surgery!

I now approach that part of the matter which has most of all occupied my attention—the substitution of some simple and always applicable remedy for these different methods of cure. I will not stop to point out the inutility or inapplicability of antiphlogistic treatment to this symptom, as any one versed in the disease must have observed cases where the chordee came on though the patient had been treated most heroically. Sedatives I utterly object to, as I have never used them in sufficient quantity to have any material effect on the chordee without finding the patient much worse afterwards. They generally disordered the stomach, produced headache and languor, very often with constipation of the bowels. The scalding and discharges were rendered worse and more obstinate, and, to crown all, the chordee was merely abated for an instant, and returned the moment they were left off; nay, even when they were again administered without increasing the dose. Nor have I ever been able to understand why they should be given, as the pain appears to depend on a spasm, and when this is removed the pain ceases; whereas the spasm does not necessarily subside when the pain is relieved.

I have tried the most powerful antispasmodics, as ether, galbanum, assafœtida, and chloroform, and can only say of them that I have found nothing equal to camphor in the fluid form. In powder, camphor is disagreeable to take, and did not appear to act so readily, I suppose from not being so equally diffused and finely divided as in solution. In fact, in spasm a liquid

* Pulv. ipecac. comp.

remedy, as admitting of a more rapid action, is always the thing to be sought for. The spirit of camphor, taken in the dose of 3j., in a small quantity of water, is equally energetic and rapid. The objection that it immediately becomes insoluble by contact with water, is sufficiently obviated by the fact, that its operation is most certain and rapid, and that esscence of camphor, in which the camphor is so dissolved that it does not separate on the admixture of water, possesses, so far as I have been able to judge, no advantage over the other.

As in many other cases, the chain of morbid actions must at once be broken, and this is done much more effectually by two or three full doses, repeated at short intervals, without the least remission, till the chordee is completely stopped, than by small quantities, however long continued and regularly taken. I therefore invariably adopt the following plan :—

A tea-spoonful is to be taken at night in water before going to bed, and *every time the patient wakes with the chordee, let him at once rise and repeat the dose.* In the milder cases, one dose for a night or two is generally enough. In the more severe ones, the symptom is generally removed at the end of the second night, becoming, in the meantime, milder and less frequent after each dose. So long as the clap remains bad, I frequently recommend the patient to take a tea-spoonful at night before going to bed, which suspends the chordee till the cure is completed. This plan of treatment also answers well in the bearing down pains to which women are sometimes subject in clap ; but as here, contrary to what it is in men, these pains are generally worst in the day-time, it is best to use the esscence of camphor largely in the medicine they may happen to be taking.

It must, however, be taken in full doses. A violent sudden pain like that of chordee requires an equally powerful remedy, and there is no use in trifling with it. A less quantity than a tea-spoonful will not always suffice to abate the pain at once, though it may materially alleviate it ; just as a moderate dose of chloroform will lull the acute pain of an operation without rendering the patient insensible to what is going on, while a smallar quantity, in one full dose, produces complete torpor. Now, as a tea-spoonful or two may be safely taken, it is best to insure success at once. In one or two cases, it has produced some sickness, and, strangely enough, this has been more the case with small doses than large ones; this was probably caused by something having been previously taken that had in some measure disordered the stomach. At any rate, the instances have been too few to make the affair of any moment. I only allude to it here, that no one might by its appearance be discouraged from giving so valuable a remedy as camphor really is.

The patient should be directed to keep the camphor in a tightly-corked bottle, and in a cool place, and to have it by his bed-side ready to take.   It is best taken in water, as, if dropped on sugar, it produces a strong sensation of heat in the mouth, occasionally preventing the patient from getting to sleep a-gain.—[*Medical Times.*

Case of Epilepsy treated by Tracheotomy.   By W. H. Cane, Esq., Uxbridge.

[In the case of a boatman, suffering under an extreme epileptic seizure, after which he was left in a state of deep apoplectic coma´ with asphyxia, inspiration being performed only by seldom and short catches, whilst the veins in the head and neck were every where visible, and greatly distended, Mr. Cane, after the patient had remained in this state nineteen hours, determined to perform the operation of tracheotomy ; acting upon the suggestion of Dr. Marshall Hall, that as the epileptic or other convulsion implied closure of the larynx with expira-tory efforts, the attack of convulsive epilepsy would be pre-vented by that operation.]

" Feeling convinced," Mr. Cane observes, "that the patient must shortly expire, and that the root of the evil was in the closure of the larynx, I at once proceeded to open the trachea, a matter of no small difficulty, on account of the twisted state of the neck, the engorged state of the vessels, and the constant action of the muscles.   The operation of tracheotomy was per-formed, and the tracheal tube is kept in the trachea to the pre-sent time.   The relief to the patient was immediate ; the air passed into the lungs, the state of spasm subsided, with the turgid condition of the head and neck, and the patient soon recovered his sensibility.   This was not the only gratifying result : although the poor man had experienced his epileptic seizures in increasing violence during seven or eight years, and recently thrice a week, he had, on April 1st, during two months, had no return of them.   More recent accounts of the patient, who is now in Staffordshire, confirm the former report ; the tube is still kept in the trachea, and the epileptic seizures have not recurred."—[*Lancet.*

Scarlatina.   By Dr. Volz.

Dr. Volz has recorded his experience of a severe epidemic of scarlatina in Carlsruhe, from which he draws the following deductions :—

1. The extent and redness of the eruption are not in direct ratio to the severity of the disease.

2. The proximate cause of the exanthem is a stasis in the cutaneous capillaries.

3. The exfoliating scales of epidermis do not transmit the contagious principle of the disease.

4. The mucous membranes undergo the scarlatinous eruption equally with the skin.

5. The lesions of the throat are of three varieties,—catarrhal, inflammatory, and gangrenous.

6. The inflammmation of the parotid which accompanies scarlatina seldom terminates in suppuration : that which follows the subsidence of the exanthem, often suppurates.

7. In the consecutive anasarca the alterations in the kidney are secondary, and depend on the change in the composition of the blood.

8. Death may occur in scarlatina from the following causes: congestive apoplexy, suffocation, pyæmia, and anæmia.—[*Prov. Med. and Surg. Journal.*

Creasote in Scarlet Fever.   By T. E. WALLER, M. D., of Pa.

In April, 1851, my three little boys were attacked with Scarlet Fever. The two youngest, though the fever was very high for a few days, recovered. without any of the sequelæ of the disease, in the course of three or four weeks. The eldest, a stout, hearty child, under four years of age, was the worse case I ever saw live through an attack in its malignant form. Though it was not followed by any of the common effects of the disease, except swelling and final suppuration of the glands of the neck, it was two months from the time he was taken, before he was able to stand on his feet. I pursued the ordinary antiphlogistic and cooling treatment, until the commencement of the suppurative stage. I was then at a loss what to do, so deeply and extensive were the mucous surfaces affected. Indeed, it seemed to me the case must, in spite of all known remedies terminate fatally. Matter (pus) was discharged profusely from the nostrils and ears, and his eyes were almost closed for several days, from the same cause. The pulse became more rapid, and other symptoms supervened, indicating extensive suppuration and the absorption of pus, and delirium was almost constant during the latter part of the day and night. I felt convinced that if something was not done very soon to arrest the suppuration, the child must certainly die.

In the absence of council, and in that state of mind natural to a parent under such circumstances, I felt bewildered and almost overwhelmed in contemplating the case of my little sufferer. But presently, under a sense of the pressing emergency, and the responsibility weighing so heavy upon me, I rallied, and resolved to make an effort to save my child. For an hour or more I examined authors, cases, remedies, and reflected, but without finding anything satisfactory.

The use of pyroligneous acid then came to my mind as something available; and then Creasote as still better, which I immediately resolved upon trying. I mixed three drops with an ounce of water, put it into a common sized tumbler nearly full of water, and directed half of it to be given during the night, as a drink. The balance was given during the following day, and continued at the same rate for three or four days. A decided improvement was perceptible before the first three drops were all taken, and by the second night he rested better; the pulse became slower and fuller, and the discharge diminished very much. I also washed out the mouth and throat as much as I could, and the nose and ears, with a solution of Creasote, six drops to an ounce water. I believe it was on the fifth day that I discontinued the internal use of Creasote, the discharge having nearly ceased; but applied it externally, three or four times a day, to the mouth and nostrils, until they were healed. He recovered, though very slowly; and I believe it was the Creasote that saved him.

I had no other cases until the spring, when I had an opportunity of trying it again in *seven* more *very* severe cases. In one of them, gangrene of the throat (or glands,) took place, so that in approaching the patient, the smell was very offensive. In two days' use of Creasote, the change for the better was truly astonishing. It seemed as if the child had been suddenly raised, from a state bordering on decay and inevitable destruction, to convalescence! I never saw a remedy act so like a charm before. All of these seven cases were as bad as any I ever saw, (and I have seen hundreds,) and I have pursued nearly the same treatment with each one, with the same result—recovery. I used water and lard externally, (sometimes a warm bath,) and to show the high degree of the fever, I will state that, after "peeling" all over, as they all did, the cuticle on the bottoms of the feet, in one case—a boy over nine years of age —came off whole, like the sole of a shoe.

In one case, I gave about half a drachm of carb. lig. three or four times a day, in connexion with the Creasote water, and in four of the last cases, before suppuration took place, I applied a solution of nitrate of silver (gr. x to the ounce,] to the throat and glands, which I think had the effect to diminish the local inflammation a good deal. But to cleanse the mucous surfaces, and check suppuration, thereby destroying its poisonous effects by absorption, *creasote,* in my humble opinion, is *the* remedy. I do not know whether any other physician has ever used it in this manner or not ; but if this brief and imperfect sketch will be the means of giving it a more extensive trial, perhaps the profession and the public may be benefited by its publication. I regret that I did not take notes, so that I could have given an exact and complete report of each case. Still, I trust the main feature in my treatment is rendered intelligible. I have thus treated eight very bad cases successfully ; five boys and three girls, ranging in age from four and a half to nine and a half years. I will therefore sum up as a general treatment of scarlatina maligna, as follows :

Open the bowels every other day with Castor oil or some mild aperient—apply cold or cool water and lard alternately to the whole body frequently—warm mustard bath, if necessary, and tepid water with vinegar—solution of nitrate of silver, in the first stage, to the throat, once a day—and in the suppurative stage, three drops of Creasote in twenty-four hours, until the discharge abates—wash and gargle the throat, &c., with Creasote water, six drops to the ounce, three or four times a day; and for the hoarseness and dry state of the larynx, before or during convalescence, give from five to ten drops of balsam copaiba on a little sugar, three times a day. After the patient gets up, great care is necessary to prevent taking cold, and the diet should be light for at least two weeks in most cases. The Pulv. Jalap Comp. will generally keep down or remove dropsical effusion or anasarca, if that state supervene.

N. B.—I forgot to state that, in one of the above cases I took blood from the arm. But no general rule can be laid down for that—the physician must be the judge, in each case, of such necessity.—[*Philadelphia Med. and Surg. Journal.*

We think the suggestion of Creasote as a remedy in the suppurative stage of Scarlatina entitled to peculiar regard, and have therefore placed the above article upon our pages. We must, however, dissent from the use of cathartics or even laxatives so often repeated in a disease which tends so rapidly to a prostration of the energies of the system. We think it of the utmost importance to husband the resources of life in Scarlatina.—[Ed. S. M. & S. J.

Syncope from Entrance of Air into the Facial Vein. By Moses Gunn, M. D., Professor of Anatomy and Surgery in the University of Michigan.

The substance of the following case was transmitted immediately after its occurrence, to the chairman of the committee on surgery of the National Association ; but no notice having been taken of it by that committee, and deeming it not entirely devoid either of interest or novelty, I now seek to lay it before the profession through another channel.

The patient appeared at the college clinic with a small, hard, oblong, tumor, lying under the base of the inferior maxilla, involving the facial vessels so as to require their division in its extirpation. Previous to commencing the operation, in accordance with my usual custom before making incisions in this region, I sought, by compression with my hand upon the lower portion of the neck, to ascertain the course of the external jugular vein, but was not able to detect the vessel. An incision was made parallel to the base of the jaw, and the tumor separated from its bed, except at a point near its posterior extremity where it involved the facial vessels. These were divided, the tumour detached, and its place occupied by a sponge, removing which, in order to secure the facial artery, I instantly noticed a movement in the open mouth of the facial vein, heard a bubbling sound, and my patient sank back in a state of syncope, from which he recovered with some difficulty by the ordinary means. The wound was immediately stopped on noticing the movement in the open mouth of the vein, and by means of a firm compress, hemorrhage and further entrance of air was sought to be prevented, and the wound allowed to heal by granulation.

This case is interesting from the fact that the accident arose from the entrance of air into a vein as small as the facial, and had it not been reinforced by some other, it would seem impossible for its division to be attended with such results. But it will be borne in mind, that the external jugular did not pass down the neck in its usual superficial course, but probably united with the facial, and emptied by a short thick trunk common to both into the internal jugular. The facial I undoubtedly divided at the point of junction. I have once met with just such a distribution of the veins upon the dead body.—[*N. Y. Journal of Medicine.*

On the Use of Muriate of Ammonia in Cynanche Tonsillaris. By A. B. McKAY, Green Bush, Illinois.

Although this disease is rarely fatal, yet it is one of the most distressing the human family is subject to. It is this which has induced me to lay before the profession a few remarks on a remedy which I have used with complete success in many cases of this disease ; in fact, in every case it has succeeded, in which I have used it. The remedy is *muriate of ammonia,* or *sal ammoniac.*

My usual method of administering it is as follows :

℞. Ammon. Mur. . . . . ℨiii.
Tinc. Opii, ... f℥i.
Aceti, ... f℥iv. Misce.

As soon as the vinegar is well saturated with the ammonia, I let the patient use it freely and often, as a gargle. In the ab-sence of vinegar and laudanum, I have powdered the ammonia and blown it on the affected parts. This remedy has succeeded so perfectly in my hands, that I am almost inclined to think it a specific in this disease. I use it with equal success in all stages.—[*Buffalo Med. Jour. and Rev.*

On the Treatment of Neuralgia. Extracted from an article in the Western Lancet, by LANDON RIVES, M. D., of Cincinnati.

" Most practitioners use opiates to produce an anodyne ef-fect ; and in this, I think, the fault usually lies in the treatment of this affection. When opiates are used with persons of good constitution, they may effect their andoyne influence, but if administered to persons of debilitated constitution and nervous temperament, laboring under neuralgia, the excitant effect will more than counterbalance all the good which can be expected from the subsequent sedative operation of the medicine.. The functional derangement in this disease is an exalted sensation—hence it is wrong to administer a medicine which excites, even in its primary action,—for, although the secondary action may be the one desired, the primary excitation will irritate the dis-eased tissue, and render the subsequent paroxysms much more violent. A more appropriate, and in my hands a much more efficient remedy to meet this indication, is small and frequently repeated doses of extract of hyoscyamus. This medicine, un-fortunately, is not always kept of a good quality in the shops ; hence, care should be taken to procure a good article. With a view to prevent the recurrence of the paroxysms, there can be nothing used more efficacious than quinine. It has been my good fortune to cure a number of cases of neuralgia, with sul-phate of quinine and extract of hyoscyamus, given in doses of one and a half grains each, at periods of from two to four hours during the intervals of the paroxysms. It is often necessary, and I may say, generally well to premise this course, by some gentle cathartic. I have sometimes relieved the pain and cut short the paroxysms by a pill of two grains of extract of hyos-cyamus alone.

" If the distinction is properly drawn between neuralgia and those affections only involving the neurilemma, and a sedative anodyne, instead of an excitant anodyne used in connection with quinine, this disease will cease to be an opprobrium to medical science, and its treatment will become much more sat- sactory to the practitioner as well as to the patient."—[*N. J. Med. Reporter.*

Letters upon Syphilis. Addressed to the Editor of L'Union Medicale, by P. Ricord. Translated from the French by D. D. SLADE, M. D.

FIRST LETTER.

My Dear Friend,—The modern doctrine upon syphilis meets the lot of every scientific discovery. For nearly twenty years I have sought by my teachings and by works to infuse this doctrine into the minds of my cotemporaries. I see, however, that it is not equally understood by all the world; certain adversaries still raise objections, which I have refuted a hundred times; and more curious still, certain others take up objections started by myself, and imagine, a little ingeniously, perhaps, to subdue me by arguments which I have introduced into this discussion. At this I am neither astonished nor indignant. I find in it, on the contrary, a new incentive to continue my task, and far from complaining of my adversaries, I shall thank them rather for not suffering my zeal to languish, by thus keeping it awakened. Therefore, I ask of you permission to give to the world, through the columns of your widely-spread Journal, the true doctrines of the "Hopital du Midi." I ought to tell you that it is more a general exposition, that I intend to make, than a special reply. Upon my path I shall meet with objections, and I shall try to answer them. I shall preoccupy myself also as far as I ought, with a recent publication from the pen of one of our fellow- laborers, who to find followers had no need of going to seek them modestly "en Province." I present to you, my dear friend, a preliminary reflection induced by the publication of which I have just made mention. Although it is not given to an obser- ver to see all the facts of one entire department of pathology, and to establish a general system, we must not conclude that this observer has not seen, done or established anything that his studies and his researches ought to be regarded as useless, and that we ought to hold his teachings as nothing.

This manner of philosophizing in medicine, perhaps a little too common at the present day, is convenient and expeditious, but it is neither true nor just. In syphilography especially, this manner of proceeding would lead to deplorable errors. A serious study of our art demands more moderation in language, more justice in appreciation. For myself, I am pleased to recognize and to say, that far from disdaining everything in syphilographic literature, those who know how to search for them can find worthy and curious observations, good precepts, even sometimes doctrinal whims which, in discrediting their source, no one thinks worthy to exhume. Certainly the long discussions upon mercury, guaiacum, sarsaparilla, are not entirely void of utility. Light can be thrown upon the history of blenorrhagia by the observations of those who have preceded us. Without doubt the spirit of charlatanism and of speculation have left too frequent traces of their passage, but you will find often the marks of judicious minds, of a true scientific tendency and praiseworthy efforts to arrive at a classification and a doctrine. These works, if they had no other interest than that of giving the ideas and opinions of past times, would not merit the disdain, in my opinion unjust, which some have wished to throw upon them. I shall say the same of modern observers. The critic, I know and I think to have proved it, finds frequent opportunities to exercise himself upon their works. But is that saying that we should hold them of no account? Far from me this unjust thought. On the contrary I hold in great estimation the works of Bell, of J. Hunter, and of Swediaur; the time has come to render complete justice to Culleriar, to M. Lagneau especially, whose reputation was legitimately popular, in fine to all those industrious and intelligent laborers in our science who by conscientious studies have with difficulty opened the road in which we can march more freely. Would I be unjust towards my cotemporaries? Heaven forbid, dear friend. Whatever may be our differences, it is with pleasure and spontaneously that I render the most sincere homage to the works of MM. Baumes, Gibert, Cazenave, Cullerier neveu, Bottex, Ratier, Puche, Diday, Reynaud, Payan, Lafont Gouzi, Venot, in France; of Wallace, Carmichael, Babington, and of my pupils Acton and Meric in England; Thiry, Herion, in Belgium; to the remarkable publications of laborious Germany and industrious Italy. I do not feel any sentiments of injustice or of hatred either towards the past or towards the present. You will excuse me from declaring this very distinctly before entering upon my subject. I explicitly say that I do not partake in any way the opinion of those unreasonable critics to whom ancient and modern syphilographic literature is but trash unworthy of attention. I believe, on the contrary, that this branch of pathology is as fertile as any other in useful works and in valuable researches. However, the labors of ancients and moderns could not preserve this portion of our science from the general

revolution brought upon medicine by the physiological doctrine.
The school of Broussais, in blotting out the past, had again
questioned everything. Was there a syphilitic virus? The
virole, did it exist? You know how physiologism resolved
these questions. The greatest confusion reigned in the science,
and was introduced into the publications of the times. Doubt
was everywhere, certainty nowhere. It was at this time, that
having become by "Concours" surgeon of the central bureau
of hospitals, chance caused me to enter the hospital "du Midi."
There I encountered a man, honest and loyal, a practitioner
earnest and strict, M. Cullerier, who abandoning the traditions
of family, so to speak, took upon himself to doubt his own observations, and appeared no longer to believe in that which he
had seen. Everywhere doubt had taken the place of belief.
The cause of syphilis was doubted, its effects also, and, in consequence, its therapeutics. And remark, that which they called
the modern doctrine was presented surrounded by much scientific display. M. Richond des Brus had written an enormous
book filled entirely with facts; M. Desruelles supported new
ideas upon statistics, which passed for being indisputable; all
exerted themselves from the desire to combat the speciality of
the disease, and the remedy. History was made to contribute
largely by a very learned writer of our century, who in one of
the most remarkable works of our time amused himself with
taking the observers " corps à corps," and placing them in opposition with themselves. An easy triumph, if the critic, in a severe
and partial analysis, does not know how to establish a marked
difference between the author's own ideas, those which result
from his researches from his own observations, and those which
he draws from the scientific medicine of his day. The former
are useful materials and worthy of preservation, the latter constitute the prejudices of the epoch, and have no historical value.
Jourdan did not make this distinction; it sufficed for him to combat the speciality of syphilis, to show the confusion in the contradictory opinion of our predecessors, and this he did with a
profuseness of learning which would have been extolled in a
sounder critic.

Such, then, was the state of minds and of science when I
entered the Hospital "du Midi." For some there was a destroyed edifice to rebuild; for others, at least, it was to be consolidated. That which was especially necessary was to take
up again the study of the cause of syphilis. Is there a special
cause, a virus? or do venereal accidents spring from a common
cause? For this research and study, two modes of investigation were offered to me. The first was the simple observation
of phenomena, that observation which our predecessor **had**

practised, and which had conducted them to opinions so different ; to observation similar to that of Devergie, analogous to
facts already reported by Vigaroux, by Bugny, &c. ; to that
observation, for example, relative to three officers, who had connection with the same young female suffering from a discharge
and who all three found themselves infected, the one with an
urethritis, the second with a chancre, and the third with vegetations. It is true that Devergie has deprived history of a slight
information—that of the precise state in which he found this
young woman, whom he had not examined with the speculum.
Evidently this mode of investigation was worn out, and could
only conduct to barrenness or confusion of results. The second
mode satisfied my mind better ; in other respects it was more
in conformity with the demands of modern science ; it seemed
to me to open a sure way to study, and to conduct to incontestable results. I mean experimentation. I proposed to myself
the following obligations : To follow the cause of syphilis to a
known source ; to place it upon a region visible and easy to
observe ; to note the effects.

You see, experimentation alone could fill these conditions.
But already experimentation had been consulted, and through
it contradictory conclusions had been arrived at. When J.
Hunter said yes—Carru, Bru, Jourdan, Devergie and M. Desruelles said no. To what could such different conclusions be
owing, after the employment of the same method of investigation. I did not know then, but I have learned since. That
which my reason convinced me then, was that experimentation
well and accurately made, ought to conduct to precise results,
and that the differences of experimenters should not discourage
me. These researches were difficult and delicate. Conviction
was necessary, and I say it also, courage, to undertake them.
It was necessary to be sure of thoroughly appreciating the conditions in which I was about to act ; it was neceseary to aid
myself by antecedent experimentations ; it was especially necessary to support myself upon the purity of my intentions, and
upon the testimony of my conscience. I was not contented, in
fact, with the great name of Hunter, with the experimenters
cited by Bell, with the work of Hernandez, although crowned
by the Academy of Besançon ; with the authority of Percy, and
other great names as recommendable : but I wished to study
the question in itself, to place myself in the condition of a true
inventor, in order to take upon myself all the responsibility of
the results.

How was it necessary to proceed to this experimentation ?
I could inoculate a healthy individual from a patient. I could
experiment upon the patient himself. The first mode, that is

the inoculation of a healthy individual from a patient, appeared
to me one that should be always rejected by the physician.   I
do not think that we have the right to make such experiments.
Not only the physician cannot make use of his natural authority to induce an individual to undergo experiments of this nature
but I think that the physician ought to resist against the wishes
of those, who seduced by a generous devotion, wish to volunta-
rily expose themselves to the risk of experimentation.   I do not
cast any blame upon those who have acted differently.   I repeat, only, that, for me, I did not wish to proceed in this way.

The experimentation upon the patient himself remained—
would this offer inconveniences and dangers for the patient?
In case it did not, would it conduct to conclusive results?
Here is what history, observation, and experience learned me
in this respect.   It was generally admitted that a first contagion would not prevent a second, and the old proverb of " virole
sur virole " had yet all its authority.   We know to-day what
this means.   As to the inconveniences and the dangers, we see
every day that it is rare that the primary accidents are isolated,
that they multiply themselves with great rapidity, and that, to
speak explicitly, the gravity of the disease is not in relation to
the number of these accidents.   Thus, to throw light upon such
an important question of etiology and of practice, art could without inconvenience, do that which nature constantly does.   A
much more important question presented itself here.   The
grave and consecutive accidents of infection being feared,
ought they to be in accordance with the number of primitive
lesions.   Strict observation, and the clinical observation of all
times, has proved and proves every day, that the constitutional virole is not in ratio with the number of primitive accidents,
existing at the same time and developed at the same epoch.   Onè
accident more does not add any more chance of infection—*if*
we know how to direct the experimentation.

The question of surface remained, to know if an extensive
ulceration exposes more to a general infection than an ulceration of small size.   Well, here again observation has shown
that a more or less extent of primitive ulceration has no influence upon the production of consecutive accidents.   A very
small chancre exposes just as much to a general infection as a
very extensive one ; and *vice versa*, a large ulceration exposes
neither more nor less than a small one.   In fine, the question of
the seat of the ulceration remained, of the place of election for
experimental inoculations.   It had been said by Boerhaave,
among others, that venereal accidents contracted in other ways
than by the genital organs, presented a very great gravity ; but
clinical observation proved to me, and it has shown me since,

that this opinion was erroneous. I well know that upon this point a great noise has been made of diseases contracted by physicians, by midwives, in consequence of examinations, of wounds, &c. There are very good reasons, but I do not wish to point them out here, why these accidents should give rise to a great commotion. What I can say without injuring any rules of propriety, is, that the men of art to whom these accidents happen, have no motive to conceal them, while common people attacked by syphilis have always strong motives to keep quiet.

I rested, then, convinced that the seat of the ulceration could have no unfavorable influence upon the production of consecutive accidents, but even that it could diminish or annihilate certain grave consequences, such as the production of buboes. Thus observation had already proved that the primary chancres of the thigh were almost never followed by enlarged glands, and in fact in my numerous experiments, I have never seen enlarged glands follow from the punctures of inoculation upon the thigh.

Thus, my dear friend, by history, by clinical observation of all times, by experimenters who had preceded me by the testimony of my own conscience strictly interrogated, I arrived at this encouraging conclusion. In experimenting upon the patient himself I did not communicate another disease. I did not increase the gravity of the accident by which he was already attacked. I did not expose him more to the chances of a consecutive infection.

These first and capital conditions being ascertained, it was necessary to search out those which offered to science and art all the guarantees to be desired. An explanation upon this point will be the subject of my second letter.—[*Boston Med. and Surg. Journal.*

On the employment of the Iodide of Sodium in the Treatment of Secondary Syphilis. By Dr. DAVERI.

Notwithstanding the great success which has attended the employment of the iodide of potassium in the treatment of venereal disease, its disagreeable taste, and the gastric irritation it sometimes gives rise to, induced Dr. Daveri to try how far the iodide of sodium might be advantageously substituted for it. In the nineteen cases of secondary syphilis affecting the bones and periosteum, in which he has employed it, he has found it equally beneficial, while it is far more palatable. It is also borne in larger doses, and these can be more rapidly increased ; so that the duration of the treatment is abridged. Some cases

which proved rebellious, or only slowly yielded to the iodide
of potassium. have been rapidly cured by the soda preparation.—[*Bulletino delle Sc. Med.   Brit. & For. Med. Chir. Rev.*

*On the mode of Termination of the Nerves in the Skin of the
    Fingers* By Dr. RUDOLPH WAGNER.

This celebrated physiologist has recently been making the
distribution of the nerves in the skin of the tactile extremities of
the fingers his peculiar study ; and has communicated the following results of his inquiries to the Royal Society of Göttingen.
What are usually called the tactile papillæ are of two kinds
—namely, *vascular* papillæ, which only contain capillary loops ;
and *nervous* papillæ, which are placed between them.   These
last have a conical form ; and each of them contains in its interior a peculiar corpuscle, also of conical form, which receives
the finest of the nervous fibrils that enter the papilla.   Each
primitive nerve-fibre divides into a great number of smaller
branches, to which these tactile corpuscles are attached ; and
thus each is connected with several corpuscles.   It is further
considered by Wagner that each single fibre conducts the impression made upon any of these branches to a certain spot in
the nervous centres ; and that thus but a single sensory impression is produced, whether the corpuscles supplied by any one
fibre are touched separately, or all together.—[*Gaz. Med.   Ib.*

*On the Influence of the Sympathetic Nerves on Sensibility, and
    on Calorification.* By M. CL. BERNARD.

This industrious experimenter has recently communicated tó
the Societé de Biologie two very remarkable results of his experiments on the sympathetic nerve, which we believe to be
altogether new.   It has long been known that section of the
cerebro-spinal nerves tends to diminish the temperature of the
parts which they supply ; and in the case of the pneumogastrics,
to lower the temperature of the body generally.   But, according to M. Cl. Bernard, when the trunk which unites the sympathetic ganglia of the neck is cut through on one side, the temperature on that side of the face undergoes a remarkable *increase*
which is not only perceptible to the hand, but which shows
itself in a thermometer introduced into the nostrils or the ears,
to the amount of from 7° to 11° (Fahr.)   When the superior
cervical ganglion of the sympathetic is removed, the same effect is produced, but with yet greater intensity.   This difference
is maintained for many months, and is not connected with the

occurrence of inflammation, congestion, œdema, or any other pathological change in the part. The effect is not prevented by section of any of the other nerves of the face, whether sensory or motor.

A not less unexpected effect is produced by division of the sympathetic upon the *sensibility* of the parts supplied by it: for this, instead of being diminished, is greatly augmented. As the appreciation of this fact, by ordinary methods, is difficult, M. Bernard had recourse to the woorara poison, the effect of which is to produce a gradual destruction of sensibility over the whole body ; and he found, that when the cervical ganglion had been removed, the whole of that side of the face retained its sensibility much longer than did any other part of the surface.

[*Gaz. Med. Ib.*

Injections of Salt in Intoxication. By M. LALAUX. .

The difficulty with which intoxication is sometimes distinguished from comatose cerebral affections, renders valuable the possession of a simple means of at once aiding the diagnosis and dissipating the symptoms. This, M. Lalaux declares, exists in the administration of an injection of warm water containing two tablespoonfuls of salt. He explains the benefit derived by the partial evacuation of the poison in the copious stools that are promptly produced. The injection also sometimes induces vomiting, when mechanical irritation of the fauces has failed to do this.—[*Gaz. de Hop. Ib.*

Wild Cherry Bark. By JOSEPH S. PEROT, of Philadelphia.

This bark being undoubtedly an important article to the physician, I undertook a few experiments with a view towards ascertaining at what season its properties (which depend principally for their efficacy on the amount of prussic acid which it will yield) exist in greatest perfection, and consequently when the bark is best adapted for collection. For this purpose I procured at intervals during the season at which it is brought to market for sale, portions of the inner bark from the same tree, (or from trees of apparently the same age,) and from portions of the largest branches of about the same age, which, being carefully dried and deprived of the epidermis, were bruised, macerated for a short time with water, and distilled in a close vessel; the product was treated with a weak solution of nitrate of silver, which, reacting with the prussic acid in the solution, formed a precipitate of cyanide of silver ; this being carefully washed, dried and weighed, the quantity of hyodrocyanic acid in each portion of bark was estimated by the ratio of chemical equivalents, The distillate was also treated with a strong alkaline solution, and afterwards with a weak solution of nitrate of silver in the manner proposed by M. Liebig, (See American Journal of Pharmacy, vol. xxiii., p. 253,) but the results coinciding very closely with those obtained by the former process, it was deemed unnecessary to enumerate them.

The results obtained from these experiments, with the dates at which the bark was collected, may be seen by the following statement.

1000 grains of Bark collected April 1st, 1851, yielded .478 grains Prussic Acid.
1000 "   "   "   May 20th,   "   .856   "   "   "
1000 "   "   "   June 18th,   "   1·007 "   "   '
1000 "   "   "   August 28th,   "   1·134 "   "   "
1000 "   "   "   October 16th, "   1·436 "   "   "

The bark used in the preceding experiments was taken from a flourishing tree in Philadelphia county.

1000 grains of bark collected May 23d, from the trunk of a tree in Jersey, yielded ·876 grains of prussic acid.

1000 grains collected June 13th, from the trunk of the same tree, yielded 1·159 grains.

In order to ascertain how the bark which has been kept on hand for a length of time compares with that freshly collected, I made an experiment about the middle of October upon some bark which had been collected during the previous spring, and found 1000 grains to yield ·567 grains of prussic acid.

It being the opinion of several eminent members of the medical profession, that this bark contained also phloridzin, a principle known to exist in the bark of the apple and of some other fruit trees, to the possession of which they supposed its tonic property might be owing, I made a number of experiments in the manner directed for the preparation of phloridzin, both upon old specimens of bark, upon fresh bark of the branches and trunk of the trees, and upon fresh bark taken from the root under ground, at several successive times, but in all instances failed completely to detect any indications whatever of the principle sought.—[*Amer. Jour. Pharm.*

On Peach-Leaf Water. By Messrs. FELLENBERG AND KÖNIG.

The authors distilled in 1847 and 1848, peach-leaves with water, and the difference in the proportions of prussic acid in these two sorts of water was very considerable. The leaves which yield the smaller proportion of prussic acid, were those of the year 1848, when the tree had an abundance of fruit, whilst in the year 1847, it had only one fruit. Mr. Konig in Bern, found in 1000 parts of a peach-leaf water, prepared by himself, 1·407 of prussic acid. That prepared by Fellenberg, in 1848, contained in 1000 parts, 0·437 parts.—[*Lond. Pharm. Journ.,* from *Central Blatt.*

[These facts are interesting in connection with the observations of Mr. Perot.—*Ed. Am. Jour. Pharm.*]

Improved Mode of Preparing Cafeine. By H. J. VERSMANN, Apothecary, Lubeck.

All the authors have prepared cafeine from good Brazilian coffee, and have operated on quantities of five, ten, and one hundred pounds. In the preparation of cafeine, the direction is usually given to boil the raw coffee-berries, to combine it with oxide of lead, and then to separate it by sulphuric acid. This plan the author has tried, but has found it rather unprofitable; and has gained but little profitable results. By the boiling, the gum, and the mucus with which the oil is combined in coffee, were dissolved, and the separation of the pure caffein is rendered difficult. On the other hand, he recommends the following process, as simple and suitable to the purpose:—Ten parts of bruised coffee are mixed with two parts of caustic lime, previously converted into hydrate of lime. This mixture is placed in a displacement apparatus, with alcohol of 80°, until the fluid which passes through no longer furnishes evidence of the presence of caffein. The coffee is then roughly ground, and brought nearly to the state of a powder, and the refuse of the already once digested mixture from the displacement apparatus dried, and ground again, and mixed with hydrate of lime, is once more macerated. The grinding is more easily effected after the coffee has been subjected to the operation of alcohol, having lost its horny quality, and the cafeine is thus certainly extracted. The clear alcoholic fluid thus obtained is then to be distilled, and the refuse in the retort to be washed with warm water to separate the oil. The resulting fluid is then evaporated until it forms a crystalline mass, which is to be placed on a thick filter and the moisture expressed. The moisture, after evaporation, still furnishes some cafeine. The impure cafeine is freed from oil by pressure between folds of blotting paper, and purified by solution in water with animal charcoal, and is afterwards obtained in shining white, silky crystals. In general, not more than three drachms were procured from five pounds of coffee, from ten pounds seven drachms, and from one hundred pounds, the largest quantity, viz: six ounces and four scruples of caffein ; a proof that a large quantity must be operated upon if, in a quantitative respect, a satisfactory result is to be obtained. Thus it is seen, that good Brazilian coffee contains 0.57 per cent of caffein.   At the same time it may be observed that it contains about ten per cent. of a green liquid oil, and two per cent. of a yellow, firm fat (Palmtin.)—[*Phar. Journ. and Archiv der Pharmacie.   Ibid.*

Extractum Lobeliæ Fluidum.   By WILLIAM PROCTER, Jr.

Having had occasion to prepare a fluid extract of lobelia at the solicitation of a druggist, the following process was employed, which is based on the fact, that in the presence of an excess of acid, the lobelina of the natural salt which gives activity to the drug is not decomposed and destroyed by the heat used, as explained on a former occasion, (vol. xiv. page 108 of this Journal.)

Take of Lobelia (the plant) finely bruised,   eight ounces, (troy)

Acetic acid	one fluid ounce.
Diluted alcohol	three pints.
Alcohol	six fluid ounces.

Macerate the lobelia in a pint and a half of the diluted alcohol, previously mixed with the acetic acid, for twenty-four hours ; introduce the mixture into an earthen displacer, pour on slowly the remainder of the diluted alcohol, and afterwards water until three pints of tincture are obtained ; evaporate this in a water bath to ten fluid ounces, strain, add the alcohol and when mixed, filter through paper.

Each teaspoonful of this preparation is equal to half a fluid ounce of the tincture.   It may be employed advantageously to make a syrup of lobelia, by adding two fluid ounces of the fluid extract, to ten fluid ounces of simple syrup, and mixing.   Syrup of lobelia is an eligible preparation for prescription use, in cases where lobelia is indicated as an expectorant.—[*Ibid.*

New Symptom of Pneumonia.   By WM. M. BOLING, M. D., of Montgomery, Alabama.

I have frequently observed in pneumonia a symptom of which I do not remember to have seen mention made by any other, and which I have never noticed in any other disease.   It consists in a deposition on the teeth, just along the margin of the gums, of a matter of different shades of colour, from a light

orange to a dull vermilion, forming a line about the sixteenth
of an inch wide, and of a deeper tint at the gums, and paler as
it recedes.   Unlike the blue line said to be found in the margin
of the gums in lead poisoning, and the line on the same part, of
a deeper shade than the rest of the gum, noticed by Dr. Theophilus Thompson in phthisis, and mentioned in the London
Lancet, for September 1851.   The appearance in question is
seated on the teeth ; from which, indeed, with care, it may be
principally removed by wiping, though, occasionally, a somewhat durable stain remains upon the enamel.

In regard to the manner of its production, I am at a loss for
an explanation, though it is probably an exudation from the
margin of the gums.   At first I thought it might be produced
by the deposition of the colouring matter of the expectoration,
but I have seen it in cases in which bloody matter was not
expectorated ; indeed, in a few cases of latent pneumonia,
where there was neither cough nor expectoration ; and, in one
instance, I was led to suspect the presence of this form of the
disease, which I ascertained with certainty by auscultation, by
this symptom alone.   Perhaps the miasmatic poisoning of the
system may, in some way, lead to its development in pnemo-
nia ; for it is likely, that, if it were of as frequent occurrence
in other localities as in this, it would have been noticed before.
Still, I do not remember to have seen it in any of the forms of
uncomplicated miasmatic fever.

I have made no note of the proportion of cases in which I
have observed it, but I think, at least, in one-third or one-fourth.
The cases in which it is present are generally severe, it being
very rarely found in mild cases.—[*Am. Jour. of Med. Science.*

Iodine Clysters in the Treatment of Dysentery.

Dr. Eimer believes that the great point to which practitioners have to direct their attention, is the enormous amount of
organic losses consequent on the continuance of this affection ;
so that according to Œsterlen,* within three weeks, more than
the entire blood-mass may pass away as albumen in the stools.
As a means of cutting these discharges short, he strongly *re*-
commends iodine clysters ; which, in recent cases, may at once
arrest the progress of the disease, and in all diminish the number of stools, and normalize their condition, whatever the individual peculiarities of the case may be.   From five to ten grains
of iodine, and as much iod. pot., are administered in two or
three ounces of water, from two to four times a-day—twice

* See British and Foreign Medico-Chirurgical Review, vol. v. p. 245.

daily usually sufficing. If the rectum is too irritable to retain
it, ten or fifteen drops of tr. opii are to be added, and a mucilaginous vehicle substituted for water. In spite of unfavorable
conditions, so constantly successful did Dr. Eimer find this remedy during an epidemic, that he believes the disease will, as a
general rule, be found curable by it, if it be resorted to before
the organic changes in the intestine have advanced too far, exhaustion become too considerable, or important complications
set up. In some slight cases it was employed alone. Generally, a simple oily emulsion was also administered, and sometimes
acetate of lead and opium.—[*B. and F. Med. Chirurg. Rev.*,
from Henle's Zeitschrift. Amer. Jour. Med. Science.

Starch in Cutaneous Diseases.

M. Cazenave has lately employed, largely, powdered starch,
pure or mixed with oxide of zinc or camphor, in various diseases of skin. In acute eczema, impetigo, herpes, acne rosacea,
after washing the parts with a weak alkaline solution, and well
drying them, some of the following powder is sprinkled, viz :
Oxide of zinc, one part ; starch powder, fifteen parts. In pru-
rigo of the axillæ, the anus, or the genitals, a quarter part of
camphor is added.—[*Med. Times and Gazette, from L'Union
Medicale. Ib.*

Solution of Nitrate of Silver in Pruritus of the Genital Organs.

Winternitz has lately recommended a solution of nitrate of
silver (grs. iii ad $\frac{3}{i}$ aquæ) in pruritus of the vulva or scrotum.
The solution is applied three times daily, and two cases are
given in which it succeeded after a fortnight's trial, when all
other means had failed.—[*Ibid.*, from *Zeitschrift der Gesell. der
Arzte zu Wien, from Ibid.*

Cauterization of the Glottis in Whooping-Cough.

M. Joubert has published the results of his experience of this
mode of treating whooping-cough. He has treated in all 98
cases in this manner, but he excludes 30 of these as not being
worthy of reliance. The remaining 68 cases he divided into
three series, according to the period at which the treatment was
commenced. Of these, the general results were, that in 40 the
cure was rapidly effected, in 21 a marked relief was experienced, and in 7 cases only the treatment failed altogether.[—*Prov.
Med. and Surg. Journ. Ib.*

Influence of Medicine on the Temperature of the Body.

MM. Dumaril, Demarquay, and Lecomte have associated themselves together for the purpose of inquiring into the effect of medicines on temperature. Their experiments were made on dogs. To state the results briefly, they found that cantharides, in doses of from one to six grains, raised the temperature in six hours nearly 4° Fahr.; canella, in a dose of from eight to ten drachms, elevated the temperature 3° Fahr.; and a second dose raised 2° more. One drachm of secale cornutum in five hours increased the temperature about 1½° Fahr. Acetate of ammonia injected into the veins augmented also the temperature; put into the stomach, it produced the same effect in a less degree. Phosphorus, in doses of a grain and a-half to three grains, lowered the temperature. Strychnine produced no effect.

Certain purgatives were tried, such as colocynth, castor oil, etc., the effects varied according to the dose; usually it was lowered, and then elevated to about 1½° Fahr. above the standard.

Emetics—as ipecacuanha, sulphate of copper—produced in small doses a little elevation; but, in large doses, lowering of temperature to the extent of 2° or 3° Fahr.—[*Med. Times and Gazette*, from *L'Union Medicale*, from *Ibid.*

On Chloroform as an Emmenagogue. By DAVID H. GIBSON, M. D., Fort Towson, Choctaw Nation.

Having nowhere seen, in the course of my professional reading, any allusions made to the use of chloroform, as an emmenagogue, I am induced to submit the following facts for publication, partly from a desire that relief may be afforded to the suffering, and partly from a sense of professional duty.

CASE I and II. Occurring in the same person. In October last, Mrs. W——, having a violent headache, to obtain relief resorted to the inhalation of chloroform. Within an hour after the inhalation (which was but for a few seconds) she was flowing freely, and continued thus for *four days*. There was no irregularity of the function of menstruation in the succeeding month (Nov.), but another attack of headache supervening, she again had recourse to the chloroform, and in a half hour the menstrual secretion made its appearance, the discharge continuing for *five* days. In both instances, the chloroform was inhaled about ten days after the subsidence of her regular periods. Since the last inhalation, she has menstruated at her usual period. Mrs. W—— is slightly inclined to plethora, general health usually good, aged thirty-five years.

Case III. In the absence of Mrs. W——, from home, her servant girl, having gotten hold of the chloroform, imitated Mrs. W.'s example. A like result was produced upon the girl, who menstruated for four days. The girl is very healthy and about thirty years of age. The inhalation was never renewed by her. In this case, the chloroform was inhaled two weeks prior to her usual period, at which time she again menstruated. Since then she has menstruated regularly.

Case IV. Miss ——, aged 19—general health excellent—no deviation having ever taken place since her first menstrual period, was, during a visit to Mrs. ——, induced to inhale chloroform, through curiosity to experience the sensations produced by it. In a half hour the menstrual fluid made its appearance and the flow continued for four days. The inhalation in this instance was ten days antecedent to the regular period, with which it did not interfere. Mrs. W——, my informant in regard to the foregoing cases, is an intelligent and reliable lady.

Case V. Came under my immediate observation. Was called to see Mrs. H——, found her suffering much from suppressed menstruation. To relieve urgent pain, ordered hot hip-bath, from which the patient experienced much relief. Waited three hours after the use of the bath, without recourse to any other means, having decided, as this was an opportune case, to exhibit the chloroform, which was done for *thirty* seconds. In *twenty* minutes after its administration, the patient was flowing freely and continued to do so for three days. Patient is of a weakly constitution, the result of much hardship. Age of the patient, about forty years. This case is the more remarkable from the fact that the patient has not menstruated for more than *eight* months.

The suppression was induced by causes not deemed necessary to relate at present. Prior to the suppression, she had been very regular for many years. Pregnancy has nothing to do with the case, as the patient is not at this time, nor for many years past has she been in that condition.

I regret that I have not a greater number of cases to submit for the consideration of the profession. Being but a young practitioner, I am desirous that more experienced physicians should give the chloroform a trial, in order more fully, than my position will allow, to test its value as an emmenagogue; and diffident of my ability to account *correctly* for the "modus operandi" of the chloroform in the above cases, I shall without comment submit them to those who have better opportunities for investigation.—[*Medical Examiner.*

Ligature of the Thyroid Arteries for Goitre.   Translated for
this Journal from the Journal des Connaissances Medico-
Chirurgicales.

Professor Porta has lately published in the Italian Journal,
Annali Universali di Medicina, a very remarkable case which
leads us to hope that Goitre will not always be incurable.   Ligature of one or the other, or even of both the superior thyroid
arteries has already been advised as a cure for this disease.
M. Porta thought that by ligating both the superior and inferior
thyroid arteries at the same sitting, success would be complete.
The following case, the first in which he had occasion to try
this plan, justifies his views.

CASE.   A young country woman of 17 years of age, presented herself at the surgical clinic of the University of Pavia, in
July, 1850, to be treated for a goitre about the size of an ordinary orange, situated upon the left side of the neck.   This
goitre had developed itself within the last two years : it pushed
the larynx and pharynx to the right ; from this resulted a fatiguing rattling in the throat and an impediment in swallowing.
The pulsations of the superior thyroid artery were distinctly
felt at the summit of the tumor, but those of the Inferior were
not.   As the tumor was circumscribed and the neck naturally
elongated, M. Porta thought that now or never was the time
to try the ligature of the arteries.

· On the 28th July, he began the operation by making a longitudinal incision about three inches in length between the sterno-
mastoid and sterno-thyroid muscles, as if for the purpose of
ligating the primitive carotid.   The inferior thyroid artery
being the most difficult to find, it was by this one he wished to
commence.   After having broken up the cellular tissue at the
inferior part of the incision with the finger, he could feel the
pulsations of the artery distinctly behind, and a little below the
base of the tumour, between the primitive carotid and the trachea.   Continuing to use his finger as a guide, he passed a
curved needle under the vessel and ligated it with a silk ligature.   The superior thyroid was discovered without difficulty,
at the upper angle of the incision, and ligated with a fine animal ligature.

The operation was followed by unexpected accidents.   There
was first an abscess, then hemorrhage, at the end of three weeks,
from the superior angle of the wound.   Cicatrization was not
complete until the end of October, that is, at the end of three
months.

The success of the operation in distroying the bronchocile
was entirely satisfactory.   As soon as the swelling from the

operation subsided, the tumour was perceived to have diminished one half, at the beginning of October, sometime before
cicatrization was complete, there remained no traces of it, that
is, there was no enlargement.

Tannate of Quinine.   By JOHN P. LITTLE, of Richmond, Va.

In the summer of 1850, I read a short paper before the Medical Society, in which I mentioned some experiments made to
remove the bitter and disagreeable taste of quinine.   It was attempted to remove this taste by giving the medicine dissolved
in strong tea ; and I was led to make these experiments by learning that coffee had been used for this purpose in France.   The
result of my experiment was that the taste was almost entirely
removed, and that the injurious effects upon the brain and nervous system, which so commonly result from the use of quinine,
did not make their appearance.   I learned subsequently, from
the experiments of Dr. Thomas, of Baltimore, that it was the
tannin contained in tea which produced this loss of bitterness.
Having for two years past prescribed tannin and quinine in all
cases requiring the use of the latter remedy ; having found this
tannate of quinine a more efficient preparation than the sulphate,
both in the treatment of intermittents and neuralgia ; and having seen none of those peculiar effects upon the head observed
ordinarily in the use of this article, I wish to call the attention
of the profession to its value.   I have by me a number of cases
in which benefit has resulted from its employment, where the
sulphate had been used without good effect, or where its use
could not be borne.   One case of intermittent, occurring in a
delicate child, in which I had used sulphate of quinine, various
vegetable tonics, iron, and finally Fowler's solution, without
any other than a temporary effect, yielded to this remedy.   In
many other cases of neuralgia occurring in very delicate women, where I was assured that quinine had been frequently
attempted to be given, and that its use could not be persevered
in becàuse of the headache and other severe symptoms that
ensued, I have given large quantities of the tannate with happy
effect on the disease and without any injurious result.   In some
very susceptible persons a slight ringing in the head was perceived, though not complained of, after a large quantity had
been taken.   My usual mode of administering the remedy is to
have it made into pills, containing two grains of quinine and
two of tannin each ; or, if the patient is very susceptible to the
action of the remedy, three grains of tannin to two of quinine.
I prefer it in pill form, because, in solution with so large a proportion of tannin, while the taste of the quinine would disappear,

that of the tannin would be very disagreeably perceived. In those cases of neuralgia where quinine and iron are indicated, I have not thought fit to combine quinine, iron and tannin in one pill, but have given on one day as much tannate of quinine alone as I would have given of quinine combined with iron in two days, and on the preceding day have also given as much iron alone as I would have given combined in two days.

This compound of tannin and quinine is also serviceable as an astringent in the dysentery of the season, and can be used as such with good effect. I mention its use, that others may be induced to try it, and that by the observation of many physicians, its claim to notice, as a compound of quinine that can be given without any injurious effect, may be decided upon. My own experience is in its favor.—[*Stethoscope.*

Miscellany.

New Theory of Tubercular Deposits.—Dr. M. Troy, of North Carolina, has written quite an interesting article upon tubercular deposits, in which, after a brief account of the opinions hitherto advanced in relation to the pathology, he adds:

"It now remains to state my own views of the nature of this deposit. It is with the greatest diffidence that I attempt what some of the greatest men who have ever adorned our profession have failed to accomplish, through a long life of patient toil and investigation, devoted to the subject. But they have cleared the way, and but little is left to do now but advance upon the smooth road they have made.

I consider tubercle to be the solid matter of the cutaneous excretion, especially of the sebaceous follicles. This secretion not being expelled by the natural emunctories, is retained in the blood until, in the attempt to eliminate it through an unnatural channel, it is deposited in some other excretory organ, where its fluid matter being absorbed, it becomes a tubercle."—[*Amer. Jour. Med. Science, July* 1852, *p.* 107.

Dr. T. then goes on to prove " that the secretion of the skin is of sufficient importance to produce this effect when retained," by a reference to its quantity, its constituents, and the acknowledged deleterious effects which follow its suppression or imperfect elimination, as well as the morbid condition of the skin in various affections in which this morbid condition is usually regarded rather as a complication than as a *cause* of the more obvious disease.

The following paragraph will serve to show Dr. T.'s conclusions:

" I think I have shown that the nature and importance of the secretion of the skin are sufficient to give rise by its deficiency of suspension to the accumulation of tuberculous matter in the blood; that in those individuals in whom consumption is hereditary, there is often a congenital deficiency of the sebaceous follicles ; that the disease can at any time be produced or aggravated by causes which depress their action ; and prevented or relieved by causes which exalt it ; that the only well-ascertained product of the secretory action of these follicles is found in large amount in tubercle ; and that it is deposited in precisely such situations as we would be led to suppose, upon general principles of physiology, that the retained secretions of the skin would be.

This theory has at least the merit of being consistent with all the phenomena of the disease ; of explaining the action of the causes which produce it upon established physiological principles ; of explaining its hereditary transmission by the same law which causes children to resemble their parents; of redeeming our practice from empiricism, and making it rational, and most important of all, of *explaining* the efficiency of hygienic means, and thus impressing the necessity of them more effectually than any amount of mere recommendation could do, even though this were founded upon the largest experience. It differs from the views of Andral and Carswell, by showing the nature and source of the " peculiar secretion, " of which they speak ; and seems, upon the whole, far more simple and definite than any other yet advanced. —[*Ibid p.* 116.

We regret that we have not room for the whole of this very original and ingenious paper.

On the Development of the Ductless Glands in the Chick. By HEN-RY GRAY, Demontrator of Anatomy at St. George's Hospital.—In this very meritorious paper, the author has demonstrated the evolution of the Spleen, Supra-renal and Thyroid gland, and the tissues of which each is composed, in such a manner as to show the place that may be assigned to each in a classification of the glands.

The *Spleen* is shown to arise between the fourth and fifth days, in a fold of membrane which connects the intestinal canal to the spine (the " intestinal lamina"), as a small, whitish mass of blastema, perfectly distinct from both the stomach and pancreas. This fold serves to retain it and the pancreas in connexion with the intestine. This separation of the spleen from the pancreas is more distinct at an early period of its evolution than later, as the increased growth of both organs causes them to approximate more closely, but not more intimately with one another ; hence probably the statement of Arnold, that the spleen *arises* from the pancreas. With the increase in the growth of the organ and the surrounding parts, it gradually attains the position that it occupies in the full-grown bird, in more immediate proximity with the stomach ; hence probably the statement of Bischoff, that it *arises* from the stomach. Later, when its vessels are formed, the membrane in which it was developed is almost completely absorbed.

The author then considers the development of the tissues of the spleen, which clearly establishes, not only the glandular nature of the organ itself, but the great similarity it bears with the supra-renal and thyroid glands.—The external capsule and the trabecular tissues of the spleen are both developed between the eighth and ninth days, the former in a form of a thin membrane composed of nucleated fibres, the latter consisting of similar fibres, which intersect the organ at first sparingly, and afterwards in greater quantity. The development of the blood-vessel and the blood are next examined. The former are shown to arise in the organ independent of those which are exterior to it. The development of the blood-globules is shown to arise from the blastema of the organ at the earliest period of its evolution, and continue their formation until its connexion with the general vascular system is effected, at which period their development ceases. No destruction of the blood-globules could ever be observed. These observations disprove the two existing opinions of the use of the spleen, as the blood disces are not formed there (excepting during its early development), as stated by Gerlach and Schäffner; nor are they destroyed there, as stated by Kollicker and Ecker. The development of the pulp tissue is next examined. At an early period, this closely corresponds with the structure of the supra-renal and thyroid glands at the earliest stages of their evolution, consisting of nuclei, nucleated vesicles, and a fine granular plasma, the former constituting a very considerable portion of its structure. When the splenic vessels are formed, many of these nuclei are surrounded by a quantity of fine, dark granules arranged in a circular form, and these increased up to the time when the splenic vein is formed, when nearly the whole mass is composed of nucleated vesicles, the nuclei of which gradually break up into a mass of granules which fill the cavities of the vesicles. The Malpighian vesicles are developed in the pulp by the aggregation of nuclei into circular masses, around which a fine membrane soon appears, in a manner precisely similar to those of the supra-renal and thyroid glands, with which they bear the closest analogy.

The author then traces out the development of the *Supra-renal glands,* and shows the close analogy that exists between them, the spleen, and thyroid, from the similarity which their structure presents at the earliest period of their evolution with those glands, and from the development of the several tissues following the same stages in all.—They are shown to arise on the seventh day as two separate masses of blastema, situated between the upper end of the Woolfian bodies, and the sides of the aorta, being totally independent (as concerns their development) of those bodies, or of each other. At this period, their minute structure bears a close resemblance to that of the spleen, consisting of the same elements as that gland, excepting in the existence of more numerous dark granules, which give to the organ, at a later period, an opaque and darkly granular texture. The gland tissue of the organ, in the form of large vesicles, makes its appearance on the eighth day, whereas in the spleen it did not exist until near to the close of incubation, an interesting fact in connexion with the function of the former gland, which is mainly exercised during fœtal life, whilst the spleen exerts its function mainly in adult

life : hence, the difference in the development of the tissues at different periods.   The manner in which this tissue is developed is similar
to that by which the gland tissue of the spleen was formed—viz : by
an aggregation of nuclei into circular masses, around which a limitary
membrane ultimately forms : these are first grouped together in a mass,
without any subdivision into cortical and medullary portions.   On
the fourteenth day the first trace of this subdivision becomes manifest,
by the vesicles being aggregated into masses which radiate from the
circumference towards the centre of the glands, in some cases complete tubes being formed by the junction of the vesicles, as indicated by
hemispherical bulgings along their walls.   At a later period, the organs
increase in size, they attain their usual position, and a more complete
subdivision into cortical and medullary portions is now observed.

The author lastly traces out the development of the *Thyroid* glands,
and shows the great similarity that exists between them, the spleen
and supra-renal glands, from the similar structure they present, and
from the development of those structures occuring in a similar manner in each.—These glands are developed between the sixth and
seventh days, as two separate masses of blastema, one at each side of
the root of the neck, close to the separation of the carotid and subclavian vessels, and between the trachea and the bronchial clefts, but
quite independent, as far as regards their development, of either of
those parts.   Their minute structure at an early period closely corresponds with that of the spleen and supra-renal glands.   Later, when
the gland-tissue, of which the thyroid gland ultimately consists, is
formed, it is developed in a manner precisely similar to the same tissues of the spleen and supra-renal glands—a fact which shows the
analogy they bear to one another.

From these observations, the author concludes that a close analogy
exists between the glands already described, so that the propriety of
their classification under one group, as the " Ductless Glands," may
be considered clearly proved.   And although the spleen by many has
been excluded from them, the author considers that its classification
with them is correct, for the following reasons :—1st. From its evolution being similar with that of the supra-renal and thyroid glands ;
2ndly, from its structure, which at an early period closely corresponds with them ; and 3rdly, from the development of its tissues following the same law as that upon which the tissues of the allied
glands are formed.—[*Proceedings of the Royal Society*, Jan. 15, 1852.

[Every contribution to the anatomy and physiology of these perplexing structures is of value, as tending to throw some light upon the
nature of their function ; and Mr. Gray has most ably filled up a la-
cuna which had been left by the many excellent anatomists who have
devoted their time and abilities to this perplexing and, as yet, profitless
inquiry.—[*Medico-Chir. Rev.*

*On the Changes producible in the Properties of Bodies by Pulveri-
zation.* By M. Dorvault.—To the present time, pharmacologists
have always considered pulverization as a mere change of form in

bodies—each particle of the divided body being regarded as a diminutive, without change of property, of the entire mass.   While admitting that, in most cases, this is a mere expression of the fact, M. Dorvault believes that there is a greater number of substances than is suspected, in which this operation induces a modification of their chemical characters and medicinal properties.   At present, he can only adduce two or three decided examples in justification of this opinion.   Every one knows that sugar, on being powdered, loses a portion of its solubility and sweetening power.   Is this referrible to an altered electrical condition of the sugar, as the phosphoresence which is developed during pulverization in the dark might lead us to suspect ?   Again, gum arabic, when powdered, possesses neither the same taste nor solubility as when entire ; and pulverization so diminishes the solubility of arsenious acid, that while a kilogramme of water will dissolve forty grammes in the vitreous state, it will only dissolve fourteen of the powder.   In the above examples, the modification is exhibited by diminution of solubility, but in other cases it may manifest itself in other directions.—[*L'Union Medicale.   Ibid.*

A new instrument for cauterizing the Urethra. By E. S. COOPER, M. D. Reported by L. C. Lane, M. D., of Peoria, Ill.—An instrument for cauterizing the urethra has been invented by Dr. Cooper of this place, which for facility of application and certainty of results is superior to all other means hitherto used, combined.

It consists of a copper catheter, with the end for half an inch a little smaller than the body, and perforated with several holes. This is introduced down to the stricture, and then filled with dilute nitric acid, which acting on the copper, soon produces the nitrate, which coming in contact with the urethra through the holes, produces cauterization to the extent desired.

The strength of the solution and the length of time the instrument is permitted to remain, regulates the degree of cauterization completely. Dr. Cooper generally uses one third of nitric acid, and two of water. and permits the instrument to remain for one and a half minutes, though a much shorter time will often answer.

The shape of the instrument may be varied to suit the case ; thus, when several strictures exist in the strait part of the urethra a strait catheter might be used, with holes at several places to correspond to their number and location.

Though great contrariety of opinion exists among medical men in regard to the degree of cauterization most valuable, this instrument commends itself alike to all ; for whether it is believed that caustics should be applied bodily so as to cause the detachment of a slough, and thus physically enlarge the canal, or by a slighter application modify the action of the lining, the variations are easily made with it.—[*Med. Exam. and Rec. of Med. Science.*

New Instrument for examining the interior of the Eye.—M. Follin, prosector of the Faculty of Medicine, in Paris, has presented to the

Surgical Society of that city, an ingenious instrument, by which the retina, crystalline lens, and different parts of the eye, may be examined. It consists simply of a wax candle placed behind a lens, by which luminous rays are thrown upon a mirror from which they are reflected into the eye. By means of an eye-glass, of varying power, placed behind the mirror, the bottom of the eye is seen, illumined and magnified. The light is mild, and of equal intensity on every part, and is of a yellowish color. The bloodvessels of the eye can thus be seen, forming a beautiful net work, and the blood within them distinguished. M. Follin has seen the vascular center of the retina, and recognized the point where the central artery and vein spread into branches. He thinks that by the aid of this instrument the different states of congestion of the retina can be distinguished, its ecchymotic and varicose states, the cancerous deposite which sometimes form upon its surface, &c., and also the condition of the crystalline lens.—[*N. Y. Med. Times.*

Test for the Purity of Cod liver Oil.—Sir James Murray, in calling attention to the numerous adulterations which are made by druggists, incidentally speaks of cod-liver oil, which is extensively falsified by the admixture of other oils, animal and vegetable. The test which he recommends was suggested to him by the knowledge that in a cotton factory the spindles which were made of brass always obtained a deposit of verdigris when a bad oil was used, which was not the case with pure spermacetti oil. The test consists in heating the suspected oil in a copper capsule ; if it be genuine cod-liver oil, no discoloration occurs, whereas the spurious oils throw up a quantity of the salts of copper, forming a green film on the surface.—[*Dublin Med. Press.*

Artificial Production of the Flavours and Odours of Fruits and Flowers.—One of the most surprising achievements of modern chemistry is the artificial production of the flavours and odours of fruits and flowers ; the imitation in the crude laboratory of the chemist of the most delicate of the productions of nature, and one which it might have been supposed was beyond the reach of art.

Dr. Playfair, in his lecture on the great exhibition of 1851, furnishes us with the following interesting information on this subject :—

" The jury in the exhibition, or rather two distinguished chemists of that jury, Dr. Hoffman and Mr. De la Rue, ascertained that some of the most delicate perfumes were made by chemical artifice, and not, as of old, by distilling them from flowers. The perfume of flowers often consists of oils and ethers, which the chemist can compound artificially in his laboratory. Commercial enterprise has availed itself of this fact, and sent to the exhibition, in the form of essences, perfumes thus prepared. Singularly enough, they are generally derived by substances of intensely disgusting odour. A peculiar fetid oil, termed " fusel oil, " is formed in making brandy and whiskey. This fusel oil, distilled with sulphuric acid and acetate of potash, gives the oil of pears. The oil of apples is made from the same fusel oil by distillation with sulphuric acid and bichromate of potash. The oil of pineapples is obtained from the product of the action of putrid cheese on sugar, or by making a soap with butter, and distilling it with alcohol and sulphuric acid, and is now largely employed in England in the preparation of pine-apple ale. Oil of grapes and oil of cognac, used to impart the flavour of French cognac to British brandy, are little else than fusel oil. The artificial oil of bitter almonds, now so largely employed in perfuming soap and for flavouring confectionery, is prepared by the action of nitric acid on the fetid oils of gas-tar. Many a fair forehead is damped with eau de millefleurs, without knowing that its essential ingredient is derived from the drainage of cowhouses. The winter-green oil, imported from New Jersey, being produced from a plant indigenous there, is artificially made from willows and a body procured in the distillation of wood. All these are direct modern appliances of science to an industrial purpose, and imply an acquaintance with the highest investigations of organic chemistry. Let us recollect that the oil of lemons, turpentine, oil of juniper, oil of roses, oil of copaiba, oil of rosemary, and many other oils, are identical in composition, and it is not difficult to conceive that perfumery may derive still further aid from chemistry."—[*Phila. Med. News.*

Bromohydric Ether—a new Anæsthetic Agent.—Some experiments have been recently made with this substance on birds, etc., and M. Ed. Robin, who conducted them, is satisfied that it will prove an excellent anæsthetic agent. This preparation of ether is without taste, and possesses an agreeable aromatic odor ; and, when taken by inhalation, produces rapid etherization, without any subsequent suffering or distressing symptoms.—[*Journ. des Connaiss. Med. Chirurg. and Charleston Med. Jour.*

Prescription for Chronic or Inveterate Intermittent Fevers.—We find in the "Journal des Connaissances Medico-Chirurgicales," the following old prescription which has been supplanted by quinine, but is now proposed to be revived in consideration of its real value in those old and inveterate forms of intermittent fever which we now and then find to return, although repeatedly "broken" with quinine. The formula was formerly highly recommended by the Montpelier School.

Pulverized Red Peruvian Bark, ... 40 scruples.
"   Rhubarb, ... 15 "
Muriate of Ammonia, ... 5 "
Syrup of Peach-tree Blossoms, ... 9 s.

Mix. Make a mass, and divide into 20 boluses, four of which must be taken daily for five days. They should be taken at intervals of one hour and so that the last will have been taken two hours before the expected paroxysm. If found to be too large the bolus may be subdivided.

Furunculoid Epidemic in England.—It appears that the great increase of "boils, carbuncles, whitlows, pustules, and superficial abscesses," in London, has attracted the attention of the Epidemiological Society, and that Mr. Hunt, at the request of the President of the Society, read a paper on this subject. Mr. H. states that he had found it prevailing in the British Isles, in France, Austria, the East and West Indies, the south of Africa, and the United States. - We have seen no notice of it in our country this year, although its prevalence last summer upon the fingers was noticed in Washington City and by ourselves in the April No. (p. 256) of this Journal. We think that whitlows are now more common here than usual. Furunculoid diseases have been on the increase in England ever since 1847. Mr. Hunt remarks, that the deaths from phlegmon have nearly trebled during the last few years, and that the fatality from small pox and pustular diseases have likewise been trebled of late. Carbuncles also have been very numerous and fatal in England.

Ricord's Letters on Syphilis.—We commence with this number, the publication of a series of Letters from the distinguished physician of the Parisian Venereal Hospital, and will furnish our readers with one in each of our subsequent issues. We feel assured that they will be read with interest, as containing the last and matured views of the best living authority on the subject. The lively and peculiar style of the letters will not detract from their intrinsic merit, but on the contrary, form a happy contrast with the very dry reading of the accompanying pages. They are being translated by different hands, for the New York Medical Times, and the Boston Medical and Surgical Journal, which saves us the trouble of doing so ourselves.

MOBILE, Alabama, July 26, 1852.

To the Medical Profession of the Southern and South-Western States :

Gentlemen—At the last annual meeting of the American Medical Association, I was continued as Chairman of a Committee, to report at its next session, on the prevalence of *Idiopathic* Tetanus, (not endemic, I as was erroneously notified by my first appointment). Permit me therefore to solicit your assistance, to the extent of your information, either from personal experience or enquiry, embracing the immediate circuit of your professional supervision. Your attention to the following queries and answers seriatim, forwarded by mail to my address, on or before the 1st day of January, 1853, will not only serve the special object of the Association, but particularly oblige,

Very respectfully, your ob't. serv't.,

A. LOPEZ.

1st. Are there any physical causes, in or about your locality, productive of Idiopathic Tetanus ?

2nd. Have changes by clearing of lands, change of culture, or any other circumstances, been the cause of such disease ?

3rd. Has Tetanus been of frequent occurrence, and if so, does it hold an analagous or independent origin of malarious diseases ?

4th. Does it follow the laws which govern climatic Endemics, in sufficient number, and simultaneous prevalence to warrant the belief of its identical origin ?

5th. Have meteorological variations governed the production and character of the disease ?

6th. The average number of deaths from Idiopathic Tetanus ?

7th. Have adults or children been most liable to its attack ?

8th. What sex ?

9th. Proportion of whites to negroes ?

10th. Duration of disease previous to fatality ?

11th. Interval between cause and development ?

12th. Does *Trismus Nascentium* ever observe an Idiopathic or symptomatic character ?

13th. Are negro or white children most liable to it ?

14th. Your belief as to its origin ?

15th. Proportion of deaths to cures ?

16th Have you found any form of treatment more successful than another, in either Idiophathic Tetanus or Trismus Nascentium ?

The Knoxville Primary Medical School went into operation on the 16th of Feb., with one pupil. Several applicants have been rejected because they did not possess the requirements designated as necessary before commencing the study of medicine by the American Medical Association. Others declined because not satisfied with the terms. —[*East Tennessee Record of Med. and Surg.*

BIBLIOGRAPHICAL.

We beg leave to return our thanks for a large number of publications received within the last two months, and regret that we have not room to give an extended notice of some of them. Among the most interesting, are " The Quarterly Summary of the Transactions of the College of Physicians of Philadelphia ;" the " Proceedings of the Medical Association of the State of Alabama ;" the " Report of the Eastern Lunatic Asylum in Virginia ;" the " Third Annual Report of the Board of Commissioners for the Georgia Asylum for the Deaf and Dumb ;" " Tableaux of New Orleans ;" and " Contributions to Experimental Physiology, by Bennet Dowler, M. D. ;" the " Proceed-ings of the 7th Annual Meeting of Medical Superintendants of American Institutions for the Insane ;" " A Lecture on Gun-shot Wounds, by R. McSherry, M. D., of Baltimore ;" " Observations on the freez-ing of Vegetables, &c., by Prof. John LeConte, of Georgia ;" " The

Topography, climate and Disease of Middle Georgia, by E. M. Pendleton, M. D., of Sparta ;" " Practicability of probing the fallopian tubes, by S. A. Cartwright, M. D., of New Orleans."

The Principles and Practice of Surgery—illustrated by 316 engravings, on wood. By WM. PIRRIE, F. R. S. E., Regius Professor in the Marischal College and University of Aberdeen, &c. &c., edited with additions, by JOHN NEILL, M. D., Surgeon of the Pennsylvania Hospital, &c. &c. Philadelphia : Blanchard & Lea. 1852. pp. 885.

Prof. Pirrie, although not as extensively known as some of the surgeons of the British metropolis, shows by the work before us that he is an able teacher and can make a good book for the use of Students and general practitioners. Being written expressly as a text-book for those in attendance on Lectures, it very properly combines both the Principles and the Practice of Surgery, instead of having separate works for each of these branches of study, as is the case with Prof. Miller's works. We predict for Pirrie's Surgery an extensive sale to students, while Miller's more elaborate productions will be most used by special practitioners of Surgery.

We agree with one of our most esteemed cotemporaries in seeing no objection to the American custom of appending notes or other matter to the reprint of British works, so long as by so doing the annotator adds to the intrinsic value of the work without increasing unreasonably its cost to the purchaser. Dr. Neill is " a growing man" and deserves well of the Profession for his talents and industry.

Pure Medicinal Extracts.—Messrs. Philip Schieffelin, Haines & Co., Druggists of New York, sent us some time since, a small collection of their Medicinal Extracts for trial, and we are happy to say that they have proved to be some of the very best we have ever used. We therefore take pleasure in recommending them. The difficulty of getting pure and fresh preparations of belladonna, cicuta, hyoscyamus, stramonium, &c., has long been felt seriously by the profession, and those who, like this firm, will contribute to remedy the evil, should be rewarded by extensive patronage. We presume that their choice extracts and powders, &c., can be obtained from any of our City Druggists.

Advertisements.—We have to remind our correspondents that no advertising sheet is appended to this Journal ; hence, the omission to attend to their requests.

SOUTHERN
MEDICAL AND SURGICAL JOURNAL.

Vol. 8.]   NEW SERIES.—OCTOBER, 1852.   [No., 10.

PART FIRST.

Original Communications.

ARTICLE XXXIV.

Typhoid Fever in East Alabama. By G. T. WILBURN, M.D., of Farmville, Alabama.

After so much has been written upon Typhoid fever, it may appear to some a labor of supererogation to attempt to add anything new, or to interest members of the profession, in a subject already exhausted. But we are fully aware that the multiplicity of articles upon this dreaded malady give evidence of the difficulty met with in its management. Every practitioner will readily testify to the embarrassment and difficulty he experienced in the treatment of typhoid and other fevers, when first he entered the medical arena. The so-called systems of Cullen, Brown, Broussais, Rasori, and a host of modern authors, seemed mere individual opinions, and calculated more to confuse than to enlighten the tyro in medicine. He examined, in vain, the "innumerable volumes of cases, and interminable heaps of insulated precedents," with the feeble hope of reconciling the inconsistencies of antagonistic systems, and of discovering the true principles of correct practice. And thus the young practitioner is bewildered by authors who write more for fame and a desire to propagate their own particular dogma than for the elucidation of truth and the advance of medical science.

It is objected to the term Typhoid, as not expressive of the anatomical lesions of the disease. A similar objection might be made to the terms designating other diseases. The terms Typhus, Intermittent, Remittent, &c., are not more happy. None of these appellations teach the anatomical lesions of the diseases they serve to designate. The term Typhoid, as applied to distinguish a certain class of fevers, we believe, first originated with Louis, of Paris. He discovered that the Parisian fevers were closely allied to each other by a uniformity of their lesions, the most constant of which were inflammation of the elliptical follicles, known as the glands of Bruner and Peyer, and a softened condition of the spleen. I do not say that the term Typhoid is the best that could have been selected, but as its signification is now sufficiently understood by the profession, medical science does not suffer in its retention.

There are some who contend that typhus and typhoid are identical, and others who even deny the existence of the latter disease. These (latter) know no other fevers than remittent, intermittent and continued—terms that express nothing, and consider all other fevers as but modifications of these types.

> 'Tis with our judgments as our watches; none
> Go just alike, yet each believes his own.

I believe typhoid fever to be a disease *sui generis*, differing essentially from all the fevers known to the world, in its attack, progress, lesions, symptoms, and termination; and requiring a treatment peculiar to itself. So long as practitioners look upon it as but a modification of remittent, intermittent, &c., or as identical with typhus, they may expect to fail in treatment, and to offer a considerable barrier to a clear knowledge of the disease and the progress of medical science. Physicians, above all others, should be free from dogmatical prejudices—their labors are continued researches after truth.

All American writers, with a careless or casual investigation, have followed English authors in the unity of continued fevers. It is as difficult to break down the despotism of literature as it was to sever the bands of political union. We yet yield a blind obedience to the teachings of our mother country.

To the identity of these fevers is due the great confusion among writers in giving the symptoms of typhoid fever. Many of the symptoms of the typhoid also belong to the typhus; but there are other symptoms which serve to distinguish these diseases. The terms Typhus Mitior and Typhus Gravior have contributed greatly to the difficulty in distinguishing the two diseases, and literally made confusion confounded. But let us examine these diseases impartially, and see if they be one and the same.

TYPHOID.

Stupor, accidental and developed slowly.

Subsultus, occasional—in many instances totally absent.

Loss of hearing slight, sometimes absent, and recollection but little impaired.

Tremors and spasmodic contractions of muscles rare, but dangerous symptoms when present.

The eyes bright, and slightly but not invariably reddened.

Congestion of the capillary vessels of the extremities slight.

The fœtor of exhalation slight even in severe cases.

Rose spots, few in number, often only six or eight, rarely more than thirty; rather larger, more elliptical, and more elevated, confined mainly to the abdomen, occasionally extending to the chest, thighs and upper parts of the arms, but not to the whole surface—not seen sooner than the eighth, nor later than the fifteenth day.

The intestinal inflammation acts as a positive disturbing cause.

Pulse, from 100 to 120, soft and compressible, often undulating so much as to become a true bis feriens pulse, varying but little during the course of each particular attack.

TYPHUS.

Stupor, a prominent symptom, almost pathognomonic—comatose at an early period.

Subsultus, present in nearly every case.

Loss of hearing considerable and almost invariable, and recollection greatly impaired—no distinct impression of what has taken place during confinement.

Tremors and spasmodic contractions of muscles frequent, but do not add to the gravity of the prognosis.

Conjunctivæ reddened from congestion.

Congestion so great as to give a bluish tint to the extremities.

Exhalation from the skin very peculiar and offensive, the smell almost pathognomonic of the disease.

Exanthema extends over the whole body, papulæ rounded, varying from a point to the eighth of an inch, occurs on the third day, continuing generally five days, occasionally twelve or fourteen days.

The intestinal disorder is limited to the indirect influence of the fever and the cerebral disturbance.

Pulse, from 100 to 140, and even 160—the variations are considerable.

Typhoid.	Typhus.
In the thorax of typhoid, congestion is limited mainly to the bronchial membrane, giving rise to sonorous and sibilant rhonchus.	In the thorax there is congestion of the substance of the lungs, as manifested in feeble respiration and sub-crepitant rhonchus.

By a careful examination of the symptoms, as presented in this tabular view, it will be plainly seen that the nervous and cerebral symptoms of typhus are much more developed than those of typhoid fever. Many points sub-judice I have purposely passed sub-silentio: one of the most important of these is the contagiousness of the two diseases. In the celebrated work of Tweedie, as revised by Dr. Gerhard, the latter remarks, that the diagnosis of typhoid and typhus fever is not often made in the United States, because the latter disease (typhus) has hardly appeared for the last twenty years, except on a few occasions in two or three large cities. He also remarks, that many of the symptoms of typhoid are similar to those of typhus fever, but follow a different order of development. To those who are not creed-bound these distinctions are sufficient to overturn the identity of these two diseases.

After having thus, as I confidently trust, thrown some doubt, at least, upon the minds of your readers as to the identity of typhoid and typhus, I would invite attention to a cursory review of the former disease and its treatment, as observed and practiced by the writer in Eastern Alabama.

The Typhoid fever first made its appearance in this section tion of country in the fall of 1850, and was very successfully treated by my co-partner, the late Dr. Thos. J. Welborn, I then being absent from the State. It continued to enlarge its circle until the first of June following, and gradually declined toward the first of July. I saw no case in the fall of 1851, though some few cases occurred, as I am informed, in the practice of other physicians around me. The first case of the fever I saw was on the first of June of the present year; the cases, however, have been few, though very malignant in character and stubborn in treatment.

This disease did not confine itself to negro cabins and the cottages of filth and wretchedness, but was a frequent visitor to the well ventilated and pleasant mansions of the opulent. In houses where cleanliness was strictly observed, yards and

under-houses well swept, the inmates well clothed and fed, excellent water, situated at considerable distances from creeks,
ponds and marshes, this fever attacked every member of the
families, as frequently and as malignantly as it did the dirty
hovels of negro quarters and cabins of the poor in marshy sections and otherwise unhealthy localities. (I do, by no means,
intend this remark as an argument in favor of filth, but as a
fact observed in my practice : perhaps, *minus in parvos morbus
furit, leviusque ferit leviora Deus.*)

The symptoms observed in these cases were nearly the
same, *cæteris paribus.* I prefer not to mention any other
symptoms, than those already stated, as peculiar to this disease, and which distinguish it from its great cousin-german,
Typhus fever.

The etiology of Typhoid fever is yet a mooted question—
the pathology somewhat settled. I have assisted in the post-
mortem examination of only one case of this fever. (Were it
not too great a digression, I should be pleased to express my
views of the superstitious prejudices of the country to post-
mortem examinations. The people need information upon this
point.) In this case, nothing new presented itself; softening
of the mucous membrane of the stomach and spleen, enlarged
mesenteric glands, thickening and ulceration of the elliptical
plates of the ilion. These anatomical lesions have been observed by nearly every one who has examined those who have
died of typhoid fever. There are other lesions occasionally
met with, which, however, are not peculiar to this disease, but
due to its complication with other maladies, such as softening
of the brain and hepatization of the lungs, &c.

Treatment.—I come now to the prime purpose of this article,—the treatment of typhoid fever. I never bleed from the
arm ;—venesection in this section is sure to seal the doom of the
patient. I see other practitioners adopting general bleeding
as a *sine qua non.* Dr. H. G. Davenport (N. O. Medical and
Surgical Journal, March 1852,) remarks: "In every case
which has come under my charge for the last five years, where
I have been called to them in the beginning, I have always bled,
having an eye to the age, constitution, etc., of the patient. I

have never seen any fatal consequences follow its use ; it lessens the frequency of the pulse ; it becomes softer and slower, and remains so during the whole course of the disease." Dr. R. L. Scruggs (same Journal, Jan. 1851,) remarks : "In Tennessee, I occasionally, but very rarely, bleed from the arm, and never had occasion to regret it. In this country, (Shreveport, La.,) however, I have not deemed it advisable to resort to venesection in any case of typhoid fever coming under my care, although, I should not hesitate to do so, at any time, even here, if the appearances seemed to justify it." This quotation from Dr. Scruggs, expresses, I think, the secret of venesection in this form of fever,—that whilst it may be a therapeutic agent of great value in some localities, in others, it is not to be relied on, but to be positively avoided. Practitioners, therefore, who reject, or adopt venesection, should not be condemned, as both may be right.

I never give quinine. In the language of Dr. Scruggs, "It was my good fortune, at the commencement of my practice, to have the advice and friendship of an old, able and experienced practitioner who had treated and become familiar with this fever, and who guarded me upon this-point, (the use of quinine,) but whose sudden and untimely death left me to my own resources, and soon I wandered from his teaching, gave the quinine to extend the morning intermissions and to lessen the evening excerbations, to, my afterwards, great regret and mortification. In no instance where I gave the quinine did I observe any benefit to the patient, but in every instance an increase of the dangerous symptoms and a hastening of the stage of collapse. I have rejected the quinine from my practice in this fever, not from prejudice, for I am of the Quinine school, Augusta, Ga., but from the repeated fact, that it proved deleterious to every case, and fatal to all, where its use was persisted in. I have lost only one case where the quinine was not used, and I have treated about fifty cases, within eighteen months, of typhoid fever. Dr. Scruggs remarks, " If I know anything of the matter at all, quinine given in typhoid fever, with the view of arresting the fever, as in the remittents, and persisted in, is as certain to result in disaster and death, as that any given cause whatever, will produce its legitimate effect."

I have generally blistered in high intestinal inflammation, but do not believe it to be beneficial. I have no doubt but many physicians have, like myself, discovered, that so soon as the blister was applied that the discharges became bloody and frequent, and most difficult to control. I agree with Dr. H. G. Davenport, that " blisters do more harm than good." There is such an intimate relationship existing between the skin and bowels as to render it highly important that the former should be preserved. Prof. Michael Levy (Medico-Chirurgical Review, Jan. 1846) says: " It will not be out of place here to point to the enormous activity of the skin, the large amount of its circulating blood, and to its close and inseparable sympathies with the more purely vital organs of respiration and digestion; nor is it necessary to recall to mind the imminent danger of alarming or fatal congestions of the bronchial and intestinal mucous surfaces, consequent upon checks to the free action of the complex glandular and vascular apparatus lodged in the cutaneous organ."

There are, however, many of the profession who consider the blister their sheet-anchor in all visceral inflammations, and from such I may reasonably expect an unconditional and relentless condemnation. I entered the profession with the same dogmatical prejudices in favor of the Herculean power of blisters to subdue intestinal inflammation, but a few winding sheets have greatly obstructed my view of their remedial efficiency, and directed my attention to other means more reliable in their action, and less dangerous in their consequences. I have generally been able to control the bowels so as to obtain two or three evacuations during the day, whilst I employed poultices, &c., but so soon as I applied the blister, the discharges were bloody and frequent, followed in almost every instance by distressing tormina and tenesmus, not to mention the great annoyance and restlessness occasioned by the supervention of strangury. A cheerful spirit is an elixir of great value in all diseases, but in none is its restorative and supporting power more to be desired than in typhoid fever. But who does not know the despondency, the despair, which patients exhibit when galled by a blister:

> " Nor does old age a wrinkle trace
> More deeply than despair."

Thus much I have thought proper to write in opposition to the use of venesection, quinine and blisters, as therapeutic agents in typhoid fever.

My treatment has not been the same in every case, but modified according to circumstances ; in other words, I usually treat symptoms rather than a name.

When called to a case proving to be typhoid fever my general plan has been to give 10 grs. of hydr. sub. muriate, or 15 grs. of blue pill, to an adult, to be followed immediately by an injection of warm water and soap, &c., and by a saline cathartic in eight or ten hours. I cannot too forcibly urge upon the profession, the propriety of injections. Their therapeutic use in affections of the bowels is certainly understood by every practitioner, but in no disease do I consider them to be more positively demanded than in typhoid fever. They unload the rectum of irritating scybalæ, and act as a quietus upon the nervous system. Given at bed time they frequently procure for the wearied patient a comfortable night's rest, a thing highly desired.

After a free evacuation of the bowels I administer the following powder every four hours.

> Hydr. Sub. Mur. . . . grs. iii.
> Ipecacuanha, ... grs. ii.
> Pulv. Doveri, ... grs. v.

Should the pulse be quick, I do not hesitate to give the veratrum viride. To an adult, I commence with six drops (Norwood's) in about half a fluid ounce of sweetened water—in ten minutes, seven drops—in ten minutes more, eight or ten drops, and wait the result ; which is free emesis, a reduction of the pulse, a soft skin, and gentle perspiration. I then continue the veratrum, giving six drops (the first dose) in four or five hours and increasing one drop every four or five hours until ten drops are reached ; I then continue ten drops every six hours and gradually increasing the period to twelve hours. Some patients cannot reach ten drops ; in such cases, the practitioner should stop at that number which produces emesis, and falling one drop below it, continue the dose every six hours, and gradually extend the period.

The veratrum should be followed in every instance by free

drinks of slippery elm or gum arabic water, as also by the following powders, every two hours, extending the time as the period of the veratrum is extended.

> Ipecac, ...   grs. ii.
> Dover's, ...   grs. iv.

I speak from experience when I recommend the veratrum viride to the profession. I am as much opposed to nostrums as any one, but I do think that when a medicine has been suggested to the profession which answers a desideratum—might I not say, wipes away an opprobrium medicorum—it is but justice—it is but a just regard to the high and noble claims of science, that it should be fairly tested. I have derived the most flattering results from its use and as yet have seen nothing in its action to induce me to discontinue it. I am no enthusiast of any remedy, and would by no means pen one line concerning any drug, which might induce practitioners to essay its virtues at the imminent peril of their patients. That the veratrum controls the action of the heart, is beyond question, and that this was a desideratum in medicine is equally undeniable. The digitalis has hitherto been employed for this purpose, but that it is uncertain and even dangerous in its action is known to every one who has used it. It frequently proves powerless, and not unfrequently like a cowardly giant, watches the auspicious moment when it may exert its feigned prowess upon a helpless and prostrate victim.

The veratrum, when properly administered, is certain in its action, and does not like the digitalis apparently sleep until it has gathered sufficient force to storm and overpower. I have employed the veratrum in other diseases beside typhoid fever. Pneumonia, pleuritis, puerperal peritonitis, palpitation of the heart, and convulsions of children, and in all with signal benefit to the patient.

It is objected that the veratrum inflames the alimentary canal. This it will not do, if given as I have advised. I should state, however, that I use the elm bark fresh from the tree, and not a worm-eaten ground Indiana elm. They who complain of its irritating qualities, gave it, probably, too frequently, or without water, or an impure preparation. I have administered the medicine in numerous instances, and attempted to watch

closely its effects, and never yet have I observed the results
spoken of by other physicians. It sometimes produces stupor in
children, resembling approaching coma, but if continued until
emesis is brought about, this symptom speedily disappears.

I have been told by some practitioners that they considered
the veratrum a humbug and never gave it., Such have set
aside a valuable remedy, and worthy to be tried, and as it is
not yet too late, I say, try it.

Some, on the other hand, are fearful to use it. These individuals give frequently a more dangerous medicine—the digitalis purpura. I have written more upon the veratrum than
I at first intended, but should what I have written prove effectual in inducing practioners to try the virtues of this medicine,
I shall feel amply compensated for my labor.

After evacuating the bowels, the use of the compound powder, the veratrum, injections, &c., as described, I cup and scari-
fy the epigastrium and right iliac fossa. I then order a poultice of corn meal and Cayenne pepper to be applied over the
bowels *every hour*, with sinapism to the spine. Should the
poultices not prove sufficient to allay abdominal heat, I put on
a sinapism over the bowels to remain ten or fifteen. minutes,
and re-apply the poultice. This sinapism should be repeated
every six or eight hours until the heat of the surface is subdued.
The poultices and injections should be kept up during the whole
course of the disease. The injection should be given at least
once, if not twice, every day. The kind of enema must vary
according to circumstances—such as warm water ; salt and
soap ; warm water, laudanum and starch ; acet. plumbi, and nit.
argenti, &c. These, as many other things, depend upon the judgment of the physician. As a diaphoretic, tonic and diuretic, I
use the seneka and spts. nitre : a free drink of the former, and
teaspoon doses every three or four hours of the latter.

In severe cases, I blister the entire spine and give ice freely.
There are many opposed to the use of ice ; more especially,
those of the Vulcan school. Some cases, no doubt, die, where
ice has been used ; but should it be rejected because a few
die under its use ? This does not prove that ice was the
cause of the death. Calomel is given, and the patient dies ;
do you then reject it from your practice? And so we

might say of any medicine ;. patients die under the best treatment.

In low muttering delirium, the ice applied freely to the scalp and given internally, in pieces, to dissolve in the stomach, will, in nine cases out of ten, arouse them to rationality. I write what I have seen at the bed-side. It relieves the heat and distress of which the patient so frequently complains whilst racked by the fever. It should be given in as large pieces as can be readily swallowed. I sometimes. give lemon water with ice, but do not order a free drink of any iced water. Its solid state is the best form in which it has been administered. Applied in iced bags or bladders to the abdomen, and given freely internally, it is our sheet-anchor (I speak positively) in dangerous intestinal inflammation. I know that there is a prejudice, with many of the profession, so deep and lasting against the use of ice and cold water, that they will not credit the treatment of any one who embodies them among his therapeutic agents. Such men add but little to the progressive march of medicine: they dare not step one side an old and routine practice, for fear of committing an error : they err, in being too cautious, and condemn because they do not experiment. I do not intend to say that practitioners should experiment upon the lives of their patients—far from it; but I do say, that when life is fast failing, the physician should do all in his power to save it, and if his usual remedies prove powerless, he should try others which have been highly recommended. Short of this, he does not perform his duty.

I have now given a short and very imperfect sketch of my treatment in typhoid fever. I have not thought it proper to write the varied changes which are so often observed in this fever, preferring to leave the treatment of them to the judgment of the physician, as no two cases will be precisely alike, but varied in their progress, by constitution, habit, vicissitude of weather, &c. My purpose has been to discuss plainly and concisely that form of treatment which I believe to be most successful in typhoid fever. I wish also to be understood as. speaking of this locality ; for I write from experience in this place alone, and do not by any means attempt to dictate to any one ; but should what I have written attract the attention of any member of the profession, and "enable him hereafter to diagnosticate correctly, and to treat the disease successfully, I shall feel amply rewarded for the little toil it has cost me to write this article, and feel, too, at the same time, that I have done the profession some service."

Addendum.—Since there are many who do not believe in the existence of Typhoid, as a distinct disease, I make the following propositions:—·

1st. That physicians of Georgia, Alabama, Mississippi, Florida, Louisiana and Texas, report their names to the New Orleans Medical and Surgical Journal and the Southern Medical and Surgical Journal of Augusta, as either for or against Typhoid fever, as a separate and independent disease.

2d. That as many as can find it consistent with their labors,. write out their views as to its independence or identity with other diseases, and the treatment found most successful.

I believe that every member of the profession is honest in his opinion ; but, if possible, we should know the truth of the matter. If there is any hope of settling these vexed questions, let it be done before they are pushed upon another age. We are probably as well prepared to discuss the identity or non-identity of typhoid fever now as we will ever be. Many consider it a modification of remittent fever—some of intermittent—some as identical with typhus. It would be proper for these to state what they consider remittent, intermittent and typhus fever, and further, to relate clearly the nature of that modification which gives rise to those peculiar symptoms known to many as typhoid fever.

I wish to see an interest manifested in the profession in diagnosis, not only in typhoid, but in every other type of fever. If typhoid be intermittent or remittent fever, its treatment is clear; if not, its nature should be ascertained, that it may be properly treated. I should be pleased to see a table of physicians' names, as to identity or non-identity of this fever, and in that table I shall risk my name as to its non-identity, and in favor of the doctrine, that it is a disease *sui generis.*

I am fully aware of the incoherency of this article, written at many sittings, caused by professional duty. This, however, could not be avoided, and should it not meet with approbation, I have the consolation to know—

"Nec semper feriet quodcunque minabitur areus."

Anomalous Cases.   By E. Y. HARRIS, M. D., of Fayette C. H., Alabama.

Every physician, of much practice, occasionally meets with cases, the peculiarities of which he never heard or read of before; these, if reported, might be interesting, if not instructive, to some of the profession. Cases similar to the following may have come under the observation of others, but as yet I have never seen or heard of anything of the kind.

CASE I.   In 1845, while I was practising on the Yazoo River, in Carroll county, Mississippi, I was called one night to see a negro woman who was in the seventh month of her fourth pregnancy. The white family had gone off the previous day and left this servant by herself in charge of the house. On my arrival, I found her laboring under uterine pains, which came on about every fifteen or twenty minutes. I learned that on the previous night a man had visited her for *carnal purposes;* that she had resisted him, at which he became incensed and struck her with his fist two or three times in the left side, when she cried out so loudly that he became alarmed and left. I bled her and gave an opiate. Next morning she expressed herself as much better, said she felt the child move. She continued to feel better up to the third day after receiving the blows, though there was some discharge of bloody mucus from the vagina with occasional pains in the uterine region. Felt heavy and sleepy, considerable soreness of the left side where the blows had been inflicted. On the third day she washed a large quantity of clothes; in the evening felt worse, uterine pain, somewhat increased; she remained pretty much in this condition up to the sixth day, feeling better during the morning and worse in the evening, declaring all this time that she felt the child move distinctly. At 10 o'clock, on the night of the sixth day after she had received the injury, she was taken with strong uterine pain.

I found the uterus in its proper place ; os tincæ thick and soft, and cool, and not dilated in the least; skin cool and moist; pulse full and a little frequent; tongue natural : said she felt the child move, and when a contraction would take place re- ferred all the pain to the left side. Prescribed 2 grs. opium and 1 gr. ipecac; warm fomentation over the abdomen. Next morning, found she had rested well during the night; com- plained of her back, and occasional uterine pain. Gave an enema of soap-suds, which operated lightly, and, as the pulse was full and strong, bled to 16 oz.—continued warm fomenta- tions, and gave a pill composed of opium 1 gr., ipecac $\frac{1}{2}$ gr. She expressed herself as feeling much easier, and desired to be left alone that she might sleep. At 10 o'clock, I returned, after being absent four hours: found her lying on her back; eyes half open, but not turned up; pulse natural; breathing regular and deep; skin moist and cool. She seemed to be in a very deep sleep, and snored loudly. I attempted to arouse her, but soon found that it could not be done: she had gone into a sleep never again to awake. I dashed water in her face, poured it on her head ; applied mustard sinapisms to her spine, extremities, and over the abdomen; but all in vain. Pulse, breathing and skin, all seemed natural; no tympanitis; every organ seemed to perform its function with regularity; the nervous system seemed only to be at fault. In whatever position she was placed, there she remained ; if the eyelids were drawn apart they remained so ; if closed, they remained closed. A large blister plaster was applied over the abdomen and bound close to the skin for thirty-six hours, but did not vesicate in the least ; one was also applied to the back of the neck, which very slowly blistered; but nothing that was done gave any re- lief.

On the morning of the eighth day of her illness, in attempt- ing a vaginal examination, my hand came in contact with the child lying at the vulva and between the thighs, with the pla- centa beside it. There was not the least hemorrhage; at what time in the night the child was born no one knew; there was an old negro with her during the night, but she could give no account of it. Upon examination, it was evident that the child had been killed by the blows received by the mother eight

days before.   The child had received two injuries ; one was on
the left side of the head ; the parietal and temporal bones were
both driven in, and the parts considerably tumefied and red ;
the other was on the left side, just below the arm, where the
cuticle was of a very dark red, and bruised ; two or three of
the ribs were broken loose from their articulation with the spine,
and driven in.   The child certainly had been dead sometime,
as putrefaction had taken place, notwithstanding the mother's
assertion that she felt it move.   This clearly shows that a woman may be mistaken as to fœtal movements,—my patient remained in this cataleptic condition five days and died.   She did
not seem to get any worse until the day before her death,
when all the symptoms became aggravated and she gradually
sank.

Here was a strange condition of the nervous system, brought
on probably by the injury she received from the wretch, who,
for a moment's gratification sacrificed two lives.   Was this
condition of the nervous system brought on by the injury ?   If
so, would the same have produced similar nervous disturbance
if she had not been pregnant ?   During the whole of her comatose state, her pulse was good, her skin natural and moist, urine
passed involuntarily until the day before her death.   I have
seen two or three cases of catalepsy in my life but none like
this.   In the Medical Examiner for 1845 or 46, there is a case
of catalepsy reported which was supposed to be consequent
upon the puerperal state ; the patient died in five or six days,
but, if my recollections serves me right, the symptoms of this
case were very dissimilar to the above.

Case II.   On Monday, 5th July, 1852, William Davis, a lad
of about 15, attended a temperance celebration in Fayetteville.
About three weeks previous to this time, he had had an attack
of dysentery, but was quite well on the day above mentioned.
He stood about nearly all day, occasionally eating ginger-bread
and drinking beer ; late in the evening he complained of a sick
stomach and slight headache, went to bed, eat no supper, but
vomited two or three times between that and midnight ; about
2 or 3 o'clock, A. M., he was moaning most plaintively, and on
being asked, by his father, what was the matter, replied, that
he felt very curious.   The after part of the night he rested

badly, sometimes lying still and apparently sleeping soundly—
then rising up and rolling about, and moaning, as though in
great pain ; at day-light, his father attempted to arouse him to
go home, a mile from town. but as he appeared to be sleeping
so soundly, thought best to let him lie awhile ; in a short time,
however, he was discovered to be completely delirious, and
went into a convulsion, which lasted but a short time : he then
sank into a deep sleep.   At this juncture, I was called in, and
found him lying on his back ; breathing deep and full ; skin
rather cool and moist ; pulse 65 to 70, weak and easily compressed ; jaws seemed to be a little stiff ; great rigidity of the
abdominal muscles, which were a little sunk in, and felt as
hard as a board and ridgy.   This rigidity gradually extended
to the legs, spine, neck, and finally to the arms, so that by 5
o'clock, P. M., he was as stiff as though he had no joints.   He
would have very restless paroxysms, during which he seemed
to suffer great pain : between these, he would be quite still,
and apparently asleep.   While his restless paroxysms existed,
he would exert himself to such a degree as to become perfectly
exhausted, and sink down to rest fifteen or twenty minutes ;
then suddenly spring to a sitting position, scream and moan
loudly, scratch his head, and rub his hands over his face, as
though washing it ; fall suddenly down, roll very quickly from
one side to the other, and at times rest himself upon his knees
and forehead—in fact, during his restless moments, he would
assume every attitude imaginable, and all this time he would
scream and moan in the most plaintive tones, indicative of the
most intense suffering.   He never spoke nor articulated a single sentence from the time he lost his mind.   These paroxysms
of pain and restlessness continued until the rigidity became
general—they increased in frequency and violence until about
3 o'clock, when the rigidity became so general that it confined
him to his back.   I could have placed my hand under the occiput and raised him to his feet without bending his body in the
least ; his head and spine were inclined to draw back a little—
in fact, during the last moments of his life, the occiput rested
upon the spine, between his shoulders ; his jaws became completely locked, so that it was imposible to prize them open half
an inch.

As to the treatment, we could do but little. From the first, he had a difficulty in swallowing, and it soon became impossible for him to take any thing at all that way. His feet and legs were bathed in warm water; mustard sinapisms were applied to his legs'and arms, over the abdomen, and along the whole course of the spine; a large warm pepper poultice was applied over the abdomen; temples cupped; back of the neck blistered; one-twelfth gr. strychnine given two or three times, though it is not quite certain he swallowed it; he was sponged all over several times with spts. camphor, and hot brandy, laudanum and spts: turpentine, in pretty large quantities, were frequently rubbed over the abdomen and spine. I commenced giving chloroform to inhale as early as 10 o'clock, and continued it during each paroxysm. It seemed to shorten the paroxysm of pain, and this was the only good I could discover. I made a liniment of chloroform, sweet oil and spirits ammomia, and applied it frequently to the spine and abdomen. I attempted to give him an injection of strong soap-suds and salt water, but so great was the contraction of the sphincter ani that it was with considerable difficulty, I could introduce the canula, and when I did accomplish this, could not force up any of the contents of the syringe. Two or three hours before he died his breathing became very laborious, and continued to increase until five o'clock, when he expired. Nothing that was done seemed of any avail. I would remark that during the whole time he was delirious he kept his eyes shut ; the pupils were dilated. His former health had not been very good ; he had been chlorotic for three years ; pale and swarthy ; appetite pretty good ; little exercise produced considerable action of the heart and quick breathing, but he had been better of this for the last six months.

Case III. On the 15th July, 1852, I was called to see a negro man, Joe, 25 years of age, stout and athletic, had never been sick before. While hoeing cotton, that day, he complained to his master that when he stooped down he felt an acute pain in his forehead, and when he raised up it moved to the back of his head. He had felt this pain. occasionally for two or three months, but at this time it was worse than usual: he had tied a string very tightly around his head, but it failed to give relief.

Not more than five minutes after Joe had this conversation with his master, he fell. His master ran to him and found him resting upon his knees and head. On being addressed he made no reply, but fell on his side, his face and mouth became convulsed and drawn to the left—he had also spasmodic twitchings of the right arm and muscles of that side, but not so decided as those of the face ; the head was so much twisted to the left that his master feared the spinal marrow would sustain some injury, he attempted with all the strength he had to twist the head back, but could not move it. In twenty minutes the spasm gave way but he remained unconscious—in this condition he was carried half a mile to the house, a vein opened in the arm and 30 oz. blood drawn, and a blister applied to the forehead, a tablespoonful of No. Six poured into his mouth, but being unable to swallow, it ran out. A spasm would come on about every hour and last fifteen or twenty minutes, during which time his head would twist around to the left side, and the muscles of the face and right arm twitch and jerk. As soon as the spasm would go off he would try to bite his fingers or anything he could get hold of; he chewed off two or three spoon handles, and his tongue did not escape receiving some injury. He would do his best to bite those who were holding him, and being very strong, it required five or six to prevent his doing himself serious injury.

When I arrived I found him in the condition above described; pulse full, strong, and a little hard, 80 to minute ; skin, natural temperature ; occasionally he would place his hand upon the occiput and moan. He had become a little calm and was covered up ; on uncovering him I discovered that there was a great increase of sensibility ; for whenever a fly would rest on any part of him, he would jerk from it as though a pin or a knife had stuck him. If I touched the hair any where over the occiput, he would flinch instantly and seemed fully as sensitive as if the whole cuticle had been pealed off; sensibility was not near so acute over the parietal, temporal and frontal regions. I had him held up and bled from the arm 24 oz., when the pulse became softer and slower—he now became more rational, called for water—I gave him a large dose of epsom salts; he complained of a lancinating pain in the back of his head, said he was much easier when sitting up than when lying.   I shaved the whole occiput and applied a blister plaster that covered it and extended down the back of the neck six inches ; in three hours gave him another dose of salts, and in three more the blister had drawn well—in a few hours the salts had operated finely, producing serous discharges ; he gradually improved and now, two weeks from the date of his illness, he is quite well.

A Case of Extra-Uterine Foetation.   By M. W. Havis, M. D,, of Minerya, Georgia.

June 28th, 1851.   A negro woman, of large frame and respectable *embonpoint*, æt. 39, the mother of nine healthy children, in second month of pregnancy, was ill of metrorrhagia ; the hemorrhage inordinate ; pulse 100, full and large; v. s. 20 oz.   Ordered, hips elevated; cloths saturated with acetic acid dil. to vulva ; acet. plumb. grs. ij. ; opium grs. j., every three hours, until relieved.

29th.   Greatly improved—convalescence rapid.

July 25th.   Similar attack ; treated as before : relieved.

August 28th.   Hemorrhage active ; uterine pains severe and expulsive—a fœtus at four months delivered.   Hemorrhage continuing excessive, ordered ol. ergotæ gtt. 20 every half hour, until sufficiently diminished.   Two doses only were given. In three weeks she was convalescent and resumed her place as cook.

Oct. 1st.   After slight pains in uterus during the day, they increased at night, and were effectual in expelling a considerable mass of hydatid-moles.   Upon the use of tannin injections, the next day, more were dislodged.   She was not confined to bed, and without inconvenience continued in the exercise of her duties.   In November, she complained to me of a bad feeling in her abdomen, amounting to pain, at times, of a dragging character.   I interrogated her relative to her former labors, and learned that, up to last April, they were all normal, at which time metrorrhagia obtained and she aborted ; fœtus four months advanced.   Subsequent to this she was troubled with partial hysteroptosis, but, conception again taking place, the prolapsus was relieved. She suffered during prolapsus, from costiveness and dysuria. I examined per vaginam, found the vaginal mucous membrane in a phlogosed condition, the cervix uteri engorged, uterus slightly prolapsed and a very acrid mu-co-purulent discharge, evidencing an extension of the inflammation to the intra-uterine superficies. With these facts before me, the indications were apparent—to reduce the inflammation and thus cut short the leucorrhœa and relieve the prolapsus. Ordered, hyd. sub. mur. et. rhei, aa grs. iij., every other night; cataplasm to sacrum; vesicated surface to be stimulated with ung. sabinæ. Inject aqua acet. plumbi, three times per diem.

At the end of two weeks, very little improved; leucorrhœa profuse; pains in loins; lassitude and cephalalgia. Ord., tinct. lyttæ gtt. xx., three times a day; aq. acet. plumbi continued. At the expiration of two weeks, declared herself well of leu-corrhœa. Uterus in "statu quo." Gave pills of carb. fer. et rhei. She improved, and for three weeks did her labor as cook.

January 2d, 1852. Was taken very ill. Found her with pains in the loins and hypogastrium; pulse 100, full and tense; bowels costive; stillicidium urinæ; cervix-uteri engorged, indurated and painful to touch: v. s. 16 oz.; hip bath; calomel grs. iij.; jalap viii. grs.; spts. nitre and flax-seed tea, *pro re nata.*

Jan. 23rd. Pulse 90, soft; three alvine dejections; micturition guttatim. Ordered, infusion of uva ursi, diosma crenata and carb. sodæ to be taken during the day; pulv. Doveri grs. vii. at night. This treatment was persevered in for two weeks. Micturition normal; no febrile condition since 23rd ultimo. Vaginal tract injected, cervix firm and of bluish tint, deep fissures of semi-crucial figure divide its substance, from which exude creamy shreds of vitiated mucus; os uteri firmly closed. Ordered, cataplasms to sacrum; pil. hydrarg. grs. iij. every other night; anodyne injections; salines, *pro re nata.*

For two weeks, gradual improvement. At this time pneumatosis abdominalis supervened and induced a despondency which, with hysteria, placed her in a very unhappy state. Amm. tinct. valerian cum assafœt. proved a veritable *sine qua non.* Upon taking a fright, she strained her muscular system violently. I found her greatly prostrated: womb at os externum; fissures deep, and the eminences firm as cartilage; pulse 110, feeble and quick. Replaced the womb; enjoined recumbent posture. Ordered, syrup ferri iod. gtt. xx., three times per day; oleum tiglii. to spine; salines; inject sol. nitras argenti, twice a day. The caustic not effecting any good, it was suspended at the end of two weeks, and the ung. iod. ferri. substituted. Under this treatment, improvement was not apparent. I now consulted with my respected friend, Dr. J. Riley. He proposed, in addition to the use of ung. iod. free scarrifications of the cervix, and the vinous sol. iod. ferri, instead of the syrup. At the end of two weeks the vinous sol. iod. ferri proved such an irritant to the stomach as to cause its suspension, and the syrup was resumed. She now, for a short time, gave evidence of improvement, but soon retrograded. In conversation with my much esteemed preceptor, Dr. G. T. Cooper, I explained the nature of the case, and, at his suggestion, resolved to apply the solid caustic. She was at this time much emaciated: tympannitic; nervous tremors quite frequent in her limbs; considerable weight in left hypogastrium; appetite capricious; cervix uteri very hard. I applied the caustic freely every other day, and gave pills composed of carb. ferri. grs. iij.; rhei and gum myrrh *aa.* grs. ij., and ext. gentian q. s.—one three times per diem; oleum tigĥi continued to spine. The day succeeding the second application of caustic, she declared her conviction of a speedy convalescence, for "she had a new feeling—a great weight was removed from her bowels, and she now felt strong there." From this time (April 23d) she made gradual progress to recovery.

May 10th. The caustic having been applied eight times, I deemed its further use unnecessary, as the cervix uteri had nearly returned to its normal size and consistency.

May 20th. I was summoned to my patient, whom I found in a kind of exstacy—delight beaming from her eyes: she extended towards me her hand, in which she held what seemed to be a PEG of dark wood, and at the same time exclaimed, "I will now surely get well, for here is the *peg* and *spiders* which have so long troubled me." I found, upon examining these wonders, that the peg was the tibia, corresponding to a fœtus of four months; and the spiders, hydatids on a large scale. She had, early in the morning, been troubled with considerable pain of a pricking character in the position of the left ovarium, and in three hours thereafter had three alvine dejections, in rapid succession. Upon examining these, found the bone and hydatids, chiefly in last dejection, consisting of a yellow aqueous fluid, with flocculi, in which the bone was imbedded and the hydatids attached. Since this, she has passed two ribs, one scapula, two bones of cranium, tibia, ten metacarpal, one carpal. She is now walking about the yard without inconvenience, performing such duties as require manipulation chiefly.

The case is surely a novel one in several particulars; and, if I mistake not, the only one reported where nature has relieved herself of so serious a freak, without a vast amount of febrile disorder, and where the skeleton made its exit through the intestines, with so little trouble, not even preventing the woman from laboring.

Candor requires an acknowledgment of my entire ignorance of the existence of an extra-uterine pregnancy, previous to the 20th of May, when I had an ocular demonstration of it. The prolapsed uterus, diseased cervix, and a fluor albus of eight years duration, satisfied me as to the disease requiring treatment.

The two last months of the woman's illness, she complained of a "knot," as she termed it, in her abdomen, just beneath the left ovarium, which at times would swell, give her much pain, and then subside. I examined her abdomen repeatedly, when its parietes were thin and flaccid, and could detect a "knot," 'tis true, but never could appreciate its swelling and subsiding, as she did.

Since the convalescence of my patient, I questioned her very closely, and find that, in October, 1851, one month subsequent to discharge of hydatid moles, her catamenia appeared, and at no time up to the present date have their periodicity been disturbed. In November, she felt symptoms which had obtained in all her previous conceptions, and was led to believe that she was pregnant, but was surprised to find her menses continue. If she conceived in November, the fœtus died several months previous to expulsion per rectum, and if such be the fact, I cannot account for the absence of febrile excitement. How the fœtus, without the uterus, enclosed by a membrane so obnoxious to the most violent inflammation upon the presence of a foreign body, (which the fœtus was after death,) did fail to induce inflammation, is to me quite inexplicable. Her tongue I scarcely ever found of an abnormal appearance. She at times had pains in the back, hips and loins; but these were nervous and easily removed by sinapisms. In the fifth month of her illness, she was troubled with a burning pain in the womb, which was attributed to the phlogosed utero-vaginal mucous membrane. Her pulse ranged from 70 to 85 beats per minute, save during hysterical paroxysms, when it would grow to 100 and 110, small and feeble. So, excepting her attack on the 2d of January, she had no febrile disorder.

As regards the time of conception, there is a doubt. It may have taken place coincident with her ninth pregnancy, and the fœtus perishing at four months, have caused subsequent abortions. But the most plausible view would be, to fix the conception in November, when all the signs of pregnancy were present, save the cessation of the catamenia.

The fœtus must have occupied a place within the peritoneum, below and posterior to the left ovarium, at a point corresponding with the commencement of the rectum, judging from the seat of the pricking and weight and amount of fæces discharged, before the dislodgement of bones, &c.

ARTICLE XXXVII.

Extracts from the Records of the Physicians' Society for Medical Observation, of Greene and adjoining Counties, Georgia. By D. C. O'KEEFFE, M. D., of Penfield, Ga., Secretary.

July 12th. *On the Use of Compound Spirit of Ether.* By Dr. A. A. BELL.—It is sometimes pleasant to turn from the more abstruse questions in our Science, and retrace paths less environed with difficulties. I have been using Hoffman's anodyne (as it is familiarly called) for several years, and from the pleasant effects I have derived from its administration, I am induced to make this report, as it corroborates the virtues that have been accorded to it.

That it has the property to produce sleep, and tranquilize the nervous system, where opium or its kindred remedies will not, I think may be verified upon trial. The first instance in which I used it, with any very notable effect, was a case of delerium tremens. Laudanum had been administered freely, with occasional portions of brandy; the latter seemed to aggravate the symptoms, and the comp. spts. ether was substituted. It had a decided tendency to calm the nervous action, and allow repose to the patient.

I have also noticed its action in hysteria. I was called to a married lady who had been laboring under this singular malady for several days: the administration of comp. spts. ether had the effect of lessening sensibly the unpleasant nervous symptoms, and ensuring a great deal of comfort to the patient. It was continued, with a cathartic, with the like happy result.

I have likewise noticed its influence upon the system in cases of morbid vigilence, which frequently occurs in the course of an attack of acute diseases, especially in individuals who are in the habit of using intoxicating liquors. Several cases of this kind have come under my care; one, in particular, in which laudanum and black drop were given freely, without the desired effect. The patient's pulse at this crisis was 115, and he had passed several restless nights. I now gave him f. ℥iss. comp. spts. ether, and in the course of two hours he had a refreshing sleep, with considerable diminution in the frequency of the pulse. It was repeated, in the course of four hours, with like effect.

The cases in which it is most applicable are those of a nervous character, not dependent upon any decided inflammation, at least, of such degree as not to require active antiphlogistic measures.

On a Case of Monstrosity. By Dr. E. V. Culver.—There has been a difference of opinion among the members of the medical profession for centuries, as to the cause of *monstrosities*, or irregular births—as to whether the fœtus in the uterus can be effected in its growth or development by external causes, acting through the imagination of the mother; if so at all, at what period of utero-gestation can a perversion of growth take place? These are questions that have excited the members of the profession time and again, and it would now be presumption in me to offer an opinion upon such a subject. Without even presuming to form any conclusion in a matter so mysterious, I will detail the following case;—at the same time I will remark, that I have been unable to learn any thing, or circum-·stance, that excited or alarmed the mother. I have carefully inquired into the particulars attending her during utero-gestation.

Mrs. —— was taken in labor on the evening of the 3rd July (inst.), with her thirteenth child. She was awakened from sleep by a discharge of water, the membranes having ruptured spontaneously, and without the least pain. Free uterine hemorrhage immediately came on. I found her very much exhausted from the flow of blood, and complaining in the usual way from its loss. As soon as I entered the room, she informed me that the "child" was dead, and gave as a reason, that she had not felt it move for the past thirty-six hours. I made an examination, and found the uterus dilated and yielding, the feet presenting. The labor progressed slowly, and she was delivered, in eight hours, of a child of common size, *still-born*, she having gone the full period of utero-gestation.

The following appearances were revealed upon examination, not being permitted, nor having the time, to make further scrutiny into the case:—The face, not more than one-fourth as large as it should have been, with no part I could call a head; the frontal bones wanting, with exception of a narrow ridge just above the orbits, only a few lines in breadth; the temporal bones the same, there being a very narrow piece articulating with the sphenoid, the piece containing the glenoid cavity for articulating with lower jaw; the parietal bones were entirely deficient; the occipital also wanting, with exception of a small piece for its articulation with the atlas. The above seemed to be the situation of the cranium, from the examination I made. Not being permitted to use the *knife*, I am unable to speak confidently as to how much the bones were deficient.

The head, commencing a few lines above the eyes, down to the vertebræ, presented the appearance of a coagulum of blood, soft to touch, the hand meeting with no resistance over the

entire surface; the mouth was right, as to position and formation; very little sign of nose, except two small openings, just
above the mouth; the eyes seemed to be in proper place, but
protruding about three-fourths of an inch from the surface, of
an unusual large size; the ears were very much out of place,
approaching too near the eye, presented the appearance of two
small horns—they were about one-third the usual size, and
very much elongated; the part called the *head*, with the face,
formed a triangle, the largest diameter not more than one and
a half inches; the vertebræ of the neck were immovable and
fixed—the face slightly inclined forwards; the fingers were
bent upon the palms of the hands, and there firmly united.
The other parts of the fœtus were well formed, and free from
any deformity.

The above are the details of the case, hastily given; and
now, in conclusion, I will again repeat that the lady is unable
to call to mind any instance in which she has been much.
alarmed, and the only thing of any note that has a bearing upon
the case, is the fact, that she has frequently experienced pain
and uneasiness in the right side whilst riding on horse back,
which she occasionally practised. She says she has no doubt
from her sensation, that the back part of the head of the fœtus
was firmly united to the right side near the stomach, and that
she knew when it separated. I merely state this as she so often
says, she is sure it is so. She is fast recovering.

*Hemorrhage from the Umbilicus after separation from the
Funis, ten days after birth.* By J. E. WALKER, M. D.—Mrs.
C., primapara, was delivered of a small but apparently healthy
male child, on the second day of March, 1849, after a somewhat
protracted labour. Both did well until the sixth day after delivery, when I was called to see the child, whom I found labouring under hæmaturia, which I treated with astringent diuretics—
buchu, &c., with entire relief. It went on well then until the
twelfth day from this, at which time blood began to exude from
the umbilicus; the cord had separated about the sixth day, and
the part appeared to be sound and healthy. I was consulted
in relation to the hæmorrhage, and as it was described as a
simple oozing of blood from the part, and by no means calcu-

lated to excite alarm, I therefore prescribed tannic acid and a compress to be applied, and requested to be notified if the bleeding should not cease after the prescription was used. This was neglected, and although the application did very little good, yet the hæmorrhage was allowed to go on for twenty-four hours before I was sent for; I arrived as early as possible to see it, when called, and such a spectacle I never saw; the bleeding had continued until the child was almost entirely anæmic. Its clothing had been often changed, all of which was completely dyed in blood; it lay almost lifeless, unable to take nourishment, and almost senseless; I regarded the prognosis unfavorable, even if I should succeed in arresting the flow. I lost no time in the trial of creosote, which had but temporary effect, as it was washed away by the blood. I applied sugar of lead, and tannin, &c., with no better success. I used lunar caustic, but still the blood poured forth. The actual cautery suggested itself, and was proposed, but the parents would not consent, as the child seemed to.be dying. I then determined to try the ligature as a *dernier resort,* as I feared the vessels were diseased—the ligature, *en masse,* was decided on, that the whole bleeding surface might be embraced and secured. It was impossible to decide from whence the blood issued—whether from the arteries, veins, or the tissues surrounding the vessels. I accordingly passed a common suture needle, armed with a silk thread, through the umbilicus, from right to left, and from left to right, and, after the third stitch was made, I drew the threads pretty tight, and secured the ends together, and had the gratification to find the bleeding arrested. During the operation, the child made not the least complaint, but was unconcious of pain. As a further precaution, I applied the sulphate of iron, in fine powder, after being heated to draw off the water of crystalization, which, uniting with the blood left around the part, formed a hard compress, over which I applied a bandage. I now sought to bring about reaction, by pouring into the mouth wine whey, in small quantities and at short intervals, which, by the following morning, had so far succeeded that the child could draw a little at the breast. I recommended the wine to be continued, until strength was restored. In about four days suppuration was established, and as the threads had become loose, I divided and gently withdrew them. There was no more hæmorrhage—the part healed kindly, and left the navel almost natural in appearance. The child has since enjoyed good health, and is now a sprightly boy.

REMARKS.—I have conversed with many physicians who had met with this accident, and have found their report unfavorable, without an exception. This, doubtless, has been owing to their depending on styptics and compresses alone; the bleeding, no doubt, is, in general, from the arteries—sometimes from the veins and arteries combined; and it is always difficult to apply compresses to that part with advantage, owing to the softness of the abdominal walls.

When I performed this operation I had seen no authority for it, and it might be said I was not justifiable in its performance; but had the actual cautery been used, sloughing and secondary hæmorrhage might have been the consequence, and the life of the child only prolonged to endure a larger amount of suffering. All other means in common practice had been tried, without exerting any influence whatever.

It is to be regretted, that so little has been said by authors on this subject; and this case has been brought to the notice of our society for the purpose of eliciting the views of its members, and directing more attention to the subject.

In my reading, since I treated the above case, I have found ligature, *en masse*, recommended by Paul Dubois and Dr. Bowdich; but their cases were not successful. Their operation differed from mine in this particular—they used the hare-lip pins, with figure of 8 suture, while I used the thread, as you have observed, alone. It has been objected, that there is danger of peritonitis. That, I admit, may be true; but the operation has succeeded where death must have been the inevitable result without it. Death has often followed upon amputation; but that is no argument against such an operation, when it so often succeeds, where death would be the certain result, if it should be neglected.

Ecchymosis of Vagina from rapid Parturition. By Dr. D. C. O'KEEFFE, of Penfield, Ga.—This occurrence happened to the wife of a much esteemed medical friend. The patient, æt.

about 20, was delivered of a mature child in the short space of one and a half to two hours from the beginning of labour. She had aborted in her first pregnancy, and was frequently threatened with abortion in the present, but with great care and occasional v. s. she went her full term.

The hæmorrhagic diathesis was strongly marked in her case, as shewn by her tolerance of bloodletting, and a very frequent discharge of blood from a nasal polypus with which she was affected.

For a short time (an hour or two) after delivery, she was very comfortable and expressed a natural pleasure when her offspring was shewn her, somewhat suddenly, however, she felt acute pain between the hip-joint and perineum on the left side, which extended down the thigh of the same side ; there was also exquisite tenderness under the slightest pressure externally in the region above designated. A sinapism was applied forthwith to the seat of pain with no benefit ; a strong morphine plaster was next applied, which mitigated her suffering considerably. Moderate pain and tenderness to the touch remained however for two days, and her pulse and other symptoms indicated a febrile condition of a moderate degree. During these two days her bowels were kept open by aperients, and the lochial discharge was normal. The period of lactation now arrived, attended with increased pain and febrile action, and the pain about the hip and perineum threatened to be as distressing as when it was first felt. It is proper to state that our friend regarded this pain to be of a neuralgic character, but lest there should be some occult cause about the uterus, he determined to explore that organ. •

A vaginal examination revealed a tumour nearly filling up the vaginal canal its entire length, the index and medius could with difficulty be passed up to the os uteri along side of it. About four inches long and one and a half inches in diameter, it extended from just within the labia minora along the vaginal wall on the left, to a level with the os uteri—a line drawn from the upper extremity of the tumour transversely across the vagina would strike the lips of the os uteri at right angle. It was painful to the touch and tolerably tense ; micturition was easy, but the bowels were disposed to be confined—defecation caused an aching sensation in the left iliac fossa.

From the knowledge our friend had of the rapidity of the labour, and consequently the illy prepared state of the parts, and moreover, an unusually compact and unyielding cranium on the part of the child, he was prompt in recognizing the tumour to be an ecchymosis produced by injury to the soft parts and treated it accordingly. For four or five days from the date of its discovery, there was high febrile action, the pulse was sometimes as high as 125 to 130. During this time she took some mercurial, was bled moderately from the arm once, and leeches were applied freely to the lower abdomen perineum and to the lower extremity of the tumour itself. These means checked a strong tendency that existed to metritis, and relieved the tumour of tenderness in a great measure. At this stage of the case, another physician and ourself were requested to see it, and found it in no-wise different from what it has been described, and we could not but concur in the diagnosis pronounced by our friend. The tumour had diminished but little, if any, from the time it was discovered, but was less sensitive to the touch ; the tongue was slightly furred, the surface pleasant, and the pulse 120 and rather feeble—there was generally a febrile exacerbation in the afternoon and a remission in the forenoon. A speculum was employed to ascertain the color of the tumour, which was found to be a deep purple ; this disclosure corroborated our diagnosis.

It was agreed, unanimously, to open it, which was done with a thumb lancet, tied to a small stick, and introduced through the speculum—the lower portion only could be brought within the field of this instrument, and here a free incision was made. The discharge from the incision was very small and consisted of very dark coagulated blood, intermingled with a few drops of pus. It was now seen through the opening in the tumour that it was composed altogether of coagulated blood, and that the main indication in treatment consisted in its removal. It was accordingly deemed advisable to inject tepid water into the tumour through the opening, in order to break down its coagulated contents which succeeded but partially. This course, (the tepid water injections,) kept up three times a day, however, for three days, nearly entirely emptied the tumour of its contents—a silver probe was worked about in the tumour freely, which doubtless aided materially in breaking up the coagula.

At the time we write, the patient is much better ; tumour nearly gone ; is free from pain ; pulse 106 ; tongue improved. From the time the tumour was opened, a dose of Quinine was given every morning, and a more nourishing diet allowed. Mercurial ointment is now being rubbed over the part with a view to produce absorption of any coagula that should be left, for it was feared the vitality of the parts was very much impaired—indeed this fact seemed evident from the circumstance, that there was not the slightest pain felt in making the incision.

ARTICLE XXXVIII.

Chloasma.   By E. F. STARR, M. D., of Rome, Ga.

This disease of the skin (known also as Maculæ Hepaticæ, Liver spots, &c.) usually makes its appearance on the chest, shoulders and arms, or neck, and extends in irregular patches, so as sometimes to spread over a large portion of the body. These patches may unite and cover a larger continuous surface of some inches across. As far as the disease extends, the skin is made to exhibit a yellowish or dull brown color. The cuticle is very slightly elevated, and minutely scaly, and desquamates to a moderate extent. It seldom produces any sensation or irritability of the skin, and its existence, in many cases, would not be known if it were not seen, though it may sometimes produce troublesome itching. It is annoying, and especially so to ladies, on account of its appearance, which, upon the whole, is dirty and repulsive, and is apt to excite a sense of shame in those who are troubled with it.

Its cause, I think, is unknown—it has been attributed, of course, to derangement of the internal organs, such as the stomach, liver, &c., but it has no established connection with any such causes, for most generally I have seen it on persons with whom there were no symptoms of bad health otherwise.

The treatment of this disgusting little affection has not, I think, generally been satisfactory and successful. My object, therefore, is to introduce a remedy which is simple and efficient. In the year 1845, from analogy of a known property of sulphuric acid, I was induced to try it in a case of this kind, and found that it effected a cure in a short time. I have since tried it in a number of cases with uniform success. The method of using it is to dilute it in the proportion of about a drachm of the acid to a pint of water, more or less, according to the sensibility and tenderness of the skin of the patient, and to apply it, thus diluted, to the affected part, by rubbing it on with the hand, or a bit of sponge; and sufficient friction should be used to rub off the *separable* scales and cuticle. The strength of the wash should be so regulated as to produce a slight stinging sensation, without much pain. The application should be made once or twice a day, until the skin resumes its natural appearance, and then occasionally, for several days afterwards, to prevent a return of the disease.

These remarks have been induced by an extract in the Southern Medical and Surgical Journal of last year, from the New Hampshire Journal of Medicine, by Dr. Gray, in which he proposes the " sulphur fume bath as a remedy " and suggests that " if any member of the profession has a remedy as certain as this and more easily applied it would be highly gratifying to have it made more public." I consider my remedy equally as certain, more simple, and much more easily applied.

ARTICLE XXXIX.

Snoring prevented by excision of the Uvula. By THE EDITOR.

CASE. A. D——, about 5 years of age, had for two or three years suffered from considerable enlargement of the tonsils, which impeded respiration so much during sleep as to cause him to snore very loudly and to seem to be on the point of suffocation. About a year ago, I excised both tonsils, after which the respiration was very much improved, and the snoring nearly ceased. In March last, his respiration during sleep had become as bad as ever, and his parents apprehending that he might actually suffocate, again requested medical aid. Upon examination, I found that the tonsils had again become somewhat enlarged; that the uvula hung flabbily between them and rested upon the base of the tongue, and that this state of things

taken in connection with the natural, yet extraordinary smallness of the bucco-pharyngeal aperture, was sufficient to account
for the impediment in respiration. It should be remarked,
however, that although the uvula appeared flabby, it was not
paralyzed, for it would sometimes retract spontaneously, and
always do so when touched with an instrument.

As the tonsils projected but slightly beyond their proper limits, and their further excision was very difficult, if not hazardous, in consequence of the smallness of the mouth and extreme
narrowness of the throat, I resolved to try the effect of simply
clipping off the uvula. The child has not snored since, and has
from that time slept without any impediment in his respiration.

Would it not be advisable to resort to this simple operation
for the relief of snoring in adults? It is certainly worthy of
trial, and might add very much to the comfort of those who
are annoyed by a snoring bed-fellow.

PART II.

Eclectic Department.

Letters upon Syphilis. Addressed to the Editor of L'Union
Medicale, by P. Ricord. Translated from the French by
D. D. Slade, M. D.

[Continued from Page 559.]

SECOND LETTER.

My Dear Friend,—I am not writing a didactic work; I have
a great desire so to do, but you know that at this moment I am
not able. I address you some letters familiarly written, and for
which I ask all the privileges of the epistolary form—that is to
say, freedom of style and spontaneousness of thought. Therefore, that which I have not said in my preceding letter, I shall
say unceremoniously in this, without a too rigid adherence to
plan, method and other restraints of composition, elsewhere so
useful.

In order that my first letter should be complete in the rapid
sketch of the attempts made in experimentation, I ought not to
omit to bring to mind the facts of the attempts at inoculation of
syphilis from man upon animals. Either to avoid the inconveniences which could result from the inoculation practised upon
man himself, or to resolve the curious problem of the transmission of syphilis to animals, Hunter and Turnbull had already

attempted in vain this inoculation from man to animals. I have repeated all those experiments, and have arrived at the same negative results. However, lately a young and industrious fellow-laborer, M. Auzias Turenne, has repeated these experiments, has varied them, has employed other methods than those which were known, and he has thought to have arrived at the experimental demonstration of the transmissibility of syphilis from man to certain animals. It was my duty, then, to renew these experiments, and I was convinced anew that syphilis was decidedly not communicable to animals, and that the facts as stated by M. Auzias were illusory. M. Cullerier, at the Hospital "de Lourcine," has studied this subject with much care, and has arrived at the same conclusions as myself. My colleague, M. Vidal (de Cassis,) has experimented in his turn, with I believe the same results.

The direct observation, the experimentation upon the patient himself, were then the only sources to which I could have recourse ; to these alone, then, I resolved to apply myself.

It was necessary, first, to seek a sure source from which I could draw the principle, towards the research of which, I wished to direct all my investigations. One could no longer rely upon the stories of patients ; it was necessary, also, to avoid the objections justly brought against the experiments of Hunter and of Harrison, against the facts stated by Bell, against the experiments of Hernandez ; and for this purpose, I first endeavored to well ascertain the state of the tissues from which I took the principle reputed specific.

It was no longer enough, as Petronius formerly said, that a woman should be considered *diseased ;* it would no longer do, to take at hazard a morbid secretion coming from the genital organs of the woman, and to make of it, according to the picturesque expression of Alexander Benedictus, a venereal dye, throwing a uniform color upon all the accidents which could result from it. No, the scientific tendencies of the minds of my day, and the demands of my own conscience, required of me the employment of a method more authentic and of proceedings more rigid.

I do not wish to lay stress upon the facility with which effects were drawn from the cause. But who would not be surprised, that in a question like that of venereal maladies, where ignorance and *fraud,* according to the expressions of Hunter, are such frequent sources of error—that in a disease which above all, and almost always, is a flagrant proof of immorality, the observers, even the most judicious, should so often trust to the reports of patients, and invoke without ceasing the moral worth of the testimony.

The testimony! under such circumstances, is there anything more deceptive? and especially as regards women? Let me, cite to you two little examples, where you will see one of the most strict observers caught in the snare of feminine testimony.

Babington wishes to destroy this law laid down by Hunter, that when there is neither pus nor puriform secretion, the disease cannot be communicated; so that the infection is not possible before the appearance of a gonorrhœa or after the cicatrization of a chancre. "This conclusion is not without danger," says Babington, " which one can see from the following facts, which are far from being rare."

" A married woman was taken with the ordinary symptoms of gonorrhœa, which much surprised her, as her husband was free from all disease. However, the husband having been questioned, confessed that he had had relations with a suspected woman, about eight days before his wife perceived herself diseased, but he positively affirmed that he had had no discharge, nor any morbid sensation, and certainly he offered no symptoms of disease. At the end of four days, that is to say, about fifteen days after the impure connection, and one week after the time when he should have communicated the disease to his wife, a gonorrhœal discharge manifested itself in him.

" A traveller exposed himself to the risks of a syphilitic infection, and arrived home at the end of three days. About four days after his arrival, his wife was attacked with gonorrhœa. It was not till ten days after the infection that he perceived, for the first time a discharge, and that he was attacked by the other symptoms of gonorrhœa."—(John Hunter's complete works, vol. xi., page 167. Notes by Babington.)

If, in presence of similar facts, Babington had not sought to obtain more-complete confessions (there are some confessions that women never make, even, as I have had the opportunity of too often seeing, under the fear of the greatest dangers,) but had assured himself by a rigid inspection of the true state of things; he would have seen that in these cases the infecting cause was not in the genital organs of the candid husbands.

It was not, then, possible to think of basing any pathological truth whatever, in syphilis, upon the morality of the testimony of the patients. I had no longer confidence in the doctrines and in the facts based upon recitals of this kind. It was necessary to be removed from the mysteries of the " *alcove*," to bring to the light of experimentation the principle which I wished to find. This principle—where ought I first to seek for it? At its source; that is to say, in the genital organs of the woman, in their external portions as well as in their deepest folds. Chance was propitious for me. The Hospital " du Midi " then received the unhappy beings that the dispensary sent there.

Here you will permit me to recall, my dear friend, that before
my entrance into the Hospital du Midi, the manner of examining a woman consisted in making her sit upon the border of a
chair, in separating the external genital organs, and if no lesion
of the tissue was found, every morbid secretion coming from
higher up, was invariably considered as a blennorrhagic discharge.   At the circle of the vulva, my predecessors appeared
to have placed the columns of Hercules of chancre.   I could
not, nor ought I, to have been satisfied with this superficial and
incomplete examination.   We were at no great distance from
the time when M. Recamier had so fortunately exhumed the
speculum from the surgical armentarium.   You are aware of
the happy applications that this celebrated practitioner had
made of it, in the diagnosis of diseases of the uterus.   But this
valuable instrument had not as yet been applied to the diagnosis of syphilitic diseases ; its employment, even in these cases,
appeared and was reported to be contra-indicated.   I did not
pay any attention to this widely-spread opinion.   I made a
general use, on the contrary, of the speculum upon all the
women in my wards.

I do not know if posterity will partake of the opinion of one
of my learned critics, who reduced to a very small compass that
which I had to do in syphilopathy.   However, my dear friend,
when I call to mind the profound obscurity which enveloped
the diagnosis of syphilitic diseases before the application of the
speculum—when I compare the embarrassment of practitioners
of that epoch in settling up their opinion, with the truly wonderful facility of modern practitioners in giving an undeniable
diagnosis ; when the recollection of all the services that the
speculum has already rendered to this part of practice comes
to my mind, I think, that should my participation in its progress
be thus limited, this opinion might appear rather severe.   The
employment of the speculum permitted me to examine with
great care all the surfaces venereally affected, and to ascertain
with precision the condition of the tissues which furnished the
secretions.

These conditions established, I had to study all the accidents
reputed venereal, and comparatively with other morbid secretions.

I commenced with blennorrhagia.   You understand, my
dear friend, that I ought to suppose the state of the question, at
the time when I undertook my experiments concerning blennorrhagia, to be perfectly understood by my readers.   Once
more, I do not here write volumes with a complete history, but
a simple and concise exposition of facts which belong to me.

I sought to resolve by experimentation that problem already

differently resolved, by the observation which you know—
Does blennorrhagia recognize a specific cause ?᜵

Hunter had taught that the pus of a chancre inoculated produced chancre. If blennorrhagia recognizes a specific cause,
said I to myself, the muco-pus which it secretes, being inoculated, will produce without doubt phenomena similar to those
which pus coming from a chancre produces.

But to well ascertain the result, to isolate it from every complication, and from every cause of error, it was necessary first
to inoculate the muco-pus coming from perfectly simple blennorrhagias ; it was necessary to take this muco-pus from tissues
completely free from all ulceration ; and you see how valuable
the employment of the speculum was to me.   Without it, these
experiments were not possible.

Now these first experiments, made in great number, and a
long time continued with perseverance, conducted me to this
first fundamental result, which I here give in the form of a proposition.

PROPOSITION.

*Every time that the muco-pus has been taken from a mucous
surface not ulcerated, the results of the inoculation have been
negative.*

All experimenters who have followed me in this course have
arrived at the same conclusion ; and this, whatever has been
the period of the blennorrhagia in which the experimentation
has been made.   Thus, it is with great surprise that I have
read in your Journal the following passage, where M. Vidal,
in his *letters upon syphilitic inoculation,* reproaches inoculation
for being very often fruitless in the question of blennorrhagia ;
"In fact." says my learned colleague, "a distinguished Interne,
M. Bigot, has tried, under the observation of M. Puche, physician at the Hospital du Midi, sixty-eight inoculations with
muco-pus coming from the urethra, and these sixty-eight inoculations have been followed by no result."   I am astonished at
the surprise of M. Vidal.   These sixty-eight negative inoculations conform entirely to the facts which I have before advanced ; they confirm and corroborate my opinion upon the rarity
of *syphilitic* blennorrhagia ; and when my opposer asks you—
" Do you believe that of these sixty-eight blennorrhagias there
were none, where virus was present, no one that contained the
seeds of a verole ?" answer him confidently, no; and for this
reason, that the inoculation has been negative.

A logician as skillful and as exact as M. Vidal, could not be
prevented from perceiving that the results of experimentation,
upon whatever subject exercised. are either positive or negative
but that scientifically speaking, the negative results are no less

valuable than the possitive. The inoculation of vaccine does
not give rise to any phenomenon upon those subjects who have
already had the variola ; is that saying that the negative result
is without importance and without consequences?

But we shall soon see how much value and force these negative results have derived from the positive results of inocula·
tion. I notice, in passing, a first objection which will at a later period find its complete refutation. Some writers on syphilis have thought with Hunter that blennorrhagia was a form
of syphilis peculiar to mucous membranes. I confine myself
for the moment to remarking that the experiments before indicated destroy entirely this opinion ; we shall see later that the
virulent virus of chancre, placed upon a mucous surface, produces there, in every respect, the chancre.

From experiments shown, I shall draw this conclusion.

CONCLUSION.

The blennorrhagia, of which the muco-pus being inoculated,
gives rise to no result, does not recognize the syphilitic virus as
cause.

This conclusion, as you know, has given rise to numerous
and grave objections. But I fear that you cannot to-day afford
me sufficient room to undertake the refutation and exposition
of these. This will be, with your permission, the subject of
my third letter.—[*Boston Med. and Surg. Journal.*

On the use of Salines and Opiates in Dysentery. By F. E.
GORDON, M. D., of Alabama.

Having made a report to the Alabama State Medical Association, by appointment, on the diseases of Marion, which was
lost through the illness and absence of Dr. Jackson, its late
Treasurer, I herewith submit the following remarks on the use
of Salines and Opiates in Dysentery.

This disease prevailed here as an epidemic during the spring
and summer of 1851, and gave rise to great diversity of opinion
and treatment. This is not strange, as its pathology and management have been, for more than two hundred years, disputed
points amongst the ablest medical writers. Chisholm, and
James Johnson more particularly, contended " that the liver
itself forms the primary seat of the disease in every instance,"
and hence urged the use of mercurials even to ptyalism, while
the more venerable opinion of Sydenham, which locates it in
the larger intestines, is more generally received in this day;
and hence a revival of his practice is likely to ensue, if it may
not be said to have done so already. With the exception of

blood-letting, Sydenham's plan of daily purgation, followed by his own potent laudanum at night, is not easily improved upon. That he would have abandoned bleeding, had he lived to this day, (to say nothing of this climate) his great practical sagacity and the example of his able successors in London, warrant us in saying.

Watson contends that the sheathing of the lancet has been the result of Cholera, which, since 1832, has modified the character of diseases, and many eminent physicians on this side of the Atlantic equally ignore the abstraction of blood, though accounting for its inapplicability in different ways.

From a glance at the various reports made to the Alabama Association, which, though conflicting in many respects, generally assign a greater mortality to this disease, we would be disposed to set down our epidemic as very mild. Indeed we think fever did not make its appearance in the onset of an attack oftener than once in ten cases. We are admonished, however, that in the beginning of the epidemic the disease did prove fatal in many cases; not, however, from its malignancy, but, as we think, from the inefficiency of the practice by which it was met. Such as died were literally worn out by the excessively frequent and painful discharges, giving rise to irritative fever and emaciation. Ulceration, we are satisfied, did not occur once in three hundred properly treated cases.

Our attention was first directed to the value of Salines and Opiates in Dysentery, by an article in the Charleston Medical Journal for July, 1848, "on the comparative efficacy of certain medicines in the treatment of Dysentery and other intestinal Fluxes of hot climates."

Dr. Papillaud, the author of this paper, made his observations in a province of Brazil, in twenty-nine degrees of South latitude, and found the usual plan of treatment adopted in Paris with success, to fail entirely in this warm region.

" He experimented with castor oil, ipecacuanha, calomel, sulphate of soda; of the vegetable astringents, he tried rhatany and simarouba; of the mineral astringents, lime, acetate of lead, alum and nitrate of silver; of narcotics, extract of opium and sulphate of morphia; from the results of these experiments he determined to abide by sulphate of soda and opium, the effects of the other medicines being variable and uncertain." He says, " The English practice of calomel and castor oil is very unsuccessful." "Sulphate of soda, he thinks, deserves the praise it received from Bretonneau and Trousseau, acting energetically and most rapidly. One or two drachms dissolved in a small quantity of vehicle, and given in divided doses, usually arrest a dysentery in twelve, twenty-four, or forty-eight hours at the

longest.". He says, " Inflammation once considered a cause, is
only one form, *alteration of secretion* another."

" The indications for local bleeding are very rare ; that for
general bleeding only as an exception." " Opium he considers
equal to sulphate of soda, and together they formed one of the
most efficacious combinations."

My first trial with this remedy was soon after its publication,
and proved highly satisfactory. In a few sporadic cases I continued to use it with success. It was not, however, until the
period referred to above, viz : the spring of 1851, that I had an
opportunity of witnessing its effects on a large scale. Insensibly I fell into using Seidlitz Powders amongst my white patients,
as being more agreeable, and finding free purgation to relieve
both tormina and tenesmus, for about six hours I usually followed it up by a dose of morphine. The fractional doses of
neutral salts and morphia were then resumed.

It was remarkable that in some cases, where hypercatharsis
had been induced, (the patient in one instance taking one powder every half hour until eight were consumed) the recovery
was most prompt.

Generally, when much opium had not been previously taken,
from two to four Seidlitz Powders at half hour intervals, freely
evacuated the bowels.

As regards pathology, I do not think inflammation of the
mucous membrane of the colon so much as engorgement of it,
can be predicated of a disease so easily relieved by a serous
drain from the bowels, and so often independent of fever.
Whether the neutral salts act also as a " *local modifier*" on the
mucous membrane, according to the French view of this subject, or as a " *sedative*," I am unable to say.

In order to establish the claims of this method of treatment,
and to vindicate it from the charge of empiricism, I subjoin
reports from two of our most intelligent and respectable physicians. Dr. England says—

" Enclosed you find a list of cases of Dysentery that came
under my care during the present year, up to date, 15th August,
1851. It comprises all ages, from infancy up to advanced age.
All were subjected to the saline treament except two in January, which were treated by mercury and opium, and but one
death occurred among them. This was a case of unusual
severity, first seen thirty-six hours after being attacked,
yet under the use of Salines the Dysentery gradually yielded,
so that in three days only slight sanguinolent discharges occasionally recurred, and these subsided entirely forty-eight hours
or more before death, which occurred from nervous exhaustion,
following the excessive excitement of the system. There were

many other cases (where a single prescription relieved the Dysentery) that required no visiting or attention, of which I made no note."

" P. S.   In addition to the above, there occurred thirty-five cases during the spring and summer in the Judson Institute, which did not come under my immediate care, yet were treated with salines according to my directions—all of which recovered."

Here follows the table referred to by Dr. England :

Months.			*Cases.*	*Recoveries.*	*Deaths.*
January,	-	-	4	4	0
February,	-	-	6	6	0
March,	-	-	8	8	0
April,			12	12	0
May,	-	-	14	14	0
June,			20	20	0
July,			14	13	1
August,	-	-	2	2	0
Total,			80	79	1

Under date of August 12th, 1851, Dr. Bryant encloses me the following statement, arranged in a tabular form.   He remarks : Agreeable to your request I send you the above list of cases of Dysentery, treated by myself during the present year."

Dys.	*Cured.*	*Died.*	*Adults over 14.*	*Children under 14.*	*Total.*
March 2,	2	0	1	1	
April 12,	12	0	8	4	
May 22,	22	0	7	15	
June 24,	24	0	10	14	
July 14,	14	0	6	8	
August 8,	8	0	3	5	82

I have Dr. Bryant's authority for saying, that with the exception of a single case, otherwise treated, these were all managed, with the highest degree of satisfaction to himself, by the use of Salines and Opiates.   In the latter part of the epidemic he sometimes used Sup. Tart. Potass in the more protracted cases, with decided benefit.

These gentlemen here cited will bear me out in saying, that Calomel given to relieve the portal circulation excites a free gush of bile, which is, to use Dr Johnson's language, like so much boiling lead, throws the irritable intestines into painful contortions, and then the tormina and tenesmus are intolerable ;" and hence, like myself, they abandoned its use for the Salines, which produced a gentle action on the liver and copious discharges from the bowels, quieting for a time all distress like a charm.   The bile in these discharges was blunted by the quantity of fluid with which it was mingled.—[*N. O. Med. and Surg. Journal.*

Practical Observations on Tetanus.   By V. H. Fugate, M. D., of Mississippi.

Dear Sir,—In the July No. for 1852 of your Journal, on page 87, I notice the following remark : " We are rather disposed to give the credit of the cure to the judicious regimen adopted by the physician, and to the lapse of time—*it being well understood* that this formidable disease is but little influenced by the most enlightened medication," etc.   From the above remark I am induced to ask your indulgence while I detail a few cases (from my scrap-book) of Traumatic Tetanus, that have occurred in my practice.

First.   Negro boy, aged about 15 years, had the balls of his first and second finger slightly split with the teeth of the ginsaw.   No inconvenience resulted until the sixth day, when he was violently attacked with painful muscular rigidity and tetanic spasm of a general character, as I learned from his master.

Saw him on the seventh day (at night) after the accident ; found him perfectly inflexible at every joint ; could bend no joint ; pulse quickened ; surface warm ; wounds on the fingers healed and dry ; spasms frequent and severe, returning as often as one per minute, when undisturbed, though the slightest touch, the softest breeze, the least noise induced the spasms at any instant, always accompanied with a fearful and suppressed scream— his jaws being firmly locked.   I applied a blister to the ends of his fingers ; a batch of carded cotton from the nape to the sacrum, wet with turpentine, to which I applied a lighted torch, blistering him the whole length of the spine in an instant ; gave him as much as a grain of Morphine, and ordered that as much good French brandy as he could be induced to swallow should be forced down him, with one grain of Morphine every hour, until some change obtained.

On my arrival next morning, twelve hours from the time I left him, no change had taken place, except that I could bend his knees slightly ; the spasms less violent, though quite as frequent.   He had had taken twelve grains of morphine, and more than a pint of brandy.   I now ordered that the brandy and Morphine be continued night and day, with the addition of 20 grains of Quinine three times a day, dissolved in the brandy, and that all the strong beef tea that he could swallow or retain by injection, be allowed him.

On my next visit the ensuing day, I was astonished at the amount of Morphine and brandy consumed, and rejoiced to find an abatement of all the symptoms. I continued this course for four days, without any variation, except as the symptoms continued to abate, the amount of dose was corrrespondingly diminished, and the time between doses increased.

I neglected to mention, that on the second day, after I saw him, he drank a quart of brandy. I saw him three days after almost entirely relieved; dismissed him; brandy and Morphine were continued three times a day for several days, however. The boy recovered rapidly.

Second Case. Negro woman, aged 50, fell in the fire and burnt her hand. When the ulcer was quite healed, she took general tetanus, assuming on the second day Opisthotonos. The spasms were violent, frequent and general; jaws so locked that I had difficulty in getting her to swallow anything. I treated her alone with whiskey, Morphine, laudanum and beef tea, as in the former case, that is, forcing down as much as possible. She recovered in two weeks and three days.

Third Case. Child, aged 11 years. Clothes caught on fire, burning nearly the whole surface; two weeks after the ulcers nearly healed, tetanic spasms made their appearance.

I saw her seven days after I had dismissed the treatment of her burns, in the most aggravated form of general tetanus, truly distressing, from her emaciated condition. I put her under the influence of Chloroform, which lasted half an hour. I then gave her a large dose of Morphine, ordering her to have as much brandy and Morphine as she could bear or swallow.

I repeated the Chloroform next morning, with entire relaxation as before, which, however, did not last long, the spasms returning in an hour, though much milder at first, and gradually increasing in severity and frequency.

After this I continued as before to prescribe brandy, Morphine and Quinine, with the most nutritious diet, for five days. Pronounced her cured.

Fourth Case. Negro boy, frost bit toes. Ulcers became dry; Tetanus supervened.

I saw him four days after he had spasms first; could bend no joint; took him by the head and set him up on end like a log; could not get one drop of anything down him; having, when undisturbed, two spasms per minute.

I gave him an enema of Chloroform and Camphor, and presently applied the Chloroform sponge to his nostrils, containing

ℨij, gradually approaching it nearer and nearer, until I embraced his mouth and nose with the sponge; in three minutes
he was as flexible as a string, and breathing stertorously.
This condition continued five minutes, when on puncturing his
ear he opened his eyes. I gave him two grains of Morphine
in this relaxed condition. The spasms returned slightly during
the day.

Next morning put him under the influence of Chloroform
again; continued Morphine and brandy several days, as in the
former cases; he recovered rapidly.

I have treated several others in the same way. What say
you?

Answer—Mayhap the cases recovered in spite of the Doctor's heroic doses. Ed.—[*Ibid.*

*On the Influence exerted by Chronic Diseases upon the Compo-
sition of the Blood.* By MM. Becquerel and Rodier.

The following are the conclusions of a paper recently read
at the *Academie des Sciences,* detailing the results of MM. Becquerel and Rodier's latest hæmatological researches:—1. The
majority of chronic diseases and various anti-hygienic circumstances induce an increase or diminution in the three principal
elements of the blood—the globules, the fibrine, and the albumen, and this either separately or simultaneously. 2. The
globules undergo diminution in the course of most chronic diseases of long duration, and especially in organic diseases of the
heart, the chronic form of Bright's disease, chlorosis, marsh
cachexia, hæmorrhages, hæmorrhoidal flux, excessive bloodletting, the last stages of tubercular disease, and the cancerous
diathesis. The same result is observed in those whose food is
not sufficient in quantity or reparative power, or who are exposed to insufficient aëration, humidity, darkness, &c. 3. The
albumen of the serum of the blood is diminished in quantity in
the third stage of heart-disease, great symptomatic anæmia,
the cancerous diathesis, and insufficient alimentation. 4. The
fibrine is maintained at its normal proportion, and sometimes
increased, in acute scorbutus. It is diminished in chronic scorbutus, as also in the scorbutic condition symptomatic of certain
chronic diseases, which is most often and most markedly observed in organic diseases of the heart. 5. In all the above-
mentioned circumstances, the quantity of water contained in
the blood becomes very considerably increased. 6. A diminution of the proportion of globules is especially accompanied
b y the following phenomena: a colourless state of the skin,

palpitations, dyspnœa, a *bruit de soufflet* heard at the base of the heart during the first sound, an intermittent *bruit de soufflet* in the carotids, and a continuous *bruit* in the jugulars. 7. The diminution of the proportion of albumen, even though not very considerable, when it takes place in an acute manner, rapidly gives rise to the production of dropsy, but it requires to be much more considerable when not appearing in the acute form. Considered in a general manner, dropsy is the symptomatic characteristic of a diminished proportion of the albumen of the blood. 8. A diminished proportion of fibrine is manifested by the production of cutaneous or mucous hæmorrhages. 9. In anæmia, symptomatic of considerable hæmorrhage or insufficient alimentation, the change in the blood is characterized by a diminution of its density, an increase of the water, diminution of globules, a maintenance of the normal proportion or sometimes a slight diminution of the albumen, and a normal proportion of fibrine. 10. In chlorosis, which is an entirely distinct affection from anæmia, there may be no changes in the blood whatever. When such are present, they consist in a diminution of the proportion of globules, an increase of that of the water, and the normal quantity or an increase of fibrine 11. In the acute form of Bright's disease the fibrine continues normal, and the albumen is diminished. In the chronic form there is a diminution of globules and albumen, and sometimes of fibrine. 12. Most of the dropsies regarded as essential depend upon a diminution of the proportion of albumen; and usually originate in a material cause, consisting in a degeneration of the solid or fluid parts of the economy. 13. In diseases of the heart the blood becomes more and more changed, as they approach the fatal termination. The changes consist in the simultaneous diminution of globules, fibrine, and albumen, and an increase of water. 14. In acute scorbutus, the principles of the blood do not undergo any appreciable modification. In the chronic form the fibrine is notably diminished, while the globules are sometimes considerably increased. In both forms, the increase of the proportion of the soda of the blood explains all the circumstances; but it has not yet been demonstrated. 15. The above modifications should influence our therapeutical management of these different morbid conditions, as each element of the blood is susceptible of special modification. Thus, when the proportion of albumen is diminished, we prescribe cinchona, and a tonic strengthening diet. A diminution of fibrine and an increase of the soda of the blood are to be met by good diet, vegetable acids, and appropriate hygiène; and by hygienic measures and the exhibition of iron, we combat the diminution of globules.—[*L'Union Médicale.* *British and Foreign Med. Chir. Rev.*

On the Reciprocal Influence of Acute Diseases and Menstruation. By M. HERARD.

M. Herard terminates a recent memoir with the following conclusions;—1. All acute diseases exert a pretty similar effect on menstruation. 2. This influence varies accordingly as the disease becomes developed during a menstrual epoch, or during an interval. 3. In the first of these cases the menses are usually suppressed completely or incompletely, when they may re-appear after some hours or days, though usually in diminished quantity. The patients regard the suppression as being the cause of the febrile disease, although the contrary is the fact: and even in the case of acute febrile disease becoming manifested after suppression, we must regard it as a consequence of the chill that has produced this. 4. When an acute febrile disease is developed in the interval, if the next epoch is near at hand, so that the fever continues to it, the menstruation is favoured by the increased hæmorrhagic congestion of the uterus and ovaries. 5. The menses are usually absent or notably diminished in quantity, at the periods which occur during the decline of a disease, or in convalescence. This secondary amenoirhœa, though sometimes persistent, usually only continues for from one to three months. 6. The menstrual eruption in nowise predisposes to disease. 7. Menstruation exerts no appreciable influence on the issue of acute febrile affections. The progress and termination of these are the same, whether the discharge appears or not, whether it is increased or diminished in quantity, is earlier or later in appearance, or whether this takes place at the beginning or end of the affection. 8. In treating acute febrile affections, it is the condition of the disease that must engage our attention ; for it is rare that any special therapeutical indication is derivable from the state of the menses ; and we must act absolutely in the same way if the menses are on the point of appearing, or are expected, as if they were not so. 9. Bloodletting does not, in general, prevent their appearance or continuance. 10. The sudden suppression of the menses by the development of an acute febrile disease, or amenorrhœa consecutive to such disease, does not, in general, call for any special treatment.—[*Ibid.*

On the Influence of Pregnancy and the Puerperal State on the Progress of Phthisis. By MM. GRISOLLE & DUBREUILH.

M. Grisolle, in reporting to the Academy of Medicine upon a memoir presented by M. Dubreuilh, observes, that the views

he formerly expressed* have only obtained additional confirmation.   In none of the thirteen cases related by M. Dubreuilh, or
in the thirty-five now collected by M. Grisolle, has the powei
formerly vaguely attributed to pregnancy of staying the progress of phthisis, been observed.   In some cases, indeed, it
seems to have played the part of determining cause, and in
others to have aggravated the condition.   According to M.
Grisolle's observation, cases in which the first symptoms of
phthisis are developed at an early period of pregnancy, and
amidst a state of health otherwise satisfactory, are more common than those in which the pregnancy is consecutive to the
early appearance of the organic disease.   Both observers are,
indeed, of opinion that phthisical women conceive with difficulty; and M. Delafond assured the reporter that cows, even at
at an early period of the disease, usually remained sterile, even
though they continued fully alive to the attentions of the bull.
He added, also, that in such as did conceive, abortion was
common about the fifth or sixth month; while in such as went
their full time, the progress of the disease was in nowise modified.   In M. Grisolle's former papers he stated that pregnancy,
in his cases, so far from retarding, hastened the progress of
phthisis; and although the rate was found to be somewhat slow
in M. Dubreuilh's cases, this probably arose from their having
occurred in private practice, while M. Grisolle's were all hospital patients.   Both sets of cases, however, amply disprove the
suspending power of pregnancy; and M. P. Dubois' experience has long since led him to a similar conclusion.   Phthisis
which has appeared at an early period of pregnancy pursues a
constantly onward course; and if improvement is to take place
at all, it never does so until after delivery.   It is rare for phthisis
thus complicated to present those intermissions or sudden sus-
pensions of progress sometimes met with in ordinary phthisis.
The children brought forth by phthisical mothers, though usually small, are plump and well-looking to an extent that would
not, *a priori*, be expected from persons suffering from so exhausting a disease.
    M. Dubreuilh expresses a theoretical opinion in favor of the
prevalent belief that the progress of phthisis is hastened by *delivery*, but his facts are against him; and so complete is the
suspension of the disease sometimes, that delusive hopes of cure
are entertained.
    In regard to the influence of *phthisis on pregnancy*, both ob-
servers are agreed that such patients *ordinarily* go their full
time; which must be regarded as a remarkable fact, when it is

* British and Foreign Medico-Chir. Review, vol. vi., p. 261.

considered that more than one-half the pregnant women attacked by pneumonia, abort.   Both also find that these women
usually have very easy labours—a fact due to the smaller size
of the child and the relaxed state of the tissues.   Both, too,
consider that the attempt to suckle exerts the most disastrous
influence upon both mother and child.—[*Bulletin de l'Acad.
Rev. Med.   Ibid.*

On Hereditary Transmission of Phthisis.   By M. GUILLOT.

Since 1825, M. Guillot has been tracing out the history of
certain cases of phthisis, in order to illustrate the laws which
regulate the hereditary transmission of this disease.   He follows
the history of the family-line, in order to ascertain whether this
does not, by successive degradation, become exhausted and
extinguished.   He refers to the case of a man who died of
phthisis, aged 66.   Before the age of 48 all his four children
died of the same disease ; all had children, but the third generation did not survive the period of the first dentition, all being
carried off either by pneumonia supervening on tubercle, or by
tubercular meningitis.   In another example, a grandfather died
of phthisis.   One of his daughters also died of it at 30.   The
other daughter is still living, but three of her children have died
either of tubercular pneumonia or meningitis.   The general
conclusion is, that in proportion as phthisis descends in the
genealogical scale, its manifestation takes place at an earlier
period of life.   A child will therefore run greater chance of
falling a victim to the consequences of the numerous accidents
of a tubercular affection, in proportion as the phthisical parents
who have given birth to it have not attained advanced age.   In
a diagnostical point of view, then, the existence of tubercular
disease in the offspring while yet young, offers a very strong
presumption of phthisis.   The practical importance of this is
especially evident in pneumonia, so common is it to find tubercles of the lungs in the bronchial glands, masked by the signs
of this affection.—[*L'Union Medicale.   Ibid.*

On Measles as observed in Idiot Children.   By M. DELASIAUVE.

The remark has been frequently made, that in certain classes
of the insane, incidental diseases exhibit a severity which is
not usually observed in persons in the possession of their faculties.   Exactly the contrary to this has been, it is true, maintained by some, and a supposed immunity asserted.   Georget

and Esquirol, however, have shown that insanity disposes the subjects of it to be more severely affected than are others by ordinary diseases; and Ferrus especially points out dementia and idiocy as unfavourable conditions in this point of view. M. Thore, also, in a special essay on the subject, adopts the same view. M. Delasiauve deduces the same conclusion from the opportunities he has had of observing epidemics of *measles* at the Bicêtre. The children of the *employes* of the establishment were recently attacked in great numbers, and from these the disease was communicated to the idiot and epileptic children. While among the former the eruption pursued a normal and favourable course, anomalous conditions complicated it among the latter, and very often rendered it fatal. In different epidemics, there has been observed a predominance of some one of these, such as engorgement of the lungs, of the brain, or the parotid, œdema, &c. Violent diarrhœa was the especial characteristic of the present one. Besides this, however, in six out of eight cases, occurring in one section, asphyxia from bronchitis occurred, endangering the lives of the whole, and terminating fatally in two.—[*Annales Med. Psychol. Ibid.*

On the Cause and Diagnostic Value of Muscæ Volitantes. By M. TAVIGNOT.

M. Tavignot assigns as the cause of this phenomenon, the passage of the luminous rays through a very circumscribed spot of the semi-transparent tissue of the iris. which has become deprived of its pigmentary matter—a fissure in the uvea. This theory explains: 1st. Why the muscæ are placed near the visual axis, but always on one side of it; 2d. It explains the fact of their disappearance in obscure light, and their especial distinctness in a bright one, which induces the contraction of the pupil, and the enlargement of the aperture in the uvea; 3rd. Also their varied form, according to the different action of light upon the eye, and the effect of this upon the size of the fissure; 4th. It explains their appearance after sudden movement of the eyes upwards, which is always accompanied by a contractile oscillation of the iris, as also their diminution or disappearance as the pupil enlarges.

If this theory be sound, the muscæ ought to disappear when the pupil is dilated by belladonna; and M. Tavignot declares that his experiments have convinced him that they do disappear in proportion as artificial mydriasis is thus produced, and that they return again with the returning motions of the iris. It is to be borne in mind that these remarks are referrible only to *essential* muscæ volitantes; M. Tavignot intending to show hereafter, that in the *sympathetic* form (as in glaucoma) an altered condition of the texture of the iris explains the appearance, and adds confirmation to the above view.

Artificial dilatation of the pupil enables us to decide whether we have to do with muscæ volitantes, properly so called, or with the spots known as *scotomata*, which are found in partial opacities of the cornea, and in incipient cataract ; for while the muscæ volitantes disappear on the production of the mydriasis, the scotomata persist, and even become more distinct.—[*Gaz. dés Hop. Ibid.*

On the Treatment of Syphilis in Pregnant Women. By M. Devilliers.

The following are the conclusions with which M. Devilliers terminates a memoir upon this subject :—1. A pregnant woman usually supports mercurial treatment pretty well during the first half of pregnancy, and even from the first week. 2. Any injurious effects that may occur during this period, seem principally to depend upon a want of tolerance in the digestive organs, and consequent nervous irritability. 3. The fœtus is more sensitive to the effects of syphilis, and to the action of specific remedies, in proportion as it approaches the perfection necessary for extra-uterine life. 4. In the application of treatment, the following circumstances in relation to the progress of syphilitic disease in pregnant women should be borne in mind—viz. (*a.*) The condition of conception may excite the external manifestation of symptoms which, for a greater or less period, had remained dormant. (*b.*) The symptoms frequently exhibit oscillations during pregnancy, and have an especial tendency to re-appear about the sixth, seventh, or eighth month. (*c.*) They generally disappear spontaneously, and rather quickly after delivery. 5. Palliatives for primary symptoms in the early months are useless, and a radical treatment should at once be resorted to. It is still more urgent to treat without delay any secondary or tertiary symptoms that may be present. 6. Active treatment undertaken or re-commenced towards the latter part of pregnancy—i. e. the period when abortion from syphilis is most likely to occur—requires greater precautions to be observed than during the early period. 7. When the treatment during the first half of pregnancy has not been completely interrupted, or has been so only for a short time, its resumption on the re-appearance of symptoms during the latter period exposes both mother and child to less chance of accidents. 8. Treatment should not be discontinued too quickly after the disappearance of the symptoms, but persevered with in very small doses as long as possible. 9. The treatment seems to be well borne both by mother and child at all periods of gestation, in proportion to the complicated and aggravated condition of the syphilitic accidents. 10. The syphilitic symptoms, whether primary or secondary, which are manifested during the latter weeks of pregnancy, require general as well as local treatment. The child is then more amenable to treatment, if this be required after birth. 11. We must not wait too long after delivery, to commence or resume treatment, deceived by the decrease of the symptoms so common at that period. If the child, suckled by the mother, exhibits any mark of syphilis, we must not wait later than the eighth or tenth day. 12. In the early period of pregnancy, internal mercurial treatment is often ill borne. This is less frequently the case in the middle and later periods. In the former, inunction should be resorted to.

M. Gibert, commenting upon the above essay, likewise says that the ill effects which several practitioners have observed to result from the administration of mercury in syphilitic women, have arisen from their giving it internally. It frequently excites vomiting and colics in the fourth and fifth months; and mercurial frictions are infinitely preferable. Abortion from syphilis ordinarily occurs after the fourth or fifth month; whence, if treatment is to be preventive, it must be commenced early.—[*Bull. de l'Acad. Bull. de Therap. Ibid.*

On Edible Earths. By EHRENBERG.

Various kinds of edible earths were known in China in very ancient times, and it may be presumed, that many of them are mixed or pure tripolitan fresh water bioliths—*i. e.* species of earths or stones, the elements of which consist chiefly of remnants of microscopic living beings. In the year 1839, Biot read before the Academy of Sciences in Paris a treatise, containing everything that was then known on this subject, to which his son, the oriental linguist, Biot, furnished translations from Chinese and Japanese works. From Schott in Berlin, Professor Ehrenberg obtained in addition the following information taken from Chinese sources. The first mention of edible earth dates from the year 744 after Christ, and is contained in the Chinese work Pen-tsao-kang-mu, where it is called Schi-miàm, Stonebread, or Mi-ànschi, Breadstone; the article in the Japanese "Encyclopædia," which Biot has translated, is taken from this work. The Pen-tsao says, according to Schott, that stones contain several substances which are edible, especially a yellow meal and a fatty liquid, which is contained in the white Yü,

(a stone,) and is, therefore, called the fat, marrow, or mucilage
of the white Yü. ˙ An earthy substance, prolonging life, and
called Schi-nas, is found in the very smooth stone Hoa-shi,.
which is supposed to be Steatite. and may, perhaps, be decomposed Steatite. The Schi miàn is only used as a substitute for
bread in times of scarcity, when it is miraculously found in
different localities, as is believed. The imperial annals of the
Chinese have always religiously noticed its appearance, but
have never given any description of the substance. The Pen-
tsao quotes, under the emperor Hiuan Tsung, of the great
dynasty Tàng, in the third year Tiàn-pao (744 after Christ) a
spring in Wujin (now Liang-tschen-fu, in the province Kan-su)
which ejected stones, that could be prepared into bread, and
were gathered and consumed by the poor. (Schott.)

Under the emperor Hian-Tsung, of the same dynasty, in the
ninth year of the period Yüen-ho (809 after Christ) the stones
became soft and turned into bread. (Biot.)

Under the emperor Tschin-Tsung, of the dynasty Sung, in
the fifth year of the period Ta-tschong-Tsiang-fu (1012 after
Christ) in the fourth month, there was a famine in Tsy-tschen
(now Ki-tschen in Ping-Yang-fu, in the province Schan-si,)
when the mountains of Hiang-ning, a district of the third rank
in the same part, produced a mineral fat (Stonefat) resembling
a dough, of which cakes could be made. (Schott.)

Under Jin-Tsung, in the seventh year of the period Kia-yeu
(1062) stone meal was found. (Biot.)

Under Tschi-Tsung, in the third year of the period Yuen-
fong (1080) the stones turned into meal. All these kinds of
stone-meal were collected and consumed by the poor. (Biot.)

Very recently, in the year 1831 to 1834, similar kinds of
earth have been found in China, and were used as food during
the great famine, as has been reported by the Chinese missionary, Mathieu Ly, who resides in the province Kiany-si. In
the year 1834, he writes:—" Many of our Christians will surely die this year from starvation. ˙ The Almighty alone can aid
them in such great distress. All harvests have been destroyed
by the floods. For three years a large number of persons have
lived upon the bark of an indigenous tree ; others have eaten a
light white earth which has been discovered in a mountain. It
can only be obtained for silver, and not every one can, therefore, procure it. The people have first sold their wives, then
their children, then their furniture, at last they have pulled
down their houses and sold the .wood. Many of them were,
four years ago, wealthy men." The missionary, Rameaux, also
reported in 1834, from the province Hu-kuang, that many Chinese Christians have sent for him to administer to them the last

sacrament, and foreseeing the hour when they were to die from starvation, actually died at that very time. The very dense population and industry which necessarily takes possession of everything, are, in cases of earthquakes and deluges, the cause of these circumstances in China.

The districts where stone-bread has been found are the northern province of Schan-si, the east provinces of Schan-tong and Kiang-nan, on the mouth of the Yellow river (Huang-hu,) the provinces Hu-kuang and Kiang-si, in the valley of the Blue river (Yantsekiang). It is very desirable to know the masses, localities, extent of occurrence of these earths, as well as their geognostic character. The analysis of the two kinds, which the author has obtained, renders it very probable that all similar substances belong to antediluvian deposits, some of which are very probably tripolitan, fresh water bioliths of infusoria, while others appear to be clay mixtures or real clays. (*Letten.*)

A. White Edible Earth of 1834, *from China.*—The author obtained in the year 1841, by Humboldt, from Paris, a sample of the edible white earth, sent to Paris by the French missionary in China. One of the two pieces measured two inches in diameter, the other one inch. It has a white colour, similar to chalk, but is as light as *Kieselguhr* or Meerschaum, is somewhat fatty to the touch, not soiling the fingers, but very brittle. The pieces having been broken in those directions which were indicated by a previous crack. some of the internal surfaces had a rusty colour, but only superficially. Acids caused no effervescence. According to the analysis, this earth is merely silicate of alumina, the peculiar lightness of which is striking. If heated, it assumes a gray colour. In fifteen samples no organic mixture could be discovered by microscopic examination, which latter shows also no similarity between this substance and Meerschaum; there is also an entire absence of magnesia. This earth has much resemblance to lithomarge-like Kaolin, but its lightness and the different form of the microscopic parts admit no identity between them. Irregular, mostly globular bodies of various sizes, with soft obtuse outlines, compose the whole mass. Perhaps it is a deposit of a precipitate from hot siliceous waters.

From the blackish mould left in the impressions of the smoothly scraped natural surface, it is obvious that the fossil has not been taken out from the midst of rocks, but was dug out from a black mould. Analysis have shown eighteen different microscopic forms, which are enumerated in the 294th analysis of the micrologeogical researches of the author.

B. Yellow Edible Earth from China.—In the year 1847, the author obtained from one of the great geological collections in

London a small sample of this earth, which from a gray passes almost into a sulphur-yellow. It resembles a very fine clay, does not soil the fingers, but is brittle, and shapeable when moistened. Acids produce no effervescence, and when heated it becomes first black, then somewhat redish. Its microscopic elements are a rather coarse, double refracting, mostly quartz sand, surrounded by a somewhat finer mould. Intermixed are isolated, small green and white crystals, mica, and Phytolitharia, with now and then traces of Polygastric shells and silicious casts of stone kernels of Polythalamia. In ten analytical examinations were found fourteen forms: one Polygaster, nine Phytolitharia, one Polythalamium, and three crystals. The substance is therefore, according to this, a loamy or clayey substance. All the Phytolitharia contained in it are in a corroded porous state, just as they occur in antediluvian tertiary layers. The presence of Polythalamia, and in particular of Textilaria globulosa in a stratum, very likely of the interior continent, indicates chalk formations in the vicinity of the place, or at least in the aquatic district of the river. This appears to prove that the clay similar to the edible Tanah ambo in Java, which it very much resembles, is a tertiary fresh-water formation in the modern sense of geognosy, incumbent on chalk, or mixed with fragments of chalk. The forms occurring in it are :—

1. Polygastria : *Trachelomonas lævis.*
2. Phytolitharia : *Lithodontium Bursa, L. nasutum, L. rostratum, Lithosphæridium irregulare, Lythostylidium clavatum, L. lœve, L. quadratum, L. rude, L. trabecula.*
3. Polythalamia : *Textilaria globulosa.*
4. Inorganic forms : *green crystalline prisms, white crystalline prisms, plates of mica.*

The sum of the discovered species is eleven organic forms and three inorganic ones; among which are ten fresh-water formations and one marine formation, Textilaria.—[*Pharm. Central Blatt* and *Phar. Jour. Canada Med. Journal.*

Chloroform Ointment for Hemicrania and Neuralgia.

M. Cazenave, of Bordeaux, recommends the above ointment, which is prepared as follows : Pnre chloroform, three drachms; cyanide of potassium, two drachms and a half; axunge, two ounces; add a sufficient quantity of white wax to make an ointment of the usual consistence.—[*Lancet.*

Miscellany.

Deaths by Chloroform and Ether.—We know not whether it be from the increased use of anæsthetics, from negligence engendered by their frequent administration, or from the manufacture of impure articles, that their fatality has became so common, but it is quite obvious that the profession is not sufficiently awake to the hazard attending their indiscriminate use. Scarcely a month has elapsed during the present year, in which the medical press has not recorded one or more deaths from chloroform or ether ; and in most of the cases the operations for which they were administered were comparatively trivial—the extraction of teeth, for example. We would not censure nor repress the laudable desire to mitigate human suffering, but we feel it a duty to take a stand against the rashness that would resort to means, the danger of which is altogether disproportioned to the necessity of relief.

It is true that chloroform has been administered to thousands of parturient women with almost uniform immunity from its bad effects. This is easily accounted for when we reflect upon the circumstances and mode of administration. The parturient woman who inhales it, does so with a free will, without reluctance ; (for if she objected, no one would urge it upon her) ; she takes it to subdue pain she already suffers, not to make her unconscious of mutilation ; she has probably taken no food for several hours ; she is in the horizontal position ; she inhales it very gradually and rarely takes more than enough to induce an agreeable state of intoxication and partial insensibility.

The circumstances are very different in cases to be prepared for surgical operations. The idea alone of an operation carries terror with it ; chloroform is proposed, but the patient is afraid that he may not get enough to make him entirely insensible before the knife is plunged into his flesh, or that he may take too much and die. Even if you satisfy him that he will neither feel the pain nor be killed, he cannot be reconciled to being mangled whilst asleep. The consequence is that in the great majority of such cases, the handkerchief or sponge has to be held forcibly to the nostrils of the patient, whose struggles to remove it increase with his intoxication, until he falls back in a comatose state, not unfrequently preceded by convulsive movements. The wonder is that there are not more accidents under such circumstances.

We find the journals teeming with *precepts* for the safe administration of anæsthetics. We are admonished not to resort to them if the

patient be disposed to affections of the brain, heart, lungs, &c., and
yet death has usually occurred when these precautions were observed,
and when there seemed to be no reason to appprehend it.   We believe
that by far the most important precepts, are : never to administer
them in any other than the *horizontal* position ; nor to persons in whom
syncope may be easily induced, as nervous and hysterical females or
anæmic individuals; nor to persons who are afraid of their effects ;
nor shortly after a meal.   We believe that syncope is most commonly the immediate cause of the mischief—for with the sensibilities
blunted by the remedy, it is then extremely difficult to produce the
impressions and actions necessary to restoration.   The horizontal position is the best protection against syncope, and it is to the neglect of
this precaution we attribute the numerous deaths in the hands of dentists.   With regard to repletion of the stomach, its danger is to be
found. in the fact, that vomiting is frequently induced by the anæsthetics,
and that the insensibility of the patient then favors suffocation by allowing the food to pass into the trachea, or to obstruct the larynx.
The patient should be immediately turned upon his side with' his head
down, if he attempts to vomit

In speaking as we do, we trust that we will not be understood as
opposing the use of so great and valuble a boon, whenever the importance of the case may require it.   We repeat that we desire simply to
lend our air in repressing its indiscriminate use, until its administration may be so regulated as to lessen the risk of fatal consequences.

Influence of Climate upon Consumption.—The value of a removal
to the south, of persons affected in the northern states with consumption, has been heretofore very generally admitted; but it is now asked
whether much, if any, advantage is to be derived from spending merely
the winter months at the south and returning to the north in the spring—
and it is added that if a temprate atmosphere be all that is needed, this
may be obtained in New England by means of a well regulated system of artificial heat.   We believe it to be an error to suppose that
the southern states owe their immunity from phthisis pulmonalis alone
to the mildness of their winters.   If such were the fact, all temperate
climates ought to be equally exempt, and all cold latitudes alike unfavorable   Yet phthisis is much more common upon the seaboard and
in the mountainous districts of the southern states than at intermediate points, and it is comparatively rare in the northern portions of
Canada and Russia, whilst it makes frightful havoc in milder England, France and our northern states.

That a temporary sojourn in the southern states is advantageous, we doubt not ; but that a permanent residence here is still more so, we feel quite certain. Every practitioner of experience and who is acquainted with the means of accurately determining the state of the lungs, must have often observed how wonderfully large abscesses will heal here, which would have certainly proved fatal in a less genial clime. The writer knows persons in this state who had tubercular abscesses as long as twenty years ago, which healed kindly and have left them ever since in the enjoyment of apparently good health. That all are not equally fortunate is too true ; yet we feel assured that it is only by remaining in the south, both summer and winter, sufficiently long to acquire the peculiarities of a southern constitution, that lasting benefit may be expected. The best locations are obviously those in which the disease *orignates* most rarely, and these are unquestionably to be found midway between the mountains and sea-board.

BIBLIOGRAPHICAL.

Records of Maculated, or Ship Fever, with suggestions of treatment : being the result of a series of observations made during the prevalence of this disease at South-Boston and Deer-Island Hospitals in 1847–48—with Plates. By J. P. Upham, M. D.   1852.

Clinical Reports on Continued Fever, based on an analysis of 164 *cases : with remarks on the management of Continued fever ; the identity of Typhus and Typhoid fever ; Relapsing fever ; Diagnosis &c.—to which is added a memoir on the transportation and diffusion by contagion, of Typhoid fever, as exemplified in the occurrence of the disease at N. Boston, Erie Co., N. Y.* By Austin Flint, M. D., Professor, &c , in University of Buffalo, &c.   1852.

The publication of works upon Typhus and Typhoid fevers at this time is quite opportune, as the extension of continued fevers into portions of the Southern States hitherto exempted from them, makes it very important that they be thoroughly understood. The interest felt upon the subject by the profession at the South is manifested by the great number of communications, on " Typhoid Fever," received and published by our periodicals, and although they all evince a spirit of inquiry that cannot be too highly commended, some of them bear unequivocal evidence of a deficiency of accurate information, both in regard to diagnosis and treatment.

The works before us are not such as most persons *like* to read, because they are dry statements of facts—yet they are just the kind that every man *ought* to read who wishes to become thoroughly acquainted with disease. They are Clinical Reports—drawn up at the bed-side ;

and whose powers of description can ever equal those of nature ? A few clinical reports of any disease will convey a better idea of it than the most laboured and skilful description framed in the closet. We need more clinical reports in our country ; it is only by these that we can establish any valuable comparison between the diseases of America and those of the old world ; it is by these alone that we can effectually study their natural history and treatment. The desire for short roads to knowledge as well as to geographical points, so characteristic of our people, has induced the translators of some of the most valuable European works to mutilate them by leaving out all their clinical cases, the very materials upon which the works were based. Who, for instance, would recognize the great monument of Laennec's genius and industry in the miserable skeleton presented by the translation. Two large volumes, full of facts, cut down to a thin octavo "to suit the market !"

In conclusion, we beg leave to recommend the works of Dr. Upham and Prof. Flint—especially the latter.

The Transactions of the third annual meeting of the Medical Society of the State of Georgia, held in the City of Augusta, April, 1852.

We congratulate the Medical Society of the State of Georgia upon the publication of so creditable a contribution to Science. The work before us contains one hundred pages, and should be regarded as an earnest of still better things, when the organization will include a larger number of members. The following are its contents :—Minutes of Proceedings ; Report on Empirical Remedies of R. Campbell, M. D. ; Report upon Surgery by H. F. Campbell, M. D. ; Report on the Diseases of Perry (Houston Co.) by G. F. Cooper, M. D. ; Report on the Diseases of Roswell (Cobb Co.) by W. N. King, M. D. ; Report of cases of Urinary Calculus by P. F. Eve, M. D. ; Observations upon the use of certain new remedies by L. A. Dugas, M. D. ; Address before the Society by H. F. Campbell, M. D. ; Catalogue of officers and members.

The Report on Empirical Remedies will attract attention, both from its intrinsic merits and from its fearless denunciation of Charlatanism and its abettors. But what avails the shaft hurled by virtuous indignation at an evil which derives its very origin and sustenance from the peculiar nature of the human mind !—unless we could blot *credulity* and *cupidity* from the psychological chart, how are we to get rid of dupes and knaves ! It is in vain that we expose one species of imposture, for, phœnix-like, another will arise from its ashes.

The Report upon Surgery is a faithful exposé of what was done in this department during the preceding year in Georgia. Its matter is judiciously arranged under the three heads of surgical injuries and pathology; surgical operations; and surgical medicine or treatment nearly all the facts, we are proud to say, are derived from the pages of the Southern Medical and Surgical Journal. It is gratifying to find that, with very few exceptions, the physicians of Georgia have evinced their State pride by making their publications in the medical periodical of their own State. The following is a list of the writers whose contributions are noticed in this Report.—F. T. Matthews, L. A. Dugas, H. Rossignol, H. F. Campbell, D. C. O'Keeffe, C. T. Quintard, P. F. Eve, R. Campbell, H. V. M. Miller, W. H. King, H. M. Jeter, J. Harriss, W. N. King, J. S. Wilson, W. W. Haws, A. C. Hart.

The Report of Dr. G. F. Cooper is admirably drawn up, and may serve as a model for works of the kind. That of Dr. W. N. King is also very good, but not as extensive and minute. We hope to find such documents multiplied. We regret that our space will not permit us to reproduce, at present, any of the papers contained in these Transactions, but may do so hereafter. Dr. H. F. Campbell's Address on "The Difficulties and Privileges of the Medical Profession," is a very chaste and creditable production.

We would take occasion to direct attention to the following extract from the minutes: "Resolved, that the Transactions of this Society, when published, be withheld from such members as may fail to remit their assessment to the Treasurer, Dr. R. C. Black, at Augusta." We understand that there are several delinquents, who have, doubtless, forgotten the passage of this resolution.

God in Disease, or the Manifestations of Design in morbid phenomena. By JAMES F. DUNCAN, M. D., Physician to Dunn's Hospital, Dublin. Philadelphia: Lindsay & Blakiston. 1852.

This is a neat little duodecimo of about 230 pages, the contents of which are divided into twelve chapters bearing the following titles:— On disease, as depending upon an active and intelligent cause; on the nature of the design which disease is intended to accomplish; on the existence of disease in general as affording evidence of design; on the varieties of disease as affording evidence of design; on the pain of disease as affording evidence of design; on the modifications of pain as affording evidence of design; on some other symptoms of disease as affording evidence of design; on processes of preservation in disease; on processes of reparation; on processes of adaptation; on the phe-

nomena of disease as illustrating spiritual truths ; on the conduct of
the physician as illustrating the dealings of God with His creatures ;
conclusion.

These subjects are treated with clearness and in an easy style, entirely free from pedantry as well as bigotry.   An attentive perusal of
the work is calculated to dissipate many erroneous ideas, and to substitute for them the rational views of sound Christian philosophy.   It
may be read with equal advantage by both patient and physician.

Hints to the People upon the Profession of Medicine.   By Wm. M.
    Wood, M D. Surgeon U. S. Navy, Author of " Sketches of South
    America," " Polynesia," &c.   Buffalo : George H. Derby & Co.
    1852.   12mo. p. 67.

We have never seen a work better adapted to the purpose of correcting popular errors with regard to the medical profession than this.
It should be procured by every physician and circulated among such
of his patrons as will not get it themselves.

The Transactions of the Medical Association of the State of Missouri,
    at its second annual meeting.   St. Louis, April, 1852.

This is decidedly one of the best productions emanating from the
State associations of this year.   It contains an excellent Address by
the President, and able Reports, by Professors Pope and Pallen, upon
Surgery and Obstetrics, besides several other articles of general interest.   The Report of Dr. T. Reyburn upon the Domestic Adulteration of Drugs and Liquors is especially deserving of attention.

The Transactions of the twenty-ninth annual meeting of the Medical
    Society of Virginia, together with the President's annual address and
    the Constitution of the society.   Richmond, 1852.

These *Transactions* consist of the minutes of proceedings—nothing
more.   The Old Dominion must do better or it will lose caste.

Braithwaite's Retrospect and *Ranking's Abstract* have been received, and contain their usual amount of valuable information.   They
are excellent works, but would be better if they contained more American matter.

Pumpkin seed for Tænia.—It appears that the use of pumpkin seed
in the treatment of Tænia. did not originate in our country as was
thought by some, but that its efficacy was stated by Dr. Mongeny, upwards of thirty years ago in a French periodical, the *" Journal Uni-*
versel des Sciences Medicales."   He used a paste composed of three

ounces and a half of fresh seed and double the quantity of Honey, given in three doses at intervals of an hour, and alleges that he thus almost invariably succeeded in expelling the worm in the course of the day.

So simple a remedy is well worthy of systematic trial. Perhaps it would be effectual in the removal of other intestinal worms.

Turpentine Frictions, &c., in Intermittent Fever.—Among the numerous remedies proposed for the purpose of dispensing with the use of quinine in the treatment of intermittent fevers, a French practitioner recommends frictions to the spine with spts. turpentine and chloroform, (3½ oz. of the former, and ȝj. of the latter,) an hour or two before the expected paroxysm. It is well known here that a few cups, or even a sinapism over the dorsal vertebræ will very often prevent the paroxysm. In cases of obstinate and recurring attacks of the disease, a fly blister to the same region has long since been regarded by us as one of the most effectual means of permanent relief.

Operation for Hare-lip —M. Guersant, the distinguished surgeon of the Children's Hospital in Paris, has recently performed with success the operation for hare-lip upon an infant *one day old.*

Professor Liebig.—This celebrated chemist has left Giessen to take up his residence in Munich at the solicitation of the Bavarian government.

The Doctorate at the St. Louis University.—We perceive that the St. Louis University requires of candidates for the Doctorate, the following imitation of the Hippocratic pledge of old.

5th. And that he publicly assent to the following promise, prior to the conferring of the degree, viz :—

" You, A B , do solemnly promise that you will, to the utmost of your ability, exert your influence for promoting the welfare and respectability of the profession ; that you will demean yourself honorably in the practice thereof; that you will not put forth any nostrum or secret method of cure, nor engage in any other species of quackery ; and that you will not publish any matter or thing laudatory of yourself, or derogatory to the profession ; and in the conferring of this degree, it is done with the express understanding that the Faculty reserve to themselves the right and privilege to revoke said degree whenever the promise here made shall be violated."

Remarkable Case of Precocity—Menstruation occurring at four years of age. By C. R KEMPER.—A servant girl, owned at this time by Mr. C. M. W., of our village, is the subject of a precocious development of the female reproductive organs and appearance of the menses. The development of the general system in this girl, from a year old, was noticed to progress rapidly, till she attained her third year, when an increased size of the mammary glands was first observed, and, shortly after, there appeared the usual growth of hair on the pubes. When she was four years and one month old, her catamenia made their first appearance, and have continued regularly to return up to this date. She is now just entering her thirteenth year.

The development of the brain seems not to have kept pace with the physical growth, but she is possessed of a degree of intelligence usual for her age. She is much larger than an older sister, and has the appearance, from the breadth of the chest and pelvis, to be a fully developed *woman.*—[*Stethoscope.*

A Curious Philosophical Experiment.

Charleston, August 25, 1852.

Gentlemen : I find the enclosed article in the New Orleans " Delta." It describes an experiment of such interest that I wish to bring the subject before the intelligent and philosophical readers of your journal. Whoever the writer may be, he has certainly proved his claim to whatever honors the French Academy may see fit to extend to M. Andraud. The latter gentleman is wrong ; and his error is clearly detected, and the true experiment shown by the real discoverer, the clerical correspondent of the Delta.

The best manner of detecting the globules is with a lens ; though the perforated hole shows an interesting spectacle. The iris of the eye is also superbly magnified and rendered beautifully visible with two lens, a small and a large one, placed five feet apart ; the larger one directed to the moon or a lamp, and looking at it with the smaller (inch focus) placed close to the eye. Indeed, the experiments may be varied so as to produce the finest effects, at once novel and beautiful. Next to a telescopic view of the heavens, I know nothing in science so interesting and at the same time so simple as this " seeing the interior of the eye" with the eye itself. The Rector of St. John's parsonage has conferred a philosophical treat upon experimenters in physical science by his discovery. Trusting that my friend, the editor of Le Courrier des Etats Unis, will notice the article which I have sent you, by giving the extract an insertion, I remain gentlemen, yours respectfully,

Beaufort.

[*From the New Orleans Delta.*]

The following interesting communication from a distinguished literary gentleman and excellent clergyman of the Episcopal Church, cannot fail to arrest the attention of the curious in optics. We have ourselves verified the experiments herein recorded, and noticed one fact which our correspondent does not allude to, viz : the image of a friend, who was standing near us and at a certain angle with our

retina, projected from that nervous expansion, as it were, into the planet-like disc, where it resembled *the face in the sun,* as we see it printed
in childish books !

The communication may be headed, " The Art of Seeing the Interior of the Eye with the organ itself !"

To the Editors of the Sunday Delta :

Gentlemen : I have recently read in some of the journals a statement in relation to a late discovery, said to have been made by M.
Andraud, an eminent French engineer. The paragraph to which I
allude reads as follows :

" Some attention has been excited by the alleged discovery, by a
French engineer of some celebrity named Andraud, of some means
of seeing the air. If, says he, you take a piece of card, colored black,
of the size of the eye, and pierce with a fine needle a hole in the middle, you will, on looking through that hole at a clear sky or a lighted
lamp, see a multitude of molecules floating about ; which molecules
constitute the air. We shall see whether the theory will obtain the
sanction of the Academy of Sciences, to which it has been submitted."

My object in drawing your attention to this extract is in order to
correct an important error touching M. Andraud's alleged discovery.

The atomic globules which were rendered visible to M. Andraud,
by means of the perforated card, are *not aerial* molecules. I have
been, for some months past, familiar with this interesting experiment.
The beautiful globules seen by means of the hole in the card are the
atomic colorless globes which constitute the crystalline fluid *within the
eye.* M. Andraud supposes they are *external* and in the air, when
the truth is they are *internal* and within the chamber of the eye.

The experiment may be tried, and the fact verified by any person,
in the following manner : Take a thick visiting-card and black it
with ink, or a piece of pasteboard opaque enough to forbid the transmission of light through it, and perforate the centre with a pin-hole.
Place the card between the eye and a candle-flame, or a globe-lamp,
and not more than two inches from the eye, and the same distance
from the light ; but this distance will vary according to the convexity or flatness of the seer's eye, who must adjust it till he finds his focus.
Instead of seeing the flame of the candle, the beholder now discerns a
circular disc the size of the iris of the eye. This disc is bright and
planet-like, and is crossed by innumerable lines like the fibres visible
on the surface of a magnified rose-leaf. It *appears to be beyond the
eye,* between the card and the light ; and it is this illusion which deceived M. Andraud, and led him to suppose that he saw a portion of
the atmosphere magnified. But this visible disc is, in fact, a spherical
section of the fluidal crystalline lens within the chamber of the eye,
strongly illumined by the concentrated pencil of light, passing from
the candle into it through the minute hole in the card ; and the veined
appearance of its surface is the recticulated *materia* of the ordinarily
transparent coat of the cornea rendered visible.

The chamber of the eye thus lighted up by the intense line of light passing into it through the minute orifice (which acts as a strongly magnifying lens,) there is conveyed to the optic nerve an image (exactly the size of the pupil through which the ray passes) of a circular section of the crystalline fluid, with its atomic particles intensely magnified. The spectable is one of surpassing wonder and beauty. Myriads of illuminated molecules distinctly appear in tremulous motion in the bright fluid ; some of them are simple globes. others are encircled bv two or more concentric rings like exquisite miniatures of the planet Saturn, as seen through a telescope. Some of them are transparent, like infinitely small soap bubbles, and float about as lightly, while others are of the white color of pearls.

By contracting the eye, or by gently moving the head from side to side, these beautiful millions of globular atoms are made to undulate within the chamber of the eye, and change places, some ascending and others descending ; while others thrown nearer the focus of the light dart across the disc like shooting stars in a lesser firmament ; while others revolve about each other in orbits of infinite diversity.

The experiment is a highly interesting as well as a philosophical one, and will well recompense whoever attempts it. It will require some practice in a tyro to adjust the card to the proper focus, so as to obtain the clearest disc ; but any one who knows how to use a microscope will easily discover when the card is in focus. If the flame of the candle is seen through it it is out of focus, and it must be advanced or drawn back until a round planet-like shape is discernible. This planet-like shape, which will appear crossed by a net-work is the corner coating of the eye magnified. The pupil of the eye must now be expanded, as when one examines closely a very minute object, when the atomic world of globules that compose the crystalline fluid will be discerned behind the net-work surface of the cornea ; and the steadier one gazes the clearer is this wonderful and beautiful spectacle perceived in all its surprising variety of form, beauty, and motion.

A better medium than the card proposed by M. Andraud I have used in making this experiment. It is a small lens, (the eye piece of a broken spy-glass,) with an inch and a half focus. This held to a solar lamp or candle, at six feet distance, or turned towards the full moon, (which is better still,) the chamber of the eye is far more intensely illumined than by means of the perforated card.

The lens of ordinary magnifying spectacles will serve equally as well as the eye-piece named. by covering the surface with opaque paper, having in the centre a clear space to transmit the light throughout into the pupil of the eye.

Trusting that this experiment for seeing the elementary molecules of the crystalline lens will afford to others the pleasure which I and many friends have derived from it, and trusting to the indulgence of M. Andraud for rejecting his theory of aerial atoms, I remain, very truly, yours,   I.

St. John's Parsonage, Aberdeen, Miss., June 7, 1852.

SOUTHERN
MEDICAL AND SURGICAL
JOURNAL.

Vol. 8.]   NEW SERIES.—NOVEMBER, 1852.   [No. 11.

PART FIRST.

Original Communications.

ARTICLE XL.

Veratrum Viride, or American Hellebore. By W. C. Nor-wood, M. D., of Cokesbury, South Carolina.

We trust that the profession will pardon our appearing so frequently under the above caption. The great incredulity of many in reference to the powers of Veratrum Viride, and the apprehension by others of its poisonous properties, as well as the imperfection of our previous communications upon the subject, must plead our apology for now giving a more minute account of our experience, and urging the great importance of the subject, perhaps, for the last time. We intend to state facts and events that have repeatedly come under our immediate observation. We shall not pretend to account for the modus operandi nor the wonderful and magical effects of veratrum viride upon the system, in overcoming and subduing disease, nor shall we attempt to specify what or which are its primary or secondary, its direct or indirect effects. But we will add the opinions of a number of medical gentlemen, with the effects witnessed by them from time to time. By this course the medical world will be put in a condition to judge how far our observations and experience have been sustained by those of others who are not so personally interested as we are. Veratrum viride, as a therapeutical agent, had excited comparatively little interest previous to June, 1850 ; and it was noticed for a

time after that date, more on account of the extravagance of
the claims set up for it as a remedial agent of superior powers,
than because of any belief that it was possessed of peculiar and
valuable properties.   We could, if necessary, in this place, name
several medical journals which noticed the article or articles
written by us and spoke of the extravagance of our statements.
If we recollect correctly, it was about the year 1835 that Dr.
Charles Osgood's interesting article on the powers and properties of veratrum viride made its appearance. The only additional information he conveyed was that it is destitute of cathartic
powers, which give it a superiority over the Veratrum Album
or European Hellebore, in the treatment of cases where active
cathartics are inadmissible. Be this as it may, it is certain, and
cannot be successfully controverted, that prior to June, 1850, it
was not known positively to possess any superiority over veratrum album ; indeed the one was supposed to answer the same
purposes as the other.

Without wasting time in the proof, or in noticing the
remarks that others have made up to the period stated, we
will simply observe, that from all we find in works upon materia
medica or therapeutics, and in the standard works on the practice of medicine, there are no claims set up for its superiority
to its "European congener."   It stands unnoticed, is not even
named as a remedy, and still less as a leading and valuable
remedy, by any of the standard authors of the day in their treatises on the practice of medicine.   Dr. Wood, of Philadelphia,
in his very able, extensive and superior practical work on Medicine, even as late as 1849, does not mention or recommend it
in the treatment of a single disease.   It does not form a portion
of the work upon New Remedies, by Dr. Dunglison, a man of
untiring industry and application, and who never slumbers
until all that is known is placed in his valuable works, nor
has it a place in his work on the Practice of Medicine.

Now, if the peculiar powers and properties we claim for the
veratrum viride had been known and established—if its peculiar adaptation to the successful treatment of typhoid pneumonia, typhoid fever, scarlet fever, puerperal fever, &c., &c., had
been known, these very learned and deservedly distinguished
authors would not have failed to notice it.   We have entered

into the above brief notice to show how little was known of the value of veratrum viride prior to the notice given of it in June, 1850. When we furnish the testimony in our possession, it will be seen what a valuable remedy it is, and what a wide spread reputation it has acquired in the short time it has been before the public. Why Dr. Osgood ceased to give further notice of its powers we are not prepared to say : whether his silence grew out of a want of confidence in its remedial powers, or from death, we are wholly ignorant. We do not wonder at the violent and drastic effects he witnessed; but we rather wonder, from the large doses given, that he obtained any beneficial effects. Be this as it may, if it possesses the powers and properties we attributed to it, and is adapted to the treatment of the symptoms and diseases indicated by us, the discovery must be eminently valuable. Greatly enlarged experience and observation have strongly confirmed us in the belief of the correctness of what we stated on a former occasion, namely, that when its powers and properties are fully known and understood, it will constitute a new era in the treatment of disease.

In July, 1844, we first used it in the case of Mrs L. She had been laboring under a severe attack of pneumonia typhoides for several days. Calomel, blisters, Dover's powders, &c., failed to afford relief. We had been informed by a friend and an eminent physician, that veratrum viride " was analogous in its powers and properties to blood-root—more narcotic and less emetic, and that a fluid drachm, or a tea-spoonful of the tincture was a dose." We had often used blood-root with marked success in pneumonia, and especially in the cases of a bilious character. This case having annoyed us by its severity and obstinacy, and opium producing unpleasant effects, without relief to the pain, we determined to make a trial of the tincture of veratrum viride. We withdrew all other remedies, and put her on tea-spoonful doses of the tincture, to be repeated every three hours. Instead of making it by using (as was directed) " one pint of undiluted alcohol, of the strength of the shops, to eight ounces of the *green* root, or diluted alcohol, if the root was *dry*," we added one pint of undiluted alcohol to eight ounces of the *dried* root. This is the formula we gave to the public, and is the one we now use. It has been said by some,

that it was an extravagant formula, that we used an unnecessary quantity of the root.   We always like to have our tinctures, of very active agents, of the same or uniform strength,
and would much prefer the waste of a little root to the uncertainty of an untried tincture.   But, if any one will read Dr.
Robert's valuable article on Veratrum Viride, in this Journal,
for June, 1852, it will be seen that he added double our proportion of alcohol, and that he had to use double the quantity
of the tincture; thus demonstrating that we were as correct in
estimating the quantity necessary to saturate the alcohol, as
we were in our representations of its remedial effects on the
system.   We would not pretend to deny that less might do, if
the root were dug at the right season, (between the 1st of September and frost,) and properly assorted and put up.   But in the
form in which it comes to us, it is rare that less can be sufficient.

But, to return to our case: We gave her a tea-spoonful at
11 A. M.   About 1 P. M. we were sent for in haste, as the
medicine, or something else, was acting drastically.   We found
the patient vomiting every few minutes; skin cold and covered with perspiration; great paleness, nausea distressing; complained of a sense of sinking and exhaustion.   After the vomiting
had ceased, the pulse was found not more than 60 per minute,
full and distinct.

In a few cases, in which nausea was great and the vomiting
frequent, we have found the pulse very slow, small, and almost
imperceptible at the wrist; but as soon as the vomiting and
consequent exhaustion subside, the pulse will be found slow,
full and distinct.   The nausea or vomiting, when in excess,
can be readily and certainly relieved by one or two full portions of syrup of morphine and tincture of ginger, or laudanum
and brandy.

In this case, before administering the tincture of veratrum
viride, the skin was hot and dry; pulse 130, small and soft;
circumscribed flush on the cheeks; pain severe; breathing hurried and difficult; cough frequent; expectoration scanty.   The
very striking effects of the medicine, the great reduction in the
frequency of the pulse, and the sudden breaking up or arrest of
the disease, in this and another case, profoundly enlisted our

attention, and led us from that period to observe more particularly its powers.

The second case in which we used the veratrum viride was that of Mrs. M., who was also laboring under a severe attack of pneumonia. Pulse from 130 to 140 beats per minute; pain violent, and extending from the right side, near the spine, to, and under the sternum; tongue red on the edges and tip, and covered in the centre with a thin, dark, dry fur; bright scarlet circumscribed flush appearing first on one cheek, and then on the other, rarely on both at the same time; the end or tip of the nose and chin frequently red; very pale around the mouth; expectoration scanty; mucus streaked with blood; cough frequent and very harrassing; great increase of pain under the sternum during a paroxysm of coughing; decubitus on the back; breathing labored and difficult. Did not see her till the fourth day : she had been bled, and otherwise treated, with little or no relief. Applied a blister, and gave a camphorated powder to allay the cough and violent pain, and to excite diaphoresis. At the expiration of three hours, to commence with the tincture of veratrum viride.

The first portion excited intense nausea, violent emesis, great paleness, coolness and a sense of sinking or of exhaustion. The patient and friends becoming alarmed, another physician who lived much nearer than myself, was sent for in great haste, but when he arrived the nausea and emesis had ceased; the patient was comfortable, pain and febrile symptoms subdued, pulse sixty-five, full and distinct. The doctor was surprised to find the condition of the patient so different from the representation given by the messenger. The disease was really broken up and a crisis and resolution brought about. Our friend, the doctor, ordered a little paregoric and quinine, in which we fully concurred on our arrival, as there was entire relief of all active febrile and inflammatory symptoms.

We would here observe that notwithstanding the complete reduction of the inflammatory symptoms and pulse, the peculiar circumscribed redness on the cheek or cheeks continued for three days. In another case of pneumonia, we observed the same peculiarity, with the additional fact, that although there had been more tendency to coma or uninterrupted and deep sleep,

the patient then became preternaturally wakeful, somewhat
flighty and disposed to get out of bed.   This continued about
forty-eight hours.   We do not know how to account for this
continuance of the red cheeks under such circumstances.   A
case occurred in Georgia, in which a corpse was kept a week
in consequence of the persistence of this redness.

Deeply impressed with the peculiar effects of verat. viride, we
determined to make farther and conscientious trial of it in pneumonitis.   The third case in which we administered it was that
of Mr. T., who was taken sick when on a visit to his friend
in this section of the country.   We ordered the tincture given
every three hours, beginning with eight drops, to be increased
one drop at each dose until nausea, vomiting or some other
visible effect was produced.   On the dose reaching twelve
drops it induced vomiting with but little nausea.   The pulse
was reduced from 135 to 78 beats per minute ; the surface, from
being hot and dry, became cool ; and the severe pain was now
but slightly felt on taking a deep inspiration.   The interval
between the doses was extended from three to five hours ; but
as twelve drops induced too frequent vomiting, the quantity
was reduced to seven drops and continued three days without
any return of the symptoms, when the case was dismissed and
the patient was soon able to return home.   This case was one
full of interest on account of the success and promptness with
which the violent symptoms were removed and the disease
cured.

We might report any number of cases, but as many of them
have already been given by others, we will confine ourselves to
such facts only as may tend to illustrate particular points.   We
continued our experimental trials with various doses from three
to twelve drops, increasing or diminishing them according to
circumstances, until we acquired a perfect knowledge of its
effects, and could graduate them at will.

We ascertained that in cases which had run on for sometime
or in which emetics and cathartics had been freely used, a very
small quantity was necessary.   Where tartar emetic has been
given, it is almost sure to act harshly and drastically.   Where
tartar emetic had been taken, we would therefore always give
a full portion of syrup of morphine, at least one hour before

entering on the use of the veratrum viride, and in such cases would not commence with more than six drops for a male adult. Free venesection increases very materially its activity, especially its unfavorable or drastic effects. No one should think of following a large bleeding with the veratrum viride, unless with the greatest caution. The depressing influence of the loss of blood upon the brain and nervous system generally, cannot fail to render the use of so potent a sedative as veratrum viride exceedingly hazardous. The administration under such circumstances of an agent capable of reducing the pulse from 130 or 140 down to 75, 70, or even 50 beats in the course of a few hours, cannot be too carefully watched.

Intending to resume and to conclude in the next number of this Journal the account of our experience in the use of veratrum viride, we beg leave now to append the testimony of some of those who have kindly written to us upon the subject.

ROSWELL, GA., May 1st, 1852.

Dear Sir—I find, in experimenting with your veratrum viride, it is *all* in *all things* you have represented it, and is certainly *the only* arterial sedative on which we may at *all* times rely with *certainty*, and *the most invaluable* agent of this class in the whole materia medica.

Very truly,
WM. NEPHEW KING, M. D.

COLUMBIA, Nov. 17th, 1851.

Dear Sir—In experimenting with the tincture handed me, (veratrum viride,) I have been very much pleased with its controlling powers over the heart and arteries. I have only given it in typhus fever, and one or two cases of pneumonia. It certainly reduces the pulse without any of those immediately prostrating and alarming symptoms which take place after the continued use of digitalis; neither does it irritate the mucous membrane of the bowels, as the salts of antimony do, when continued for days. I have given it in several cases of typhus, in which there was dry red tongue, great thirst, delirium, frequent dejections from the bowels, with soreness and distension of the abdomen, without the least aggravation of any of those disagreeable symptoms. I have not found it immediately to arrest the disease, or cut it short at once, after fully formed, but certainly to make it assume so mild a form as to require very little in the future treatment. I have, in several cases, broken up the forming stage of the disease, by keeping the heart below a natural and normal action for two or three days. In fact, I regard *your tincture* of every importance in the above diseases, and fully meeting the expectations of its warmest advocates. It certainly is the very article to fill the place (a thousand times better and safer) of the tart. emetic in the contra-stimulant treatment of the "Italian school." * * *

I remain yours, most truly,
SAMUEL FAIR, M. D.

NEWBERRY COURT HOUSE, Nov. 16, 1851.

Dear Doctor—I have given the medicine you sent me,. (veratrum viride,) to two patients labouring under typhoid fever, with the best effect. In both cases the pulse was reduced from 120 and 140 to 70 and 74 beats in the minute, by giving from three to four doses, there was no return of fever afterwards. The medicine was continued five days in one case and seven or eight in the other. I was sent for two weeks ago to visit a patient in consultation with an eminent physician, labouring under pneumonitis. I saw her on the ninth day from her attack—her physician had used all the remedies usual in such cases—she seemed to grow worse. When I was called in, he said he had no hope of her recovery—all the symptoms were unfavourable. I proposed giving Dr. Norwood's medicine, as I called it; he smiled, and said he was afraid it was a humbug, but consented, as he considered the case hopeless. We gave her (a young lady fifteen or sixteen years old) five drops; increased one drop each dose until we gave eight drops to the dose. It produced nausea of the stomach by this time; her pulse was reduced from 120 to 88 beats in the minute. Her physician remained with her during the night; he stopped giving the medicine. The next morning I saw her again and found her with a pulse of 110 beats in the minute. I asked the doctor if he had discontinued the medicine; he said he had. We commenced giving it again, in eight drop doses; by the third dose her pulse was reduced to 74 beats in the minute; said she felt much better. The doctor discontinued the medicine again for eight or ten hours to see the effect. The pulse rose again to 108 or 110 beats in the minute. We resumed the medicine again—about the third dose the pulse was reduced to 70. We kept it from 70 to 74 beats for several days, some six or seven. She is now convalescent. I will say to you, however, that the doctor has sent to me a second time for a small vial of the medicine, as he is giving it to some two or three cases of typhoid fever, and says he is very much pleased with its effects.

Your friend,
J. B. RUFF, M. D.

BAINBRIDGE, GA., June 5th, 1851.

Dear Sir—Since receiving the veratrum viride, I regret that I have had but one favorable opportunity of giving it a trial; in that, however, it succeeded beyond my most sanguine expectations. The case was one of Pneumonia, complicated very decidedly with typhoid symptoms. The patient being four years old and the pulse 130, I proceeded after trying all other modes of treatment unavailingly for ten days to give the tincture in common doses. The first was ejected as soon as swallowed, but was repeated instanter and was retained. The little patient now becoming tranquil and not anticipating any very sudden change,

I suffered myself to engage in common fireside conversation for some thirty minutes, when my attention was attracted to my patient by the extreme palor of his countenance, and upon examination found his pulse reduced to about 80, the skin bathed in perspiration, and, as far as one could judge, the disease gone, and the patient sleeping sweetly. But in order to assure myself that these results were produced by the medicine and nothing else, I withheld the second dose and the result was that the fever rose in five hours. The dose was then repeated and the same results followed as in the first instance. The portion was again withheld, whereupon the fever rose again in eight hours. But a repetition of the remedy subdued it as promptly as before, and by continuing it at intervals of six hours, there was no return of the symptoms : thus conclusively showing that the favourable results obtained could not be ascribed to the agency of any other article.

Yours, very respectfully,

E. R. RIDLEY, M. D.

WAYNESBORO', BURKE Co., GA., August 4th, 1852.

Dear Sir—I had intended, as a matter of great gratitude, at an early day to write you an acknowledgment of your prompt kindness in sending me a specimen of your tincture of American Hellebore, as well as to congratulate you upon your discovery of the controlling powers of that article over abnormal organic reaction. * * * I am satisfied with the display of its magical powers, as presented for my consideration. I am satisfied that a great desideratum has been accomplished. I am proud of it as an achievement of American medicine—I am proud of it, particularly, as a triumph of Southern experiment and observation, and believe that it will weave for the brow of the discoverer a chaplet of green, and with the lancet, win a partition of empire in the domain of practical medicine. * * * * I will further, and more familiarly, say, that price shall be no bar to my keeping a supply in my office. I will never be without it, if money can get it. Deprive me of it, and I verily believe I should " throw physic to the dogs." I still have a small portion of the specimen you sent me. I intend to keep it until I am satisfied I can obtain a supply of equal purity and power. * * * * Dr. Montgomery requests me to say that he is every way satisfied with the article—that it has furnished him with a number of beautiful cases and subject matter for a communication for the Journal ; but he must plead laziness in extenuation of the omission. To use his emphatic language : " Take it from me, sir, and I'd quit the practice of physic." Before you dispose of what you have on hand, root or tincture, I must get some. I must be sure it comes from your hand—I dont care what the price is.
* * * *   I remain,

E. L'ROY ANTONY, M. D.

[To be Continued.]

[Dr. Norwood informs us that he has been at considerable expense of time and money in procuring the fresh and genuine

Root of Veratrum Viride, in order to supply the many calls upon him by physicians who were unable to obtain it. He still has some on hand which he would like to dispose of, so as to be refunded, in part, at least. The Doctor certainly deserves the thanks of the profession for his exertions to supply the article, until it is generally kept by the druggists. He will keep it no longer.]—EDITOR.

ARTICLE XLI.

Operation for the Removal of Calculi in the Urethra. By D. W. HAMMOND, M. D., of Culloden, Georgia.

Professor Pancoast, in treating of strictures of the urethra, has most truly observed that, "no class of surgical diseases demands more attentive study on the part of the practitioner than that which involves, as one of its consequences, a retention of urine." My remarks, on this occasion, will be entirely confined to retention from impacted calculi in the canal of the urethra, and requiring the knife for their removal. It may be proper here to observe that, in each of the following cases, the ordinary means were used for the removal of the calculi, prior to resorting to the knife.

The operation is usually performed in the following manner: The median line is opened directly over the urethra, which is deepened until the foreign body is reached and extracted; a catheter is then introduced into the bladder, and the external wound closed with stitch and adhesive plaster—this is the plan now recommended by Dr. Mütter. There are many objections to this operation, which will be pointed out in the sequel.

In my first case, I performed the operation as recommended by this distinguished surgeon, and in consequence of a fistulous opening remaining in the urethra for some considerable time, and which required much trouble and pain for its eradication, I determined, should ever another similar case occur in my practice, that I would perform the operation in a different manner.

CASE I. In the fall of 1829, my associate in the practice of medicine, Dr. Richard Banks, the distinguished surgeon now of Gainesville, was summoned in haste to see the son of Mr. Wm. Sodlers, of Elbert county, about 5 years of age. He being absent, I was requested to visit the case. The messenger having apprised me of the condition of the patient, I fortified myself with the necessary instruments. I found the little boy in the most intense agony from retention of urine; the bladder was very much distended, reaching nearly or quite to the umbilicus. On making an exploration of the urethra, I detected a calculus lodged in the canal, just anterior to the bulb. Making some abortive efforts to remove it, I cut down upon it, and readily extracted it through the opening; the urine gushed from the wound with considerable force, to the great relief of the little sufferer. A catheter was introduced, and the wound approximated, and confined by stitch and adhesive plaster. From the constant stillicidium of urine through the opening, the plasters were soon washed away, and the pain and irritation produced from the presence of the catheter becoming so insufferable that I was compelled to withdraw it. Considerable tumefaction of the penis and scrotum ensued; this, however, subsided in a few days by appropriate treatment. The patient recovered from the operation, with the exception of a fistulous opening, as before stated; this was, in the course of five or six weeks, closed by frequent applications of the nitrate of silver.

Case II. In the year 1831, (as well as I now recollect, for I kept no notes of the case,) my co-partner and myself were requested to visit the son of Mr. Wm. Alexander, a child about three years of age, near Ruckersville, Elbert county. He had retention of urine, from the lodgment of a stone in the membranous portion of the urethra. The operation was performed in the following manner:—The patient was secured as for the operation of lithotomy; an assistant, placed on the right of the patient, with the fingers of the right hand forcibly drew the skin across the perineum from left to right, and held it firmly against the ramus of the ischium—by this procedure the raphe or median line of the perineum was from a half to three-fourths of an inch from its natural position, and to the right of the urethra; an incision was now made in an oblique direction down to the stone, which was readily removed by a small pair of forceps. The assistant removing his hold upon the skin, it at once assumed its normal state. The orifice through the skin was now found from a half to three-fourths of an inch from the median line, and on the left side of the urethra. The wound healed by the first intention.

CASE III. On the 15th of August last, I was requested to see the child of Mr. Orlando Holland, about one mile from Culloden. The little patient had been laboring under a difficulty of micturition for several days, for which he had taken diuretics and mucilaginous drinks, without relief. On the introduction of a silver probe, a small calculus was found lodged just behind the glans penis, about midway between the glans and front of the scrotum. Making some effort to force it out of the urethra, and failing to accomplish it, I proceeded to remove it by the knife. The penis was grasped by the left hand, twisting the skin from the left to the right side, and holding it firmly—a scalpel held in the third position completed the operation. The penis being released, the skin at once retracted, throwing the orifice made by the scalpel on the left side of the penis, and one-half inch from the median line beneath, presenting the appearance of the operation having been performed through the corpus-cavernosum instead of the corpus-spongiosum urethræ. In this case, union took place by the first intention; not a drop of urine ever passed through the wound.

REMARKS.—In the first case, we had a troublesome fistulous opening to contend with for several successive weeks, caused, no doubt, by the manner in which the operation was performed. When the opening is made through the integuments, directly over the urethra, the wound has a natural tendency to *gape*, from the traction constantly kept up by a contraction of the skin in a lateral direction—superadded to this, a portion of the corpus-spongiosum is almost certain to protrude through the lips of the wound; the presence of the catheter in the urethra causes great pain and irritation, and at the same time distends the *calibre* of the canal beyond its natural size, which keeps open the rent in the urethra; and, in addition, the *stitch* recommended to close the wound, developes, in a majority of cases, still more irritation, and not unfrequently ulceration is the consequence. Many other objections might be urged, but I think it would be an unnecessary consumption of time to do so at present.

In the plan I propose, as detailed in the second and third cases, neither of the foregoing objections obtains. The opening through the skin is some distance from that in the corpus-spongiosum urethræ, consequently the external integuments immediately over the wound are entire. After the operation is performed, all that is necessary to complete the cure is proper pressure. The slight tumefaction which always succeeds the operation, produces a rigidity of the integuments—this thickening and immobility of the parts institutes a steady and constant pressure, and this, too, being so accurately applied, and steadily maintained, that there cannot be any impediment to union by the first intention; whereas, in the old plan of performing the operation this seldom ever takes place, for reasons already stated.

ARTICLE XLII.

Cases of Typhoid Fever. By J. A. Williams, M. D., of Pike county, Ga.

Case I. Called 7th June, 1851, to see Mr P., aged 25 years, who had been complaining some ten days, the last three or four of which he was confined to his bed with a dull headache, indisposition to exercise, indolent stupid feeling, no appetite, and a slight diarrhœa. I found him somewhat emaciated, skin hot and dry, pulse from 100 to 110, some deafness, tip and edges of tongue red, centre covered with a white fur, bowels tender to pressure, with the usual gurgling noise and other less prominent symptoms, characterizing a simple case of typhoid fever.

Treatment.—A blister to the nape of the neck, a pepper poultice to the bowels, gum or elm water to be drank constantly; no other food allowed; laudanum when necessary, to control the bowels.

June 11th. Patient in the same condition—the symptoms a little aggravated: ordered treatment continued, laudanum increased.

June 20th. Patient doing well, no pain, pulse 90, skin moist, slight diarrhœa: ordered small portions soup or gruel. Patient dismissed with instructions to keep within doors, guard the appetite and continue the laudanum if necessary.

CASE II. Mrs. W., aged about 40, the mother of eight children, a woman who leads quite an active life, of stout and robust habit, somewhat inclined to corpulency, was attacked about the 1st of July, 1851, with a dull headache, a disinclination to exercise, no appetite, unpleasant taste, in which situation she remained until the 4th, when I saw her ; emaciated, skin hot and dry, tip and edges of tongue red and parched, a brownish fur on the ·centre with distinct papillæ appearing through the coating, pulse ranging from 120 to 140 rather full, bowels tender, a little distended, slight diarrhœa. In connection with the above, Mrs. W., had a slight cough, and upon exploring the chest detêcted some irritation in the right lung.

Treatment.—A small blister over the occipito atloid articulation to combat tenderness, a pepper poultice to the bowels, gum or elm water drank constantly, squills occasionally, a Dover's powder at night, laudanum if necessary.

July 10th. Little or no alteration in patient; treatment continued, squills increased.

July 17th. Sent for in haste to see patient. No abatement of fever, bowels distended and very irritable, tongue red: applied a blister plaster to the abdomen, former treatment continued, with instructions, should strangury ensue.

July 20th. Blister acted like a charm, swelling in the bowels subsided, some abatement of fever ; treatment continued. Ordered a little rice water, in a day or two with instructions to increase the diet as the stomach could bear.

July 25th. Patient convalescent; skin moist and cool, pulse nearly natural, tongue cleaning off, sharp appetite. Dismissed.

CASE III. January 6th, 1852. Called to see Archer, a negro boy, the property of Mr. R., who had been sick about a week. Mr. R., had given him salts once or twice, and a dose of Cook's pills ; all ineffectual. Archer presented the usual symtoms of typhoid fever with a slight attack of pneumonia.

About this time, Dr. Norwood's preparation of hellebore made its appearance ; thinking I had a proper subject for its use, commenced by giving five drops every three hours until nausea was induced, which occurred in ten hours, with vomiting, at which time I left, ordering the veratrum viride again in five hours, to be repeated as before. This practice was continued until the 10th, with the effect of reducing the force and frequency of the pulse during its administration, but upon its discontinuance that symptom would resume its former station. Being satisfied of the inefficacy of veratrum viride in this case, my patient was put upon the palliative plan and recovered in a few weeks, the fever having run its course uninterrupted by any therapeutic agent.

Cases IV and V. April, 1852. Called to the family of Judge E.; found his son, a youth of 15 or 16 years old, with headache, hot and dry skin, tongue red and pointed, bowels regular, with other characteristic symptoms of typhoid fever.

Treatment.—Elm water, a Dover's powder at night, laudanum if necessary. While attending the above, my attention was directed to a negro woman in the same family, who presented the same symptoms as above. Treatment the same; both were relieved in four or five weeks.

Remarks.—The object of reporting the above cases is to induce some one more competent than myself to experiment, note and publish the result of the palliative treatment in typhoid fever. In looking over the Journals of the day, we see that some rely on mercury as the sheet anchor, others on veratrum viride, and a few on stimulation ; all of which (according to my experience) are useless, if not detrimental. In general, mercury only serves to debilitate, and in some instances aggravates the already irritated bowels ; veratrum viride merely exercises a temporary control over the vascular system, and of course leaves the alimentary canal in an irritated state, and more subject to colliquative diarrhœa ; stimulants cause increased nervous and arterial excitement about the brain, inducing nervous derangement, subsultus tendinum delirium, coma, &c. So, upon the whole, our main dependence in typhoid fever are, palliatives, good nursing, and the vis medicatrix naturæ.

Vicarious Menstruation. By A. W. KNIGHT, M. D., of White
Springs, Hamilton Co., Florida.

Mr. Editor—The following case may, perchance, interest
some of your readers, or, at least, it will go to prove our text-
books correct, when they assert that an evacuation may take
place at various parts of the body, vicarious of the normal
uterine periodical secretion.

On the 8th of February of the present year, I was called to
visit Mrs. W——, of Columbia county, who was much alarmed
at a hemorrhage from the *left eye*: she is about 30 years of
age, and the mother of six children. Reported to me, that for
four or five nights past, she had perceived that her left eye had
been bleeding about a table-spoonful during the night, as near
as she could judge, from the stain upon the pillow, and that the
eye was suffused with blood during the day. During the same
period, she had a slight hemorrhage from the nose, and had
discovered traces of blood in the expectoration. Feeling no
pain in the eye, and having never received any injury from
blow or otherwise, she was at a loss how to account for it.

Making particular inquiries into the case, I learned that she
had menstruated in the usual manner only three times in twelve
years, and that this was the proper time for the menses to appear. Her general health, during this time, has not been good,
and her appearance, at the time of my visit, was decidedly
anæmic, with some tendency to anasarca.

On careful examination of the eye-lid, I could detect some
slight congestion of the minute blood-vessels; otherwise not different from the other. With a view to the improvement of her
general health and to the re-establishment of the uterine function, I prescribed mineral tonics, chiefly the preparations of
iron, for the interval, and special emmenagogues for the week
on which the menses ought to return. Up to the present month
she has had no return of the vicarious menstruation.

She followed my prescription for about one month; but the
normal discharge not taking place, she became discouraged,
and discontinued the medicine. Having understood that, some
years since, her menses appeared after a few days bathing in the

sulphur spring at this place, and as there has been no return of the regular menstruation, I have advised her to try the bathing again.

A few weeks since, I was called to treat her for intermittent fever, and was struck with a remark of her's—that the side on which the vicarious discharge appeared "felt *numb* when the fever was on." Does this throw any light upon the state of the nervous system in "intermittents?" Could the peculiar condition of the uterine system cause any loss of sensation in the nerves of one side more than the other? Here is a point worthy of investigation by older practitioners than myself.

The "intermittent" yielded readily to treatment; and once since the convalescence she says that symptoms have induced her to think, that the vicarious discharge may again return from the eye.

August 24th, 1852.

ARTICLE XLIV.

Case of Extensive Sloughing of the Foot from Frost Bite; Amputation below the Knee. By B. M. Thompson, M. D., of Danielsvile, Ga.

It is not uncommon to see cases of frost bite of more or less severity in this climate; but it is rare to see a whole limb destroyed by congelation alone. Such accidents are of much more frequent occurrence in the higher latitudes. The following case is interesting on account of the extent of the injury sustained and the consequences resulting from it—the loss of the entire foot and leg. My object in reporting it for the Journal is merely to record it, to furnish a link for the great chain of medical statistics.

The patient, a Negress, about 25 years of age, a native of Virginia, the property of Mr. J. W. H., of this county, ranaway from her master about the 18th January last, and was out during the very cold weather experienced here about that time. She was out some three weeks, and when found near her master's plantation, was unable to walk from the swollen and painful condition of the left foot and leg. The foot, however, was

neither much swollen nor very painful, but a considerable portion of its skin was off, and there was a good deal of redness in
the denuded part. This redness, as I was informed by her
owner, was soon succeeded by a bluish colour; there was very
little sensibility in the part. There was a good deal of soreness
about the ankle, which was greatly swollen. There was no
sloughing of the soft parts, except of the integuments, as before
mentioned, when she was brought home. The foot was dressed
with poultices wet occasionally with spirits of turpentine. This
treatment had but little effect other than to stimulate the efforts
of nature to cast off the lifeless foot. In the course of a few
days the soft parts around the ankle joint began to slough, and
when I was called to the case on the 29th of February, I found
the sphacelated foot almost ready to drop off at the ankle joint.
It was black, dry and hard, not unlike dried beef in appearance.
The sloughing was extensive, especially on the inner side of the
articulation, the tarsal bones were more or less exposed. The
foot was only prevented from dropping off by the tendo-achilles,
a small portion of the skin and some of the ligaments on the
outer side of the joint. The other tendons, the nerves and
bloodvessels were completely severed, and the arteries occlu-
ded. The leg for some distance above the ankle presented a
very unhealthy appearance—it was nearly twice as large as
the other, œdemetous, of a bluish or livid hue, the integuments
appeared to be thickened, and it resembled elephantiasis. The
lower ends of the tibia and fibula could not be seen on account
of the swollen condition of the tissues which covered them. A
considerable quantity of very offensive pus was discharged from
about the joint; there was a number of pale and exceedingly
unhealthy looking granulations shooting out from the stump,
which would slough upon the least handling. There appeared
to have been very little constitutional disturbance amid all
this local disorder. Her constitution was good, she was greatly
emaciated, but was free from symptoms of organic disease of
any vital organ.

Amputation of the diseased member seemed the only mode
of relief and the circular operation was performed on the 5th
day of March, by Dr. Benjamin V. Willingham, of Lexington,
who at my request kindly consented to operate, assisted by his

brother and associate, Dr. Willis Willingham, of the same place,
Dr. William Johnson and Mr. Howard, medical student, of
Oglethorpe county.   The limb was taken off about three finger's
breadths below the tubercle of the tibia, the patient being under
the influence of chloroform.   It was performed in the usual
manner, and with much skill and dexterity by my friend, Dr.
Willingham.   I had some apprehensions as to the final result
of the operation, as the patient was at times stubborn and refractory, but she convalesced rapidly and satisfactorily and is
now (June 1st) entirely well, with a good looking stump.   It
may not be amiss here to state that this patient had her right
foot frost bitten in the early part of last winter, (being runa-
way at the time,) which was followed by considerable sloughing
of the skin and subcutaneous tissue of various parts of the foot;
these ulcers healed slowly and had not entirely cured up when
she went off in January: they are now, however, well—there is
slight contraction of the flexor tendons of that foot together
with a little stiffness of the ankle joint.

The chloroform had the happiest effect in this case; about
three drachms of this article poured on a piece of sponge and
enveloped in a handkerchief folded into the shape of a hollow
cone, were applied to the patient's nose, which produced complete suspension of sensation in less than two minutes.   She remained under the influence of this wonderful " pain killer" in
all about twenty minutes, perfectly unconscious of what was
going on during this time, and awoke after the operation was
over as from a pleasant slumber.   It produced no unpleasant
symptoms in this case, the pulse was as full, soft and regular,
and the breathing as easy and natural as that of a person in the
most perfect health.

ARTICLE XLV.

A Simple Instrument for Operating upon Hare-lip.   Described
in a letter to the Editor, by E. F. STARR, M. D., of Rome,
Georgia.

Dear Sir—Enclosed I send you a small plate made of pew-
ter, with eyes, or loop-holes, on the back, which, if you will
adjust upon one prong of your long straight dressing forceps,

will make (should it fit well) a convenient instrument for operating for hare-lip. To have the lip firmly clasped the entire
distance it is to be cut—to have it well supported by a substance which will not destroy the edge of the knife when cut
upon, and to have a guide for the knife in making the cut—are
objects to be desired. These may all be obtained by this instrument, thus arranged, in *one cut.* It might be well, perhaps,
to have a thin piece of leather pasted upon the face of the plate.
The opposite blade of the forceps should be rough like a file,
longitudinally, to prevent slipping. An instrument might be
made for the purpose with plate attached, and the edges or
sides of the opposite prong should be made straight, as guides
for the knife. In using it, the operator should take hold of just
so much of the lip as he wishes to remove, then cut along the
edge of the outer prong, next the body of the lip, down to the
plate on each side. You will readily perceive its application,
however. The plate may be made wider or narrower, to suit
individual cases. I used this one not long since in an operation, and found it quite a help.

ARTICLE XLVI.

Observations upon the use of certain New Remedies. By
L. A. DUGAS, M. D., Professor, &c.

Believing it to be the duty of members of associations of this
kind to make known such results of their observation as may
be useful, I will beg leave to offer a few remarks upon the use
of some of the remedial agents recently brought into notice.

Chloride of Sodium or *common salt* has been, at various periods, proposed as a valuable remedy, but has attracted more
than usual attention during the last twelve months.

I have long been in the habit of prescribing it alone, or in
combination with the Bi-carbonate of soda, in certain forms of
dyspepsia and general debility. From 10 to 30 grains of salt in
a tumblerful of cold water, taken every morning on rising from
bed, is highly promotive of appetite and digestion when the
dyspepsia is unattended with organic lesion of the gastric surface and seems to be rather dependent upon a state of atony.
The soda, in an equal quantity, constitutes an useful addition

where there is a tendency to acidity, and also when the kidneys do not secrete freely and properly. The remedy appears to be especially applicable to the cases of general debility and nervous irritability so common among our ladies of sedentary habits. It may be sometimes necessary to commence with a smaller dose than just mentioned ; but I have stated that suited to the majority of cases.

In Acute Dysentery, I have found common salt often of striking usefulness, but it must in general be given early in order to realize its value. It is now ten years since I first witnessed its efficacy in this disease. I had been attending a mulatto boy, eight years of age, for four or five days without being able to ameliorate his condition. The onset of his attack was attended with high febrile action, which, however, gradually subsided as he became exhausted by the continuance of the countless, bloody, mucous stools, and painful tenesmus. The rectum rejected anodyne enemata as fast as they could be administered. Nothing I could suggest seemed to bring any relief; and I left him one night, thinking his case hopeless. On the next morning I found him wonderfully relieved, and was congratulating myself with the idea that my last prescription had " done the deed," when the boy's father announced that he had taken the liberty to omit my prescription and to give his son last night, in lieu of it, a cupful of strong fish brine, which afforded so much relief that he had just again repeated it. The stools became watery and less frequent, the tenesmus was entirely relieved and the patient convalesced rapidly.

I have ever since that time resorted to salt and water ; when the high febrile excitement conter-indicated the immediate resort to anodyne enemata ; and when the administration of these failed to give relief. In the early and high febrile stage, it will often subdue the fever and tenesmus most admirably, and the patient will rapidly recover.

The efficacy of this and perhaps of other saline purgatives in dysentery, probably depends upon its combined depletory and revulsive operation. The depletion is derived from the *small* intestines in the form of serous stools, and this action must also relieve, by revulsion, the morbid condition of the *large* intestines. The case loses the painful and alarming character of dysentery and assumes that of ordinary diarrhœa, which will either gradually subside or yield to vegetable astringents combined with opiates.

In the spring and in autumn, when the causes of periodical or paroxysmal fevers combine with the vicissitudes of temperature to produce diseases in which the phlegmasiæ and the neuroses are so commingled as to re-act injuriously upon each other, we often find dysentery prevailing to so great an extent as to constitute an epidemic. If the febrile excitement be then closely observed, it will often be found to present daily exacerbations, which must be prevented by the use of quinine during the remissions, in order that the remedies directed to the local affection may have time to prove beneficial. If the quinine be withheld each febrile exacerbation will aggravate the intestinal inflammation, and this, in its turn, will make the next paroxysm more alarming—until it be too late to avert the fatal result. The same may be said of the so-called epidemics of pneumonia, which are most prevalent in mild winters and in remittent fever districts.

In cases unattended with fever, I am in the habit of resorting, as soon as the bowels are *thoroughly emptied*, to enemata consisting of a teaspoonful of laudanum, or half a grain morphine suspended in half a gill of thin starch or mucilage, repeated until retained long enough to give complete relief. This plan will be found to succeed in the great majority of such cases. Yet, we occasionally encounter one in which the anodyne will not be retained, and it is then that I resort to the salt and water.

The dose I administer is a teaspoonful of salt in a cupful of water, to be repeated every three or four hours until the stools pass off freely and without tenesmus. If the tenesmus returns, the salt should be again given, but at longer intervals.

I am aware that the sulphate of soda in similar doses has been highly recommended, and I have sometimes used it, as also the sulphate of magnesia, with decided advantage. Common salt, however, is less disagreeable, more convenient, and, I think, more efficacious.

Common salt has been of late urged in France, especially by M. Piorry, as a valuable substitute for quinine in Intermittent

Fever ; and if it can be thus used advantageously, the discovery would be one of great importance to those who cannot afford to purchase the more costly article. I have prescribed it in only two cases of Intermittent fever ; in one of which it proved successful, the patient having had but one paroxysm after its use was commenced. In the other, which was complicated with tubercular disease of the lungs and intestines, it increased the diarrhœa so much as to cause its discontinuance after the second dose. In these cases a teaspoonful in a tumblerful of cold water was ordered three times a day. It is to be hoped that this application will be fully tested by the Profession.

Lemon Juice in Rheumatism.—There is perhaps no disease, for the relief of which more remedies have been and are still being continually suggested, than Rheumatism. The last in the list is lemon juice, of whose efficacy the British Journals are full. It may be known to some of those present, that I have for many years advocated the theory (first suggested by Prof. J. K. Mitchell, of Philadelphia,) of the Spinal origin of Rheumatic affections, and consequently the use of counter-irritants in the vicinity of the origin of the nerves leading to the seat of pain. My views upon this subject were published in the Southern Medical and Surgical Journal in 1837, and I have seen no reason to change them since. We however, not unfrequently, meet with cases of acute Rheumatism of great intensity, in which the spinal treatment cannot be energetically carried out on account of the inability of the patient to rest in any other position than upon his back. In these cases it is difficult to cup the spine often, and very painful to apply blisters to this region. We are then compelled to resort to other means. I should also add that the spinal treatment is by no means so speedily effectual when large joints are much affected with acute inflammation, as in cases of less violence. This is of itself an additional reason for the use of internal medication, than which I have found nothing more useful than repeated emetics of tartarized antimony, followed in the evening by full doses of opium or morphine.

Within the last few months, however, I have been induced to try the Lemon Juice in a number of cases of acute rheumatism and in the exacerbations of the chronic form of the disease, and always with most decided advantage. The remedy is very grateful to the palate, and the patients own that they feel better as soon as they begin its use, and worse when it is omitted. I usually order a tablespoonful of the lemon juice of the shops to be taken every four, three, or two hours, according to the violence of the case and the toleration with which it is received by the stomach and bowels. It seems to promote the action of the kidneys, to keep the bowels solvent, to lessen general excitement, and to diminish pain.

So simple and pleasant a remedy in so formidable an affection is well worthy of farther and systematic trial.

Collodion and its kindred preparations, the solution of *Gutta Percha in Chloroform* and *Gum Shellac in Alcohol,* are agents which promise to be useful. Collodion has been much lauded as an application to Erysipelas, and it is, therefore, proper to hear the testimony against it as well as that adduced in favor of its efficacy. Having recently had charge of a case of this disease, I applied the collodion very early to the part affected and a little beyond the inflamed surface. But the disease extended rapidly from the ear to the face and scalp, and in a few days invaded the entire head and a portion of the neck. The collodion was persevered in to the last without appearing to exercise any controlling influence whatever. My patient recoved, it is true, but I cannot attribute this result to the local application. This is the only case of erysipelas in which I have used it.

Solution of Gutta Percha in Chloroform.—This is made by dropping into a vial containing chloroform small fragments of pure gutta percha until the solution acquires the consistence of thick mucilage. It is then applied with a camel hair pencil, which should afterwards be repeatedly dipped in pure chloroform and carefully wiped with paper or old linen so as to prevent its becoming stiff and unfit for farther use.

I will now relate the result of its application in two cases of cancerous affection.

Mr. L. had been troubled with an epithelial cancer of the lower lip which had resisted all applications for eighteen months. There existed, upon the right side of the median line and at the junction of the skin and mucous surface, a small and thin scale

or scab, which would occasionally fall or be rubbed off, leaving
a raw surface of exquisite sensibility exposed to irritation until
another scab would be formed.   Beneath this surface there was
an induration about the size of a common pea, or rather a little
larger, in which the patient frequently felt a very annoying
sense of burning, and sometimes darting pain.

At this stage of the case, as the patient was averse to the
knife, he was advised to try the application of collodion, which
he diligently persevered in for about six months, applying it
three or four times daily.   This arrested the farther growth of
the disease, relieved its itching and burning, protected its
surface from ordinary irritants, but did not heal the denuded
surface.   He then substituted the solution of gutta percha in
chloroform in lieu of the collodion.   In a letter to me he thus
describes its effects:—"In a few days I saw and felt a change
in the color of the sore and in the irritation; in a week or ten
days, the lump disappeared and the irritation subsided, and in
three weeks it was almost entirely healed over; in less than a
month it was well, leaving an indentation on the lip."

In a note dated the 1st of this month, (April,) my patient
writes me: "I begin to feel a return of it in the same place the
cure was made eighteen months ago.   Recently a lump has
appeared in the lip; it is *hard* and sometimes a little sore—it
gives me no trouble yet, but I am afraid of it."   I will advise
him to use the gutta percha and chloroform again.

The next case was that of Maria, a negress, about 50 years
of age, who was sent to me from the country on the 3d of November last, with a cancerous ulceration of the mamma of several months standing.   Both mammary glands were very much
atrophied, but the affected one was the smaller of the two,
presented nothing but a mass of schirrous induration which
seemed adherent to the thoracic walls, and in the depressed
centre of which the remains of a nipple were to be seen drawn
back and ulcerated.   The ulcer covered a surface equal to the
areola.   The axillary glands were much enlarged, and the patient a prey to continual pain, especially at night, which deprived her of sleep.

Feeling satisfied that the knife promised no relief under such
circumstances, yet unwilling to send her off without trying

something, I put her upon the use of the gutta percha and chloroform, thoroughly coating the whole breast daily with it. The discharge from the ulcer would at first cause the pellicle of gutta percha to become loosened in twenty-four hours, so that the surface had to be cleansed before the re-application of the remedy. The suppuration, however, gradually lessened until the coating would remain a week—the painting still being made each morning. Under this treatment, the patient was gradually relieved of all pain about the breast and even in the axilla. She slept quietly at night, enjoyed her meals and felt quite well. Her general health improved, and she left at the end of one month, with instructions to continue the treatment perseveringly, and to get her master to inform me of the result. I have had no report from her since, but have learned incidentally that she never applied the remedy after she left here, and placed herself under the charge of some one who professed to be able to cure cancers—with what result, I know not.

These two cases are narrated with the simple purpose of directing attention to an application which may stay, if it does not cure, so formidable an affection as cancer.

Solution of Shellac.—The costliness of the solutions of gun cotton and of gutta percha renders it desirable to have a cheaper article that may be used as a substitute in cases which require the consumption of a large quantity of such plastic materials. A solution of shellac in alcohol has therefore been proposed for this purpose. This may be prepared by adding successively small bits of shellac to the alcohol of commerce until enough be dissolved to make a mucilaginous solution.

Some of the French practitioners having attributed to collodion extraordinary antiphlogistic properties when applied over afffected joints and other inflammatory affections, even more deeply seated, I determined to try, during last winter, the shellac solution in an old case of Rheumatism, in which most of the joints of the extremities were being successively invaded. The toes, ankles, knees, fingers, wrists and elbows were nearly all alternately implicated—becoming very painful and rapidly swelling, so as to be almost doubled in size in a day or two. I furnished the patient a bottle of the shellac solution and ordered it to be painted over and around the joint as soon as it would commence to be painful, and to repeat the application several times a day until a thick coating remained, after which it might be applied only once a day. Under this treatment I was gratified to find that the patient could, in a few hours, arrest the pain and prevent the swelling of the joints to which he made the application. He stated that he never had any thing to give him such prompt and effectual relief, although he had been suffering such attacks every winter for the last ten years. One joint or another continued to annoy him for a month, during all of which time he resorted to the shellac with the same success.

This is the only case in which I have tried this solution.

[*Trans. of the Med. Soc. of the State of Georgia.*

PART II.

𝔈𝔠𝔩𝔢𝔠𝔱𝔦𝔠 𝔇𝔢𝔭𝔞𝔯𝔱𝔪𝔢𝔫𝔱.

Letters upon Syphilis. Addressed to the Editor of L'Union Medicale, by P. Ricord. Translated from the French by D. D. SLADE, M. D.

[Continued from Page 618.]

THIRD LETTER.

My Dear Friend,—The conclusion which terminates my last letter,—*The blennorrhagia of which the muco-pus being inoculated gives rise to no result, does not recognize the syphilitic virus as cause,*—this conclusion, deduced from undeniable facts, again places the history of blennorrhagia at the same point from which it has been transmitted to us in the book of Leviticus. Old as man, older than he, for animals created before him are subject to blenorrhagia, and not to the verole, this disease has nothing in common with the syphilitic infection.

In spite of those, who, since Paracelsus, Bethencourt and Fallopius, have wished to make of blennorrhagia, not symptomatic of chancre, a new disease identical with syphilis, the researches that I have made, corroborating the descriptions so exact of Alexander Benedictus and of Cataneus, have given to the doctrines of Balfour, of Todus, and of Duncan, the value and the solidity that Bell would have given them himself, if he could have explained the facts supposed to be exceptional, as we can explain them at the present day.

But blennorrhagia, as I understand it, absolutely different

from syphilis in its causes, in its form, and in its consequences, does it depend upon a special virus?

There would be nothing repugnant in admitting a special cause having the power specifically and constantly of producing blennorrhagia and its consequences. Nothing is more apt, in fact, to determine a blennorrhagia, than the muco-pus furnished by certain inflamed mucous surfaces. But when we go back in the strictest manner, and with the most rigid observation, to the causes determining *the best characterized blennorrhagia*, we are forced to see and to confess that the blennorrhagic virus ordinarily has no share in it.

Nothing is more common than to find women who have communicated blennorrhagia the most severe and the most obstinate, with the most varied and the most serious *blennorrhagic* consequences, and who were only affected with uterine catarrhs, sometimes scarcely purulent. Quite often the menstrual flow appears to have been the only cause of the communicated disease. In a great number of cases, in fact, we do not find anything, or only some errors in diet, fatigue, excess in sexual relations, the use of certain drinks, such as beer, or of certain articles of food, such as asparagus. From these circumstances spring that frequency of belief very often correct, that a gonorrhœa has been caught from a woman perfectly healthy.

Upon this point I am certainly aware of all the causes of error and I pretend to say that no one is more careful to guard against the frauds of every kind sown upon the steps of the observer than I am. It is, therefore, with full knowledge of the causes that I sustain this proposition.

PROPOSITION.

Women frequently give blennorrhagia without having it.

Blennorrhagia, such as some individuals persist in understanding it, that is to say, as the consequence of a contagion, is as rare in women as it is common among men. I do not believe that I advance too much when I say that women give twenty gonorrhœas where they contract one. And this is easy to understand, for women so subject to discharges not syphilitic from the genital organs, are the most frequent source of discharges which in the man cannot be considered as an effect of contagion.

It has been impossible for me to consider as serious the doctrine of my learned colleague, M. Cazenave, who admits very readily that many women under the influence of chronic utero-vaginal catarrhs, can have sexual relations without communicating any thing, provided that they are not "*echauffées*" to the

degree of virulence, or that they are not raised, so to speak, to
a red heat. Is it not more simple to understand and more rational to say, that with a less degree of excitement, the secretions
are less irritating, and that the being habituated to these secretions, would produce an immunity for some persons, and a sort
of acclimation.   It is thus, as I have frequently seen, that a
married woman can cohabit with her husband without communicating any thing; but should a lover come, this last contracts
a blennorrhagia.   The husband was acclimated, the lover was
not.   When one studies blennorrhagia without prejudice, without preconceived ideas, he is forced to acknowledge that it is
often produced under the influence of most of the causes which
determine the inflammation of other mucous surfaces.

The experience of Swediaur is here to prove this.   This
observer injected volatile alkali into the urethra, and produced
a blennorrhagia.   Does this experience show that a blennorrhagia can be always produced, and at will, by irritating injections?
No, certainly not, no more than a coryza or an ophthalmia
could be produced by the same means.   For a blennorrhagia,
as for every other inflammation, the pre-existence of predisposition, that great unknown influence which dominates over all
pathology, is necessary.   This is proved by the fact that a blennorrhagia is not always taken in those same conditions where
it is the most evidently communicable.   Without this fortunate
immunity which the absence of predisposition gives, blennorrhagia, already very common, would be still more so.

An experience of twenty years has taught me, and permits
me to affirm, that excepting blennorrhagic discharges symptomatic of chancre, it is often perfectly impossible to recognize
the cause of a blennorrhagia.

I know that many of my colleagues obstinately refuse to admit this opinion ; every blennorrhagia awakens in them the idea
of syphilis, and their therapeutic prescriptions are but the logical result of their prejudices.

Here, my dear friend, I ought to make to you a confession,
and I shall make it publicly.   This persistence of some of my
honored and learned colleagues, to always consider and to
treat blennorrhagia as an accident of a syphilitic nature, has
often astonished me.   Thus it has many times happened to me,
not to satisfy a frivolous curiosity, much less to yield to a culpable, slanderous motive, but to enlighten and re-assure my
mind, to have recourse to a stratagem of which I wish to make
the avowal with all the reserve and the delicacy that I owe my
honorable brethren.

It was under the following circumstances:—A man presented himself at my consultation with well-marked blennorrhagia.

He stated to me that he had had relations with but one woman, and that this woman was his wife or his mistress. This man was uneasy or alarmed. He brought with him the woman the cause of his trouble, and the latter, protesting her innocence, along with the patient, supplicated me to submit her to the most rigorous examination. This examination, made with all the attention and care of which I was capable, showed me the sexual organs of this woman in a perfectly healthy state. There was nothing, absolutely nothing, in the most profound folds of those organs which could explain the blennorrhagia of that man. I begged the woman to pass into a neighboring room, and alone with the patient, I made use of all the means possible, of which I spare you the details, to arrive at this certainty, that the patient had had no sexual connections but with this woman; it was in these alone that he could have contracted the disease which he had. I reassured the husband or lover; I acquitted the wife or the mistress; but I begged them both to be accomplices in a little stratagem, which it remains for me to indicate. I sent them both and separately, let it be well understood, to such of my learned colleagues whom I know to be direct antagonists to me upon the question of blennorrhagia. I said to the patient, demand clearly this question: is my blennorrhagia syphilitic? I said to the woman, demand distinctly, could I give a blennorrhagia to a man? The couple returned to me, the man with a diagnosis thus written—"*syphilitic blennorrhagia;* the treatment followed *ad hoc.* The woman returned with this—"*the perfectly healthy state of the organs permits me to affirm that madam could not communicate a malady which she has not.*"

It is not an isolated fact that I point out to you, my dear friend; this experiment I have often renewed, and sufficiently so, with some variations, to corroborate my convictions, and to re-establish my ideas.*

What do these facts signify? That the cause of a blenorrhagia cannot be always known; that this disease can be pro-

---

* There are some facts more curious still than those relating to blenorrhagia contracted with healthy women. A case analogous to the following has not been presented, perhaps, to the notice of M. Ricord, but of its authenticity it is not possible for me to raise the least doubt.

A man of thirty years of age, a physician, had been continent for more than six weeks, and his last sexual relations were not of a suspicious character. A fortuitous circumstance permitted him to pass almost an entire day in company with a young woman whom he loved. From ten o'clock in the morning until seven o'clock in the evening, he made vain efforts to overcome the resistance of this woman, whose virtue did not yield. But during all this time, this physician remained in a constant state of excitement. Three days after, he was taken with a blennorrhagia of the most violent and painful kind, which lasted forty days. Most assuredly here is the form of a blenorrhagia not syphilitic.—*Note of the Editor.*

duced by causes common to all inflammation, if there is a predisposition ; but that the most special agent of blennorrhagia
is the muco-pus furnished by the inflamed genito-urinary surfaces.

This manner of regarding it appears to me more rational
than that which would attribute the blennorrhagia called venereal to a sort of half virus imagined by our very learned brother
and ingenious writer on syphilis, M. Baumès. To this practitioner, blennorrhagia is a degenerated kind of chancre ; it can
give rise to a constitutional syphilitic infection, more feeble
however, than that produced by chancre, but without being able,
nevertheless, to reproduce this latter by means of contagion or
inoculation. "One can then foresee," adds M. Baumès, "the
greatest similarity between the constitutional symptoms which
are the consequence of the one and of the other of these diseases ; and in fact experience proves that the difference between
these symptoms lies not in their nature, but only in their degree
of intensity, in their gravity, and in their situation, which after
blennorrhagia extends generally to fewer tissues, and to a smaller number of organs, than after chancre."—*Baumès, Précis
théorique et pratique sur les maladies vénériennes, tom. i., page*
259.

Here is a true half-way doctrine. This mere theory is neither justified by facts, nor by observation or experience ; one condition is alone wanted to it—the proofs.

Hitherto, then, and it is certainly my present opinion, that
simple blennorrhagia is completely stranger to syphilis as to the
causes which can produce it.

But it has been objected to this, that the pus of chancre, that
is to say the syphilitic virus, can produce blennorrhagia. This
opinion is very old ; it has been sustained since the appearance
of the verole in Europe, and it can be very legitimately still
sustained. But what does this mean? Are the observations
of the ancients to be relied upon ? They are incomplete and
insufficient; it is impossible with these to proceed scientifically
from the effect to the cause. Would you appeal to experiments similar to those of Harrison, who drew his conclusions
from the production of a blennorrhagia by the introduction into
the urethra of pus furnished by a chancre, without knowing
what it had physically determined. No, we shall arrive more
simply and more logically at the conclusion of the possibility of
the production of a non-virulent blennorrhagia, by the pus of a
chancre, in considering this pus as having the power to act in
the manner of simple irritants. A woman having chancres at
the inoculable period, could thus produce a blennorrhagia in a
man which could not inoculate. We can thus understand the

observations of Swediaur and others, in supposing that they had
not committed some error in diagnosis, inasmuch as these observers made use of neither speculum, nor inoculation—observations which prove that men affected with chancre, have communicated blennorrhagia to women.

Here is what clinical observation teaches, and that which
experiment can demonstrate. It is not rare to see patients with
a chancre of the glans or of the prepuce, successively taken
with balanitis or with balanoposthitis, determined by the irritating action of the pus of the chancre. But while the chancre
furnishes pus inoculable, the pus furnished by the balano-pos-
thitis is not so. (We shall see later that in order that the virulent pus should act specifically, some conditions are necessary
which are not always met with.)

Faithful to my first conclusion, reducing to their just value
these first objections, I affirm that when Harrison produced
blennorrhagia with the pus of the chancre, either this pus acted
after the manner of simple irritants or it produced an urethral
chancre which was not ascertained. We shall see also later,
than when Hunter produced a chancre with some pus supposed
to be blennorrhagic, it was with the product of a true urethral
chancre that he had operated.

But if inoculation has proved that the cause or the causes of
blennorrhagia, *whatever may be its seat* in the two sexes, differ
from the specific principle, from the virus which chancre *fatally* produces, the consequences of blennorrhagia ought always
to differ from those of chancre ; and yet many constitutional
veroles are attributed to blennorrhagia. These are the questions which will make the subject of my next letter. We shall
see, also, if it is possible to establish a differential diagnosis
between two affections which some wish systematically to confound. You will permit me first to speak a word upon the inoculation of blennorrhagia.   Yours,   RICORD.

FOURTH LETTER.

My Dear Friend,—As I promised, I shall say a few words
upon the incubation of blennorrhagia. Incubation has been
made a condition of virulence. Every virulent disease ought
to present a period of incubation. Thus those who admit that
blennorrhagia is a product of a virus, admit equally that this
virus does not produce its first effects till after a time of incubation more or less long.

I say more or less long, and it is not without reason. The
authors, in fact, as well for the incubation of syphilis properly
called, have admitted for that of blennorrhagia a period the
most convenient. The term of the incubation has been fixed

between some hours (Hunter and others) and fifty and some days (Bell.) What shall I say? MM. Cullerier and Ratier have reported the history of an incubation which lasted during five months. Assuredly a very elastic incubation. You know that matters are far from passing thus in the virulent diseases where the incubation is incontestable. The limits of the period of incubation can be more accurately fixed in the variola, in vaccinia, in scarlatina, in the measles, and in hydrophobia. The fine works of M. Aubert Roche have ever told us the certain limits of the incubation of the plague, which never exceeds eight days. For blennorrhagia, it is a far different thing, as you will see; here there are no certain limits.

What is, then, this incubation of blennorrhagia, which they have made me again very recently deny? We must understand this matter; it is a pure question of words. I do not deny the evidence; and consequently I do not deny that between the action of the cause, and the appearance of the first phenomena of blennorrhagia, there is a period more or less long; but is there present an incubation properly called, an incubation similar to that of the variolic or vaccine virus? I contest this, and I explain that time, more or less long, which exists between the action of the cause and the appearance of the phenomena, by the disposition and by the particular susceptibility of the tissues which have undergone the influence of the cause. There is no more incubation present in this case, than there is between the action of an exposure of the feet to cold, and the appearance of a coryza. One does not blow muco-pus immediately from the nose after such exposure to cold; there exists a certain period between these two actions. Do you call this period the incubation of the coryza? Why then make use of a similar expression for blennorrhagia?

In those cases where blennorrhagia does not appear till long time after one is exposed to the suspected cause which produced it, is it not more rational to admit another cause which remains unknown, than that pretended incubation which nothing explains, nothing justifies? Is it not so in almost all inflammations? Can you always go back to the direct cause of a pneumonia, of an arthritis, of a phlegmon? Without doubt, in man the sexual relations are the most direct cause of blennorrhagia; but we should fall into strange errors, if we wish to refer all blennorrhagias to a virulent cause. I could give you some very singular examples which prove the contrary, but I refer the reader to the interesting note with which you have accompanied my preceding letter.

From this exclusive manner of considering the etiology of blennorrhagia, there results often, in practice, a singular manner of interpreting facts. A man affected with blennorrhagia has had connection with several women ; he hastens to make a sort of moral choice among these women, and by means of elimination he happens to fall often upon the most innocent. This sort of application of the law of suspicion has caused strange errors to be committed, of which I have often been witness.

Let us then conclude upon this point that the effects of blennorrhagia can follow at some distance from the cause which produces them, but that nothing proves that the period which exists between the action of the cause and the appearance of the morbid phenomena, is the result of a true virulent incubation.

I should prefer, my dear friend, not to make too frequent digressions from my programme, but how can I avoid deciding incidental questions when they present themselves beneath my pen ? Such is that of the specific seat of blennorrhagia. You know that the question of this seat has been much agitated. In man it has been made to travel from behind forward, from forward backward ; to advance or to retreat, at the will of the fertile imagination of writers upon syphilis. From the spermatic passages, in passing successively by the glands of Cowper, the fossa navicularis and the follicles of Morgagni, the seat of blennorrhagia has travelled a good deal. It is true that Bell, in establishing different degrees in blennorrhagia, has made its seat retrograde from before backwards. But it is not with these questions, so well known, that I wish to detain you. I will call your attention, however, to a singular prepossession of Hunter. This great observer admitted, as you know, a virulent blennorrhagia to be identical to chancre ; he placed the seat of it in the fossa navicularis ; but he inquires if the inflammation which propagates itself by degrees towards the posterior portions of the urethra, continues to be virulent beyond the fossa navicularis. We must confess that the genius of Hunter yielded to the spirit of system. Besides, in studying Hunter, we see his observing genius constantly in contest with his theory of blennorrhagia. He started with a false idea ; facts come constantly to prove it to him, but theory is there to obscure his intellect, and in place of dismantling his theory by facts, he endeavours, on the contrary, to make facts agree with his theory—an excellent example of the dangers of pre-conceived and systematic ideas in the cultivation of the sciences of observation.

In the female, Graff placed the seat of the virulent blennorrhagia in the follicles in the neighborhood of the urethra. One of our brother physicians of Bordeaux, who died a few years since, Moulinié, thought he had seen in the glands of the vulva (so well described by Bartholin, and of which Boerhaave has traced

the pathological history, resumed and completed in our day by
M. Hugenier) a sort of organ of virulence in a blennorrhagic
point of view.

In the midst of all these opinions, strict observation shows that
those portions of mucous surfaces the most exposed, are those
which are the most easily affected.   Nevertheless, we must
allow that the mucous surface of the urethra in the two sexes is
more often affected after sexual intercourse than the other mucous surfaces of the genital organs.   This fact is an argument .
for the partisans of the virulent contagion.   I will corroborate
it, if they wish, by this proposition, which appears incontestible,
that a woman attacked by blennorrhagia of the urethra can be
considered as having the most commonly contracted it from a
man suffering from blennorrhagia; and you see that this proposition could have its importance in legal medicine.   Thus, for
me, I should be ready to admit that a woman in whom I discovered ·a blennorrhagia of the urethra had taken it from a man.
But does this fact come in aid of the existence of a virulent contagion?   No, and I explain it by this other fact, alone true and
incontestable, that pus furnished by the urethra is the most irritating of all pus for certain mucous surfaces.

While certain writers on syphilis contest the existence of
blennorrhagia of the urethra in the female, others do not admit
in her of a blennorrhagia except when it has its seat in the
urethra.   These two extreme opinions are erroneous.   Observation has led me to admit all the varieties of blennorrhagia upon
all mucous surfaces.

Whilst I am here, will you permit me to disembarrass myself
of some other incidental questions relative to blennorrhagia?   I
shall proceed more freely and more rapidly afterwards, on the
great questions which remain for me to treat of.   If I examine
the lesions of tissue which blennorrhagia produces, whatever
may be the mucous coat affected, I do not find anything that
simple inflamation cannot produce.   There is sometimes a slight
erythematous condition without secretion.   It is the dry blennorrhagia of some writers, a denomination ridiculous and absurd,
introduced into the writings upon syphilis, and in view of which
we can admire the persevering efforts of M. Piorry to bring a-
bout a reform in the nomenclature.   Sometimes we have to do
with a mucous element, catarrhal, and with all its products at
different degrees, mucous, mucoso-purulent; in fine there are
some true phlegmonous complications which we meet with, from
which result in man for the urethra, the blennorrhagia accompanied with chordée, and the quite frequent production of abscess upon the course of the urethra.

But neither in the state of the tissues nor in the nature of the

products do we find anythihg which can be compared to the accidents of syphilis properly called.

Are the consequences of blennorrhagia comparable to those
of syphilis ? It has been said so, but it has not been proved.
There are some analogies, without doubt, but some notable differences also. Thus one of the first accidents which blennorrhagia can produce, and which resembles one of those produced
by syphilis, is bubo. But in the first place, enlarged glands are
. infinitely more rare as the consequence of blennorrhagia, than
of chancre. In the next place, the bubo is never met with except in blennorrhagia of the urethra, in the two sexes, the other
varieties never giving rise to enlarged glands. I well know that
one of our fellow medical men of Belgium speaks of buboes
peri-auriculaires, which ought to manifest themselves in blennorrhagia of the eve, but I must confess that I have yet to look
for an example. In fine, the blennorrhagic bubo has this speciality, that purely inflammatory, it has very little tendency to
suppuration, and when this happens *it is never inoculable.*

Do you wish to follow out that which blennorrhagia can produce ordinarily upon the two sexes ? Take blennorrhagic
ophthalmia, which never manifests itself but during *a blennorrhagia of the urethra ;* in good faith, is it possible, unless we
wish to confound everything, to establish the least comparison
between this ophthalmia and syphilitic iritis ?

With regard to blennorrhagic rheumatism, is it reasonable to
establish the least difference between this affection and the accidents produced by syphilis upon the osseous system ? Is there
anything in the world more unlike than blennorrhagic arthritis
and exostosis, for example ?

What should I say of the cutaneous affections, except that I
am profoundly astonished that some physicians have wished
to discover a resemblance between the cutaneous affections produced by certain remedies employed in the treatment of blennorrhagia, and the special affections of the derma that syphilis
produces. The previous holding of a false doctrine has here
produced some very strange confusions. Blennorrhagia, it has
been said, produces cutaneous affections like the chancre ; and
the roseola which succeed the use of copaiba and of cubebs
have been cited as examples. I assure you that these roseola
do not appear but when these resins are given. They answer
me—but they do not appear except when there is a blennorrhagia existing. I answer, in my turn, that copaiba and cubebs
are not given, but when there is a blennorrhagia. I add, and
this is important, that I have administered copaiba in cases of
vesical catarrh, and I have often seen these exanthemata make
their appearance.

But these *resinous* exanthemata have characteristics so marked, that with the strongest disposition in the world, it is impossible to confound them with genuine syphilitic exanthemata. They are developed generally with great rapidity; they are very *acute*, of *rubeolic* form, or often connected with lichen urticarius ; if they are not very confluent, they are grouped preferably in the neighborhood of the articulations, and in the sense of extension, such as about the wrist, elbow, knee, instep, and around the ears ; they are commonly accompanied with much itching, which is the contrary of syphilides, and a most important condition ; so that we can say of them—*sublatâ causâ tollitur effectus.* In fact, they rarely survive a week the cause that produced them.

These exanthemata bring to mind a curious fact, which I ask you to permit me to relate in the form of an episode; it has also its instruction. Two or three years since, one of our most distinguished brother physicians presented himself at my house very much frightened. Until now, said he to me, I have had faith in your doctrine, but I find it at fault, and in my own case, that is truly hard. So saying he took off his clothes and said, " What is this?" showing me his chest and back. I examined and said, " That is a beautiful syphilitic roseola," " Syphilitic, do you say ; and are you very sure of it ?" "Perfectly sure !" "Ah, well, you convict yourself. I have never had in my life any other venereal accident than a blennorrhagia, and that was twelve years ago." " On your side are you very sure of that ?" "Just as sure as of my existence. I examined my friend from head to foot, and having done so, I said to him gravely, and with a certain air of solemnity, " Friend, you have *recently* had a chancre upon the right hand, and the chancre was situated neither upon the thumb, nor upon the index finger, but upon one of the three last fingers." " You are joking," said he. " I am joking so little," I added, "that you still carry a bubo,"—and I made him feel, in fact, an axillary gland still enlarged. Then my friend, recalling his thoughts, told me that some months before he had attended and dressed a woman who had chancres ; that an ulceration had come upon the middle finger, that he had not taken care of it, and that this ulceration had cicatrized. There is the source of your roseola, said I, and act accordingly.

Finally, what physician at the present day could confound the blennorrhagic epididymitis with the syphilitic sarcocele ? It is no longer possible, since the time of Bell, still less possible since the works of Astley Cooper, and since what I myself have done in regard to this subject.

You will permit me to pass in silence the pretended tuberculous diathesis invented in Germany as a consequence of the blennorrhagic virulence. The question of tubercles in general is already sufficiently obscure, without adding to it any new darkness.

You see, dear friend, that I approach at last the programme that I had traced out for myself. In my next letter I shall enter upon it resolutely.—[*Boston Med. and Sur. Journal.*

Elephantiasis Arabum of the right inferior extremity successfully treated by Ligature of the Femoral Artery. By J. M. Carnochan, M. D., Professor of the Principles and Operations of Surgery in the New-York Medical College, Surgeon to the State Emigrants' Hospital, Opthalmic Surgeon to the same Institution, &c., &c.

Case.—Charles Roller, of lymphatic temperament, and short stature, æt. 27, born in Aix-la-Chapelle—occupation, merchant, left his home in December, 1849, landed in New-York in February, 1851, went thence to Connecticut, where for eight months he worked in a factory, standing during his hours of labor ; thence went to Virginia, where he worked on a farm for about six months, at the expiration of which period he was taken with fever, of an intermittent character. Up to that time, he had always been in good health.

During the fever, the inguinal glands became swollen and painful ; the swelling and pain extending in the course of the femoral vessels as far as the knee. The pain was followed by swelling and redness of the thigh down to the knee. From the knee, the pain and swelling continued to extend downwards as far as the toes ; being, at this time confined chiefly to the portions of the limb along the course of the saphena vein, and also of the posterior tibial vessels. The redness and tumefaction here, as in the thigh, was preceded by deep-seated pain. The tumefaction of the limb continued to increase ; while, at the same time, febrile exacerbations occurred at intervals, varying from two to six days. After a period of about six weeks from the commencement of the disease, the fever entirely disappeared, and by this time, also, the pain and redness had entirely ceased ; the limb, however, remaining hard, swollen and rough, and presenting, in a marked degree, the peculiar characteristics of elephantiasis Arabum, in the chronic period of the disease. From this time forward, the hardness and intumescence gradually increased, and the limb became so cumbersome, that the patient was obliged to give up all business, and confine himself chiefly to a recumbent posture. In this condition, the patient left Virginia for the purpose of seeking medical relief at the New-York Emigrants' Hospital, into which he was admitted

the fifteenth of January, 1851.   The appearance of the patient
upon entering the Hospital was somewhat emaciated.   He had
no febrile symptoms, and the chief difficulty, under which he
labored, arose from the enlarged and hypertrophied condition
of the right inferior extremity.

The limb was enlarged from the toes to within a short distance below Poupart's ligament.   The thigh, although enlarged,
was not much indurated ; while, from a short distance above
the patella, downwards, the limb presented a dense, hypertrophied, hard, scaley, shapeless mass, the appearance of which
will be best apprehended by referring to accompanying plate.
the morbid condition of the tissues pervaded the foot and toes,
there presenting groups of tuberculated growths.   The circumference of the limb around the ankle, was nearly as large as
that of the calf; measuring fifteen and one-half inches, while
the circumference of the calf measured nineteen and one-half
inches.

The patient was put under treatment upon entering the
Hospital.   The recumbent posture was enjoined, and for some
time various discutient lotions were used.   Bandaging was
resorted to, with frictions of ung. Potass. Iod.; the Iodide of
Potassium being also prescribed internally.

At times, also, the limb was painted with strong tincture of
Iodine; local and general baths were used, regular bandaging
of the limb, from the toes upward, being the while carefully
observed.

This plan of treatment was perseveringly adhered to from
the fifteenth of January to the twenty-second of March, a period of a little over two months, without any amelioration.
Having thus tried, without success, the method of treatment
most approved of, I proposed to place a ligature upon the femoral artery, with a view of changing the morbid condition of
the structures supplied by the branches of this arterial trunk.
A consultation was held, and my proposition was acceded to as
preferable to amputation, the usual alternative resorted to in
this stage and extent of the disease.   Accordingly, on the
twenty-second of March, 1851, I secured the femoral artery, a
short distance below the origin of the arteria profunda.   Upon
exposing the femoral artery, this arterial tube was found to be
changed, so as to present an appearance somewhat like the
color of the aorta of the ox, and to be larger than the common
iliac of the human subject.   In consequence of this appearance
of the artery, after some hesitation, I applied the ligature, preferring to do this, ratner than to expose the external iliac, of the
soundness of which I could not be certain.

The ligature came away from the femoral artery on the

eleventh day, accompanied by secondary hemorrhage, the occurrence of which I had expected as probable. For the purpose of arresting the hemorrhage, the *external* iliac artery was
secured by ligature, by Dr. A. E. Hosack, who happened to be
on duty at the time in the Hospital. The external iliac was
found to be about the size of the brachial artery. This, for a
time, apparently had some influence upon the hemorrhage;
but on the following day, bleeding was again renewed from the
orifice, in the femoral artery, with as much profusion as ever.

The hemorrhage was now restrained by the prompt application of a tourniquet, on the *cardiac* side of the bleeding orifice,
by the house surgeons, Drs. Thompson and A. K. Smith.

This even failed to stop permanently the hemorrhage, and
the blood recommenced oozing copiously at intervals. The
patient was now sinking fast, and the ligature of the common
iliac, or amputation at the hip-joint, appeared to be the only resources left. But the hemorrhage now being evidently reflux,
it was suggested to apply the tourniquet, so as to produce compression on the *distal* side of the bleeding orifice: this was
done, and was followed by a complete cessation of the bleeding.

From this time, (April fourth, 1851), the house surgeon kept
an instructive record of the case, which record I have now
before me. For several days, the pulse ranged from 115 to 108:
the dressings were carefully attended to, and light diet prescribed. On the twelfth, the leg was found to be considerably
reduced in size, and the ligature of the external iliac, came
away. On the seventeenth, brandy and quinine, with good
nourishment, were ordered. On May the first, finding the leg
still more reduced and the lower wound healed, I ordered tincture of iodine to be painted on the leg, and the bandage to be
continued; I also ordered a solution of chloride of soda to be
used as a wash on the upper wound, which continued to discharge freely.

The patient now went on gradually improving in strength
and appearance, and left the Hospital in the latter part of
June, completely cured of his malady. At this date, sixteen
months after the ligature of the femoral artery, the patient is
in robust health, and presents no indications that the disease
will return.—[*New York Journal of Medicine.*

On the Therapeutic Properties of Arnica Montana. By M.
MARTIN LAUZER.

Contusions, Ecchymosis, Sanguineous Tumors, etc.—The
efficacy of arnica in these affections was first discovered in
Germany; and gained for it the name of *Fallkraut,* or *herba*

lapsorum. It was formerly applied as a topical remedy ; but at present it is more usual to trust to nature, and to employ rather camphorated spirits and saline lotions. It is not unreasonable, however, to give arnica internally after a fall, if the patient has, as often happens, undergone violent concussion amounting to stupor; but when reaction has set in, medicines of another class must be used.

Pulmonary Diseases.—Murray extols the power of arnica in a host of various diseases ; and, in the first place, we have pulmonary affections, of which the names have in the present day changed : such as pain in the side with dyspnœa, false pleurisy, humeral cough removing in the summer and autumn ; cachectic and œdematous cough ; asthma arising from sudden chill, with rheumatism of the chest and back; asthma following delivery, with alteration of the voice and pain in the nape of the neck; peripneumonia. The tonic and stimulant properties of the arnica would evidently be far from always serviceable in these diseases, some of which correspond to pneumonia and pleurisy, others to catarrhs, or to convulsive coughs. But, according to Dr. Roques, the nauseating properties of arnica have several times triumphed over obstinate catarrhs. In these cases, the arnica should be combined with pectoral medicines, and its use must be persevered in for some time. Arnica is no less useful, according to the same author, in cases of pneumonia of an ataxic character. In these cases, the arnica is given with extract of cinchona ; this combination excites the powers of the system, reanimates the action of the lungs, and favors expectoration.

M. Martin Lauzer remarks that M. Guitrac gives large doses of tartar emetic in chronic catarrh ; and Professor Broussonet and Cruveilhier give large doses of ipecacuanha in the same affection and in the pneumonia of old persons ; and suggests that arnica might produce similar effects, in such cases, to those of ipecacuanha.

Arnica has been recommended by various authors in inflammation of the liver with petechiæ, suppression of the menses or lochia, uterine hæmorrhage, congestion of the spleen, nodosities of the breast, general atony, hectic fever, atrophy, calculous nephritis, and contractions of organs.

Paralytic Affections.—The writers of the last century have chiefly pointed out the effects of arnica in cases of paralysis. Juncker states, that he cured more paralyzed and contracted limbs with arnica alone, than with combinations of remedies. Collin states, that he cured tremblings, convulsions, palsies, and other nervous affections. Under the influence of this remedy, the patients had pain in the eyes, creeping and tickling sensations in the limbs, and a sense of heat; and these phenomena almost always were prognastic of benefit. These effects are precisely those produced by strychnine; hence arnica would be a succedaneum for this formidable agent; and why should it not be employed before having recourse to the preparations of nux vomica? Collin says that, in cerebral affections, arnica is contra-indicated until the fever has ceased, or has diminished; and then nitre must be added to it. Kornbeck extols the action of arnica in mercurial paralysis: it would evidently be only useful in asthenic palsies, in whatever situation. Dr. Roger relates the case of a woman who, after fever, had a sense of weight and loss of power in the lower limbs. Under the use of powder of arnica flowers, she experienced creeping sensations and pain, followed by complete restoration of motion and sensation. According to Collin, Murray, and Conradi, arnica has also cured cases of asthenic amaurosis; but M. Martin Lauzer believes, with Schumucker, that it always fails in cases of amaurosis which have slowly gained their highest degree of intensity.

Spasms and convulsions: convulsive cough.—Arnica, according to Murray, has cured tremblings of the limbs or tongue, opisthotones, convulsive movements of the head, and twitchings of the limbs. If these affections are nervous, of asthenic origin, and consequently calling for the employment of tonics and stimulants, arnica may be of use.

Intermittent Fever.—Collin, Stoll, Aaskow, Deiman, and Voltelen, praise arnica as a remedy in ague. Stoll was very successful in the treatment of a quartan, which resisted cinchona. He made an electuary with flowers of arnica and syrup of orange peel; and gave a piece as large as a nutmeg four times a day. This dose caused severe pain in the stomach, and cold clammy sweats, with a large, full, and very slow pulse; but opium calmed these symptoms, which, however, were the forerunners of a rapid cure of the fever.

Typhoid Fever.—It was in the treatment of this disease that arnica enjoyed its best days; but here its fame also suffered dire shipwreck, thanks to its abuse by the Brownians, who almost used it as a specific in continued fevers. Collin said that arnica, by its cardiac power, removes stupor, somnolence and delirium, in putrid fevers, brings back the eruption of suppressed exanthemata, and resolves metastatic swellings. But Murray judiciously adds that, in order that the desired result may be produced, we must take account of the season and of general conditions;—words full of justice, a reflection on which would have prevented the abuse of using a single remedy in a disease so variable in its form. Stoll, who introduced the use of arnica in putrid fevers, gave it only in those cases in which, the pulse remaining nearly quiet, the patient was feeble, stupe- fied, prostrate, in a state of somnolence, or muttering delirium. Arnica is also particularly indicated where the pulse is small, weak, and fluttering, with torpor and prostration of the muscu- lar system. Dr. Roques says that it should be used especially in the enervating diarrhœa, in the obstinate dysenteric flux which, in the third stage of typhus, threatens to entirely destroy the vital powers. Murray recommends it, combined with cam- phor, when gangrene has supervened on other adynamic symp- toms.

In the campaigns of the empire, the good effects of arnica in the army-typhus have been observed and recorded. Dr. Ca- zin, who used it successfully in the army hospitals during the campaign in Germany in 1809, has since that time frequently employed it in the adynamic stage of typhoid fevers, combining it with the roots of valerian and angelica, which dilute its emetic and cardialgic properties.

Gout.—Barthez has recommended arnica in the treatment of gout. Dr. Roques was of opinion that the best treatment of gout is to torment the patient as little as possible with medi- cine.

Summary.—Arnica is an energetic excitant, which is far from meriting the oblivion into which it has fallen. Its tonic, excitant, and emetic action, allies it to ipecacuanha; and the nervous symptoms which it secondarily excites, give it some relation to the preparations of nux vomica. Gilibert considered it tonic and aperient in small doses: and in large doses emetic, purgative, diuretic, sudorific, and emmenagogue. When given alone, it is liable to produce more or less severe pain in the stomach. This may be prevented or assuaged by combining the arnica with a small dose of opium or some aromatic, such as angelica, canella, or ginger. But if its nauseating effects be desired, it must be given alone.

Doses and mode of administration.—The *infusion*, accord- ing to the formulary of the hospitals of Paris, is made by in- fusing for an hour, a drachm of the flowers in a quart of water, and straining. The *decoction* is made with the same propor- tions: it is more powerful. The dose of the infusion may be as much as an ounce, sweetened with syrup.

The *powdered flowers* may be given in doses of from ten grains to three or four drachms, in electuary or bolus; this form is preferable in cases of paralysis. The *powdered root* may be given in the same manner.

The dose of the distilled water is from an ounce and a half to three ounces of the alcoholic tincture (one part of the root to

eight of alcohol) from fifteen minims to five drachms; of the
ethereal tincture (one part of flowers to four of ether) from fifteen minims to two and a half drachms; of the aqueous extract
·(one part to five of water) from seven grains to a drachm, in a
draught or in pills; of the alcoholic extract (one part of flowers
to eight of alcohol and one of water), the same quantities.

For External Use, the leaves and flowers may be used as a
poultice: and the powder may be employed as a sternutatory.

Compound infusion of arnica flowers. (Roques.)—Take of
arnica flowers, valerian root, each two drachms; infuse them
in a closed vessel with half a pint of boiling water; then strain,
and add, of peppermint water two ounces, simple syrup one
ounce, ether a drachm, tincture of opium from fifteen to twenty
drops; to be given by spoonfuls in the adynamic period of
typhoid fever.

Compound preparations of arnica.—The above-named preparations are advantageously combined with wine, cinchona,
camphor, and valerian.

Compound powder of arnica root. (Roques.) Take of arnica root in powder fifteen grains; camphor three grains; to
be given every three hours in dysenteric typhus, to combat the
prostration of the vital powers.

Stimulant bolus.—Take of camphor, arnica flowers, and trea-
cle, each fifteen grains; divide into twelve boli, and give one
every hour.

Stimulant electuary.—Take of powdered arnica root an ounce
and a half, crude opium three-quarters of a grain, syrup a sufficient quantity. Divide it into six doses; one to be given every
two hours in case of purulent absorption.

Aromatic tincture of arnica.—Take of arnica flowers an
ounce and a half; cloves, canella and ginger, each two and a
half drachms; anise, three ounces; alcohol, a quarter; macerate
for eight days. and strain. A spoonful in water two or three
times a day in contusions.—[*London Jour. of Med. Ibid.*

---

*On the Effects of Anæsthetic Agents in Operations for Gunshot
Wounds.* By J. B. PORTER, M. D., Surgeon U. S. Army.

In our former paper, the case of Williamson was presented
with some remarks in relation to the use of sulphuric ether for
producing anæsthesia in operations in the General Hospital at
Vera Cruz, in 1847. In the summer of that year, an amputation
of the thigh was performed, the patient having been put under
the influence of ether, in which the hemorrhage was almost uncontrollable. The blood spouted in all directions, and I have

never seen an operation where it was necessary to secure so·
many bleeding vessels. Even after every small vessel that
could be got at was secured, it was necessary to use cold water
freely to suppress the general oozing of blood. At the time, I
imputed the obstinate hemorrhage to the pernicious influence
of the ether. In gunshot wounds anæsthetic agents are almost
universally unnecessary, and are almost universally injurious.
It was for this reason that they were entirely given up in the
hospital at Vera Cruz.

It may be well questioned whether anæsthetics are not calculated to produce injurious effects in all important amputations; but they certainly do so in operations performed for
gunshot wounds. M. Velpeau says: "Chloroform evidently
depresses the nervous system, and as great prostration always
exists in patients who have received gunshot wounds, it is advisable to refrain from any anæsthetic means."—*Ranking's
Abstract*, 1848. Mr. Alcock refers to the cases of soldiers
wounded in battle, where the excitement is such as to carry
them through almost any operation. I regret that Mr. Alcock's
paper is not before me. These are the cases spoken of by Mr.
Guthrie: "Soldiers in general are anxious to undergo an operation when they find it inevitable, and frequently press it before
the proper time; that is, before they have sufficiently recovered
the shock of the injury."—*Gunshot Wounds*, p. 232. These are
the cases which require a little more time, some "encouraging
words," and perhaps a little wine or brandy and water; but
no anæsthetics, for the patients are already sufficiently depressed.

There are two sets of cases; in one (Velpeau's), the shock
to the nervous system is great, from which the patient may
not recover, and the use of anæsthetics would be awfully destructive; in the other class, they are unnecessary, and would
prove useless and injurious. In the flap operation they must
prove more injurious than in the circular; from the fact that
muscle forms almost the entire covering for the stump; and the
contractility of the muscular tissue is for a time almost annihilated, to be recovered irregularly at irregular intervals. Further, after the use of these agents wounds do not heal so readily
by the first intention.

M. Jobert, on the use of ether, states that the local inflammation has proved less, and that union by the first intention has
been prevented. I am able to bear testimony to the correctness of M. Jobert's statement.

I must be permitted to refer to the *Transactions of the American Medical Association* for 1851, pp. 271, 272, 315, 323. In
the Massachusetts General Hospital:—

"It does not appear that the fatal results of amputation have at all diminished by the introduction of anæsthetic agents."

New-York Hospital :—

" The general mortality has been for three years and a quar‑ ter forty *per centum.* As regards the method of operating, we observe that the amputations of the thigh, in which the fatality was as high as thirteen in seventeen, were all flap operations. Eleven of the leg were removed by the circular, one died ; while of four by the flap, two died."

That is, nine *per cent.* in one set of cases, and fifty *per cent.* in the other.

"In almost every case chloroform or ether was employed ; but while it is admitted that anæsthetics may have had some influ‑ ence in the increased mortality in the New-York Hospital over preceding years, since union by the first intention was now much less frequently observed ; still it is to be remembered that hos‑ pital gangrene, entirely unknown before and purulent cache‑ xia and erysipelas, extensively prevailed there during the past three years."

Could the anæsthetics have had an influence in producing the " hospital gangrene, entirely unknown before," and the " puru‑ lent cachexia and erysipelas," as well as prevent union by the first intention ?

Dr. Lent, Resident Surgeon of the New-York Hospital, says :

" In almost every case, however, either *chloroform or ether* was employed ; generally the former until the occurrence of a fatal case from it in this hospital ; afterwards the latter, from which we have never had any bad consequences, and which has never failed to prove effectual. * * * Anæsthetics came into general use about the period of the commencement of these sta‑ tistics. May not the employment of these have had its influ‑ ence upon the mortality ? This is a very important question. We do not deny that it may have had some influence in aug‑ menting the facility of operations ; but we have seen no reason to infer that it has, except perhaps the fact that *union by adhesion* seems to have been much less frequent since the introduction of anæsthetics into this hospital than before. Whether the two are in the relation of cause and effect, it is, we fear, impossible to determine at present."

In an unhealthy atmosphere or climate, the healing of wounds by adhesive union is doubly important for obvious reasons ; and I have often regretted that etherization was so much resorted to in capital operations at Vera Cruz during a portion of 1847 ; nor can I avoid congratulating both the patients and myself that before the summer had passed away, its employment was wholly abondoned. Anæsthetics poison the blood and depress the ner‑

vous system; and in consequence, hemorrhage is much more apt to occur, and union by adhesion is prevented.—[*American Jour. of Med. Science.*

Wound of the Liver—Excision of a large portion of the right Lobe. By J. C. MASSEY, M. D., of Houston, Texas.

Some three weeks since I was summoned, in great haste, to visit a son of Mr. Simmons, at a distance of some thirty miles from this city. A brother of the unfortunate youth wounded, had a gun lying across his lap, picking the flint; it went off, the contents of the whole load passed into the right hypochondrium, and mostly out about the region of the epigastrium. The youth, who is about seven years of age, was standing close to the gun, and it was charged with large shot; a portion of the liver protruded through the external wound. A physician in the neighborhood was sent for, who reached the case about four hours after the accident. After examination, he viewed the case as hopeless, and consequently declined doing any thing; he visited the case, however, on the next day, and advised that I should be sent for. On the fourth day after the accident I visited the patient, accompanied by my friend Dr. Black. We found him in a very deplorable situation; the anterior margin of the right lobe of the liver was protruding through the cavity on the right and a few lines above the umbilicus; it was in a gangrenous condition, with a portion of the omentum attached; the substance of both was so much altered, that it was really difficult to tell what the protruding portion was; the abdomen was very tense and hard, the least pressure giving severe pain; there was great arterial excitement, accompanied by a high inflammatory fever. This is a brief and very succinct account of the condition of the little patient, and my friend Dr. Black, as well as myself, regarded the case in a hopeless condition. I informed his friends, after making known to them the danger of the operation, that I would operate, remove the gangrenous portion of the liver, and give him all the possible chance there could be left for his life. From the external character and appearance of the wound, I was fearful gangrene had extended within the abdominal parieties.

I commenced the operation by enlarging the orifice about four inches; on examining the substance of the liver, I found two shot had passed at least two and a quarter inches from its inferior border, penetrating through it; the substance of the liver which was in juxtaposition to the wounds had a thick, grumous appearance, with sphacelated portions. Under the circumstances, I determined to excise every portion of the liver which had the appearance here described.

Blanchard, in his *Anatomica Practica Rationalis, says,* " A small portion of the substance of the liver may be removed without necessarily inducing a fatal result ; and Dr. Henen, (Mil. Surg., p. 439) says, " A deep wound of the liver is as fatal as if the heart itself was engaged."

I felt great apprehension in excising the amount I was necessarily compelled to do, and when I inform you that I excised quite one half of the right lobe, equal to twice the amount of the left, you will then see how easy it is for persons high in the profession to make statements without proper data.

When the operation was finished, I passed a strong suture through the abdominal parietes, closed the wound, and subsequently a vigorous antiphlogistic treatment was adopted. I will not encumber your pages with a long detail of the daily treatment of this case. Nothing very remarkable, except for about ten days his discharges were passive, and he could exert no control whatever ; at the present time he is able to exercise in his room, secretions natural, wound nearly healed up, and I consider him entirely out of danger.

This is an instance among many which may occur, and which may serve to prove to the profession, that a case, however desperate it may appear, should never be given up without an effort ; and I do deem it very reprehensible, when professional men retreat, if I may use the term, in desperate cases. An operation once undertaken, should always be concluded *secundem artem*—according to the circumstances of the case, however desperate may be the supervening results, or the obstacles that may seem to render the operation unavoidable. Sometimes he will find in spite of all opinions, the patient recovers. I had a patient to lie apparently lifeless, in Grimes County, which is well recollected, under my own Scalpel, and under this embarrassing situation I finished the operation, and my doing so is the means of his present enjoyment of health, and his friendship to me. I was kindly assisted by my friend Dr. Black.

[*New Orleans Med. and Sur. Journal.*

On the Jaundice of Infants. By M. Duclos.

Although this frequent affection of early infancy does not, in the great majority of instances, present any danger, it occasionally gives rise to important occurrences, and indeed, when complicated with other affections, may sometimes prove fatal.

Besides the yellow colour, the icterus of infants may be attended with fever, somnolence, tension of the belly, and colic, with constipation or diarrhœa. Its causes may be ranged under five different heads, which it is of importance to distinguish.

1. *Retention of the meconium* is the most frequent of all. If it be not evacuated within twenty-six hours, colicky pains are set up, and the skin becomes yellow. The *colostrum* is in this case the best purgative. When the child cannot or will not suck, a tea-spoonful or two of the syrup of rhubarb, chicory, and peach-flowers, equal parts, may be given. When, after the meconium has been passed, a considerable degree of tympanitis remains, together with what is called "windy colic," preventing sleep, M. Duclos administers small doses of rhubarb and calcined magnesia. 2. The next in frequency is *spasm of the digestive organs.* The child suffers from cardialgia and colic, is in a state of fever, is constantly trying to suck, and has few or greenish stools. Sometimes convulsions occur. Purging and vomiting aggravate in place of relieving the condition. As retained meconium is usually the origin and cause of the symptoms, that must first be obviated, and then recourse had to emolient baths, mild anti-spasmodics, linseed poultices, friction with camphorated oil, and mild *lavements.* If the milk is too old, the nurse should be changed ; and when an anodyne is required to relieve the violent colic; a little lettuce-water should be added to some sugared water. This description of medicine, however, requires care, and opiates in any form are inadmissible. Narcotism, which induced death in one child and was nearly fatal in another, was brought on by a clyster containing ten drops of laudanum. 3. *Engorgement of the liver* is another cause, and one especially acting after compression of that organ by the uterine contraction in foot and breech presentations. When this condition is present, purging the child is not sufficient. It must be kept warm, and its skin rubbed with hot flannel; with gentleness, however, lest erysipelas be induced. When the skin is rough and hot, emolient tepid baths are useful adjuvants. 4. *Bad nourishment* is a frequent cause of icterus, the milk disagreeing with the child, or improper food being given to it when brought up by hand. 5. *Cold and humidity:* young infants are very susceptible to changes of temperature—too great heat or cold being alike injurious to them ; but as regards the present affection, cold is especially mischievous.—[*Rev. Med. Chir. Med. Chir. Rev.*

Burns and Scalds.

There is no practical subject in our profession, in which the disastrous and fatal effects of mal-treatment by medical men, as well as the mischiefs of popular ignorance are more apparent, than in the remedies resorted to in the cases of scalds and burns, now unhappily so frequent in our country, by reason of the murderous recklessness of human life in the men entrusted with our public conveyances, in which steam is employed.

So long ago as 1830, in the first American edition of Cooper's Surgical Dictionary, published by the Harpers, of this city, we took occasion to urge upon the profession and upon the public the importance of a better philosophy and practice in the medical management of the mischiefs resulting from such accidents, than that usually in vogue. We then stated the results of our experience for ten years in the treatment of scalds and burns by the instant application of wheat flour, an article always at hand, and the perseverance in this application alone until all the acute inflammation had subsided. Our theory and practice thus promulgated, was approved and recommended in the then forthcoming edition in London, by Mr. Samuel Cooper himself, and has since found its way without credit into numerous publications at home and abroad. Even in the late Therapeutical work of Dr. T. D. Mitchell, of Philadelphia, this identical practice is ascribed to Dr. John Thomas of *England!* who in 1832 called the attention of the profession thereto, as we are told, in the Ohio Medical Lyceum; two years after our publication as aforesaid, and twelve years after our testimony to its efficacy had been published.

But waiving the unimportant subject of priority, we are grieved to learn from the public press that such multitudes are annually perishing by scalds in steam-boats, and from burns by camphene, spirit gas, and otherwise; nearly all of whom, however severely burned, we do not hesitate to say might be preserved from a fatal result if this simple practice were adopted immediately after such accidents. Instead of this, however, we hear of the application of *cold water, lead water, molasses, oils, cotton, "pain extractors,"* &c. &c. accompanied almost uniformly by the death of the sufferer, and often " after lingering in excruciating torture" for days or hours.

Now it ought to be promulgated to the profession, and for humanity sake to be known to the whole people, that in any case of burn or scald however extensive, all the acute suffering of the patient may be at once and permanently relieved, and that in a moment of time, by sprinkling over the injured surface a thick layer of wheat flour by the hand, or what is better, by a dredging box. Every vestige of pain produced by such injuries is instantly removed, and the sufferer not only escapes the shock to the nervous system accompanying such torture, but will generally fall into a quiet sleep the moment the atmospheric temperature is thus excluded from the wounds.

Why then should persons thus injured be allowed to die with intense agony, occasioned by burns and scalds, as they often do, if not without treatment by the applications so often made, many of which augment their sufferings, and render such injuries irreparable ?   Even in the late explosion on board the Reindeer, it is said that many of the scalded lived for hours, suffering all the time from their external injuries, and then treated with raw cotton, lime water, and linseed oil, &c. &c· until they were dead.   Not a pang need have been endured beyond the time necessary to apply the flour, which must have been at hand, if the ignorance of their friends, and the antiquated prejudices of their medical advisers, had not led them to rely upon the miserable substitutes which superstition has canonized for centuries.   And so, we affirm of every case of burn and scald, even if the entire surface has suffered.

In the New York and Bellevue Hospitals this mode of treating burns has been long in use; until recently, as we learn, the same object has been effected at the former institution by the analagous method of covering the injured parts with a mucilage of Gum Arabic, so as to protect the denuded surface from the atmosphere, and which the surgeons there prefer to the flour in some cases, where the weight of the latter becomes an inconvenience.   To this method we make no objection, but having for so many years employed the flour alone, to the exclusion of all other agents, and in every variety and extent of injuries by fire, we have thus reiterated our testimony, and as this agent is found in every house, and can be instantly procured with more readiness than any of the other articles named, we give it the preference over all others.   And we repeat our full persuasion that not one in a hundred of those perishing by burns and scalds, need succumb under their injuries if they were at once, or as soon as may be, covered with wheat flour.   We have applied it successfully, after numerous other remedies had been unsuccessful, and when many hours had elapsed after the accident. To give this suggestion to the people, and scatter it broadcast over the land, will save a multitude of lives in a single year.

[*New York Medical Gazette.*

Poisonous Chloroform.

To the Editor of the Boston Medical and Surgical Journal.

Sir,—The numerous deaths which have recently taken place from the inhalation of chloroform, seem to require that I should state what I know upon this subject, without waiting for more extended researches which I have now in progress ; for a word in time may save human life, and I shall therefore present my views, even though some may think that I ought to wait until my work is completed to its full extent before publication.   I have

formerly been charged with dilatoriness in presenting my discoveries to the public, and wish to avoid a repetition of this
accusation, even though my work, in its present state, is not so
complete as would be required for scientific purposes.

I have long had a strong suspicion that the very sudden deaths
resulting from the inhalation of chloroform, must have been produced by the presence of some poisonous compound of amyle,
the hypothetical radical of Fusel oil or the oil of whiskey ;
and I began a series of researches upon this subject several
years ago, but was called off from my work by unexpected per-
secutions. This work I have resumed, and I will now state
what facts and inductions I am able to lay before the public.

1st.   When chloroform, and the alcoholic solution of it called
chloric ether, was made from *pure* alcohol diluted with water,
no fatal accidents took place from its judicious administration.

2d.   When chloroform was made, as it now too frequently
is, from common corn, rye, and potato whiskey, deaths began to
occur, even when the utmost care was taken in its administration.

3d.   In the Chelsea case, where this kind of chloroform was
probably contained in the alcoholic solution incorrectly called
chloric ether, death took place in a very sudden manner, and
the post-mortem appearances of the subject indicated the usual
effects of poisoning by chloroform.

From these data, it might justly be inferred that some poisonous matter exists in the cheap chloroform of commerce, and I
suspected that it arose from the Fusel oil which exists in whiskey.
This opinion, at my suggestion, was published by two of my
friends, to put the public on their guard, and those gentlemen
urgently advised that physicians and surgeons should return to
the use of pure sulphuric ether (oxide of ethyle,) as originally
prescribed by me.

It is well known that I have always preferred my original
anæsthetic agent to all the substitutes that have been proposed
since ; but still I have always been willing to give the proposed
substitutes a fair trial, and did try them all, first upon myself, and
then upon such of my pupils as felt willing to allow the experiment to be made upon them.   I also in a measure compromised
with that powerful anæsthetic agent chloroform, by mixing small
proportions of it, about one fourth or fifth part, with sulphuric
ether, so as to concentrate the anæsthetic agent into a smaller
bulk, and I have extensively used this preparation in the production of anæsthesia, and without producing any dangerous
or even unpleasant symptoms in any case, but I always took
care to ascertain that the chloroform used by me was pure.

Having, during the last month, succeeded in procuring some

very pure Fusel oil (of whiskey), I undertook the researches
which have resulted in the conviction that it is this amyle compound that produces the poisonous matter of certain kinds of
chloroform.   When mixed with hyperchlorite of lime (bleaching powder) and water, in the same way as we prepare alcohol
for the production and distillation of chloroform, I found that
the mixture in the retort, after agitation and standing some time,
became warm, indicating that a re-action was taking place between the Fusel oil and the hyperchlorite of lime.

After some hours the retort was placed in a water-bath and
distillation was effected, the volatilized liquid being condensed
by means of one of Liebig's condensers.   A clear colorless
liquid came over, which was at once recognized as having the
peculiar *odor of bad chloroform.*   It is perhaps a *ter chloride of
amyle,* but has not yet been submitted to analysis.   It is so powerful that merely smelling of it makes one dizzy, and working
over it made me so sick that I was obliged to go out of doors for
fresh air several times during my operations on it.   In order to
make sure that the Fusel oil was all decomposed, I again mixed
the product of the distillation above mentioned with a new lot
of bleaching powder, and water ; and after three hours, with
frequent agitation, it was again distilled, and gave what I regard
as the pure unmixed poison.   This I am now to test on such
animals as have proved good ether subjects, and shall make
report of my results in this Journal.

If my views are correct, it follows :—

1st.   That all chloroform intended for *inhalation as an anæsthetic agent should be prepared from pure rectified alcohol,* to
be diluted with water when used for distillation from hyperchlorite of lime.

2d.   That no druggist should sell for anæsthetic uses any
chloroform which is not known to have been properly prepared
as above suggested.

3d.   That the mixture of chloroform and alcohol, commercial-
ly known under the name of strong chloric ether, must be made
with the same precautions as chloroform.

There is less danger of the existence of Fusel oil in sulphuric
ether, which is always made from strong rectified alcohol.

There is more danger of the existence of sulphurous acid in
this liquid, and that is a dangerous poison, but it is one readily
detected ; and persons will object to inhaling ether containing it,
on account of its wellknown disagreeable odor of burning sulphur.

Fusel oil itself, according to the microscopic researches of
my friend Dr. Henry C. Perkins, of Newburyport, appears to
act as a poison.   His experiments were suggested by an article

published by Mr. Henry A. Hildreth, imputing the poisonous qualities of some kinds of chloroform to Fusel oil contained in it.

It is important now that this Fusel oil has been introduced into medicine as a remedy in phthisis, that the profession should know that when it is inhaled it may produce fatal results, and that great caution is necessary in the use of so powerful an agent. Administered, a few drops at a dose, by the stomach, it does no harm, but is undoubtedly useful in some forms of disease. Experience will soon show how far it is remedial in tuberculous diseases; and this remedy is in good hands at present—Dr. Morrill Wyman and Dr. Perkins having engaged in the researches as to its medicinal use.

I annex a letter which I have just received from Dr. Perkins, deeming it an interesting contribution to physiological science.

Respectfully your ob't serv't,   C. T. JACKSON, M. D.
Assayer to the State of Mass.
Boston, Sept. 1, 1852.   *and to the City of Boston.*

NEWBURYPORT, Aug. 27, 1852.
My Dear Friend,—Noticing the other day, a paragraph in one of the papers, which attributed the evil effects of chloroform to the Fusel oil it contained, I tried an experiment upon a frog with a few drops of this oil dissolved in ether, and found that after inhaling it for a short time the same effects were observable under the microscope as appear when chloroform is used, viz., an *almost entire* suspension of the circulation in *all* the bloodvessels ramifying upon the web of his foot; there was in fact, only a *very slight backward* and *forward* motion to be seen in *one* single vessel; in *all* the others the blood was *perfectly stagnant.* The frog was insensible for a much longer period than when the ether alone is used. He is now bright and ready for another experiment—to which I proceed.

I exposed him to the vapor of a few drops of Fusel oil dissolved in about a drachm of New England rum, for about six minutes, when he closed his eyelids and seemed under its influence. He was then placed upon the stand of the microscope, but not the slightest appearance of circulation was to be found in any of the vessels of the web; it was unusually pale and exsanguinous. He removed his foot twice or thrice from the stand, and gasped several times. I was now called away, and was absent about half an hour. Upon my return, the frog was found *dead.*

Several queries suggest themselves, which you will allow me to propose :—

1st.   Is there any Fusel oil in sulphuric ether?

2d.   Can the Fusel oil be removed from the chloroform?

3d.   Would the vapor of New England rum, rot-gut whiskey (which contains this oil,) produce anæsthetic effects?

4th.   In what cther liquors is this oil found?

5th   Does it in small doses. as administered by our friend, Dr. M. Wyman, and as I am now trying it upon his recommendation, diminish the pulse and act as a direct sedative?

To the third and fifth queries I shall direct my attention. The others I leave for your investigation.

Very truly your sincere friend,   H. C. Perkins.

Statistics of Hernia. By M. Hutin.

At a recent examination of the pensioners at the Hotel des Invalides, M. Hutin found that among the entire population of 3177 pensioners, there were 670 who had hernia. These were distributed as follow:

631 Inguinal (213 double, 418 single.)

  6 Femoral (5 left, 1 right.)

 18 Umbilical.

 11 Superumbilical.

  2 Subumbilical.

  2 Near spine of ilium.

670.—[*Rev. Med. Chir. Med. Chir. Rev.*

Miscellany.

Should the Use of White Lead as a Paint be forbidden by Public Authority?—This question is exciting considerable interest in France, one of the few countries in Europe where a due regard to the public health is part of the business of government. In England, and this country, we are too jealous of individual rights, too independent, if you please, to allow our rulers to watch over the well-being of the community.

We shall therefore merely present facts, without comment, as given to us in a memoir of Dr. H. De Castelnau :—

"In his remarkable memoir on *Painting with White Zinc*, Dr. Bouchut advised the government, if it had due regard for the health of workmen, to forbid the use of white lead as a paint on all the public buildings, and that an example should be presented for imitation by the substitution of an article less deleterious. The favorable manner in which this proposition was received by the Academy of Medicine, at its session on the 4th of November, 1837, indicates their full accord.

ance in the idea, although they were necessarily restrained from entering into the merits of the question of economics, and we derive a
similar indication of opinion in the large premium bestowed by the
Institute, in 1849, on M. Le Claire, for his essay on the means of
rendering occupations less unhealthy.

All these circumstances have doubtless tended to aid in diffusing a
report that government is about suppressing the manufacture of white
lead.   To aid such a measure, a few details on the point of sickness
and mortality will be of use.

In accordance with a requisition from the prefect of police, the administration of hospitals demanded an annual return of all cases
admitted into them of diseases from lead.   It thus appears, that during
ten years (1838 to 1847,) 3142 were admitted, and that 112 of these
died, being an annual mean of 314 sick and 11 dying.   There can,
however, be scarcely a doubt but that the first number is too low.
There is very frequently a doubt as to the nature of the complaint on
admission—indeed lead affections take some time to develop themselves
and thus cases are frequently referred to other diseases.   It is highly
probable that at least 400 cases are annually admitted, and that fifteen
deaths occur.

Of the gross number (3142,) three-fifths (1898) were cases of workmen engaged in the manufacture of white or red lead, and the remaining two fifths were persons employed in using these products, as paint-
ers, grinders, makers of porcelain cards (so called,) &c.

Then again, there are many cases treated at their own dwellings,
but unfortunately we have no data exactly to estimate their number.
It is quite probable that they are at least equal to those treated in hospitals, and if this be conceded, we have annually 400 cases of lead
disease in those who are strictly manufacturers of the preparations of
lead, and of which 14 die.   It would be too extravagant to carry this
proportion throughout France.   Reducing it ninetenths, and with a
due regard to the statistics of provincial hospitals, we are certainly
safe in stating the total annual result at 2000 cases of disease and 80
deaths.   These would be at an end with the suppression of the manufacture.

But there is another matter to be also considered.   The average
sojourn of a patient with saturnine disease in a hospital is 16 days. .
Add to this, the illness and loss of time that precedes, and the debility,
broken health, and loss of business that follows so many of the workmen.   Even if we do not estimate this last, still, the hospitals will be
relieved annually of sixteen or seventeen thousand days of sick persons,
not to take into account the permanent residence of many incurables.

Can there, then, be a doubt that the public health will be greatly
improved by the suppression of these manufactories?   Still, however
powerful may be the arguments in favour, it would hardly answer to
attempt their suppression, unless we could find a proper substitute,
both in the healthiness of its manufacture, and its value in the arts-
Can both of these objects be accomplished by the employment of the
white oxide of zinc (*le blanc de zinc ?*)

As to the first, Dr. Bouchut, just at the time of concluding his memoir, in July, 1851, received the following return from the company
manufacturing zinc at Asnieres.   Up to the date named, they had
employed 151 workmen, who together had performed labour during
31,585 days and had been in the factory 36,156 days.   In other words
the average was 209 labour days, and 344 days of residence for each
person.

It is scarcely possible to present a more fevourable bill of health.
Who ever heard of a manufacturer of white lead remaining in its manufacture during 344 successive days?   Besides, most of the above
workmen still remain, and are able to count upwards of 1000 labour
days.

Dr. Bouchut has carefully studied what should be called the *effects*
rather than the *diseases* caused by this species of manufacture.   They
are as follows :—

1.   Pains in the throat and slight cough occur during the first
days of labour, until the mucous membrane becomes accustomed to
the exhalations from the white zinc.   But they disappear very soon,
and the workmen there are no more subject to cough or throat affections than the same given number of any other persons.

2.   Many of the workmen are at various periods subject to a curious
species of innervation shown by febrile or non-febrile restlessness at
night.   But this does not affect the general health, and they return in
the morning to their labour.   Occasionally, there is a species of excitement, temporary, such as Delaroche and Barbier ascribe to the
oxide of zinc, but with most it is the short feverish feeling just described.   It is always of short duration, never dangerous, and disappears
after the system has been accustomed to the employment.

3.   Occasionally eruptions appear on the skin, of reddish papulæ,
which readily disappear with proper treatment.

Having thus noticed the effects, Dr Bouchut proceeds to mention
three cases of slight disease, ascribed to this cause.   But a careful
analysis proves that they were not owing to it.

Here, then, we have results which are frequently produced by
emanations from the *most harmless substances,* when inhaled in the
form of powder.   The difficulty only extends thus far.   But while
white lead as powder causes its severe results also, we must recollect
that it is equally noxious when manipulated in the humid form.   From
this, however, white zinc is totally free.   It is only the powder of it
that affects the workmen.

We should also remember the large doses that have for many years
been administered of the white oxide as a medicine, without causing
any accident.   M. Orfila, the highest authority in toxicology, gave 20
grammes (   ) to small and feeble dogs, with only the result
of gentle vomiting, and a subsequent perfect recovery.   How very
different are the consequences of administering white lead.

As to the economic value of white zinc.   It can be manufactured
for exactly the same price as white lead, and being much lighter, a
larger quantity can be sold for the same sum of money.   It cannot be

adulterated. This, indeed, has been made a formidable objection to it. White lead is very commonly mixed with sulphate of barytes, and not unfrequently with chalk. White zinc can be used with equal facility as a paint. It does not dry as readily as white lead, but the difference in time is small. It has been objected that it does not set well as a paint, but this is altogether a mistake. Two coats cover wood *very nearly* as well as white lead, and there is this further advantage, the vapours of sulphuretted hydrogen do not affect it, whilst all the preparations of lead turn black from them.

M. Leclaire, an eminent house-painter, and others, have verified its use, on more than two thousand buildings, some of them public ones, to the satisfaction of the community.

The results, then, of suppressing the use of white lead by public authority will be—to save annually the lives of eighty workmen—to prevent 2000 cases of disease, some of them, indeed, incurable—and to enable active industry to continue its labours uninterrupted.

[*Abridged from La Lancette Francaise (Gazette des Hôpitaux)*
American Jour. Med. Sciences.

The influence which Daguerreotyping exerts upon the Health of Daguerrean Artists, together with some Observations on Light and Actinism. By CHARLES W. WRIGHT, M. D., of Cincinnati.

It is stated by Chevalier, in the Annals of Public Hygiene, that the vapors of iodine exert no injurious effect upon the health of the workmen engaged in its preparation; but this observation does not appear to hold good in other pursuits, where persons are compelled to inhale the vapors of this substance. Thus, there are some phenomena presenting themselves in the art of daguerreotyping, that would seem to indicate that the vapors of iodine, when inhaled for a considerable length of time, produce all of the peculiar effects of that agent when administered by the mouth. It must, however, be borne in mind, that besides iodine, the chloride of iodine, bromine and hydroflouric acid are employed in the photographic art, and that the vapors of these bodies are floating in the atmosphere along with that of iodine; and as these substances belong to the same class, and when administered produce similar effects on the system, may contribute also to the appearances observed.

The influence which these vapors exert on the respiratory aparatus.— The most striking effect is the continual clearing of the throat. This the operator is frequently not aware of himself, until his attention is called to it. This symptom appears not to result from irritation or inflammation of the respiratory passages, but seems to be caused by thickening of the bronchial mucous. The same symptom is frequently induced by inhaling chlorine. Occasionally there is considerable difficulty in dilating the chest, but where the rooms are well ventilated, this is rarely observed. Inflammation has never been observed as a result of the inhalation of these vapors, as they are ordinarily diffused in the operating room. Some operators mix their compounds by the sense of smell, and not by weight or measure.

Effects on the Brain and Nervous System.—These vapors frequently produce determination to the brain and vertigo. Sometimes a species of intoxication is observed, where the fumes are very strong, but this is not common. These effects speedily disappear by exercise in the open air.

Effects on the Sight.—Irritation and chronic inflammation of the conjunctiva are sometimes observed. This membrane is so sensitive to the vapor of iodine, that many operators can detect its presence in the operating room more readily by its effect on the eyes, than by the sense of smell. It exerts no influence on the sense of hearing and touch.

On the appetite.—It very frequently diminishes the appetite, and in no case have I ever known it to be increased.

On the bowels.—It exerts no perceptible influence on the condition of the bowels.

On nutrition.—It has not been observed to cause emaciation, nor any decided increase of flesh.

On the salivary secretion.—In no case was salivation observed, but very frequently dryness of the mouth and fauces was complained of; at the same time the secretion of the nose was diminished.

On the kidneys.—The urinary secretion did not appear to be either increased or diminished. The urine passed when the operator is actively engaged in coating plates, always contains iodine, and by operating on a considerable quantity at a time, I never failed to detect its presence. In some cases there is considerable irritability of the bladder, and in one instance the individual could not retain his urine for a longer period than two hours.

On the skin.—The skin does not appear to be much affected by these vapors. In one instance, however, the eruption which is sometimes observed to result from the use of iodine, made its appearance. This person was sent to the country, when in the course of three weeks the eruption disappeared, but in returning to the same pursuit, it again developed itself, and the individual is at the present time affected with it.

On the genital organs.—These vapors sometimes act as an excitant to the genital organs. In some instances this excitement was followed by an almost total extinction of the sexual appetite. In one case there was an absorption of one of the testicles, with atrophy of the other.

It will be observed that all of the foregoing appearances are those that can be produced by the administration of iodine alone, and it would seem to be the active agent in these cases; but the bromine and chloride of iodine may, and probably do, contribute to the same result.

The mercury which is employed to bring out the image, is so small in quantity as never to produce the symptoms of mercurial poisoning; at least I have never noticed it, or heard of its producing a bad effect.

In galvanizing the silver tablets, the fingers are sometimes plunged into the solution of cyanide of silver, which induces a painful ulceration around the nails, which, however, speedily disappears by proper treatment.

The above is the result of three years investigation of this subject, and the facts are gathered from the history of forty-three daguerrean artists, who have been in the business for periods, varying from two to twelve years.

Before leaving this subject, I would call the attention of the profession to the subjects of *Actinism* and *Light*, as these promise, above all others, to give us a clearer insight in regard to the influence which the atmosphere exerts upon health and disease, than any other branch of the natural science.

It is found that the actinic force is influenced by the seasons, temperature, the quantity of light which is transmitted through the atmosphere, and other causes which are not well understood. Thus the quantity is greater in March and April than at any other period of the year; and Prof. Draper states that in his progress from New York to the Southern States, he found it to diminish; and this is in accordance with the experience of daguerrean artists. The extinction of actinism in the atmosphere is not the same as that of light. Thus on certain dark, close days in the spring, the actini force is much less than it is when the air presents a more hazy appearance. There is also a very marked difference in the atmosphere of the city compared to that of the country, in regard to extinctive power. When a given amount of change is produced on a sensitive surface in the country in two seconds, it will frequently require thirty seconds to produce the same effect in the city, under the same circumstances. The extinctive power of the atmosphere of Cincinnati is about twice that of Louisville; and the atmosphere in the vicinity of Harrodsburgh Springs, Ky., possesses less extinctive power than that of any other locality which has been examined in the West.

Electrical action is quickened by actinism, and I found by making a sensative plate a part of the galvanic circuit, that the action of actinism was favored by the electrical current.

It is to be hoped that some one who has the proper apparatus, will investigate the magnetic properties of oxygen in its relation to actinism, as these subjects must have a very important physiological bearing.

The following is a summary of our knowledge of solar radiations, by Prof. Hunt:

1. The rays having different illuminating or colorific powers, exhibit different degrees and kinds of chemical action.

2. The most luminous rays exhibit the least chemical action upon all inorganic matter. The least luminous and non-luminous manifest very powerful chemical action on the same substances.

3. The most luminous rays influence all substances having an organic origin, particularly exciting vital power.

4. Thus, under modifications, chemical power is traced to every part of the prismatic spectrum; but in some cases this action in positive *exciting*, in others negative *depressing*.

5. The most luminous rays are proved to prevent all chemical

change upon inorganic bodies, exposed at the same time to the influence of the chemical rays.

6. Hence, actinism, regarded at present merely as a phenomenon different from light, stands in direct antagonism to light.

7. Heat radiations produce chemical change in virtue of some combined action not yet understood.

8. Actinism is necessary for the healthful germination of seed; light is required to excite the plant to decompose carbonic acid; caloric is required in developing and carrying on the reproductive functions of the plant.

9. Phosphorescence is due to actinism, and not to light.

10. Electrical phenomena are quickened by actinism, and retarded by light.—[*Western Lancet.*

Lucifer Match Making and Amorphous Phosphorus.—The announcement of Prof. Shrotter's discovery of the mode of preparing amorphous phosphorus, derived much of its practical interest from the supposition that the phosphorus in this state would be less dangerous and injurious to the persons engaged in the manufacture of lucifer matches. A medal was awarded to Mr. Albright for the introduction of the prepared phosphorus as an article of commerce, and it may now be obtained at a moderate price of Messrs. Sturge, of Birmingham. The dreadful disease to which the makers of lucifer matches are liable, from inhaling the fumes of ordinary phosphorus, having been described and brought under public notice, it might have been supposed that no time would have been lost in ascertaining the value of the above discovery as a means of alleviating so much human suffering. Matches prepared with the amorphous phosphorus were shown in the Great Exhibition, and it was stated at the time that in the manufacture of these matches, the evils arising from the inhalation of deleterious fumes were obviated, while the result of the experiment was satisfactory.

It is, however, difficult to introduce any innovation of this kind into an extensive branch of manufacture. A series of experiments must be made to test the efficacy of the new preparations, the most advantageous mode of employing it, the quality of the goods, and the economy of the process. In the mean time the several departments of the manufactory are progressing like clock-work. All hands are busily employed, the proprietor is fully occupied with superintending the operations and the accounts, and a large box of amorphous phosphorus remains in the office unpacked, waiting for a convenient opportunity to complete the experiments.

Such was the state of affairs at Mr. Dixon's manufactory at Newton Heath, near Manchester, on the occasion of a recent inspection. Outside the building large piles of timber were stored up ready for use. A machine worked by a steam-engine was reducing blocks into the form of matches. A block previously cut the length of the match, and pressed against the side of the machine, disappeared in a few seconds. The sticks being removed into the next room were tied into bundles

about eight inches in diameter, ready for dipping in sulphur. This
was done in another room in an iron vessel over a furnace. Immediately after the dipping, the workmen give each bundle a slight pressure with a rotatory movement to separate the matches from each other
at the moment of solidification, otherwise the sulphur would cohere
into a solid mass The matches are next transferred into a room
where they are arranged, so as not to be in contact with each other,
in frames about two feet by one foot, ready for the phosphorus
dipping. The composition used for this purpose consists of chlo-
rate of potash, phosphorus, and glue, and it is spread in a thin layer
on a stone or marble slab, heated below by steam or hot water.
The operator holds the frame lengthways, and dips the ends of the
matches in the composition, taking care that all of them are coated.
Sometimes the sticks are in the first instance cut twice the required
length, dipped at both ends, and afterwards bisected. In the process
of cutting they occasionally ignite, occasioning loss and also vitiating
the atmosphere. When the dipping is completed, they are taken to
the sorting room and packed in boxes. In another room the boxes are
labelled and sent to the packing room. The boxes are made on the
premises, the shavings cut, and the tops and bottoms stamped by machinery, cut to the proper size, glued, and fitted, which operations
are performed in separate apartments. Each box of lucifer matches,
price retail one halfpenny, passes through the hands of seventen persons, chiefly children. The Factory Act is not applicable to these es-
tablishments, and the children, averaging from seven to twelve years
of age, work twelve and sometimes thirteen hours in the day. They
earn (by piece work) from 3s. to 5s a week, and the adults from 9s. to
12s.

The cases of disease occur chiefly in the phosphorus dipping room,
sometimes in the room where the matches are sorted and packed in
boxes. but seldom in other parts of the establishment. The nature of
the disease is described in the *Dublin Quarterly Journal of Medical
Science,* for August, page 10, by Mr. Harrison:

" An affection ensues which is so insidious in its nature that it is at
first supposed to be common tooth-ache, and a most serious disease of
the jaw is produced before the patient is fairly aware of his condition.
The disease gradually creeps on until the sufferer becomes a miserable
and loathsome object, spending the best period of his life in the wards
of a public hospital. * * * * Many patients have died of the
disease ; many, unable to open their jaws, have lingered with carious
and necrosed bones ; others have suffered dreadful mutilations from
surgical operations, considering themselves happy to escape with the
loss of the greater portion of the lower jaw."

Mr. Harrison's paper contains much interesting information, with
the medical reports of several cases.

It would be foreign to our purpose to enlarge upon this view of the
subject ; but the disease being of chemical origin, the *modus operandi*
of the poison may involve a chemical enquiry. Does the phosphorus
when inhaled destroy the vitality of the bone by chemical action on its

substance? or does it operate merely as an irritant on the tissues, causing inflammatory action? The bone in its diseased state has a spongy cellular appearance, with excrescences of a similar character adhering to it. The teeth generally continue sound and white, while the jaw which contains them is altered in texture, dead. and discolored. We believe the diseased bone has not been chemically examined. Whether such examination would throw any light upon the subject is a speculative question; but we think it not unworthy of consideration.

There are at this time in the manufactory several persons who have suffered severely from the disease, and who, on recovery, immediately returned to their work—not however to the dipping department. In the Museum of the Manchester Infirmary is the lower jaw of a young woman who is now at work Her face is much disfigured by the loss of her chin, and in looking into her mouth the root of the tongue is seen connected with her under lip, the space formerly occupied by the jaw being obliterated by the contraction of the cheek. A young man who has lost his jaw is also in the factory. They are not isolated cases.

It is stated in the factory that the workpeople have sometimes applied the phosphorus paste to decayed teeth, under the idea that it was a cure for the toothache, and to this imprudence some of the early cases of the disease are attributed. The frightful nature of the disorder is now sufficiently understood to serve as an incentive to greater precautions Increased attention has been paid to ventillation and cleanliness, and the practice of taking meals on the premises is not allowed. It appears, however, from the statements of some of the workpeople who are engaged in the phosphorus dipping room, that their clothes become incandescent in the dark, and although the cases of the disease are less frequent than they have been formerly, a security against its recurrence is not attained. The proprietor of one factory states that he has had no cases in his establishment on account of a more careful method of dipping the matches, by which the face of the operator is further removed from the source of danger; but we are informed that some patients, from that factory have applied for medical relief in the neighborhood. Mr. Standring informs us that there is now in the Manchester workhouse a young woman suffering from a "phosphoric jaw." She worked three years in a match manufactory; she then went to a silk mill, where she had been about a year and a half before the disease first made its appearance. Eleven months since she was was admitted into the infirmary and remained there eighteen weeks, since which time she has been an inmate of the work-house. The disease at present affects only one side of the jaw—a portion of which is likely soon to be detached.

Various means of prevention have been tried, and others suggested. In a manufactory in Dublin, camphor is added to the composition, which masks the smell, and is said to act as a prophylactic. This latter opinion requires further proof. Mr. Taylor of Nottingham, suggests the use of a mask with a tube communicating with the outside of the building. Mr. Stanley of St. Bartholomew's Hospital, recommends the exposure of oil of turpentine in saucers about the workrooms, as a solvent of the fumes of phosphorus. Dr. Baur recommends the use of a sponge or handkerchief moistened with a solution of soda or potash and applied to the mouth. The proprietor of the factory above referred to states that he has diminished the quantity of phosphorus to less than a third of that which he formerly used, and that by this and other precautions the prevalence of the disease has been greatly diminished. He has tried the amorphous phosphorus on a small scale, by way of experiment, and says that it is more expensive than the ordinary kind, as a larger quantity is required. But the chief objection appears to be that the composition now in use answers quite well. The matches never fail; the mode of preparing the composition is understood; the result is known, and the demand for the matches unceasing. The amorphous phosphorus requires further trial; the makers are not yet accustomed to it. If it should fail their trade would be injured; the experiment would interfere with the habits of the factory ; therefore the operations are continued in the usual way, the box of Sturge's phosphorus remains unopened in the office, and the value of the discovery is not fairly put to the test.—[*London Pharmaceutical Journal.*

American Medical Association.—At a meeting of the Association held at Richmond, Va., May, 1852, the undersigned were appointed a committee to receive voluntary communications on medical subjects, and to award two prizes of $100 each to the authors of the best two essays.

Each communication must be accompanied by a sealed packet, containing the name of the author, which will be opened only in the case of the successful competitors. Unsuccessful communications will be returned on application after June 1st, 1853.

Communications must be addressed, post-paid, to the Chairman of the Committee, Dr. Joseph M. Smith, 56 Bleeker-st., New York, on or before the 20th of March, 1853.

JOSEPH M. SMITH, M. D.
JOHN A. SWETT, M. D.
W. PARKER, M. D.
GURDON BUCK, M. D.
ALFRED C. POST, M. D.

New York, Sept. 17th, 1852.

Another Medical School.—We perceive by the newspapers that our Savannah friends are about to establish a Medical School in that city, and that the Faculty has already been organized, as follows:

R. D. ARNOLD, M. D., Professor of Practice.
P. M. KOLLOCK, M. D., Professor of Obstetrics and the Diseases of Women and Children.
WM. G. BULLOCH, M. D., Professor of Surgery.
C. W. WEST, M. D., Professor of Chemistry.
J. G. HOWARD, M. D., Professor of Anatomy.
H. L BYRD, M. D., Professor of Materia Medica.
E. H MARTIN, M. D., Professor of Physiology.
J. B. REID, M. D., Professor of Pathological Anatomy and Demonstrator of Anatomy.

SOUTHERN

MEDICAL AND SURGICAL

JOURNAL.

Vol. 8.]   NEW SERIES.—DECEMBER, 1852.   [No. 12.

PART FIRST.

Original Communications.

ARTICLE XLVII.

Morbid Sensibility of the Stomach.   By G. T. Wilburn, M.D.,
of Ridge Grove, Alabama.

In writing a treatise upon Dyspepsia, no important result can
be anticipated if the same old beaten track is to be pursued, or
if the same accustomed tale of woe is to be repeated. But,
young as we are in physic, how dare we brave the long-received
opinion of the anacks in medical lore ! Shall we stand alone
against a host of medical philosophers, and attempt to teach
sages truth and science ? Shall all the labor of physicians to
discover the nature and cause of dyspepsia prove to be naught,
and the proud monuments which have been erected to their
genius be hurled to the dust ? Yes, let it all go, if science can
be advanced thereby. We have a right to our opinion, and,
should it be correct, let it be received; should it, however,
prove erroneous, let others prevail: we adopt your motto—'*Je
prends le bien où je le trouve.*'

Works on Practice contain much upon dyspepsia—journals
likewise have their pages frequently filled with essays upon
this popular theme. Dyspeptics write the history of their
own feelings and spin out a long theory of their cause and progress. These writers have been our teachers upon this dreadful malady, because we take for granted, what is far from being
true, that a sick man can tell the nature of his disease.

We have read many of these essays, and confess, honestly, that we have not, as yet, seen one word concerning what we consider the true cause of dyspepsia. Inattention to diet—luxurious indulgence in aliments indigestible by quality or quantity—sedentary habits—mental application—the habitual use of coffee, tea, tobacco, liquors, &c.—have all been arraigned as the cause of this vexatious disease. The pathology is almost universally considered to be a morbid condition of the gastric nerves.

Before stating what we believe to be the true cause of Dyspepsia, let us examine the situation of the stomach and its relation with surrounding parts. We shall here avail ourselves of the views of Cruveilhier.

The stomach is situated at a juncture of the upper tenth with the lower nine tenths of the alimentary canal, between the organs of deglutition and those of chylification. It occupies the upper part of the abdominal cavity, almost entirely fills the left hypochondrium, and advances into the epigrastrium, as far as the limits of the right hypochondrium. It is maintained in its place by the œsophagus and duodenum, and also by some folds of the peritoneum, which connect it with the diaphragm, the liver and the spleen. The stomach is directed obliquely downward to the right side, and a little forward.

The anterior surface of the stomach is directed forward, and a little upward. This surface is in relation with the diaphragm, and is separated by it from the heart; with the liver, which is prolonged upon it to a greater or less extent; with the last six ribs, being separated from them by the diaphragm; and with the abdominal parietes in the epigrastrium.

The posterior surface of the stomach is directed downward and backward, and is seen in the sac of the omentum, of which it forms the anterior wall. It has relations with the transverse mesocolon, which serves as a floor for it, and separates it from the convolutions of the small intestines; with the third portion of the duodenum, called the pillars of the stomach, (ventriculi pulvinar;) and lastly, with the pancreas. The duodenum, the pancreas, the aorta, and the pillars of the diaphragm, separate it from the vertebral column, upon which it rests obliquely.

Such is a short account of the position and relations of the stomach. We have given the natural position of this viscus when empty; when distended, its position is somewhat altered : for instance, the great curvature is directed almost vertically downward in the empty condition of the organ, and almost directly forward when it is full. Again, the lesser curvature is directed upward when the viscus is empty, upward and back- ward when it is full; and it then embraces the vertebral col- umn in its curvature, being separated from it by the aorta and the pillars of the diaphragm ; it also embraces the small lobe of the liver or the lobulus spigelii, the cœliac axis and the solar plexus of nerves.

The great *cul de sac* is in close relation with the spleen, and when distended is moulded upon that viscus. This portion of the stomach corresponds in the greater part of its extent to the left half of the diaphragm, which is in accurate contact with it and separates it from the lungs above and from the last six ribs in front. It is more or less elevated, according to the de- gree of distension of the stomach, and from this we can easily understand that difficult respiration may be caused by two large a meal. The great extremity of the stomach has rela- tions behind with the pancreas, and with the left kidney and supra-renal capsule.

The human system is accurately made. Every organ has its own locality and relations, and its position is mathemati- cally exact in each individual.

We do not say, that all the organs are located mathematical- ly the same in all persons, comparitively, but we do say, that each organ in each human being, is mathematically adjusted with the remaining organs.

So long as each organ maintains its mathematical relation with surrounding organs, the system is in a state of health, (we here speak only of position,) but any permanent deviation from this mathematical relationship is productive of disease, acute or chronic. We wish to be understood here as discussing mal- position alone as a cause of disease, we are not now examining the multiplicity of causes which *may* produce disease.

Let us apply the rule to the stomach—a wheel in the great and complicated machinery having its place to maintain and its relationship to observe in order that it may perform its proper function.

712 Wilburn, on Morbid Sensibility of Stomach. [December,

We select an individual whose stomach is located as we have
previously described. Now, the important questions are—What
will be the result upon that viscus and surrounding ones, should
its position and relations be altered? and would the functions
of each organ, now, as before, be properly performed? Suppose (and it is sometimes the case) the great extremity of the
stomach to be dragged downwards in a displacement of the
spleen? In this case, we must necessarily have an altered relationship of the abdominal viscera. Every part connected
with the stomach must undergo a corresponding change in position. Now comes the questions—Will each organ during this
displacement perform its proper function?

The watch is a beautiful machine. Its parts are admirably
adjusted for the purpose for which the machine was intended.
But if the several parts had been differently shaped from what
they are, (we speak of an individual watch) of a different size
from what they are, or placed in any other order than that in
which they are placed, either no motion at all would have been
carried on in the machine, or none which would have answered the use that is now served by it. (Paley.)

Is not the argument equally potent when applied to the
human organism? The machinery is transcendently more
important in its structure and purpose; the parts are more nicely adjusted; and, consequently, derangement of any organ must
be productive of consequences proportioned in mischief to the
importance and relations of the organ thus altered in position.
There is, however, one point of difference between a deranged
wheel in a watch and a deranged organ in the human system.
The altered position of a wheel does not necessarily imply an
injury to the wheel, per se, but an altered position of an organ
must imply an altered function of that organ.

This we believe to be particularly true of the stomach. It
is located in each system, with a hair's-breadth nicety. The
space through which it may play in the act of digestion, without mischief to itself or other organs, is mathematically circumscribed. Its limits of distension are exactly fixed, and its
motions necessary for digestion are governed by immutable
laws. No other position than its original one—no other motions and play than such as were primarily given it—no other

space for action than that which was first assigned it, can be consonant with its healthy and proper function.

This, to some, may appear a *petitio principii*—an assumption of the question originally intended to be demonstrated and proved. We cannot stop to discuss minor points, but must content ourselves for the present with the statement of general propositions whose ultimate deductions are clear and intelligible.

There is a separate screw to each string of a violin, and each string depends for its tension and tone upon its own individual screw. Should that screw be broken or altered in position, to which is attached the base, that string must evidently suffer in proportion to the damage done.

So in the human system, though in a greater degree, if an organ is altered in position, the nerves, blood-vessels, &c. must suffer a proportional injury, and the result of their action, as in digestion, chylification, &c., must be correspondingly altered. To suppose otherwise, would be to affirm omnipotent action in any organ, and that its peculiar and individual ends could and would be accomplished, under any and all circumstances, irrespective of position or relationship with other organs.

We lay down, then, this broad affirmation: That morbid sensibility of the stomach is primarily due to displacement of that viscus, and that the morbid sensibility of the gastric nerves is a secondary affection supervening upon or originating from the visceral displacement.

Professor I. P. Garvin, in a communication published in the Southern Medical and Surgical Journal, in Dec., 1846, gives as the "most prominent cause of" dyspepsia, "food of an improper quality, or in undue quantity." We admire the professor and sincerely regret that we cannot endorse an opinion so honestly entertained.

If the sensibility of an organ be an index of its liability to disorder from outward agents, which seems to be the case in the eye and in serous membranes, certainly this test is wanting in the stomach, which bears the presence of substances such as no other organ undefended by epidermis could tolerate. Here the ingesta are, as it were, suddenly deprived of their active properties; for the scalding liquid, the pungent spice, the acrid medicine, the frozen sweetmeat, nay, the mechanical irritant, are often forgotten, when the impressions which they left upon the tongue, the fauces and the gullet, have been effaced. The necessity for such an organization that neither pain nor the derangement of which it is the criterion, should be easily excited, is obvious from a moment's consideration of the difference between its circumstances and those of every other hollow viscus. The heart, the bladder, the intestines, all receive substances, more or less chemically prepared for them, and differing but little in their composition at different times; but into the stomach are carried the most heterogeneous agents, which have received only a mechanical adaptation to the organ which they visit. (Tweedie.) This organ escapes injury, from a wise provision of its organization, the copious secretion of mucus, and the capability possessed by this organ particularly of accommodating itself to varying quantities of blood. But, independent of the adaptation of the stomach for the reception of its varied ingesta, it would somewhat puzzle the learned Professor to account satisfactorily for all the symptoms he relates in his own person.

We have not space nor leisure to copy his article, but we will group together the symptoms as he relates them. (Med. & Surg. Journ., Dec. 1846.)

Discomforture after eating.

Fulness and distension—acid eructations.

Flatulence, headache, excitement of circulation.

Burning heat in the stomach.

Bowels costive—scybalæ.

Liver occasionally disordered.

Heart deranged in action.

Functions of the brain disturbed.

Distressing malaise.

An indiscribable sensation radiating from the stomach to the surface, resembling aura epileptica. This is succeeded by a general trembling. At the close of these attacks there is always a copious discharge of colorless urine.

The above constitute the principal symptoms found in the article alluded to.

We submit the question to every candid reasoner: From the anatomical position and relationship of the stomach, would not its displacement give rise to every symptom related?

Why discomforture—distension—fulness after eating, and its subsidence in a few hours? Evidently, because, the free and original action of the organ cannot take place during displacement, and hence an uneasiness is felt when this viscus attempts to perform its accustomed duty, due to resistance from, and pressure upon adjacent parts. The affections of the heart, bowels, liver, kidney, lungs, brain, &c., are easily explained according to the theory of displacement.

The malaise—aura epileptica—morbid condition of the gastric nerves, &c., are probably due to a deflection of the nerves of the stomach from their original and proper direction. We are aware that here we stumble upon a new theory of nervous action, but it is not to our purpose at present to discuss it. We would suggest, however, that neuroses can probably be more easily explained upon the principle of deflection of the nerves from their original direction, than upon the theory of nervous lesion.

The stomach derives its nerves from the eighth pair and from the solar plexus. By means of the eighth pair this organ is connected with the œsophagus, the lungs, the pharynx, the larynx and the heart. Through the nerves, from the central epigastric plexus, it is connected with the ganglionic system, and is brought into relation with the numerous viscera of the abdomen.

This extensive and intimate connection of the stomach with the entire system is a proof of the importance of the organ, and its displacement cannot result otherwise than deleterious to the whole organism.

No one will deny skill and design in the Creator, in the order of parts—their positive and sympathetic relationship, and their separate and peculiar function. If each part was thus particu. larly and mathematically adjusted, no other arrangement of parts—no other order—no other location—no other connection or relationship can answer fully the ends of the original design. To reason otherwise would be an imputation upon the wisdom of Deity.

We submit what we have written to a heartless and relent. less criticism. We are fully apprised of the meager garb in which our subject must go dressed before the world, but under existing circumstances the evil could not be remedied. The object of the present article has been more to state clearly our views than to discuss them. We have not thought it proper to anticipate and answer objections, neither have we propped our assertions by cases and logical deductions, as these did not come within the sphere of our original design in writing this article. We have discussed briefly such points only as were essential to render our views intelligible.

ARTICLE XLVIII.

Remarks on the Topography and most Prevalent Diseases of lower East Tennessee. By J. A. LONG, M.D., of Tennessee.

That portion of country familiarly known as lower East Tennessee is a high, broken, and well watered country; the spring water is mostly impregnated with lime, but is occasionally found pure. Most of the tillable land lies in valleys, and is rich and productive, especially along the water courses. The banks of the streams are high, and always sufficient to prevent overflows, so that we never suffer from inundations at any season of the year. Nearly all our water courses, from the smallest tributary branch, to the largest rivers, are swift running and shoaly streams, with good banks, as above stated; consequently the creeks are blocked up, from head to mouth, with numerous mill-dams. This, no doubt, is a fruitful source of fevers in this section. The climate is extremely variable, so much so, that sudden and severe changes take place even in twenty-four hours—hence our great liability to influenzas, inflammations, and diseases of the *respiratory organs in general.* We are subject, in this section, to all the diseases (with but few exceptions) that are common to the United States. Up to the present, we have had no cases of cholera, small-pox, congestive, nor yellow fever. The natural growth of this country is oak, hickory, poplar, ash, gum, walnut, chesnut, pine, &c. The diseases of this season are pretty much as in former years, though they seem to be undergoing a gradual change, especially the fevers.

Fevers constitute, probably, one-fourth of the whole sick-

ness in this region; next in importance are the diseases of the
respiratory organs, with occasional epidemics of measles and
scarlatina. Diseases peculiar to women, should occupy a
prominent place in the consideration of the diseases of this section, as they are probably as numerous in this as in any other
rural district; and this, I think, is satisfactorily accounted for
by the fact, that, parturient women are almost entirely in the
hands of uneducated *midwives*, and also by the variableness of
our climate. Puerperal diseases, and especially *puerperal fever*, have been very rife in past years; so much so, that parturient females have looked for it as an unavoidable or necessary
consequence. Notwithstanding its prevalence, it has never
yet appeared to me to present any of the features of an epidemic, nor has it appeared to be contagious or communicable,
in any way, from patient to patient, through the medium of
the practitioner, or otherwise. This disease (notwithstanding
it has presented all the characteristics of general puerperal
fever, as laid down in the books) has not been that formidable
monster spoken of by the older writers, but has, in a great
majority of cases, yielded promptly to remedial measures,
when timely administered. These remarks on the prevalence
of puerperal fever, are more especially applicable to my own
immediate bounds of practice. My patients invariably recovered under a moderately antiphlogistic treatment—such as,
bloodletting, purging, fomentations, blisters, &c. Venesection,
however, was found necessary only in a small proportion of
cases. Calomel and opium was used, with the happiest effects,
in all the cases that came under my care, in the proportion of
from 6 to 10 grs. of the former, with 1 to 2 grs. of the latter,
and this, too, in cases of obstinate costiveness, as well as when
diarrhœa was present. The medicine, in obstinate cases, was
afterwards continued in smaller doses, with a view to its constitutional effects. There never was any more difficulty experienced in procuring free alvine discharges, when the opium
was used in connection with calomel, than when it was withheld; on the contrary, it seemed to relax, and materially aid
this desirable end. Fomentations, followed by large blisters,
were invaluable auxiliaries in the treatment of puerperal fever;
nor was it necessary, in all cases, to use blisters, as the abdom-

inal pain and soreness seemed readily to abate under the persevering use of hot fomentations in conjunction with other
appropriate remedial measures.   Most of the cases convalesced
slowly, and relapses were very common and dangerous.

An epidémic influenza has prevailed here, more or less, for
the last few years, of a typhoid type, and often mistaken for
genuine *typhoid fever*, especially when both diseases existed
simultaneously in the same family, or the same neighborhood.
They had many points of resemblance, but were sufficiently
distinct, in their modes of access and general course, to be
readily and properly diagnosed by the attentive observer.
The greatest points of resemblance were, that both *typhoid
fever* and *influenza* were seen attacking whole families, or
neighborhoods, as if from contagion : both were attended with
diarrhœa, continued fever, great weakness, restless jactitation,
&c., especially at night.   These symptoms were common to
all cases of typhoid fever, from the mildest attacks to its gravest
form—whilst, in influenza, they were only noted in the graver
forms of the disease.   The onset of the two diseases was
strikingly different ; that of typhoid fever was almost invariably slow and gradual, whilst that of influenza was as uniformly
sudden.   The former continued several weeks, and was not
controlled by treatment—whereas, the latter was of short duration, and readily yielded to proper remedial means.   Both
were attended with a cough, but this was mild in typhoid fever,
whilst, in influenza, it was severe and troublesome, constituted
one of the leading symptoms of the disease, and was most generally accompanied with a severe pain in the side.

Dysentery, is another disease that claims a place in this
report, whether it be considered in reference to its frequency,
or to the severity of its symptoms.   This disease has also partaken of the prevailing typhoid type, and required to be managed with great prudence.   The treatment almost uniformly
successful in my hands was the free use of mucilaginous drinks
and injections, suppositories of opium, fomentations to the abdomen, &c., with the occasional use of small doses of calomel,
acetate of lead, and opium, or its equivalent in Dover's powder ;
but this internal medication was not often repeated, nor given
to induce constitutional effects.   Blisters proved, in some cases,

highly beneficial, especially in the chronic form of the disease. The oil of turpentine was extensively used and greatly lauded in many portions of the country. Having had no experience in its use in this disease, I can say nothing of its effects, but am inclined to oppose its administration, unless it be in an extremely advanced chronic stage, and then with great caution and distrust. Oil of turpentine has been recommended by Dr. Wood, in his Practice of Medicine, in the chronic stage of *typhoid fever*, to excite a more healthy action in the *intestinal ulcers*, known to be so common and obstinate in that disease : hence, probably, its introduction in the treatment of dysentery. I have no hésitancy in saying, that in all cases of dysentery, in which the patient recovers after the use of calomel, oil of turpentine, and other similarly irritating drugs, he does so, in spite of both disease and treatment ; and that he would have recovered much more readily, if left to nature and a good nurse. When the patient is robust, and the inflammatory symptoms run high, venesection may be resorted to with benefit, if cautiously done with the finger on the pulse, and with an eye always to the prevailing *typhoid type.* Then it is only necessary to clear the alimentary canal, by the use of castor oil, preceded or not by from 2 to 5 grs. of blue pill, with from $1\frac{1}{2}$ to 2 grs. opium; after which, nothing of an irritating or indigestible character should be taken, either in the form of medicine or food.

Pneumonia is a very common disease in this region of country, and for the last few years, or since the prevalence of typhoid fever, there has been a good deal of that form denominated *pneumonia typhoides.* Nearly all diseases have become less inflammatory, and partake more of the low or typhoid form, than in former years, in this section of country. The lancet is not used half so often as formerly. Fevers have undergone an almost entire revolution since I commenced the practice of medicine, nine years ago. The prevailing type then, was almost universally *intermittent* and *remittent*, with occasional cases of inflammatory continued fever, wholly different from the typhoid of the present day. Typhoid fever became more prevalent, and periodical fevers less so ; as the former increased, the latter diminished, and periodical fevers were rarely seen until, the present summer and autumn, in

which we have had nearly an equal number of periodical and
of typhoid fevers.   I shall not remark further in this place on
the subject of typhoid fever, as I have already given my views
of it in this Journal.   (June No., 1851, p. 324.)

Consumption has prevailed here considerably of late years.
The great prevalence of influenza, and of the typhoid type in
all diseases, combines two circumstances which tend to produce it—viz., irritation of the respiratory apparatus, and an
asthenic condition of the whole system ; the former acts as an
exciting cause, and the latter perpetuates it.   Three deaths
take place in this section from *consumption* where one did five
years ago, or prior to the prevalence of influenza and typhoid
fever.   Nearly as many deaths have taken place from *phthisis
pulmonalis* here, in the past spring and winter, as from all other
diseases combined together, and I do not recollect a single
case, under my care, or that of others, that could not be traced
to a severe attack of *influenza*, or to *typhoid fever*.   It is hardly necessary to remark on the treatment of consumption ; it is
sufficient to say, that the patients invariably died.

Worms are very common in this locality, especially the *lum-
bricoid;* it is not uncommon for them to be discharged in great
numbers, by the use of domestic remedies or in the course of
the treatment of other diseases, both in children and adults, especially when calomel is given.

Diarrhœa, in children, has been prevalent and obstinate
during last summer; it seemed to be very little under the control of medicine, especially when chronic, as was the case in
a majority of the instances I saw.   The discharges were not
difficult to check by fractional doses of *calomel* and *ipecac*,
sometimes combined with small doses of pulv. Doveri, or what
was better, acetate of lead ; but this appeared only to sicken and
prostrate the little sufferers.   Having derived decided benefit
from the use of chalybeate waters, in a case in my own family,
I have since prescribed a weak solution of sulphate of iron
with advantage.

ARTICLE XLIX.

Additional Remarks upon the Treatment of Dysentery. By
E. F. STARR, M. D., of Rome, Ga.

In a former number I offered a few remarks upon Dysentery,
and the use of large doses of opium in its treatment. I now
propose to direct attention to a plan of treatment which differs
somewhat from that in general use. I would do this, because
I believe there is some room for improvement, and that the
want of success is not to be charged altogether to a fault in the
resources of the materia medica. It is a fact worthy of some
notice, that, of late years, while medicine has been triumphing
in so remarkable a manner over some forms of disease, dysentery has not been shorn of its terrors, and its treatment now is
little more successful than it was many years ago. As we
have certainly not arrived at a point beyond which we may not
advance, we are justifiable in casting around us to see if there
be not means as efficient for the relief of other diseases as
quinine is for the cure of autumnal fevers. Is there no reliable
remedy for dysentery?

If I am told there is a vast weight of authority in favor of
the calomel treatment, and that it has been the established
practice for scores of years, I appeal to the number of deaths
by the disease at the present day. Comparatively but a few
years ago, calomel was considered the great remedy for autumnal fevers; yet the physician who knows no better now is
far behind the times. I esteem calomel very highly as a remedy; nor is my design so much to wage war against it, as to
place it in the back ground, compared with opium, in the treatment of dysentery. I am disposed to "retain the mastodon in
harness," and to make it useful by judicious and cautious administration whenever necessary, which will rarely be the
case in dysentery. A patient with sound bowels may perhaps
take a full purgative dose of calomel with impunity, but that
one with inflamed intestines can do so with entire safety admits
of much doubt. Unfortuuately, from the word bile has been
derived bilious, and from this, bilious attacks, and bilious fever,
and bilious colic, and bilious dysentery, and bilious every thing
else to which the term could be applied; and to this prevalence

of the *bilious idea* is to be attributed the belief, that to cure these affections there is little more necessity than to purge out the bile and "regulate the secretions," with calomel, of course.

Dysentery is a primary inflammation of the parts ostensibly affected, and it is not to be expected that it can be promptly and certainly cured, without directing attention to the condition of the diseased locality; nor need we hope to obtain success in the use of an irritating and motor-exciting treatment: for an inflamed organ needs rest, and to place it in the most favorable condition for a restoration to health, it must have rest. The hazard to which a little untimely exertion may subject a patient suffering with acute inflammation of any important organ is well known—how certainly then must undue action in an organ, itself inflamed, produce injurious effects. The value of opium, therefore, and the danger of a different class of agents, must be apparent under this view of the subject.

With regard to the use of cathartics, I would not be misunderstood: they are sometimes useful and necessary, but should, in such cases, be cautiously used, and, in general, be combined with opiates. I think there is often too much anxiety among practitioners upon the subject of scybalæ, and too great a passion for producing discharges of fœcal matter; yet I would not produce the impression that the contents of the bowels are to be left entirely without attention, but, that they are of little importance compared with the *intrinsic features* of the disease. In confirmation of this view, I will quote a fact from Dr. Brandon's article, in the March No. of this Journal. In describing some violent cases, which came under his notice, he says, that he "seldom observed fœcal matter in the discharges until a change for the better had occurred." The improvement, then, could not have been produced by the feculent discharges, but these must have been the result of an amelioration of the disease—showing that the disease may be first subdued by opium and other remedies, and the bowels afterwards emptied more safely.

In the treatment of dysentery, our object should be to effect, promptly, the cessation of spasm and pain, and the reduction of inflammatory and febrile action. These indications are all under the control of the therapeutic properties of opium, to a greater or less extent, and if these indications and these properties are properly weighed and considered, in connection with each other, the tendency will be towards the establishment of the treatment which I am endeavoring to urge upon the attention of those who may notice these suggestions. The reason why so little reliance has been placed in opium, is, that it has not been given in sufficient quantities—in doses large enough to overcome the force of disease, and to produce its legitimate and peculiar antiphlogistic and antifebrile effects. There is no confidence to be placed in an ordinary or medium dose of opium when the patient is suffering the effects of violent inflammatory action, the tortures of pain, or the depressing adynamic influences of malignant disease. The dose must be proportionate to the emergency of the case. I suggested from two to four grains, but this should not be considered the limit; this quantity is rather the minimum than the maximum—circumstances must determine the precise amount. In dysentery, if the pain, fever, and flux persist, they are sufficient evidence that enough has not been given—six grains are not too much in such cases. The antiphlogistic virtues of opium seem generally to be imperfectly known or understood, or if known, not appropriated and applied. All agree in admitting its usefulness as an anodyne, as a soother of pain and promoter of sleep, etc.; but who administers it with a view of overcoming fever, or who looks to it principally to subdue some severe forms of inflammation. Yet, what diaphoretic will produce such certain and general opening of the pores and genial moisture of the surface?—what will so equalize the circulation?—what so control the heart and arteries? and what afford such suspension of pain, thereby breaking the *chain* of the morbid actions of inflammation? Fever and inflammation cannot well persist under such circumstances—under the effects of full doses of opium.

To carry out more effectually the suggestion above made, in relation to the indications of treatment, it may be often proper to resort to one efficient bloodletting, in cases where there is much fever and no want of strength. This will render the system more susceptible to the favorable influence of opium,

which now, if properly administered, will never fail to mitigate,
and seldom to relieve entirely, the sufferings of the patient.
When this is done, the use of opium is not to exclude other
substances as auxiliaries ; such, for instance, as calomel or oil,
when they are needed, or sugar of lead and other astringents,
when, after the subsidence of the inflammatory symptoms, the
discharges remain too frequent and watery.   These, with fomentations, blisters, enemata of watery solution of opium and
starch, &c., may be resorted to ; but opium in large doses,
given either by the mouth or rectum, in the early stage of the
disease, should be the leading remedy and chief reliance.

ARTICLE L.

Dysentery treated with Sulphate of Magnesia. By PETER-
FIELD TRENT, M. D., of Richmond, Va.

June 18th, 1852, I was called to see Polly Gentry, a colored
woman, of robust constitution, aged 50 years; found her suffering
with acute dysentery.   Prescribed : 2 grs. calomel, 2 grs. acet.
plumbi and ½ gr. opium, every two hours; enema, night and
morning, of 10 grs. acet. plumbi and 30 drops tinct. opii. in 2 oz.
of starch-water; diet, milk thickened with arrow-root, or rice
and milk ; drink, toast water, or the water in which rice had
been boiled, to which a little salt was to be added.   6, P. M.,
visited my patient again; found her no better.   The tormina
still excruciating ; the tenesmus constant and harrassing ; the
fever slightly abated ; the dejections frequent and blended with
blood and lymph, with a great deal of water.   Ordered a continuance of the treatment directed in the morning—patient to
be allowed to dissolve small particles of ice in her mouth, to
relieve the urgent thirst.

June 19th.   Patient no better.   Same treatment to be continued.   4, P. M., a little better—the discharges having more
of a fœcal appearance.

June 20th.   Patient easier, but no decided improvement in
the evacuations.   In hopes of procuring some action from the
liver, ordered 5 grs. calomel and 5 grs. acet. plumbi every two
hours ; enema, as at first, omiting the tinct. opii.   6, P. M.,
evacuations very dark, but watery, no appearance of blood ;

tenesmus harrassing; epigastrium very tender upon pressure—to relieve this, a mustard-plaster to be applied. No change in the other treatment.

June 21st. Patient apparently better—discharges more fœcal. Thinking I had given mercury enough, I ordered no medicine this visit: her diet to be the same as heretofore. 4, P. M., sent for in haste: patient in every respect worse. Ordered 5 grs. tannic acid and 3 grs. acet. plumbi every two hours. 11, P. M., evacuations consisting entirely of bloody mucus. Repeat prescription ordered in the morning; give an enema ℨss tinct opii to ℨij starch water.

June 22d. Again sent for me in haste. Patient evidently worse and sinking—passing her evacuations involuntarily. Ordered wine whey—requested consultation. In the meantime, directed enema of 20 grs. acet. plumbi, 60 drops tinct. opii., to ℥ij starch water, to be given immediately. My friend, Dr. Bolton, met me, at 2, P. M. We found her complaining of dryness of the throat and violent thirst; the tenesmus being very violent; epigastrium very sore, evacuations of pure blood, though frequent, yet small. We determined to try the following:—℞. Sulph. Magnesia, ℥i.; Tinct. Opii. ℨi.; Aq. Menth. Pip. ℥iv. Dose, ℥ss. every two hours. Enema, of Əj. Argent. Nit. Crystal. to ℥i. Aq. Dist. (I may here state, that by mistake the enema was not given.) 10, P. M., no better.

23d. Patient a little better; had vomited first dose of saline mixture. Treatment continued. ' P. M., evacuations more consistent; patient easier.

24th. Patient better; tenesmus but slight; no epigastric tenderness; evacuations appearing like those of diarrhœa. 6, P.M., patient improving, discontinue saline mixture. If tenesmus is annoying, use acet. plumbi and tinct. opii. enema, as before.

25th. From this time until I ceased visiting her, she slowly improved, and is now (July 10th) well enough to resume her duties as a washerwoman.

I have treated some ten cases since the above successfully, with the salts and laudanum, not having given any other medicine from my first visit to the last.

The case just reported is a fair example of one of the most intractable forms of the disease, and requires all the physician's

skill. The intense suffering of the patient and the probability
of a fatal termination, unless the disease be arrested within a
short period, appeal strongly to his humanity. He applies
active counter-irritation—he administers mercury, opium, astringents and demulcents, per orem et rectum—an amendment
takes place—the patient is convalescent—at the very next
visit his hopes are dashed by the recurrence of all the worst
features of the case: the treatment has been palliative—it has
not effected a radical cure. Let us consider the pathological
condition in such a case. There is inflammation of the mucous
membrane of the rectum and perhaps of the adjoining colon;
or it may be still more extensive. The tenaceous bloody mucus, tenesmus, tender abdomen and symptomatic fever, tells
us this. We want then to eject thoroughly all scybalæ or
other local irritants; we want to deplete the hyperæmic surface—we want to change the character of the secretions, from
a thick, tenaceous matter, which requires wearisome and painful efforts to dislodge it, and produce instead, a loose, watery
matter, which will run off almost insensibly. Such are precisely the effects of sulphate of magnesia—a refrigerant purgative reducing the fever and cleansing the intestinal canal—
effecting local depletion by drawing off the serous portion of
the blood from the over-distended vessels, changing the unmanageable dysentery to a manageable diarrhœa. Opium and
calomel are highly valuable as adjuvants—the former quiets
the spasmodic action of the muscular coat of the intestines and
obtunds its excessive sensibility—by composing the whole
system, it relieves the sense of weakness and exhaustion. The
latter keeps the portal circulation flowing freely, and thus relieves the congested vessels, which pour their contents into it;
at the same time, by its specific action, it aids in restoring a
healthy secretory process.

ARTICLE LI.

On the Circulation of the Blood. By A. R. WELLBORN, M. D.,
of Newton county, Ga.

Having noticed a great deal said in the Boston Medical and
Surgical Journal, since last January, in regard to Mrs. Wil-

lard's Theory of the Circulation of the Blood, it was our intention to write an article proclaiming the merits of a theory
much more satisfactory; professional engagements, however,
have prevented our doing so, and we only give an outline of
Dr. Draper's theory, to those who have not examined the subject, hoping it will call forth remarks from some more able pen,
and thus justice be done the author.

It was for a long time supposed that the circulation of plants
was carried on by the forcing power existing in the spongioles
or extremities of the roots, aided by a kind of suction power
in the leaves. This, though a plausible reason, does not account for the downward flow of the sap. By means of the
spongioles, the water holding the different saline properties derived from the earth is taken up, and by means of capillary
attraction is carried through the body of the tree or plant to
the leaves. On the surface of the leaves, a change in the
chemical constitution of the watery solution takes place. It
obtains, on coming into contact with the air, a portion of carbonic acid gas, and is, by the agency of sunlight, decomposed,
and a mucilaginous solution ensues. This mucilaginous solution, containing the nutritive material, is then forced back
through the proper vessels to the bark of the tree. This
elaborate sap, in its descent to the root of the plant, moves
through a system of vessels which anastomose with each other,
and imparts nutrition. If we take a capillary tube of such
length and diameter that when one end is immersed in water
the fluid will rise to the top—break off a portion of that tube,
and again immerse one end, the fluid will rise to the summit,
and remain stationary, unless there is something to produce an
exhausting effect. We see, then, it is owing more to the exhausting action of the leaves that the capillary movement is
continued, and not to their suction power, and that the chemical changes account for the elaborate sap being driven forwards to the under side of the leaf, thence to the bark of the
tree. The circulation, then, of the nutritive juices, both in the
vegetable and animal kingdoms, rests upon this physical principle, "that if two liquids communicate with one another in a
capillary tube, or in a porous or parenchymatous structure,
and have for that tube or structure different chemical affinities'

movement will ensue, that liquid which has the most energetic
affinity will move with the greatest velocity, and may even
drive the other fluid entirely before it, that this is due to common capillary attraction, which, in its turn, is due to electric
excitement."

Dr. D. remarks, that even gaseous substances, as is shown
experimentally in the appendix of his work, pass into one another with a force greater than the pressure of a column of
water seven hundred feet high, so that to elevate the sap in a
tree, or to drive the blood in an animal, is an insignificant demand on the energy which this force could put forth. Let
us then apply these principles, to account for the circulation
of blood in the higher animals. The arterial blood passes
from the left ventricle, to the capillaries, burning out the effete
carbonaceous matter of the tissues, and perhaps converting its
hydrogen into water. Having obtained carbon, venous blood
is formed, and is driven forward along the capillaries of the
veins; the affinity which then exists between the venous blood
and the oxygen of the lungs, causes it to rush forward, driven
by the momentum received by the chemical change in the
tissues. In the first place, the intense affinity which the oxy-
genized or arterial blood had for the carbon of the tissues,
causes it to rush toward the extremities; it then undergoes a
chemical action, and the condition of the affinities is changed.
The venous blood is now driven toward the heart by means of
the affinity existing between the carbon of the moving mass of
blood and the oxygen existing in the lungs.

We see, then, the two forces which are brought to bear—
the one expressed by the intense affinity existing between
oxygen and carbon, the other arising from the physical principle before mentioned, that if two liquids communicate with
one another in a capillary tube, or in a porous or parenchymatous structure, &c.

It does seem to us clear, that the *primum mobile* of the circulation cannot reasonably be attributed to the caloric evolved
in decarbonizing and oxydizing the blood, but that the chief
force lies in the chemical affinities, as illustrated by Dr. Draper.
We do not say that caloric has no influence, but if it has any
propelling power, it is merely a subsidiary or resulting action.

Neither do we deny that the heart has an important agency in keeping up the circulation of blood—it certainly does have ; but we must agree, with Dr. D., that this central organ is given us more to act as a regulator between the pulmonary and systemic circulation.

To strengthen the view here taken, it is to be considered that *plants* are wholly destitute of a heart, yet the sap flows, and their juices circulate. In many animals the circulation is carried on without a heart. In *insects* no such central organ exists. But we are asked, how do you account for the circulation in the fœtus ? Let us consider the fœtal circulation for a moment. We find here, the blood passes from the placenta through the umbilical vein, a large branch of which having passed into the liver, the blood from which is driven into the hepatic vein, and thence conveyed to the ascending vena cava, the principal branch conveying the blood immediately into the vena cava. From the vena cava ascendens, it passes into the right auricle, guided by the eustachian valve through the foramen ovale into the left auricle ; from the left auricle, it passes into the left ventricle, and from the left ventricle, into the aorta, whence it is distributed by means of the carotid and subclavian arteries, principally to the head and upper extremities ; from the head and upper extremities, it passes through the descending vena cava to the right auricle ; from the right auricle, it is propelled into the right ventricle ; from the right ventricle, into the pulmonary artery, and through the ductus arteriosus into the descending aorta. It is then distributed to the inferior extremities, whence it returns to the placenta through the umbilical arteries. We find here a circulation, commencing in a capillary system and terminating in a capillary system. How, then, can we say the heart is the cause of such a circulation being produced and kept up? Why cannot the same principle apply here that did in the adult circulation? If we say the placenta has the power, as some believe, of vivifying the blood, then precisely the same affinities are applicable, and act in the same way. If, as others believe, the placenta has not this power, still the same reasoning applies ; for we find the fœtal circulation similar in many respects to that of the portal circulation in the adult, and we bring in the same general principles

explaining the mechanical causes of circulation in this case.
" That, for the physical reasons which have been assigned, a
pressure will always be exerted by the fluid, which is ready to
undergo a change upon that which has already undergone it;
a pressure which, as there is no force to resist it, will always
give rise to motion in a direction from the changing to the
changed fluid."

We will remark, in conclusion, that for some time past, since
typhoid fever has been prevailing in its malignant form in this
section of country, we have noticed an irregular pulse in the
majority of cases.   How to account for this we are at a loss.
The blood, no doubt, is vitiated, and contains a poison—what'
that poison is, we are not prepared to say : it may be *hydro-
sulphate of ammonia,* according to the experiments of M. Bon-
net, or it may be carburetted hydrogen.

In those cases which proved fatal, we are not aware that any
lesion of the brain existed; nor have we detected any pressure
of the brain from symptoms during life; nor have post-mortem
examinations revealed any to the eye.

May it not be that the poison in the blood produces more
or less derangement in the chemical affinities, that a languid
circulation is the result, and that in consequence of the abnormal stimulus the heart receives, this irregularity of pulse
is produced.

ARTICLE LII.

Sudden Rupture of an Ovarian Tumor—peritonitis—recovery.
By L. A. Dugas, M.D.,

Mrs. D., aged about 42, the mother of thirteen children,
had always enjoyed good health until the birth of her last
child in March, 1851. Her delivery, although natural, was
followed by considerable hemorrhage, and she has ever since
felt a fixed pain or soreness in the left iliac region. At the end
of a few months a distinct tumor could be perceived by
pressing firmly over the painful region, and this gradually acquired a volume equal to that of a fœtal head. When turning
over in bed upon the right side, a sense of dragging would
always be experienced to so unpleasant a degree as to prevent

her sleeping upon this side. The left lower limb would some-times be swollen, and often feel benumbed. Sitting upon a very low seat became so uncomfortable, from the pressure of the thighs upon the abdomen, (the patient being corpulent,) that the night-glass for ordinary use was placed in a chair of usual height.

Such was the state of the patient when, on the 5th January last (1852), she was taken with uterine hemorrhage. She was in the habit of menstruating during lactation, and had done so ever since her last confinement, with the exception of the two last periods, which induced the belief that she was now two months pregnant, and was about to miscarry. The hemorrhage did not yield to ordinary means, but rapidly increased and be-came attended with uterine contractions. Ergot was now freely administered—a mole or false conception was expelled ; but the loss of blood continued so excessive that fatal exhaustion appeared inevitable. A tampon was introduced and the ergot continued, which arrested the flow, but she remained pulseless, with often recurring syncope, and a cold sweat during ten or twelve hours, notwithstanding the additional free administra-tion of brandy. The hemorrhage was effectually stayed, and did not return upon the removal of the tampon.

The patient recovered very slowly ; the anemia continued very great, and the painful annoyance in the iliac region increased. At the end of a month she was still unable to walk about the house without fatigue, and on the 4th of February was carried down stairs to a room below for a change of scene. General debility and distressing tenderness in the region of the left ovary were now the prominent features of the case. On returning to her bed-chamber in the afternoon of the 4th of February, she inadvertently sat upon a night-glass to urinate, instead of using the chair, as heretofore. As she did so, she suddenly felt a most excruciatiug pain throughout the entire abdomen, swooned, and fell upon the floor. On recovering, she attributed her suffering to intense cramp colic, and said she felt as if all her intestines were violently constricted or " drawn up." There was no discharge per vaginam. Enemata and warm fomentations were resorted to, and the bowels were evacuated, but without the least relief. I saw her about two hours after the accident : she had not yet been able to have her garments taken off to get into bed, but was lying upon a couch. She felt a "burning, drawing pain" throughout the entire abdomen, which was exceedingly tender to the touch, but not at all tense. Her pulse was frequent, and her respiration short and thoracic. She had thrown up the contents of the stomach, but felt thirsty. The tumor could no longer be recognized by the touch. She thought she had bruised it with her thighs, in sitting upon the vessel to urinate. The fact was evident, that she had not only bruised, but actually ruptured the tumor, and that its contents had escaped into the abdominal cavity, inducing peritonitis, which, in her enfeebled condition, could not be otherwise than extremely dangerous. 40 drops of laudanum were immediately administered, and a large blistering plaster applied over the abdomen; the laudanum to be repeated in two hours, unless relieved.

5th Feb. The blister is well drawn; the tr. opii. had to be repeated in the course of the night, and again this morning. Abdomen still very sore and somewhat full; pulse small and very frequent; surface hot and dry; eructations and occasional vomiting; great thirst; breathing short and thoracic; coughing very painful. Ordered, the lateral surfaces of the abdomen, or flanks, to be covered with blistering plasters, and the anodyne to be repeated as often as necessary to mitigate the intensity of the soreness. Bi-carb. soda and lime water, alternately, in small quantities of cold water, for beverage.

6th. Local symptoms about the same, with the exception of a little increase in the volume of the abdomen. General state, better. Continue same treatment.

7th. Abdominal tenderness less marked: passed a comfortable night; nausea relieved; pulse not so frequent. Continue same beverage—take a little chicken broth occasionally.

12th. The peritoneal inflammation gradually subsided, but the abdomen is still tumid. No fever—patient convalescent.

May 1st. Mrs. D. is now in her usual health, but still feels a soreness in the iliac region. No tumor can now be detected. She has menstruated regularly at each period since the attack of hemorrhage, with the exception of that which came on at the time of the rupture.   •

It will be observed that the details of this case are given with considerable minuteness. This was necessary, in order to convey a correct idea of its nature, and to show the reader the grounds upon which the diagnosis was established. One cannot be too minute in describing cases of such rare occurrence as one in which an ovarian tumor has been ruptured by violence and emptied into the abdominal cavity, without causing death.

PART II.

Eclectic Department.

From the Transactions of the Medical Society of the State of Georgia.

Report of the Committee on Surgery. By H. F. Campbell, M. D., Chairman.

The resolution under which the Committee on Surgery was appointed having contemplated in its plan, only Surgical facts occurring to practitioners in the State during the past year, leaves a very restricted field for a report. The only practical mode of collecting these facts, viz: by a review of the journals and by calling on the Profession throughout the State in a published card has been adopted. The result of our efforts with this mode of procedure will, we fear, present but little of interest to the Society.

We find that most of the Surgery published in the State during the past year has been transmitted to the Southern Medical and Surgical Journal, there being, so far as we know, but one case published elsewhere.*

In presenting their review of the journals during the past year, the Committee have adopted as their system, that of classing the matter under three heads, viz: Surgical Injuries and Pathology; Surgical Operations; and lastly, Surgical Medicine or Treatment. We have placed reports under these three heads, according to the respective importance presented by these three features. Thus, cases published on account of the interest attaching to the pathology, on account of some peculiar mode of Treatment or remarkable surgical operation, have found their places accordingly under these respective heads.

In thus classing these cases, the Committee have taken the liberty of exercising their own judgment as to the particular

---

* Charleston Medical Journal and Review. Case of Injury of Cranium, by F. T. Matthews, M. D., herein reported.

head under which such cases should appear, and it will be seen by a reference to the journals from which our collection has been made, that we have sometimes found it necessary to dwell upon points as interesting in these cases, which their original re- porters appeared to view as of minor importance, and *vice versa.*

In making our collection, the Committee has in view of the paucity of the published reports, determined not to exclude any that have come under their observation; our object has been to present a faithful resumé of the Surgical facts, of the past year, throughout the State, and to show as far as we were able, the amount of Surgery practiced or reported in the State du- ring that period. In doing so, we have used the space between January, 1851, and the present time, which, though the time is somewhat more than twelve months, we have still felt author- ized in doing.

Of the three departments of Surgery arranged by the Com- mittee as heads, we have found a greater number of cases occurring under that of *Surgical Pathology* than under either *Operations* or *Surgical Medicine.*

SURGICAL PATHOLOGY.

Under the head of Surgical Pathology we have placed all those cases which have come under the observation of the Committee in which the pathological condition of the patient appeared to be, in our judgment, the most remarkable feature.

The following case has been deemed appropriate for this re- port from the fact that, though it comes more properly under the domain of general practice, still the Surgeon is more fre- quently consulted for the relief of such affections than the ordinary practitioner.

Progressive Muscular Atrophy.—L. A. Dugas, M. D., Pro- fessor of Surgery in the Medical College of Georgia, in some favorable editorial remarks upon the Treatise of Dr. F. A. Aran, of Paris, on this subject, coincides with Dr. A. in the opinion that such cases are often mistaken for nervous diseases, and incidentally relates the following case from his own prac- tice as corroborative of this opinion:

"The case was that of a much esteemed professional brother, who, in the prime of life, and the possession of a vigorous constitution, perceived that he was gradually losing the power to flex the thumb of one hand. The loss of the use of the thumb having become complete, the finger next to it began to weaken also and became useless; the middle finger followed next, and thus, successively all the fingers of that hand became powerless. The loss of voluntary motion invaded the wrist and then the elbow, and finally all the muscles of the shoul- der. When it reached the elbow of this limb, the thumb of the other hand began to give way precisely as the first had done and the disease progressed in this limb as it did in the other until both arms were left as dangling appendages to a robust frame. It is worthy of remark that such was the slow progress of the malady, that its ravages were not complete, I think, until the lapse of two years; that during the whole of this time the patient's general health was perfect; that the sensibility of the affected parts was entirely normal; that he suffered no pain; and that the loss of motion regularly coincided with the complete atrophy of the muscles. The limbs and the shoulder-blades appear completely emaciated and are soft and flabby to the touch. Although about ten years have elapsed since the occurrence of this affliction, he still enjoys fine health and unimpaired mental powers, and is enabled to discharge the duties of an active practice in the country. Sensibility being yet perfect he judges of the pulse as accurately as ever, when his fingers are placed upon the artery by the assistant who accompanies him.

"Our friend was not only treated by ourselves, but also sought the advice of most of the distinguished practitioners of the United States in vain. He submitted patiently to the trial of every remedy and mode of treatment, that had ever been recommended in paralytic affections without any modification or check of the disease. M. Aran thinks that Galvanism will sometimes arrest its progress, but it proved unavailing in our case."*

As the Doctor remarks, the subject is eminently worthy of further investigation, and it is on account of the novelty of the case, this being the first, so far as we know, related in the United States, that the Committee have here recorded it. Dr. Aran's views on this subject, a synopsis of which has been given in the Journal, are well worthy the attentive consideration of the Profession.

Anæsthesia from Turpentine.—In the same volume of the Journal, among other Surgical cases, Dr. Henry Rossignol reports the following as having occurred under his observation in the practice of his associate, Dr. L. A. Dugas. The notes taken by us of the case are the following:

The patient, a negro man aged 60 years, an old drunkard by habit, had of late resorted to Spirit of Turpentine whenever alcoholic liquors could not be procured; on one occasion, after a large potation of Turpentine, he fell asleep before the fire, with his feet resting on the burning wood. He required to be aroused by another person after the shoe, stocking, and a large portion of the pantaloons had been consumed. He then got up, walked about, said he felt no pain, and did not believe his foot burnt at all. The limb was so extensively injured that amputation was necessary. The patient having evinced symptoms of mania a potu, died ten days after the operation, the stump having partially healed.

In the same report we find two cases given to show the un-

* Southern Medical and Surgical Journal, vol 7., N. S., p. 244.

certainty which attends the injury produced by falls. In one, the patient fell from the fourth story of a cotton-factory, a distance of fifty feet, and yet sustained but little injury, being perfectly well in a few days, while in the other case the patient sustained very extensive injury, as excessive concussion of the brain and its accompanying effects, (even temporary insanity) which continued nearly two weeks. Here the patient had fallen but twelve feet.

In connection with these cases the reporter would beg leave to refer to a case occurring in his own practice, wherein a child of six years of age was precipitated over a banister to the ground, a distance of nearly twenty-five feet, and yet no injury was sustained with the exception of slight bruises on prominent portions of the ileum and greater trochanter of the side upon which she alighted.

In the same paper, we find also a case of Encephaloid Carcinoma of the Thigh, wherein the patient recovered after amputation. A case of extensive sloughing from an old burn. The patient was affected with Epilepsy at the time of the receipt of the injury, but never after did he have a convulsion.

Upon this case we may make the remark, that although the Epilepsy was *here* relieved *apparently* by the revulsion occasioned by the burn, still this is by no means the invariable result in cases of this character ; for how common is it to see patients horribly disfigured by burns received during their convulsions, and yet the Epilepsy continues in unabated severity. It is but seldom that we can effect a compromise with this terrible malady, even at the expense of scorched bodies and mutilated extremities.

Also, a case of Ulcerated Lipoma of the Occiput, and one of Fibrous Tumor of the Mamma. For a minute detail of these we refer to the Journal.

In the Charleston Medical Journal and Review, we find an interesting case of Extensive Fracture of the Cranium, reported by F. T. Mathews, M. D., of Muscogee county, Ga.

"The blow which had inflicted the injury was received while riding on the coupling pole of a timber wagon. The chain confining the lever gave way, and the latter, impelled by the weight of a heavy green pine log, swept through its full course and descended violently upon his head.

"The patient exhibited very severe symptoms of compression, which continued unabated after purgation and venesection. The patient was trepanned seventeen hours after the receipt of the injury. The cranium was found extensively fractured in the frontal and parietal bones, and the pieces removed, left a space the size of a dollar. Consciousness and speech gradually returned, after the operation, and the case, with but little exception, progressed regularly to complete recovery."

At the conclusion of this report, the Doctor remarked that "this case is strongly confirmatory of the general opinion that fractures occasioned by a rounded body, though the force applied be very great, is not so fatal in its consequences, as in those instances where it results from a more pointed one, impelled with much less violence."

That this is a common opinion, we may perhaps admit, but certain it is that we frequently see cases which are very strangely confirmatory, of the very reverse of this proposition, while at the same time our knowledge of the anatomy and relation of the cerebral mass to its containing structure, would make this converse opinion most rational.

Among the cases militating against the review of the reporter, we would adduce Dr. Harlow's celebrated case, reported by Professor H. J. Bigelow, wherein an iron crowbar, a pointed instrument, passed through the centre of the cerebrum, and yet the patient scarcely lost consciousness, and finally, entirely recovered with the loss only of an eye.

Another case, somewhat similar, is that of Dr. H. F. Campbell, wherein the patient, a negro man, had the cranium deeply cleft with an axe, a sharp-edged instrument, and the chop extended deeply into the cerebral mass, and yet, like in the former case, the patient did not lose his consciousness and had no bad symptoms during the whole treatment, the wound healing kindly after trephining.

We would explain the escape of the patients, in these instances, by the fact that in the case of the sharp-pointed and edged instruments only the portion of the brain infringed upon is affected, whereas in the case of the fracture by blunt instruments, the whole brain must be affected or compressed, as the instrument does not enter readily as in the other case, but presses before it the cerebral mass and thus compresses it in *all* its parts against the walls of the cranium.

Although we have deemed it expedient to signify our difference of opinion with Doctor Mathews on the above points, we would here remark, that we consider his case quite an interesting one, and one in which he does himself credit, both as an operator and a reporter.

In the September number of the Southern Medical and Surgical Journal, D. C. O'Keeffe, M. D., of Penfield, details the particulars of a case of Uterine Polypus, and accompanies the report generally, and the difficulty attending their diagnosis, by some reflections on uterine tumors, which we consider very judicious and worthy the attention of the Society.

Prof. C. T. Quintard reports a case of Glossitis in the Southern Medical and Surgical Journal, page 77. This is quite a rare disease in this section of our country, that is, to occur idiopathically. The treatment pursued in this case was bleeding, active purgation, and the application of cups ad nucha, and the administration of sedative doses of morphine to relieve pain.

There are reported iu the 7th volume of the Southern Medical and Surgical Journal, the notes of a post-mortem examination by Prof. Paul F. Eve, in which the patient died of a Stricture of Œsophagus. The subject was extremely emaciated from long continued abstinence previous to death. The stricture had been caused by the accidental swallowing of a piece of caustic potass, by a child three years old. The autopsy was made about five months after the receipt of the injury, and "revealed a permanent contraction with thickening of the tissues of the œsophagus. The diameter of the strictured portion being reduced to about a line, for an inch and a quarter, and which was quite tortuous. The stomach was contracted in its capacity, but the ileum was largely distended with feces.

Dr. Eve has also furnished us with the particulars of an extensive injury of the cranium, in which a large portion of the frontal bone was removed, together with a portion of its orbitar plate and also the crista galli of the ethmoid bone, so extensive was the injury. The patient lived, we think, about one week after the receipt of the injury. As we understand fiom the Doctor that this case will be published shortly in detail, we forbear further remark, as they would be anticipations of his own report.

In the April number of the Southern Medical and Surgical Journal, for the present year, we find an interesting account of a very unusual epidemic—Paronychia, by the Editor, Dr. Dugas, a part of which account we here insert. After some very pertinent remarks in relation to the mystery and inscrutability investing the advent, progress, and departure of epidemics, the Doctor thus relates the result of his observations in this disease.

"On returning to our post, about the first of October last, we were surprised at the frequent occurrence of sore fingers among our employers, and on enquiry found they were equally common in the practice of other physicians, and had been so for several months. In some families, nearly every inmate suffered more or less. Upon a large plantation in this vicinity they were so numerous as seriously to interfere with working the crop, and to lead to the suspicion that they were designedly induced in order to furnish an excuse for idleness. We learn from physicians residing at various points between this city and our northern frontier counties, that they also saw an unusual number of Whitlows during the same period. The cases commenced in July and continued to present themselves until the beginning of November. We are not informed whether such a state of things existed in the counties south of this.

"The disease generally assumed some one or other of the forms of Paronychia or Whitlow—the majority of them being superficial, and the smallest number affecting the theca of the tendons and periosteum. Although occurring spontaneously in most instances, the slightest abrasion or irritation of the finger or hand would terminate in suppuration more or less troublesome. Erysipelas complicated some of the cases, and proved fatal in one of them here.

"The season was one of the warmest and driest ever known in Georgia. The health of the city, and indeed of the whole State, is represented as having been unusually good. The supervention of cold weather put a stop to the sore fingers, and the writer has not seen one since."

It appears that this tendency to Epidemic Whitlow has existed elsewhere than in Augusta; for in the January number of the American Journal of Medical Sciences we also find a short article on the subject, by James E. Morgan, M. D., Demonstrator of Anatomy in the National Medical College at Washington. "Paronychia," says Dr. Morgan, " has, without doubt, existed in Washington this summer as an epidemic. Scarcely a day passes but that I am called upon to prescribe for several cases of this apparently trifling but always painful and sometimes fatal disease." He details the particulars of a fatal case, with the autopsy. The bronchiæ and air cells of the lungs were found infiltrated with a thick bloody mucus. The Doctor regarded this as a case of spasmodic asthma, caused by the same pathological condition of the pneumogastric nerves, which exists in the spinal nervous system in Tetanus, its mediate cause being Paronychia.

The case which terminated fatally in Augusta, it will be observed, was entirely unlike the above—here Erysipelas was the fatal complication, and not anything of a nervous character.

On the subject of this Epidemic the Reporter would beg leave to add his testimony to the prevalence of Whitlow during the time specified, it having been necessary to amputate more than one finger on this account during the past season.

Robert Campbell, M. D., Assistant Demonstrator of Anatomy in the Medical College of Georgia, has given, in the Southern Medical and Surgical Journal, the account of a case of Senile Gangrene. The patient was a white man aged about 50 years, of spare habit and in extremely bad health from intemperance. Amputation was performed by the Doctor, but the patient died five days after the operation.

This case was reported by Doctór Campbell on account of

the rareness of the disease in this region, and he has handed to the Committee the notes of two unpublished cases occurring in the practice of his brother, Dr. Henry Campbell, and himself, during the same year. The first case, was an old man aged 60 years, who first evinced symptoms of the disease by the formation of a small blackened patch on the bottom of the heel. This continued for several weeks, when the foot and limb became swollen, and finally œdematous. The disease continued to progress—delirium and fever supervened, and in consultation, amputation was decided on and accordingly performed. The delirium continued for nearly a week after the operation—but the appetite gradually returned. Brandy was freely allowed, and after the lapse of nearly eight months, the stump healed and the patient is now in the enjoyment of tolerable health, for an old drunkard, as he will be probably, to the day of his death.

In this case, the use of brandy proved highly beneficial; without it, it is our opinion, the case certainly must have terminated fatally.

The other case was that of a negro woman aged about 72 years, who, on the receipt of a slight abrasion on the ankle evinced symptoms of mortification and œdema; amputation was performed but the patient died the day succeeding the operation.

In all these cases, ossification of the arteries was without doubt, the cause of the disease.

H. V. M. Miller, M. D., Prof. of Physiology and Path. Anatomy in the Medical College of Georgia, has contributed an elaborate and highly creditable article to the pages of the Southern Medical and Surgical Journal, on Phlegmasia Dolens, and its Pathology. And the conclusion to which his observations on this subject have led, are the following: That Phlegmasia Dolens or Phlebitis is caused by the introduction of diseased matter, usually pus, into the blood—that inflammation of a vein is not an essential part of the primary affection, which precedes constitutional symptoms, *even when morbid matter has found its way into the circulation through a vein,* and that when the veins are inflamed, it is an *effect* and not the *cause* of the reception of diseased foreign matter into them.

This view of the subject, Doctor Miller strengthens by a reference to the known effect of the introduction of foreign matter, and especially pus, into the blood, as has been established by the experiments of John Hunter, and more recently of Mr. Henry Lee, of London.

This view of the Pathology of Phlegmasia Dolens is original so far as we know. The application of the effect of pus on blood is ingenious and certainly very rational.

Doctor D. C. O'Keeffe, the Secretary of the "Physicians Society for Medical Observation of Greene and adjoining counties," reports a case of uterine polypus which occurred in the practice of Doctor H. H. King, of Greenesboro. The disease occurred in the person of a negro woman, and the weight of the tumour after removal was three pounds. The tumour had been extruded from the vagina by uterine contractions previous to the operation for its removal.

A tumour of a similar nature was removed in this city during the past year, by the Reporter, though in this case, the most difficult part of the operation consisted in extracting the mass, which was the size of a child's head, from the vagina.

Robert Campbell, M. D., Assistant Demonstrator of Anatomy in Medical College of Georgia, details the particulars of a case of Ovarian tumor occurring in a child about ten years of age. This child presented an excessive abdominal protuberance, attended with general emaciation. She was attacked with fever, suffered from obstinate vomiting and in a few days died.

Post mortem examination revealed the following condition of organs: Spleen very much enlarged, peritoneum injected, especially around the tumor, which was found in the cavity of the pelvis, in the situation of the ovarium and attached to the uterus and Fallopian tubes. This tumor weighed 36 drachms and was of the color of ordinary liver. It was nodulated and slightly reniform in shape; soft almost fluctuating in its consistence. The Doctor considers it a case of encephaloid cancer. The lymphatic glands in the mesentery and in the lumbar region being very much enlarged favors somewhat this opinion.

We know that encephaloid cancer is apt to occur in any region or organ of the body, and that in youth it is more apt to . manifest itself, all the circumstances attending this case appear to establish the opinion of its encephaloid character.

Doctor O'Keeffe also reports a case occurring in his own practice, wherein urethral inflammation was produced in a female by continued use of the catheter in paralysis of the bladder.

Lastly, under the head of Surgical Pathology, we find an unusual case of Amaurosis, reported by Henry F. Campbell, M. D., of Augusta. In this case the retinæ were partially paralytic. The whole of one nerve being diseased, both eyes were consequently affected. The following is an extract from this article to the Southern Medical and Surgical Journal, vol. 7:

"At the time of our observation, the patient frequently remarked that he was very often unable to see at all with his right eye, and that when he caught a glimpse of objects they were such as were passing before him; but, as a general thing, vision was extinct in that eye.

With the other eye, exactly the reverse obtained : here, the faculty, though much impaired in its distinctness, was still generally present, but occasionally he lost sight of objects for a moment, when they would re-appear as they changed their position on the field of vision.

" In order to test the correctness of his views in regard to his case, we passed the hand slowly before each of his eyes successively, the other being closed; on the left side, he could see the hand until it reached a certain point to the right, when it would suddenly disappear, but by continuing the movement it would become again visible.   On the right side, the hand, on being passed as above, was *not* perceived till it had attained a point on the *left* exactly corresponding to the point on the *right*, at which he could not distinguish it.   This experiment we repeated frequently and invariably with the same results.

"To explain this very singular feature in this case, viz., that in the right eye vision was confined to a small portion of the retina, while the generality of this membrane was entirely amaurotic ; and that at the same time the reverse obtained in the left eye, which had most of its retina sensible to luminous inpressions, with only a small amaurotic spot, corresponding to the healthy spot in the amaurotic eye, we will review some of the peculiarities in the anatomy of this important pair of nerves.   Firstly, we know that the nervous filaments, which are to compose the optic nerves, arising on either side from the geniculate and quadrigeminal bodies, proceed through the optic tract to the chiasm. Here all of them, with the exception of a few fibres, cross over to constitute the optic nerve of the eye on the opposite side, into whose retina they are finally expanded, forming by far its greater portion ; but the few fibres which do *not cross* and only *approach* the chiasma, pass on with those from the opposite side to expand into the retina on the side from which they originate, yet from their paucity, they can supply only a very small portion of this membrane.   And, secondly, the retina of each eye is produced out of fibres from both sides of the brain—consequently the destruction or injury of either nerve behind the chiasm would affect vision in both eyes, though much more extensively in the eye opposite to the tract injured.   This is the fact illustrated in the present case.

" On a careful consideration of our case, we think the following facts in the anatomy of these nerves may be considered, in a great measure, corroborated by it : Firstly, that the theory of chiasm in the fibres of the optic nerves, is correct, and also that each nerve is engaged in the production of the retina of both eyes ; secondly, that the fibres are very unequally divided, one eye receiving by far the greater number ; and thirdly, that in their distribution to the retina the two sets of fibres, viz., the crossing and continuous, are not intermixed together forming *all* parts of the retina, but are engaged in the production of separate and distinct regions of this membrane."

SURGICAL OPERATIONS.

Under the head of *Surgical Operations*, the Committee have deemed it advisable to report those cases in which the *operation*.

has been the most important feature, either on [account of its novelty, the skill with which it was performed, or the success attending its result. A review of the journals will consequently show a somewhat greater number of operations performed during the past year, than are recorded under this head of the report, for the Committee have placed many cases in which operations have been reported, under the head of Surgical Pathology, and injuries as better deserving that position than the present.

C. T. Quintard, M. D., Prof. of Physiology and Pathological Anatomy in the Memphis Medical College, has reported a case of trepanning, in the Southern Medical and Surgical Journal, the circumstances of which are the following:

"The patient had received an injury by a stone of two pounds weight on the frontal bone near the coronal suture which produced fracture and depression followed by hæmorrhage. Coma soon supervened which lasted several days and suddenly subsided, and the patient was able to walk about—seemed conscious of surrounding objects, but had lost the power to articulate distinctly. The wound healed but there remained a fistulous opening discharging matter. Audition was much impaired, this symptom being attended with 'a constant roaring in the head.' General health good at time of operation.

"The operation of trephining was performed and the depressed bone, together with several spiculæ, removed. *Immediately—instantly* —on the removal of the bone the noise in the head ceased, and all disagreeable symptoms subsided. The wound was dressed, adhesion rapidly progressed and the case resulted in entire recovery.

"The remarkable feature in this case is the immediate and sudden relief obtained by the operation."

In the same Journal, Doctor Quintard relates the particulars of another operation, viz., Exsection of a portion of the inferior maxillary bone for the removal of an osteo-sarcomatous tumor.

The patient, a young woman aged about 14 years, in her general health, bore all the unpromising features of the cancerous cachexia. The operation was performed in the usual manner. The bone was divided with Hay's saw, first above the angle and afterwards at a point to the right of the symphisis, and the piece removed. The wound healed rapidly. Eight months had elapsed since the operation; at the time of the report no disposition to a return had been evinced. A member of this Committee had an opportunity of examining this case some months after the operation. The deformity was but trivial, and the general health of the patient appeared remarkably good.

H. M. Jeter, M. D., of Buena Vista, Ga., reports a case in which he successfully performed the Cæsarian operation. The patient was a very delicate woman, aged about 30 years; was in labor with her sixth child. She had been confined to bed for two months previous to the operation, and was affected with *general anasarca of the whole system.* After using every possible means of delivery, as turning and embriotomy, for a portion of the fœtus was delivered, and waiting as long a time as the safety of the woman would permit, finding that she was rapidly sinking, Doctor Jeter proceeded to perform the cæsarian operation, which he thus describes:

"Having given the patient a stimulant, 'I made an incision along the linea alba six inches in length, cutting down carefully to the peritoneum, upon dividing which, the head of the foetus presented, showing that my apprehensions were correct in the womb having been ruptured sometime previous to the operation. The head of the child was so large that the incision had to be extended to ten inches in length to admit its passage. The head measured twenty-nine inches and four lines in its longitudinal or occipitofrontal circumference, and twenty-eight inches two lines in its perpendicular circumference. It was hydrocephalic.' The head and remaining portion of the body being removed the placenta was also found without the uterus within the cavity of the abdomen. This was removed and the womb was found contracted down to the size of a small cocoanut, and the cavity of the abdomen filled with coagulated blood, from the hemorrhage which took place at the time of the rupture. Having carefully removed the blood, the wound was dressed by the interrupted suture and adhesive straps, leaving a space of two inches at its inferior extremity for the discharge of fluid."

The patient was extremely weak, stimulants were freely administered. Vomiting and fever gave much trouble, but these were finally relieved; the soreness in the abdomen gradually subsided, and the patient, when visited for the last time, on the 29th day after the operation, was sitting at the fire and directing the domestic affairs of her family.

Lithotrity.—Professor L. A. Dugas reports a case of Lithotrity in the Southern Medical and Surgical Journal. The patient had suffered in early childhood from Phymosis. The orifice in the prepuce being only large enough to admit a small knitting-needle, the prepuce was always distended during micturition. His general health was bad in consequence of the concomitants of retention of urine. He was relieved of all these symptoms by circumcision in his twentieth year, after which his health rapidly improved. Though he was still troubled with severe nephritic pains, he continued to attend to his usual occupation, and on urinating one day, he felt a stone fall into his bladder—a short time after, on attempting to urinate, the water was suddenly arrested by the engagement of the calculus in the urethra. These details have been given in order to establish that he did know the exact time at which the stone came into his bladder. He was shortly afterwards examined by Dr. Banks, at that time his attending physician, who readily detected the stone.

On the arrival of the patient in Augusta, Dr. Dugas, finding the stone small, determined to crush it. Dilating bougies, slippery elm tea, with the hip baths, and rest, in reclining position, were used for a week preparatory to the operation.

Heurteloup's Brisepierre, as modified by Charriere, was the instrument used. The bladder was filled with tepid water. The stone was readily seized and crushed three times on this sitting without pain. Fragments of stone passed away during that evening and next morning with the urine. There being but little irritation produced by this operation, it was repeated on the next day, and all the remaining fragments passed out during the night. The man said he was entirely relieved next morning, and Dr. Dugas could detect no fragment on the most careful examination.

The dimensions of the stone, as ascertained by the crushing instrument, were about one inch in length and half an inch in thickness. Analysis, by Prof. Means, proved it Oxalate of Lime. It was very hard.

" The features in the above case, which I deemed most interesting, are : 1st. The existence during twenty years of a Phimosis attended with almost a complete closure of the prepucial orifice, and which seriously implicated the general health of the patient before he applied for Surgical relief. 2d. The occasional recurrence of nephritic pains during ten years after circumcision, which pains finally became confined to the left side. 3d. The accurate indication by the patient of the precise moment at which the stone came into the bladder. 4th. The passage of the stone into the bladder just after micturition ; and lastly, the circumstance that a stone entered the bladder *three months* after the last nephritic attack. These are facts which, although already, perhaps, within the domain of Science, are not of very frequent occurrence. Such may be on record, but I do not remember a case in which the knowledge of the precise moment at which the stone came into the bladder, is so well established."

Lithotomy.—In the same volume of the Southern Medical and Surgical Journal, we find recorded three cases of Lithotomy ; one performed by W. Nephew King, M. D., of Roswell. subject a child 7 years of age. Bilateral operation perfectly successful. The stone measured in its greatest diameter two-thirds of an inch, and in its shortest one-third of an inch, and was composed of the Oxalate of Lime.

The two other cases are reported by Henry F. Campbell, M. D., of Augusta. The first patient was a young man 18 years of age. Bilateral operation. Amount of calculous matter removed, one ounce and a half. Composition, Uric Acid deposit, formed into three separate calculi of nearly equal size.

The second case was a child 8 years old. Bilateral operation. Here there was but one calculus composed of the Oxalate of Lime, the largest diameter of which was one inch and three-tenths, the shortest diameter seven-tenths of an inch. Weight, two drachms and one scruple immediately after the operation.

The reporter will also here refer to another case unpublished, operated on in this State by himself during the last month. The patient, a child 4 years of age, a native of Ireland, had been troubled with symptoms of Stone from a very early age, shortly after birth. We made the Bilateral operation; removed three calculi of about the size of a chestnut. The case progressed regularly, and like the other two cases referred to, was followed by entire recovery. The great peculiarity of this case, is the extremely tender age at which the patient began to evince symptoms of the disease. We know of not less than three children who are Irish immigrants, all of whom have been affected with stone from a very early age—two of them were of one family. We cannot attribute this to the change of climate entirely, as two of them were subjects of the disease before leaving the land of their nativity.

Juriah Harriss, M. D., of Augusta, has contributed to the pages of the Southern Medical and Surgical Journal, a valuable article on Fissure of the Anus, in which he develops the treatment by sudden dilatation of M. Maisonneuve, of Paris, which, as he remarks, is really a revival of Recamier's treatment; the only difference between the two being, that Recamier recommended the gradual, and Maisonneuve the rapid dilatation of the Sphincter ani in those cases which depend upon its permanent contraction. The Doctor thus describes the operation as performed by M. Maisonneuve:

" The process he recommends is to introduce the index fingers of both hands into the anal orifice and to dilate forcibly the contracted muscle, first in the antero posterior diameter, and then transversely. This simple and almost instantaneous operation removes the cause or the most important feature of the disease."

As the Doctor remarks, this operation possesses many advantages over other modes of operation : 1st, no cutting instrument is used ; 2nd, no wound is left to heal ; 3rdly, there is no

danger of Phlebitis, and lastly, the pain, which is but momenta-
ry, can be entirely avoided by the use of Anæsthetics.

We would certainly recommend this mode of treatment, except in cases complicated with hemorrhoids, as occurred to the
reporter of this committee a few months since. Here the case
was relieved by repeated cauterization with the Nitrate of
Silver.

The same gentleman also reports a case of Phymosis in
which he operated upon Ricord's plan with Phymosis forceps.

Doctor King, of Roswell, reports a case of Comminuted
Fracture of the Leg, wherein he amputated for mortification,
which afterwards attacked the stump and produced a fatal termination. The patient was of a Cachectic Diathesis and quite
anæmic.

SURGICAL MEDICINE AND TREATMENT.

Under this head, the Committee have reported all surgical
cases coming under their notice in which the treatment presented any thing of novelty, or was attended with any marked
degree of success.

John S. Wilson, M. D., of Muscogee county, has furnished
to the pages of the Southern Medical and Surgical Journal, a
short treatise on the internal and external application of the
Nitrate of Silver, in which he details the particulars of several
pertinent cases. The surgical applications of the remedy recommended by Dr. Wilson are its application to Ulcers of the
Leg, Stomatitis, Metritis and to Anginose and Herpetic affections. And also in Ophthalmia, Opacity of Cornea, &c.

Tetanus.—W. W. Haws, M. D., of Houston county, reports
a case of undoubted Tetanus, treated by himself with success.
The disease resulted from frost-bite, attended with loss of the
toes—therefore came under the class Traumatic—was quite
violent. Treatment consisted in the administration of calomel, opium, quinine, with veratrum viride, and Indian hemp,
together with the application of general bathing and extensive
revulsion. Case lasted from the 11th to about the 23d of Janu-
ry. " He rested on his nates and occiput all the time of his
illness, except one day and night, and then, opisthotonos was
complete. The Indian hemp which I used," says the Doctor,
" presented all the physical qualities of a fine article, but was
certainly devoid of all the fine action ascribed to it by Doctor
O'Shaughnessy. The quinine seemed entirely out of place; it
proved rather conservative of the spasm, than otherwise, and
I attribute the sudden increase in the violence of the disease on
its administration, to this drug alone. The veratrum viride

effected such sedation as to give unwonted potency to the Dover's powder, and it was for this I stopped it, feeling confident
I could continue the sedation as well with the Dover's powder
alone, as with the hellebore, and secure a more decided action
upon the gastro-enteric function."

Our attention has been called to a similar case of Traumatic
Tetanus, treated by Dr. Hart, of this city.   Cause, injury from a
plank falling on the occiput.   Treatment, which was successful,
principally consisted in large doses of morphine in combination
with chloroform.   Indian hemp was also used without any
known good effect.

Dislocations and Fractures.—In the Southern Medical and
Surgical Journal, Professor Dugas has given the report of seven cases of Dislocation of the Radius and Ulna backwards at
the elbow.   His remarks on the extreme difficulty of the diagnosis of this injury are very pertinent, but more especially
would we call attention to his suggestion in the application of
forces, for the reduction of the bones, for these, we think, in
certain particulars are original and peculiar.   Referring to Sir
A. Cooper, Liston, Miller and Druitt, the Doctor says, "with
due deference to these high authorities, I think a very important element in the mechanism of this process has been overlooked, which, if borne in mind by the surgeon, will materially
increase the chances of success.   I allude to the *lever power*
secured by using the olecranon, as a fulcrum for dislodging the
coronoid process from the posterior fossa of the humerus.   This
effect will be readily perceived if the reader will place the
bones of a skeleton in the position they would occupy in this
dislocation, then gradually extend those of the forearm, making
at the same time gradual traction.   It will be found, that the resistance offered to reduction is principally produced by the
lodgment of the coronoid process in this fossa—but that as soon
as the extension is carried *a little beyond the straight line*, the
olecranon will rest upon the humerus ; the coronoid process
will rise from the fossa and the bones will promptly slip down
into their proper position.   The surgeon should therefore carry the forearm a little farther back than the straight line, with
the humerus, if he wishes to derive all the advantages of this
method of reduction.   It is scarcely necessary to say that if
the dislocation resist a certain degree of force, whether applied
with the arm flexed or extended, prudence should dictate a
cessation of our efforts rather than hazard the consequences of
such lacerations as might be produced, especially in old cases
and with pullies."

In the February number of the Southern Medical and Surgical Journal of the present year, there is also an article on Fractures of the Clavicle, by Doctor Dugas, in which the Doctor gives his mode of treatment, which, on account of its simplicity, as well as efficiency, we think worthy of attention. In the following we find embodied all the important points of his treatment:

"The sling bandage is that to which I have given a decided preference for the last fifteen or twenty years. It is unnecessary to describe the numerous modifications of this simple bandage, proposed by surgeons of all countries, and I will therefore proceed to describe at once the one I habitually use, without, for a moment, pretending to originality, lest perhaps some book-worm might discover that *precisely* the same had been proposed by others.

"The displacement having been carefully reduced by movements of the shoulder in various directions, according to the particular case and by direct action upon the fragments themselves, let an aid maintain the reduction by placing the ends of the fingers of the affected limb upon the top of the opposite shoulder by bringing the elbow against the side, and by pressing up the elbow so as to carry the shoulder upwards, outwards and backwards, as will be done under those circumstances. The next step will be to secure the limb in this position. For this purpose, I procure a square yard of cotton fabric, (unbleached shirting, for example, as this is softer than the bleached, which is usually starched,) and cut it diagonally, so as to obtain a triangular bit; to the acute angles of which should be sewed slips three inches wide and three or four yards long.

"Apply the middle of the base or long side of the triangle beneath the elbow, leaving a margin of about two inches behind, and carrying the obtuse angle towards the fingers. One of the acute angles with its strip, will now be carried between the arm and chest, up to the fractured clavicle, around the back of the neck over the shoulder, in front and beneath the axilla and finally around the chest including the arm just above the elbow. The other end and strip will be carried in front of the forearm, up to the sound shoulder, behind and beneath the axilla, and around the chest and arm so as to meet its fellow, and to be tied to it firmly. The margin left projecting behind the elbow should then be elevated, doubled, and so secured with stitches as to prevent the elbow from sliding out of the sling in that direction. The portion of the triangle situated along the forearm should be also folded around it, and thus secured. Lastly, the strips encircling the chest and arm should be stitched, to prevent the upward and downward displacement. If it be necessary to press down the sternal fragment, this can be effectually done by interposing a little pad between the bone and the bandage which passes over it.

"The advantages of this bandage are to be found in its perfect adaptation to the necessities of the case, in its great simplicity, in the facility with which it may be made secure, and in the very slight inconvenience to which it subjects the patient. Children as well as

adults bear it without murmur ; and if it becomes necessary for purposes of cleanliness to remove it, any intelligent mother or nurse may
re-apply it, if the physician be not accessible. Whilst it cannot be
denied that under any plan of treatment, there will occasionally remain some unevenness or deformity at the seat of fracture, I must say
that I have very rarely seen any thing of the kind in cases treated on
this plan, notwithstanding the fact that I have not unfrequently, after
applying the bandage once in the presence of the mother, left the subsequent management entirely to herself."

In closing this part of their Report, this Committee would
express their regret that they have found the contributions on
the important subject of Fractures and Dislocations so few ;
for here, it is well known, rests the opprobrium of American
Surgery, and here the French and English practitioners have
been, to the present time, our superiors. It appears—and we
should confess it with much regret—that the treatment of these
injuries have been regarded as of secondary importance by our
countrymen. The broken bone, when properly mended, tells
no history of the skill with which it was managed, but the mutilated and useless limb through which the knife has passed,
marks, on a glance, that here has been the Surgeon, the brilliant
and bold operator. Hence less attention has been paid to them
than they actually deserve, and their treatment is therefore often
unsatisfactory in its results. It seems that unless there is something to *cut*, something to destroy and leave a memento of our
exploits, we do not regard the affection of the first importance
surgically. We would therefore take this occasion to urge,
most respectfully; on the practitioners of our State, a greater
amount of attention to this important and much neglected department of Surgery.

> HENRY F. CAMPBELL, Ch'n.
> J. M. GREEN,
> GEORGE F. COOPER,   Committee.
> R. J. RODDY,
> J. M. SIMMONS,

Augusta, Ga., April 14, 1852.

On the Value of Local Treatment in Traumatic Tetanus.
By Mr. Eddomes.

[Mr. Eddomes narrates the case of a man in whom tetanic
symptoms supervened upon a wound of the thumb with a packing needle. The symptoms came on three days after cicatrization. The treatment consisted in removing the cicatrix, and
applying morphine to the wound. A blistered surface was
also made in the opposite hand, which was also sprinkled with

morphine. He stated that the spasms never became general, and that the stiffness of the jaws did not entirely subside till the eleventh day. The author appends the following remarks:]

There are many points of interest in this case, and I would wish to call attention to one or two of them.

1. *This man's symptoms first came on after the healing of the wound,*—a circumstance by no means unusual, though I am not aware that any reasons have been given why such should be the case. I think that one of Dr. M. Hall's experiments, showing that the extreme terminations of nerves possess the excito-motory power in a much higher degree than the trunk, will help us to furnish an explanation. "If," says he, "after removing the head of a frog, we divide the integuments along the back, and raise them by means of the forceps, we observe the *trunks* of many cutaneous nerves. Now, if we irritate these trunks no movements follow; but if we irritate the cutaneous texture on which they ramify, movements of a *very energetic nature* are produced." Now, in the healing process of a wound it must be evident that the extreme distributions of the cutaneous nerves would only be involved when that process was nearly or wholly completed. And may it not be the involving these, the more easily excited terminal branches, that is the starting point of the disease. Another point of interest in this case is—

2. *He had spasm of the wounded hand and arm as one of the earliest symptoms; it continued throughout, and at last was the only remnant of the disease.*—This condition is not a reflected one, but the result of disease in the reflex or motor nerve; while, on the other hand, the trismus, with the affection of the abdominal muscles and legs are reflected, resulting from injury to an incident or exciter nerve. Had the spasm been a reflected action, we should have had the opposite extremity affected in a similar manner; and it would not have occurred till later in the disease. I merely mention this as being a curious and interesting circumstance, showing that the injury to a reflex nerve is more persistent, and less easily influenced by remedies, than an injury to an incident nerve.

3. *The treatment of traumatic tetanus.*—It is needless to say what a formidable and intractable disease it has always been found; but I believe that the ill success has in some measure resulted from not acting upon proper principles in the treatment. Look over the melancholy records of this affection, and what has been the treatment? Venesection, narcotics, antispasmodics, mercury, cold bath, warm bath, and a hundred other plans—all given to affect the system *generally;* while the seat of irritation, the primum mobile of the disease, is en-

tirely passed over, or receives only a secondary share of attention.

I would suggest that such plan of treatment is most unphilosophical, and that the treatment should *begin* at the seat of
irritation, to allay which should be our first and most strenuous
effort.

In conclusion, I would remark that, in the treatment of the
present case, all I claim is, that it is simple and rational. Is it
not simple to apply a soothing remedy to an irritated part? Is
it not rational, when a *morbid stimulus* is transmitted from one
extremity of the spinal cord, to be reflected on the system at
large, to transmit a *sedative influence* to the spinal cord at the
opposite extremity; a morbid stimulus from the left hand, and
a sedative influence from the right, meeting at the same portion
of the cord.—[*Medical Gazette.*

Total removal of the Collar Bone. By A. J. WEDDERBURN,
   Prof. of Anatomy, in the University of Louisiana.

Michael Foggerty, age 21 years, a labourer, was admitted
into the wards of the Charity Hospital on the 21st of January,
1852, with caries of the clavicle, so extensive as to require its
entire removal, by disarticulation at both extremities. The
operation was made whilst the subject was under the influence
of chloroform.

OPERATION.—An incision was made down to the bone over
its entire length, and sufficiently far beyond its articulating
points, to enable the disarticulation to be effected. The soft
parts attached to the upper surface and the anterior border of
the bone, were separated—next the separation from the acromion effected—the dissection was then continued close to the
bone beneath, whilst the parts were kept on the stretch, by elevating the bone from the point just indicated. During the dissection the bone broke, from its diseased condition, about one and
a half inches from its sternal articulation, which rendered the
dissection connected with this portion of the bone more tedious
than it would have been, had there been a sufficient length of
bone left to have given a purchase. For the removal of such
a diseased part as this, there can be no established mode of
operation. Circumstances must always govern. Caution and
a thorough knowledge of the region, is all that is necessary to
make such operations simple and easy. The result of this
operation was perfectly successful—recovery was rapid, and
the case was discharged cured, towards the last of April, in
something less than three months after the operation. When
the case left the hospital, the use of the arm was perfect, the

shoulder occupied its natural position ; it was neither depressed, projected forward, or drawn nearer the sternum, and no other evidence presented that a operation had been made, than the cicatrix.   He was discharged on the 8th of April.

TREATMENT.—The cavity from which the bone was removed was filled with lint saturated with a solution of quinine, and kept in this condition for twenty-four hours.   The next day the cut surface was brought together with adhesive plaster, over which was placed a compress of lint, wet with a solution of quinine, about 5 grains to the ounce of water.   No other treatment was resorted to during the cure.   The shock from the operation was so slight, that he was sitting up in twenty-four hours after the removal of the bone.   The solution of quinine was chiefly used in this case for its prophylactic effects against erysipelas, which was prevailing in the hospital at the time.

The total removal of the collar-bone has been done but twice before in this country.—By Dr. Valentine Mott, in its successful removal for osteosarcoma of the left clavicle, in 1828, and also, by Dr. Warren, in 1833.   In Europe, it has been made by Meyer and Roux, on account of caries; by Travers, "on a boy of ten years of age, who, in consequence of a fall probably broke the collar-bone, without rupturing the periosteum, had large effusions of blood within it, which formed a tumor, that by degrees involved and destroyed nearly the whole bone, except at its sternal end."—[*New Orleans Med. Register.*

Case of Hermaphrodism, involving the Operation of Castration and illustrating a new principle in Juridical Medicine. By S. D. GROSS, M. D., Professor of Surgery in the Medical Department of the University of Louisville.

The following case, which came under my observation in 1849, will, if I mistake not, prove both novel and interesting to my professional brethren.   So far as my information extends, there is no account of any operation for a similar object upon record.

The subject of the case, at the time I first saw her, was three years of age, having been born on the 10th of July, 1846.   She had always, up to this period, been regarded as a girl, and had been so pronounced at her birth by the accoucheur.   At the age of two, however, she began to evince the tastes, disposition, and feelings of the other sex; she rejected dolls and similar articles of amusement, and became fond of boyish sports.   She was well-grown, perfectly healthy, and quite fleshy.   Her hair was dark and long, the eyes black, and the whole expression most agreeable.   A careful examination of the external geni-

tals disclosed the following circumstances :—There was neither
a penis nor a vagina; but, instead of the former, there was a
small clitoris, and, instead of the latter, a superficial depression,
or *cul-de-sac*, covered with mucous membrane, and devoid of
everything like an aperture, or inlet. The urethra occupied
the usual situation, and appeared to be entirely natural; the
nymphæ were remarkably diminutive; but the labia were all
developed, and contained each a well formed testis, quite as
large and consistent as this organ generally is at the same age
in boys. Her hips and chest, thighs and superior extremities,
were perfect.

It being apparent, from the facts of the case, that it was one
of malformation of the genital organs usually denominated
hermaphrodism, the question occurred whether any thing could
or ought to be done to deprive the poor child of that portion of
the genital apparatus which, if permitted to remain until the
age of puberty, would be sure to be followed by sexual desire,
and which might thus conduce to the establishment of a matri-
monial connection. Such an alliance, it was evident, could
eventuate only in chagrin and disappointment, if not in dis-
grace, ruin of character, or even loss of life. Certainly, impregnation could never occur, and even copulation could not
be performed, except in the most imperfect manner.

I need not say that I gave the subject all the consideration
and reflection that I was capable of bestowing upon it. I was
deeply sensible of the responsibility of my position. A new
question involving the rights and happiness of my little patient,
and the dearest interests of her parents, was presented to me.
I examined the case in all its bearings and relations—moral,
physical, and juridical; I appealed to the records of my profession
for a precedent, and I sought the counsel of medical friends.
The parents were anxious for an operation; they were intelligent, kind, and tender-hearted, and were willing to sacrifice
everything for the welfare of their child. Their only object
was to save it from future suffering and misfortune. My own
mind was made up; but, before I proceeded to take any further
steps, I determined to consult my excellent friend and colleague,
Professor Miller, in whose judgment and integrity every one
who knows him has the utmost confidence. He saw the child
and examined her. He viewed the case, as I had previously,
in every possible aspect, and his conclusion was, that excision
of the testes was not only justifiable but eminently proper under
the circumstances; that it would be an act of kindness and of
humanity to the poor child, standing as she did towards society
in the relation, not of a boy or a girl, but of a neuter, to deprive
her of an appendage of so useless a nature; one which might, if

allowed to proceed in its development, ultimately lead to the ruin of her character and peace of mind.

Backed by such authority, I no longer hesitated what course to pursue. I performed the operation of castration on the 20th of July, 1849, aided by my pupils, Dr. D. D. Thompson, of this city, Dr. Greenburg R. Henry, of Burlington, Iowa, and Dr. William H. Cobb, formerly of Louisville, now of Cincinnati. The little patient being put under the influence of Chloroform, I made a perpendicular incision, about two inches in length, into each labium down to the testis, which was then carefully separated from the surrounding structures, and detached by dividing the lower part of the spermatic cord. The arteries of the cord being secured with ligatures, the edges of the wound were brought together with twisted sutures, and the child put to bed. Hardly any blood was lost during the operation. About two hours after, the left labium became greatly distended and discolored; and, upon removing the sutures, the source of the mischief was found to be a small artery, which was immediately drawn out and tied. No unpleasant symptom of any kind ensued after this, and in a week the little patient was able to be up, being quite well and happy.

The testes were carefully examined after removal, and were found to be perfectly formed in every respect. The spermatic cords were natural.

I have seen this child repeatedly since the operation, as her parents live only a few squares from my office, and have carefully watched her mental and physical development. Her disposition and habits have materially changed, and are now those of a girl; she takes great delight in sewing and housework, and she no longer indulges in riding sticks and other boyish exercises. Her person is well developed, and her mind uncommonly active for a child of her years.

I would fain present this example as a precedent in similar cases. The reasons which induced me to recommend and perform this operation in the instance before me have been already mentioned, and now, after a lapse of three years, I have no cause to regret the undertaking, or to think that I acted harshly and inconsiderately. If the records of surgery and medical jurisprudence are silent upon the subject; if the learned doctors of the Sorbonne, the fathers of the Royal Academy of Paris, and the Fellows of the Royal College of London have left us no precepts; and if the experience of the present day furnishes no examples; all this, and much more, does not prove that the practice here recommended is not perfectly just and proper, and vindicated upon every principle of science and humanity.

A defective organization of the external genitals is one of the most dreadful misfortunes that can possibly befall any human being. There is nothing that exerts so baneful an influence over his moral and social feelings, which carries with it such a sense of self-abasement and mental degradation, or which so thoroughly "maketh the heart sick," as the conviction of such an individual that he is forever debarred from the joys and pleasures of married life, an outcast from society, hated and despised, and reviled and persecuted by the world. Nothing but the most perfect resignation, and a well-founded confidence in the mercy and justice of the Creator, can render the lot of such a being at all supportable.—[*Amer. Journ. of Med. Sci.*

We doubt that many of our readers will agree with the distinguished Professor in the validity of the reasons assigned for the above operation. This will certainly not obviate the evils so forcibly set forth in the last paragraph by the author.

[Ed. s. m. & s. j.

Extract of Belladonna in Hooping Cough.

Dr. H. Corson, of Pennsylvania, recommends (Am. Journ. Med. Sc.) very highly the use of Belladonna in Pertussis, and states that he rarely fails to arrest the disease in from one to three weeks. This remedy was proposed nearly 20 years ago by Dr. Jackson of Northumberland, and has since that been occasionally referred to in the periodicals. We have frequently tried it alone, and in combination with camphor and carbonate of iron, but have seldom succeeded in arresting the cough, except in cases which had already existed several weeks, and which had therefore nearly run their usual course. Dr. Jackson prescribed it in doses of 1 gr. to a child 2 years of age; but Dr. Corson thinks this too much, and gives, of a solution of 8 grs. in 1 oz. water, to those under one year of age 9 drops every 2 hours until the pupils are dilated, the face flushed, the mouth dry, and vision confused. The dose to be increased or diminished according to effects—but to be given daily. [Ed. s. m. & s. j.

Nitric Acid in Rain-Water.

M. Barral has lately found, after very careful and well-conducted experiments, which stretched over more than six months, that the rain-water collected at Paris contains appre-

ciable quantities of nitric acid.   This discovery has been confirmed by a committee appointed by the Academy of Sciences,
and composed of Messrs. Dumas, Boussingault, Gasparin,
Regnalt, and Arago.   It is supposed that the presence of nitric
acid in rain-water will explain certain hitherto ill-understood
telluric phenomena, and lead to some practical applications.
It is due to Dr. Bence Jones, of St. George's Hospital, to say,
that he had already pointed out the fact, in the *Philosophical
Transactions* of 1851, as to the rain-water collected at Kings-
ton (Surrey), Melburg (Dorset), the neighborhood of Cork, and
in London.   Dr. Bence Jones was herein in opposition with
Liebig, who has denied that rain-water contained appreciable
quantities of nitric acid.—[*Lancet.*

Yeast in the treatment of Boils.

Mr. Mosse, in a communication in the *Lancet*, July 31, 1852,
states that, "During a period of eight years and more, being
in practice in the West of England, where these annoyances
rather raged, and were known by the name of 'pinswills,' I
was induced to try the efficacy of common yeast (having failed
to give relief in general modes of treatment), in doses of a
tablespoonful with some water three times a day, for an adult,
and smaller doses for children.

"I have now practised in this town nearly six years, and
have had frequent opportunities also here of witnessing the
good effect of yeast in these troublesome affections, easily con-
summating a rapid and complete cure without further recurrence, and by a most simple remedy, within reach of all."

[*Medical News.*

Lateral Hermaphroditism.

Dr. Banon brought before the notice of the Surgical Socie.
ty of Ireland (May 1, 1852) a very remarkable instance of
lateral hermaphroditism—a fusion of the generative organs of
both sexes.   The subject of it had died of phthisis.   Dr. B.
had not become acquainted with the sexual peculiarities of this
individual until shortly before death.   Dr. B. ascertained, however, that at the birth of the individual there was considerable
doubt as to the predominant sex, but that at length it was pro.
nounced to be a female, and baptized by the name of "Anne."
In a year subsequently, however, the organ representing the
penis had so increased in size that a different conclusion was
arrived at, and the name changed to "Andrew," since which
period he had been always treated and looked on as a male ;

and as he grew up, even excelled in many of the manly exercises. His predilections were, according to his own statement, for females, and it was ascertained that he had never
menstruated.

Dr. Banon gave a full and minute description of the external
and internal organs of generation which were present in this
individual, by which it appeared that he possessed a penis of
the usual size in the male adult, and provided with glans and
prepuce, but that it was imperforate, a rudimentary opening
only existing in the site of the orifice of the urethra. The individual had himself stated that it was, during life, subject to
erections. On raising up the penis, Dr. Banon observed that
the female external organs were present in a nearly perfect
condition. The labia were well marked, but terminated behind
rather abruptly, the fourchette being absent. Within these the
nymphæ were seen occupying their usual situation, and between them there was a longitudinal opening which led directly to the bladder. Behind this urethral opening was observed
one of a more circular form leading to a canal in the direction
of the uterus, and separated from the bladder in front and the
rectum behind by distinct septa. This orifice was so small as
to admit only of a No. 8 catheter, and was surrounded posteriorly by a distinct hymen. The mons veneris was not developed, which might have been owing to the great emaciation
present. Many of the secondary characters of the male were
observed. The hair, arms, hands, lower limbs and feet, the
larynx, all partook of the male character. The voice, during
life, was decidedly masculine.

On the other hand, there was a feminine character in the
features of the upper part of the face, and the pelvis and skull
were decidedly those of the female. The occipital regions of
the latter were unequally developed on each side, which point
was dwelt upon by Dr. Banon as illustrating, in this instance,
the interesting physiological fact, that the development of the
reproductive organs is influenced by this portion of the brain,
these organs being, as he afterwards pointed out, situated principally on the side of the body opposite that of the increased development in the posterior lobes of the cerebrum and cerebellum.

On dissection, the penis was found to be composed of cruræ,
uniting in the usual manner to form the body. A substance
similar to the corpus spongiosum urethræ, could be traced anteriorly to the glans, and behind becoming bifurcated to inclose
the longitudinal opening leading to the bladder. The prostate
and Cowper's glands were absent. The spermatic cord on the
right side was large. On the left, it rather deserved the name
of the round ligament of the female.

On dissecting the parts within the pelvis, a well-formed but small uterus was found in its normal position between the bladder and rectum. It was supplied with but one Fallopian tube, which passed from its left cornu backwards and inwards, between the rectum and uterus, to the right side of the latter, where it terminated in a well-marked "corpus fimbriatum," being permeable throughout its whole course.

The corpus fimbriatum rested on an ovary which, as well as the Fallopian tube, was single, no trace of a second being visible. Not far removed, however, from the ovary already mentioned, was observed a testis, pendulous into the true pelvis, in front of the right sacro-iliac synchondrosis, and immediately behind the internal iliac artery, as it decends into the pelvis. Applled to its anterior surface was seen the epididymis in a partially unravelled state, and the spermatic artery and vein were traced into close connection with it. The vas deferens was plainly seen emerging from the epydidymis, and taking a remarkable course—at first, forwards and outwards, in the direction of the right internal abdominal ring, to which it had reached about half way, when it turned back, forming a loop, with the convexity towards the ring: it then took its course inwards and somewhat backwards in the direction of the uterus, to which it was finally conducted by the broad ligament of the right side. It could be traced into the substance of the uterus, into the cavity of which Dr. Banon proved that it opened by pressing mercury gently through it. Dr. Banon could not find any trace of vesiculæ seminales, nor of a second testicle. Dr. Banon here gave a minute description of his dissection of the different organs, and of the appearances of some of them under the microscope, which enabled him to speak with confidence of their identity. He then entered at some length into the discussion of the means of discriminating between the spurious forms of hermaphroditism and those which are entitled to be considered as a real blending together of the reproductive organs of both sexes, or the "true hermaphroditism;" and cited some remarkable cases, both in the human subject and the lower classes of animals, in which both forms had been observed. In the present instance, he came to the conclusion that it should be placed under the division of "true hermaphroditism," termed "lateral," by Professor Simpson. Dr. Banon also alluded to some of the most interesting of the physiological changes which take place in the earlier development of the embryo, and explained how an error of function at this period in the corpora Wolffiana, by which both the male and female reproductive organs, the testes and ovaries, are originally formed, would be likely to cause subsequent anormalities and malformations to appear. He also entered into the question—How far the conditions necessary for self-impregnation were present in the case of Andrew R. ? And although he was obliged to admit that were the testis by any means so excited as to cause its secretion to pass through the vas deferens into the uterus, there was nothing to prevent the semen from proceeding farther, through the Fallopian tube, to the ovary ; still, from the absence of the procreative elements (the spermatozoa) in the seminal fluid, as proved by the microscope, and also of the germinating elements of the ovary, self-impregnation in this instance could not have occurred. Dr. Banon concluded a highly interesting paper by stating that it was his intention to publish it in full, and bring it before the profession in a form rendered complete by the addition of lithographic plates of the drawings and casts which he had now the pleasure of exhibiting to the Society.—[*Dublin Medical Press.*

Miscellany.

A Case of Doubtful Paternity.

By W. L. SUTTON, M. D., Pres't. of the Med. Society of Kentucky.

What distinguishes a child of pure White blood, from one tainted with that of the Negro ? About a fortnight ago, a child was brought to Georgetown by its reputed father, accompanied by his physician, a gentleman of some forty-five or fifty years, for examination by the physicians of the town, partly with a view of ascertaining whether any course could be suggested which would insure the continuance of its life, and partly to silence some neighborhood talk which had arisen on account of its color. The physician believed that the color of the child was occasioned by the foramen ovale remaining open; in proof of this, he alleged that when the child cried he became much darker— decidedly blue—and thought that the imperfect aëration of the blood consequent upon the patent condition of the foramen, was sufficient to account for the permanent dark color of the skin. Another physician who had seen the child at two months old, believed then that he labored under inflammation of the brain, and, from some cause, suspected the foramen ovale was open. Among other things he suggested a trial of the advice of Prof. Meigs, respecting position.

The moral testimony in the case was, that up to the birth of the child, the mother had been entirely above suspicion. In fact, she was considered a very modest woman. She was said to have fair complexion, light hair, and blue eyes. The husband, who accompanied the child, had nothing remarkable as to complexion ; hair of the ordinary brownish color. His mother reported to be very dark, with black hair.

The child is a boy of four months, with black, straight hair, the fine hair on the forehead black ; rounded forehead, broad nose, partic-ularly expanded at the alæ, skin dark, yet not darker than purely white children are sometimes seen. Near the extremity of the coccyx, and rather to one side, was a spot, oval in shape, about three-fourths of an inch long, decidedly dark. No other dark spot perceived. There is a popular notion that when a child is tainted with African blood, the scrotum and a streak down the back are always dark. Nothing of that kind existed.

Three physicians (the one who had seen the child at two months, among them,) were unanimous that the color did not depend on cyano-sis, and that there were appearances about the child of very suspicious tendency ; but declined any expression as to admixture of blood, without a better acquaintance with the relatives of the husband and wife. One, however, could not believe that two parents of the temperament of the husband and wife, could produce a child of that color. Another thought it possible that with a grandmother decidedly dark, a child might be even that dark ; but could see no good reason why a child purely white should have such a nose. The third thought that although the appearances were suspicious, they were not enough so to give an opinion unfavorable to a woman as free from suspicion as the mother had been.

The family physician, who had unshaken faith in the chastity of the woman, expressed his unfeigned astonishment that any hesitation should be felt in giving an opinion tending to exculpate the mother from all suspicion. Not satisfied with the result of this consultation, he procured the attendance of some five or six others at the residence of the parties. These last, I understand, took very much the same view of the case that had been taken in the consultation.

Subsequently it is reported that the woman acknowledged that she had had occasional connection with two negro men in the neighbor-hood.

As this is a point which has been but little investigated, (some little discussion in Beck's Medical Jurisprudence being all that I am aware of,) it may not be amiss to make a few comments. Many persons think nothing would be easier than to "tell a white child from a black one;" but like a great many other things, the more it is studied, the more difficulties start up. From the nature of things, our European brethren give us no authority upon this point. Beck, vol. 1, p. 485, gives us a case which occurred in New York. In this case, a mulatto woman swore a child to a black man. On trial, when the child was one year and seven months old, it appeared in evidence "that the child was somewhat dark, but lighter than the generality of mulattoes ; and that its hair was straight, and had none of the peculiarities of the negro race. Many of the most eminent members of the medical pro-fession were examined, and they all, with the exception of Dr. Mitchill, declared that its appearance contradicted the idea that it was the child of a black man. Dr. Mitchill, for various reasons, placed great faith in the oath of the female, and persisted in his belief of its paternity, although he allowed its appearance was an anomaly. The Mayor

(Hon De-Witt Clinton) and the Court decided in favor of Whistelo,"
i. e. that the child was by a white man.

Dunglison ridicules the opinion of Dr. Mitchill. But Mitchill was altogether as respectable in the profession, and probably as cautious as Dunglison. Beck comments upon the above case as follows: "It will not do, however, to extend this rule too positively with what may be called *mixed breed.*"

Parsons gives an account in the Philosophical Transactions of a black man married to an English woman, of whom the offspring was quite black. In a similar case, the child resembled its mother in fairness of features, and indeed the whole skin was white, except some spots on the thigh, which were as black as the father.

White, in his work on the *Gradation of Man,* mentions a negress who had twins by an Englishman. One was perfectly black, its hair short, woolly, and curled; the other was white, with hair resembling that of an European.

So, also, Dr. Winterbottom knew a family of six persons, one-half of which were almost as light colored as mulattoes, while the other was jet black. The father was a deep black, the mother a mulatto.

"The offspring of a black and white," says Lawrence, "may be either black or white, instead of being mixed, and in some rare cases it has been spotted."

I have made the above extensive extract from Beck, (which is all he says on the subject,) because of the liability of such cases to arise in this community, where we have not only the white and black races, but every conceivable degree of mixture. In a note to the above extract, Beck adverts to the fact that, "At birth it [the new-born black infant] cannot be always distinguished from the white; its hair has not yet its peculiar make, and we can only notice the tendency to dark on some parts of the body. In a few days, however, the change commences on the countenance, and gradually extends over the body." This is rather too positive. In many cases, a child of purely black parents is so white at birth as to exhibit no "tendency to dark" on any part of the body; and like other changes, this sometimes takes place much more slowly than in others.

There is much truth in the extracts made by Beck above, as careful examination of our mulattoes will shew. In this town there is a family—the father half white, the mother three-fourths—whose children vary very much in color. Some being pretty good samples of the negro, and others, at five or six years old, not only as white as most white children, but having straight and light-colored hair.

The spots spoken of in the above extracts are certainly rare; nor do I know to how much consideration they are entitled. There was one on the child which gives rise to these remarks. On the other hand, without being able at this time to refer to any particular case, I am certainly under the impression that I have seen persons, entirely free from suspicion of admixture, who had a dark spot on some part of the body. I, some time since, owned a negress who clearly had no white blood in her, yet she had a large spot on the forehead and temples greatly darker than her skin in other parts.

The hair, although a very important feature, is not conclusive in determining our judgment. It does not necessarily begin to assume its distinctive character in a few days, as we might infer from the expression of Beck. In half-breeds, generally, it is only curly, and not knappy, as in the negro; frequently it is no more curly than occurs occasionally in persons purely white; whilst again it is as knappy as in the negro.

It seems that no reliance can be placed upon the popular notion that the scrotum and skin over the spine are dark in children having an admixture of African blood. I have examined several children of six to eight years old without finding it in any of them; they were however, more than half white—some two-thirds, some three-fourths.

We must pay some attention to what is called moral testimony, but that like other considerations, must be watched. The above case shows how guilty a woman may be, and yet escape suspicion.

In stating facts, I have gone upon the presumption that they were really as they appeared. For instance, in the family referred to as living in this town. Some of the children *may* be by fathers purely white, and others by those wholly black. I can only say that no suspicion attaches.

The case cited in which an Englishman impregnated a negress, one child being white and the other black, may be as reported, yet we have a case reported of a woman in Virginia having connexion with her husband, and very soon afterwards with a negro man, and becoming impregnated by both.

There is, perhaps, no subject connected with our profession which presents more knotty points than this. For this reason—and because no one knows when he may be consulted upon such a case, and further as we have so little authority on this point, and because the country South of Mason & Dixon's line could and ought to furnish the facts and authority upon this subject—I have thrown together the above facts and suggestions, in hope that they may be a means of drawing others out on the same subject.—[*Western Med. and Sur. Journal.*

Report on Variola and Vaccination.

[The following Report relates to a subject of so much interest both to the profession and the community, that we think we shall be performing a useful service by giving it an insertion. The facts therein set forth should be extensively circulated.]—*Med. News & Library.*

The Committee appointed at the last meeting of the Medical Society of the State of Pennsylvania, to investigate the accuracy of certain views relative to smallpox and vaccination, recently put forth by Drs. Gregory, of London, and Cazenave, of Paris, and referred to in a communication made to the Society at its last session, REPORT:

That, considering the high authority heretofore attached to the names mentioned, the opinions in question, if erroneous, are calculated to unsettle the views of physicians, and shake the confidence of the public in regard to the protective powers of vaccination, more than any promulgated since its adoption. The Committee think these grounds sufficient to justify them in treating the subject with particular attention.

The principal points and questions calling for consideration, are:—

1. Whether persons vaccinated, lose, through lapse of time, any of the protective power once afforded against smallpox?

2. Whether the prophylactic powers of vaccination performed during infancy, are restricted to the first fifteen years of life, and of no avail afterwards?

3. Whether the accumulated evidence of the present day is calculated to sustain Dr. Gregory in his belief, that the efficacy of cowpox as a protection against smallpox has diminished, and a large increase of smallpox resulted from the extension of vaccination?

4. Whether, as asserted by Drs. Gregory and Cazenave, inoculation after the fifteenth year of age, of persons previously vaccinated, produces a specific papular eruptive disease of a non-contagious character, unattended with danger, and giving protection in after life against smallpox?

5. Whether circumstances exist which render it most advantageous to substitute inoculation for vaccination, after the fifteenth year of age, as proposed by Dr. Gregory?

The morbid miasm, or agent productive of smallpox, seemed for a long while kept in check by the prophylactic power of vaccination, which, indeed, at one time, promised the complete extermination of variola. But it cannot be disputed, that of late years variolous attacks have been common among those hitherto considered as completely protected. A new form of disease has, in fact, become known, designated "*varioloid*," from its resemblance to variola, or smallpox, of which it is generally regarded a milder form, as if modified and rendered less formidable, through some remaining prophylactic influence. This, of course, long before Dr. Gregory promulgated his peculiar views, furnished grounds for believing that the protection once relied upon from vaccination, was diminished by lapse of time, or that the potency of the smallpox miasm had increased.

Dr. Gregory's views, when first promulgated in England, were well calculated to rouse the attention of the medical profession, and elicit inquiry. The Epidemiological Society of London, appointed a special committee to investigate the important subjects of vaccination and smallpox, and this committee has recently collected and placed before the public, some highly important facts, through its chrirman, Mr. Grainger. As the information thus derived is so highly valuable, and directly calculated to meet the points started by Dr. Gregory, the committee think they cannot do better than give a short abstract from Mr. Grainger's statements.

In the evidence brought forward by the committee of the Epidemiological Society, we have the results of the experience of a large number of medical practitioners in different parts of England; and it is interesting to find that, out of 430 replies to questions issued by the

Society, one, only, expresses any doubt of the protective power of smallpox vaccination; and this one doubt simply amounts to this: that having been inoculated during infancy, this gentleman felt himself more secure than if he had been vaccinated.

With regard to opinions founded upon observations prosecuted in hospital practice, the committee would remark, that the results are so often influenced by the existence, here and there, of modifying circumstances, that an appeal to the experience of any single one would certainly afford most incorrect data, on which to found important conclusions, as these should always rest upon, multiplied facts, and observations extended through long periods.

In a table presented by Dr. Gregory and published in his paper, given in the London Medical Times, for 1849, we find the following statement of the results exhibited in the Smallpox Hospital, over which he presided:—

	Total.	Deaths.	Percentage of Deaths.
Unprotected cases	254	103	40
Vaccinated with cicatrices	365	38	10
Vaccinated, without cicatrices	63	25	39
Total vaccinated	428	63	14
Previously inoculated	3	1	33

Now the rate of mortality here presented is so much greater than that generally met with in other institutions, or in common practice, as to leave little doubt that the patients had been subjected to some of those malign influences, such as defective ventilation, &c., which have so often operated most injuriously in rendering mild cases severe, and originally severe ones almost inevitably fatal. If we compare the results exhibited in Dr. Gregory's Hospital practice, with those presented in 30 returns received from medical practitioners, by the London Epidemiological Society, taken without selection, we shall find the contrast most striking:

	Total.	Deaths.	Percentage of Deaths.
Natural smallpox in the unprotected	1756	361	20.85
Smallpox after vaccination	927	32	3·44

Previous to the introduction of vaccination, the annual mortality from smallpox amounted to 40,000 per annum, in the British Islands alone, being about 1-10th of all the deaths from every source. The average number of deaths per annum in London from smallpox, a century ago, namely, during a decennial period ending in 1750, was 2036; which presents a proportion strongly contrasted with the annual average of a decennial period ending in 1850, which is 498. This shows a mortality four times greater during a period when the population was not a fourth of what it was at the time last named.

Dr. Casper, of Berlin, shows in his statistics that the deaths from smallpox, in Berlin, during the eight years, from 1814 to 1822, were 535 out of a general mortality of 51,389, being only one death from smallpox in 1000 from all diseases. This exhibits either an almost total absence of epidemic influence, or a very general diffusion of protective means. It is stated in a publication containing the regulations for medical and other officers, issued in Berlin in October, 1803, that smallpox caused, on an average, 40,000 deaths a year in Prussia, in a population of about 10,000,000, during a period when inoculation was the only protection relied upon. In 1849, when the population had increased to more than 16,000,000, the average mortality from smallpox was 1760; showing that during the first period, when inoculation was the sole reliance, the proportional mortality from small pox was 37 times greater than when vaccination became generally diffused. These striking facts are, we think, very far from sustaining Dr. Gregory's opinion that an extension of vaccination has resulted in an increase of smallpox ; nor do they offer any encouragement to those who would restore the former practice of inoculation.

The frequent occurrence, of late years, of smallpox after vaccination, with instances of mortality, have been much commented on, and occasioned no small alarm. Hence, the great value af such accurate information as the following, furnished in 356 replies sent by physicians to the Epidemiological Society.

Of these, 182 state, expressly, that *they have never seen a death* from smallpox after vaccination.

44 state their experience in numbers, and give an aggregate of 70 deaths.

127 give no statements of their experience.

From the same source we gather the results of the experience of thirty physicians on the respective degrees of mortality of natural smallpox, smallpox after smallpox, and smallpox after vaccination.

	Cases.	Deaths.	Percentage of Deaths.
Natural Smallpox	1731	361	20.85
Smallpox after smallpox	58	22	37.92
Smallpox after vaccination	929	32	3.44

It is remarked, in reference to the 32 deaths reported after vaccination, that in 7 cases the evidences of vaccination were not satisfactory, whilst in six other cases the deaths were owing to superadded diseases. Deducting the 13 deaths, the ratio of fatal cases occurring after vaccination would be scarcely 2 per cent., whereas that of smallpox after smallpox is nearly 38 per cent.

To these statements of results of very extensive experience abroad, we are glad to have it in our power to subjoin evidence equally conclusive as to the protective power of vaccination, obtained among our own practitioners. In the report on varioloid, the protective power of vaccination, &c., presented to the College of Physicians of Philadelphia, in Nov. 1846, replies to interrogatories of the committee were received from 51 practising physicians of the city and districts, who reparted 776 cases of varioloid as having occurred in their practice during the epidemic of that period. Forty of these cases occurred after inoculation or a previous attack of smallpox in the natural way, and the remaining 736 after a reputed vaccination. Of the whole number of 776 cases, but 12 deaths occurred, or less than 2 per cent., and of these cases several were attended with serious complications. These cases all occurred in private practice, except two, which took place at the Smallpox Hospital at Bush Hill.

It is worth noticing, among the evidence from abroad upon this subject, that Mr. Marsden, resident physician of the London Smallpox Hospital, has, within the last sixteen years, vaccinated no less than 40,000 persons, not one of whom had returned to the hospital with smallpox. Had there been any considerable number of the vaccinated attacked subsequently with smallpox, there is reason to believe that very many would have found their way to an institution which receives multitudes of patients from the same ranks in which the vaccination took place.

Statements made by Dr. Grainger, prepared from official returns received from all parts of England to the Poor-law Board, show a greater neglect of vaccination than could be well imagined to exist among civilized people. In London, 13 unions, exhibiting 21,598 births, report the number vaccinated at only 4641, or 21 per cent.; whilst 31 unions in the country give only 9.2 per cent. of vaccinations under the first year of life. In many others, the proportion of infants vaccinated in the first year of life is much less, being occasionally as low as 1 per cent. Whilst such is the sad case in the country boasting a national vaccine institution, and acts of Parliament for the promotion of vaccination, things seem to be even worse in Ireland. In a very valuable report, made by Mr. Wilson, of Dublin, contained in the report of the census of Ireland for 1841, it is stated that, of the 56,000 deaths from smallpox which occurred in that country in the decennial period from 1831 to 1841, no fewer than 79 per cent., or 45,824 were of children under 5 years of age. Dr. Gregory gives results for England very nearly the same. He states that of 9762 persons who died of smallpox in that country during the years 1837-38, the deaths under 5 years were 7340, or about 75 per cent. of the whole. If, as Dr. Gregory asserts, in his valuable lectures on eruptive fevers, the protective power of cowpox may, for all practical purposes, be considered as complete, at least till the eighth year of life, the frightful infantile mortality here exhibited from smallpox, proves a neglect of vaccination almost equal to that which prevails to such a lamentable extent in Ireland.

In Prussia, Sweden, and some other countries, legislative authority has been brought into play with considerable efficiency in promoting the general extension of vaccination. But still, in despite of every precaution and exertion yet made, it would seem there are every where to be found thousands of unprotected persons, among the improvident, ready to become victims to smallpox whenever this may be introduced through epidemic or contagious influences.

In estimating the protective powers of vaccination, the public mind often seizes upon individual and isolated cases of death occurring after vaccination performed in childhood, without forming, at the same time, a just estimate of the vast number of individuals who are thereby enjoying immunity from the ravages of variola. Persons are not given to reflect that such deaths constitute the *exception* to the general law of exemption, and that they happen only among a very few individuals peculiarly susceptible to the variolous poison. It is also highly probable that the limited class upon whom vaccination appears to exert little or no protective power, are rendered no more safe by inoculation or an attack of smallpox, as we find occasional instances of death from a second attack of genuine smallpox, even in persons who have had the disease so severely as to be extensively pitted.

As to the new form of eruptive disease asserted, by Drs. Gregory and Cazenave, to be developed by inoculation performed upon those vaccinated previous to the fifteenth year, the Committee has been prevented from testing its verity by actual experiments, penal laws existing against inoculating within the city and adjoining districts, embraced within the limits of the Board of Health. A few experiments have, however, been made during the past year, by Dr. D. F. Condie, of Philadelphia, on persons situated beyond the jurisdiction referred to, the results of which were by no means calculated to sustain the views of Drs. Gregory and Cazenave. Although such limited experience cannot be regarded as furnishing evidence sufficiently conclusive upon the subject, we think it proper to place the results before the Society.

Ten cases were experimented on by inserting variolous matter in the arms of individuals, six of whom had been previously successfully vaccinated by Dr. Condie, and of the successful vaccination of the other four he had the most unquestionable evidence.

In *three* of the cases, between seven and eight years had elapsed since the period of the vaccination.

In *five*, between thirteen and fourteen years.

In *two*, between fifteen and sixteen years.

In *one* case, a local variolous pock appeared upon the arm at the place of inoculation—attended, between the eighth and ninth days, with a pretty smart fever. The scab separated on the twentieth day, leaving a decided cicatrix. The remaining portion of surface was entirely free from any form of eruption. This individual had undergone successful vaccination seven years and two months previously.

In *four* cases, the local disease was attended with a general eruption of acuminated pocks—with hard base and slight areola—sparsely disseminated over the surface. In different cases, from twenty to one hundred pocks appeared. In these cases, the pustules on the arm and over the body were attended with a very slight fever about the fifth day—after this period they desiccated very rapidly, forming small, light brown conical scabs, which commenced failing off on the eighth day, leaving no cicatrix. The periods which had elapsed since vaccination in these cases were, thirteen years in two, fifteen in one, and fifteen years seven months in another.

In *five* cases a local inflammation, but no pustule, occurred at the part where the matter was inserted, which disappeared within four or six days, leaving no cicatrix. These cases were unattended with fever, or any form of cutaneous eruption. These patients had under-gone vaccination seven years and five months, seven years and nine months, thirteen years and six months, and in two between fourteen and fifteen years.

These experiments were performed without the jurisdiction of the Board of Health of Philadelphia, with the consent of the parties and their friends, and with due precautions to prevent the individuals operated on from becoming foci of contagion.

It certainly appears strange that the poison of smallpox, which, when taken the natural way by persons previously vaccinated, produces the disease in its regular, pustular, and contagious form, should when introduced by inoculation into the systems of persons similarly situated, develop an entirely different form of disease, such as that described by Dr. Gregory as a specific papular eruptive affection of a non-contagious character, unattended with danger, and giving the most perfect protection in after-life against smallpox. Even supposing the result to be as stated by Dr. Gregory, the production of such a mild and benignant train of symptoms as those he describes from the introduction of the smallpox virus, affords one of the strongest evidences of the inestimable protective power exerted by cowpox.

In regard to the fifth and last point of inquiry, your Committee have no hesitation in expressing it as their belief, that no circumstances exist to justify the general substitution of inoculation after the fifteenth year of age, as proposed by Dr. Gregory. And they regret that, at the present time, whilst strenuous efforts are making through individual exertion, occasionally helped forward by judicious legislation, statements calculated to lessen confidence in the protecting power of vaccination, should have been promulgated. Happily, however, abundant evidence exists to show that although the hopes of complete exemption from smallpox, once fondly indulged, have not been fully realized, vaccination still offers the only dependence for protection against a disease, the fearful ravages of which have tended so much to darken the pages of history previous to the precious discovery made by Jenner.

As the neglect of vaccination, especially among the poor and improvident, may, we think, be regarded as the principal cause operating to promote the extension and mortality of smallpox, the Committee would urge it upon the State Medical Society to continue their efforts to obtain from the legislature the passage of a law providing for the gratuitous vaccination of the poor, and calculated to secure, as far as practicable, the fullest extension of vaccination in every portion of the commonwealth.

> G. EMERSON,
> SAMUEL JACKSON,
> JOSEPH WARRINGTON,
> ISAAC PARRISH,
> JOHN D. GRISCOM.

Ice as a Local Anæsthetic. By W. A. BERRY, M. D. Washington, D. C.—I propose to make known to the many readers of your valuable Journal the application of a new local anæsthetic agent, which probably is not familiar to a large majority of them. This agent is applicable to but a very limited part of the frame, but its efficacy is such as to cause its use in all like cases. I refer to the local anæsthetic effect of ice in the removal of the nails of the toes or fingers. This most painful operation is disarmed of all its terrors by this simple means, and the patient witnesses it with as much composure as his operator. The agent was first made use of in the wards of M. Velpeau, during the past summer, in Paris, by one of his internes, and afterwards successfully applied by himself in a number of cases. The ice is powdered finely, and mixed with a sufficient quantity of salt ; next enveloped in a thin cloth, and the two phalanges of the great toe or thumb enveloped in it ; the application should not be continued over five or six minutes, this time being sufficient to produce the most perfect anæsthesia. M. Velpeau proceeds with the operation in the following manner : Immediately upon removing the ice, the nail is divided in its length with a common sized bistoury from its free extremity to the root, then seizing each half successively with a strong forceps, it is removed with a moderate *jerk*. The frequent necessity for the performance of this operation, and the great pain attending it when removed under other circumstances, is sufficient to cause its universal application by the profession. M. Velpeau directs the application of compresses of cold water to the part during the first twenty-four hours ; and the simple cerate dressing for a few days is all that is required.

It may be objected that the reaction under the application is such as to prevent its use ; I will simply say that of the six patients that I saw operated upon by M. Velpeau, no such accident occurred to any one of them ; and to the one case in which we applied it but a few days since, (and which has suggested this communication,) we have reason to believe that the agent is free from any unhappy results.

The simplicity and efficacy of this piece of minor surgery, and the so frequent necessity of some surgical interference in these cases, has induced me to send you this communication.—[*Medical Examiner.*

New mode of applying Leeches.—Dr. Sloan, of Ayr, says, that by covering leeches with a cupping-glass and exhausting the air moderately by means of an air-pump, they suck much more rapidly, and soon become fully distended and fall off. A sufficient quantity of blood may be obtained by continuing the exhausting process afterwards. The erysipelatous appearance which usually follows leech-bites, is thus prevented.—[*Monthly Journ. of Med. Sciences.*

Mineral Springs.—Doctor John Bell, (Philadelphia,) who is preparing a work on mineral springs, more especially on those of the United States, is desirous of procuring, at an early day, all accessible information on the subject. With this view, he requests his professional brethren to transmit to him all the facts in their possession, which may throw light on the chemical composition and curative powers of the waters of the springs, in their respective neighborhoods.

Proprietors of these waters, would oblige by sending to Dr. Bell authentic accounts, on these points; and also, of the topography of the springs, and the roads by which they are approached.—[*Medical News and Library.*

Medical Classes.—It would seem that the classes in some of the Northern Institutions are unusually small this year, and that the circumstance has been attributed to the emigration of young men to California in search of more profitable employment. We are happy to say that the youth of "*these diggins*" have been more considerate, and that they have preferred to remain at home. The class in attendance at the Medical College of Georgia this session is unusually large.

Death of Daniel Drake.—The Profession of our country will learn, with profound regret, the demise of Professor Daniel Drake. An accomplished physician, scholar and gentleman, Dr. Drake was an honor to his profession and to his country. We hope that his biography will be written by an able hand, and that the queen city of the West will erect a suitable monument to the memory of her most gifted and patriotic citizen.

A new Syringe.—Dr. Mattson, of Boston, has made improvements to the syringe so as to adapt it to various purposes. It is represented as much better than those in common use.

BIBLIOGRAPHICAL.

On Syphilis, constitutional and hereditary ; and on Syphilitic Eruptions. By ERASMUS WILSON, F. R. S., &c.—with 4 colored plates. Philadelphia: Blanchard & Lea. 1852. Pp. 284.

The writer of the work before us has been favorably known as the author of a Treatise on Diseases of the Skin, and of other interesting papers. We believe that his reputation will not suffer in the present instance, and that his contribution to the study of so important a class of affections as the Syphilitic, will tend to the elucidation of points already too long within the domain of controversy. The work is divided into eight chapters, comprehending The syphilitic poison, Primary syphilis, Secondary or constitutional syphilis, Evolution of the syphilitic poison by the skin, Local affections of syphilis, Congenital syphilis, Hereditary syphilis, and the Treatment of syphilis—

the whole judiciously interspersed with cases illustrative of his conclusions.

We would recommend the book to the attentive perusal of general
practitioners.

A practical treatise on Diseases of the Skin. By J. MOORE NELIGAN,
    M. D., M. R. I. A., &c., &c., Lecturer on the Practice of Medicine
    in the Dublin School of Medicine. Philadelphia: Blanchard &
    Lea. 1852. Pp. 330.

Diseases of the skin are so little understood, that we ought not to
hesitate to read anything that may be published upon the subject by
so judicious an author as Dr. Neligan—especially when he tells us
that his object is to simplify their study and treatment. The work is
small, concise and well written, and will doubtless amply compensate
for a more minute inspection than we have as yet been able to give it.

General Pathology, as conducive to the establishment of rational princi-
    ples for the diagnosis and treatment of disease; a course of Lectures
    delivered at St. Thomas's Hospital in 1850. By JOHN SIMON, F.
    R. S., one of the surgical staff of that hospital, &c. Philadelphia:
    Blanchard & Lea. 1852. Pp. 211.

These Lectures were originally published in the London Lancet,
and met with much favor. The profound attainments of Mr. Simon
have enabled him to comprehend in a comparatively brief volume
much of most valuable matter, especially in reference to the morbid
conditions and products of the blood, Tumours, Scrofula, Nervous diseases, and morbid poisons. The author is one of the ablest pathologists of the age, and his writings should be studied by all who wish to
practice medicine with proper discernment.

A practical treatise on Dental Medicine, being a compendium of Medi-
    cal Science, as connected with the study of Dental Surgery; to
    which is appended an inquiry into the use of Chloroform and other
    anæsthetic agents—second edition, revised, corrected aud enlarged.
    By THOMAS E. BOND, A. M., M. D., Professor of Special Patholo-
    gy and Therapeutics in the Baltimore College of Dental Surgery.
    Philadelphia: Lindsay & Blakiston. 1852. Pp. 366.

Professor Bond's work is deservedly popular with the Dental Profession, and has already reached its second edition in less than two
years. It is an excellent book, both as regards manner and matter.

To Correspondents.—We are compelled, for want of space, to defer
until our next issue the publication of several valuable papers—among
which is one from the pen of Dr. Charles T. Jackson, of Boston, upon
Anæsthetic agents.

INDEX TO VOL. VIII.

Lightning Source UK Ltd.
Milton Keynes UK
UKHW020243070119
334855UK00012B/2042/P